Inborn Metabolic Diseases: A Clinical Approach

Inborn Metabolic Diseases: A Clinical Approach

Editor: Bradley Alba

AMERICAN
MEDICAL PUBLISHERS
www.americanmedicalpublishers.com

AMERICAN
MEDICAL PUBLISHERS
www.americanmedicalpublishers.com

Cataloging-in-Publication Data

Inborn metabolic diseases : a clinical approach / edited by Bradley Alba.
p. cm.
Includes bibliographical references and index.
ISBN 978-1-63927-119-1
1. Metabolism, Inborn errors of. 2. Metabolism--Disorders. 3. Genetic disorders.
4. Metabolism--Disorders--Treatment. I. Alba, Bradley.
RC627.8 .I53 2021
616.390 42--dc23

American Medical Publishers,
41 Flatbush Avenue,
1st Floor, New York,
NY 11217, USA

ISBN 978-1-63927-119-1 (Hardback)

Contents

Preface

The purpose of the book is to provide a glimpse into the dynamics and to present opinions and studies of some of the scientists engaged in the development of new ideas in the field from very different standpoints. This book will prove useful to students and researchers owing to its high content quality.

The disease or disorder that disrupts normal metabolism is known as a metabolic disease. It affects the procedure of conversion of food into energy on a cellular level. It also influences the ability of the cell to perform critical biochemical reactions that involve the processing of proteins, carbohydrates and starch. Metabolic diseases are typically hereditary. Some of the symptoms that can occur in metabolic disorders are lethargy, weight loss, jaundice and seizures. Tandem mass-spectrometry is a new technology that helps in the detection of multiple abnormal metabolites. However, gene therapy is successful in the treatment of some of these metabolic diseases. Screening of metabolic diseases in newborns can be done via blood tests, skin test and hearing tests. If the metabolic disease is detected at an early stage, it can be treated by nutrition management. This book provides comprehensive insights into the field of metabolic disease. It consists of contributions made by international experts. Researchers and students in this field will be assisted by this book.

At the end, I would like to appreciate all the efforts made by the authors in completing their chapters professionally. I express my deepest gratitude to all of them for contributing to this book by sharing their valuable works. A special thanks to my family and friends for their constant support in this journey.

Editor

Beta-Ketothiolase Deficiency: Resolving Challenges in Diagnosis

Elsayed Abdelkreem, MD, MSc[1,2], Hiroki Otsuka, MD[2], Hideo Sasai, MD[2], Yuka Aoyama, PhD[3], Tomohiro Hori, MD, PhD[2], Mohamed Abd El Aal, MD, PhD[1], Shaimaa Mahmoud, MD, PhD[1], and Toshiyuki Fukao, MD, PhD[2]

Abstract

Beta-ketothiolase deficiency is an inherited disorder of ketone body metabolism and isoleucine catabolism. It typically manifests as recurrent ketoacidotic episodes with characteristic abnormalities in the urinary organic acid profile. However, several challenges in the diagnosis of beta-ketothiolase deficiency have been encountered: atypical presentations have been reported and some other disorders, such as succinyl-CoA:3-oxoacid CoA transferase and 2-methyl-3-hydroxybutyryl-CoA dehydrogenase deficiencies, can mimic the clinical and/or biochemical signs of beta-ketothiolase deficiency. A final diagnosis of beta-ketothiolase deficiency requires an enzymatic assay and/or a molecular analysis, but some caveats must be considered. Despite the reported missed cases, screening programs have successfully identified an increasing number of patients with beta-ketothiolase deficiency. Early diagnosis and management of beta-ketothiolase deficiency will enable prevention of its serious acute and chronic complications and ultimately improve the prognosis.

Keywords

beta-ketothiolase deficiency, diagnosis, challenges, screening, management

Introduction

Beta-ketothiolase deficiency (Online Mendelian Inheritance in Man [OMIM] 203750) is an autosomal recessive disease caused by a defect of mitochondrial acetoacetyl-CoA thiolase (T2). This disorder affects ketone body metabolism and isoleucine catabolism. Beta-ketothiolase deficiency is also known by other names including T2 deficiency, mitochondrial acetoacetyl-CoA thiolase deficiency, 3-oxothiolase deficiency, 3-ketothiolase deficiency, and 2-methyl-3-hydroxybutyric acidemia.[1-3] In this review, beta-ketothiolase is abbreviated as T2.

T2 and 3-hydroxy-3-methylglutaryl-CoA (HMG-CoA) lyase (OMIM 246450) deficiencies are the most common disorders of ketone body metabolism.[2] Since the first description of T2 deficiency in 1971,[4] more than 100 cases have been reported worldwide, with no ethnic predisposition.[1] T2 deficiency is estimated to be a very rare disease with an incidence of less than 1 per 1 million newborns.[5]

In this review, we provide an overview on T2 deficiency, illustrate challenges in diagnosis, and clarify ways to overcome these challenges; a diagnostic flow chart for T2 deficiency is provided.

Biochemistry

The ketone bodies acetoacetate (AcAc) and 3-hydroxybutyrate (3HB) are important substitutes for glucose. They are produced in the liver and can be utilized as energy sources by most tissues except the liver itself. They are especially important for the brain as the only substitutes for glucose.[1,2]

[1] Department of Pediatrics, Faculty of Medicine, Sohag University, Sohag, Egypt

[2] Department of Pediatrics, Graduate School of Medicine, Gifu University, Gifu, Japan

[3] Department of Biomedical Sciences, College of Life and Health Sciences, Education and Training Center of Medical Technology, Chubu University, Kasugai, Japan

Corresponding Author:

Elsayed Abdelkreem, Department of Pediatrics, Faculty of Medicine, Sohag University, Nasser City 82524, Egypt.

Email: d.elsayedmohammed@med.sohag.edu.eg

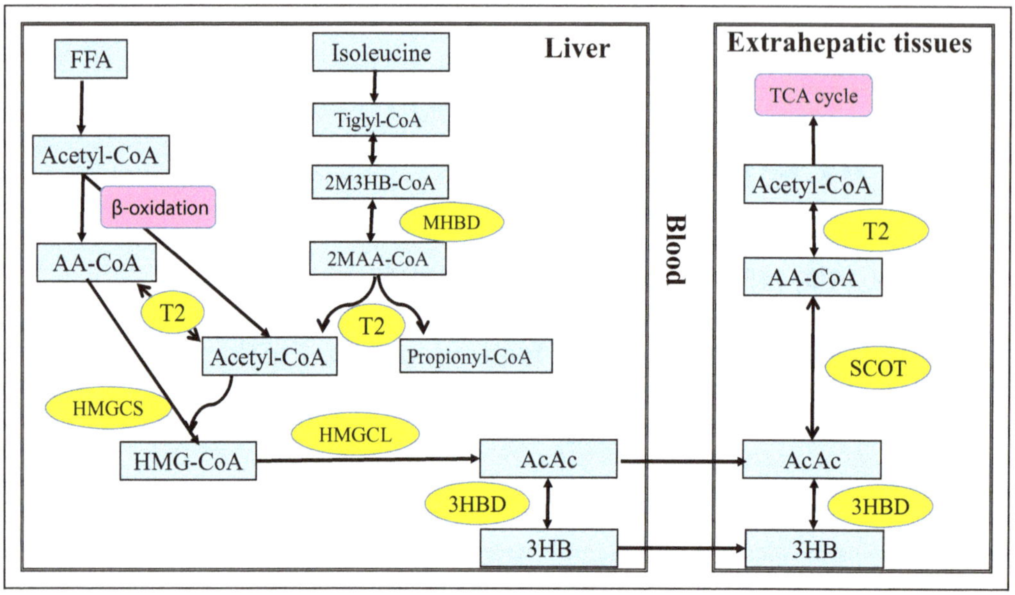

Figure 1. Summary of ketone body metabolism and isoleucine catabolism. 2M3HB indicates 2-methyl-3-hydroxybutyryl; 2MAA, 2-methylacetoacetyl; 3HB, 3-hydroxybutyrate; 3HBD, 3-hydroxybutyrate dehydrogenase; AA, acetoacetyl; AcAc, acetoacetate; CoA, coenzyme A; FFA, free fatty acids; HMG-CoA, 3-hydroxy-3-methylglutaryl-CoA; HMGCL, HMG-CoA lyase; HMGCS, mitochondrial HMG-CoA synthase; MHBD, 2-methyl-3-hydroxybutyryl-CoA dehydrogenase; SCOT, succinyl-CoA:3-oxoacid CoA transferase; T2, mitochondrial acetoacetyl-CoA thiolase; TCA, tricarboxylic acid.

As shown in Figure 1, ketone body metabolism starts in the hepatocytes with β-oxidation of free fatty acids (FFA), supplied from adipose tissues, to produce acetyl-CoA and acetoacetyl-CoA (AA-CoA). T2 can convert acetyl-CoA to AA-CoA and vice versa. Mitochondrial HMG-CoA synthase condenses acetyl-CoA and AA-CoA to form HMG-CoA. HMG-CoA is converted by HMG-CoA lyase to AcAc, which is partially reduced to 3HB by 3-hydroxybutyrate dehydrogenase. AcAc and 3HB are transferred to extrahepatic tissues via the bloodstream, where 3HB is converted back to AcAc. Succinyl-CoA:3-oxoacid CoA transferase (SCOT) activates AcAc to AcAc-CoA, which is then cleaved by T2 into acetyl-CoA.[1,2] Hence, T2 is important in both ketogenesis in the liver and ketolysis in the extrahepatic tissues. Another thiolase, mitochondrial 3-ketoacyl-CoA thiolase, can compensate for T2 deficiency in ketogenesis but to a lesser extent in ketolysis. As a result, deficiency of T2 leads to ketosis.[1-3] Monocarboxylate transporter 1 (MCT1), a transmembrane transporter, has been shown to transport monocarboxylates, including ketone bodies, into extrahepatic tissues. This is essential for ketolysis, particularly during periods of catabolic stress.[6]

In isoleucine catabolism, T2 is responsible for thiolysis of 2-methylacetoacetyl-CoA (2MAA-CoA) to acetyl-CoA and propionyl-CoA. The 2 upstream reactions, conversion of tiglyl-CoA to 2-methyl-3-hydroxybutyryl-CoA (2M3HB-CoA) and conversion of 2M3HB-CoA to 2MAA-CoA, are reversible; the latter reaction is catalyzed by 2-methyl-3-hydroxybutyryl-CoA dehydrogenase (MHBD). Consequently, T2 deficiency leads to accumulation of 2MAA-CoA, 2M3HB-CoA, and tiglyl-CoA, whereas MHBD deficiency results in accumulation of only the latter 2 metabolites.[1-3]

Clinical Presentation: Diagnostic Challenges

Clinical Presentation

Typical presentation. T2 deficiency classically manifests between 6 and 18 months of age with recurrent ketoacidotic attacks; patients are generally asymptomatic between attacks. Ketoacidotic episodes are often triggered by fasting, fever, infections, or other ketogenic stresses. Coma, convulsions, and even death are possible acute complications, whereas neurodevelopmental impairments are possible long-term complications, mainly as sequelae of severe metabolic decompensations. The severity of the disease varies among cases, but the overall prognosis is usually good.[1,3,7,8]

Atypical presentation. Some patients with T2 deficiency having atypical presentation exhibit signs and symptoms at an earlier age, even in the neonatal period,[1] whereas others experience their first attack at an older age.[8] Furthermore, some patients present with neurological symptoms before the onset of ketoacidotic attacks.[9] In contrast, some asymptomatic patients with T2 deficiency have been identified by screening, either because of the existence of an affected family member or as a result of newborn screening (NBS) programs.[10-14]

Diagnostic Challenges

Metabolic disorders should be suspected in ketoacidotic patients. Therefore, critical samples (blood, serum, and urine) should be collected, and routine laboratory tests should be performed before treatment is started[3]; however, unwary pediatricians may not do so. Symptomatic management of dehydration, acidosis, and hypoglycemia (if present) may lead to improvement in the condition. The patient may then be discharged without receiving a final diagnosis.[15] There are many examples in the literature of failure to diagnose patients with T2 deficiency during their first presentations. Such patients received attention only when they had a second episode or when there was a similar presentation in another family member.[16-18]

A second possibility is that the patient will be seen by a consultant who will order many metabolic investigations (if applicable). Such investigations may lead to the diagnosis of a metabolic disorder, but T2 deficiency might be missed (discussed later).[19] Conversely, the patient may die during the acute attack. An important finding in many cases of T2 deficiency is a positive family history of unexplained sibling deaths.[20-23] The siblings might have had undiagnosed T2 deficiency as well.[3]

The following are some possible solutions for the aforementioned clinical challenges:

1. Education of health-care staff, especially those working in emergency wards, to improve their knowledge of T2 deficiency, ketone body disorders, and metabolic disorders in general, and provision of diagnostic guidelines that identify the circumstances in which ketone body disorders should be suspected and what should then be done.[1,3] T2 deficiency should be considered in the following situations: (a) infants and children with an acute attack of metabolic acidosis following prolonged fasting, acute gastroenteritis, respiratory tract infections, or other febrile states and (b) patients with severe ketosis exceeding predicted values in the context of the clinical circumstances (discussed later); and (c) sick neonates with metabolic acidosis.[1]
2. Establishment of 1 or 2 metabolic centers in countries with a highly consanguineous population, where the incidence of genetic and metabolic diseases, including T2 deficiency, is expected to be high.[24,25]

Investigations: Diagnostic Challenges

Investigations

Routine laboratory investigations. During ketoacidotic attacks, a blood total ketone body (TKB) concentration >7 mmol/L is the major finding. Blood sugar is typically normal, but hypoglycemia or hyperglycemia has been reported.[3] Blood ammonia is usually normal, but it may be slightly elevated in some cases.[1,3]

Urinary organic acid and blood acylcarnitine profiles. T2 deficiency is usually suspected during acute ketoacidotic attacks when there is increased urinary excretion of 2-methylacetoacetate (2MAA), 2-methyl-3-hydroxybutyrate (2M3HB), and tiglylglycine (TIG). Blood acylcarnitine analysis usually reveals increased tiglylcarnitine (C5:1) and 2-methyl-3-hydroxybutyryl-carnitine.[1]

Diagnostic Challenges

When ketosis is associated with hypoglycemia, several disorders are considered, including ketotic hypoglycemia, endocrinal disorders (eg, Addison disease), and metabolic disorders of glucose and glycogen metabolism (eg, glycogen synthase deficiency).[3] The severity of ketoacidosis in T2 deficiency may distinguish this disorder from other causes of ketotic hypoglycemia (Figure 2).[2] The highest reported plasma glucose level in patients with T2 deficiency is 14.1 mmol/L.[15] Ketoacidosis with hyperglycemia, mimicking diabetic ketoacidosis, has been reported in some organic acidemias, although diabetic ketoacidosis is usually associated with much higher plasma glucose levels than ketoacidosis caused by organic acidemias. In such cases, glycated hemoglobin or glycoalbumin levels may help distinguish them (Figure 2).[26] When ketoacidosis is associated with hyperammonemia, organic acidemias are suspected. Such suspicion can be excluded by urinary organic acid analysis.[1,3]

Individuals with SCOT deficiency (OMIM 245050) may present with ketoacidotic attacks mimicking T2 deficiency.[3] SCOT deficiency has 3 important characteristics: (1) neonatal onset in 50% of cases, (2) permanent ketosis, even postprandially, and (3) lack of a characteristic urinary organic acid profile.[1,2] Given that (1) T2 deficiency may manifest in the neonatal period,[1,2] (2) permanent ketosis is not a feature in all cases of SCOT deficiency,[2] and (3) some cases of T2 deficiency show only subtle biochemical abnormalities in the urinary organic acid profile,[1,19] the 2 conditions may be very similar at both the clinical and biochemical levels. Actually, both conditions should be suspected and investigated in cases of unexplained and/or recurrent ketoacidotic attacks. The conditions can be differentiated by enzymatic assay and/or molecular analysis.[1-3]

MCT1 deficiency (OMIM 616095) is a novel disorder of ketone body utilization. After confirmation of the diagnosis in the index patient, pathogenic mutations, both homozygous and heterozygous, in the MCT1 gene (*SLC16A1*) were identified in an additional 7 of 96 patients who had unexplained recurrent episodes of severe ketoacidosis. The extent of ketonuria varies during episodes, and the blood pH is normal between episodes.[6]

Regarding urinary organic acids, several caveats must be noted: (1) the aforementioned characteristic abnormalities, which are typically present during acute attacks, may be subtle in stable conditions, especially in individuals with mild mutations.[1-3,19] This can lead to the usual scenario described earlier, in which undiagnosed T2 deficiency is neither suspected nor investigated during the first acute attack.[16,17,27] The results of any subsequent investigations might be inconclusive if samples were obtained after stabilization of the patient's condition.[2,19,28] (2) In some reported cases, there were only subtle abnormalities in urinary organic acid and blood acylcarnitine profiles during the acute ketoacidotic episode.[10,19] (3) Even in the presence of increased urinary excretion of 2M3HB and TIG, a diagnosis of T2 deficiency cannot be confirmed.

MHBD deficiency (OMIM 300438) is a neurodegenerative disorder with a variable clinical presentation that is usually

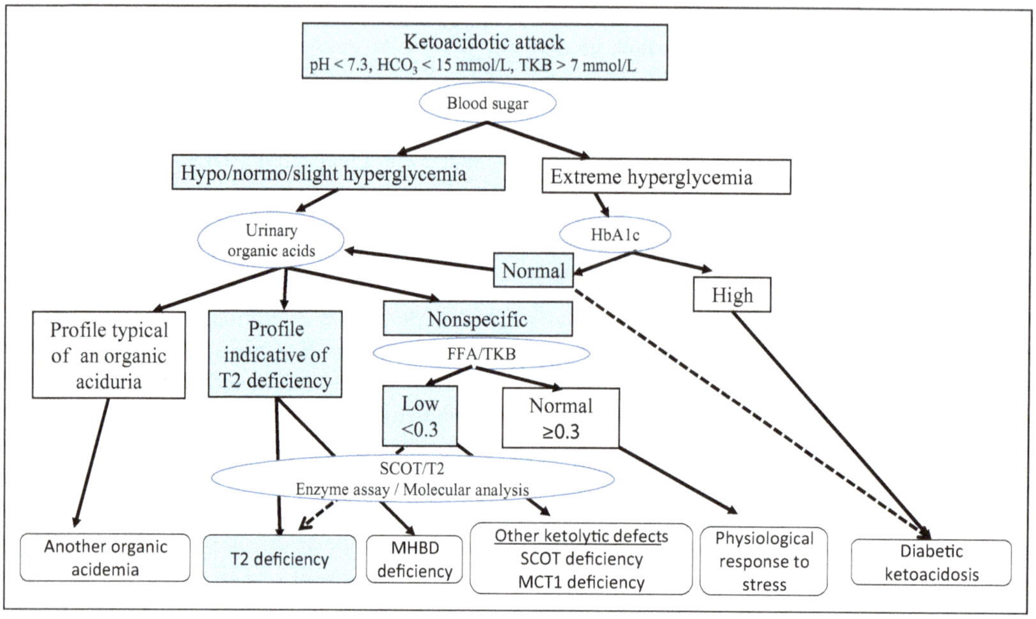

Figure 2. Diagnostic flow chart for beta-ketothiolase (T2) deficiency. An FFA/TKB cutoff of 0.3 is not an absolute value. Fasting for too long may decrease the ratio, and glucose infusion reduces FFA faster than TKB, also decreasing the ratio. Dotted lines indicate rare but possible consequences. Extreme hyperglycemia with elevated HbA_{1c} is usually diagnosed as diabetic ketoacidosis; however, ketoacidosis mimicking diabetic ketoacidosis has been reported in some organic acidemias. Hence, although HbA_{1c} is a good marker for diabetic ketoacidosis, normal HbA_{1c} levels cannot exclude diabetic ketoacidosis conclusively (indicated by a dotted line). If the urinary organic acid profile is nonspecific during ketoacidosis, T2 and SCOT should be analyzed by enzyme assay or gene analysis, since patients with T2 deficiency could have a nonspecific urinary organic acid profile (indicated by a dotted line). FFA/TKB indicates free fatty acids/total ketone body; HbA_{1c}, glycated hemoglobin; MCT1, monocarboxylate transporter 1; MHBD, 2-methyl-3-hydroxybutyryl-CoA dehydrogenase; SCOT, succinyl-CoA:3-oxoacid CoA transferase; T2, mitochondrial acetoacetyl-CoA thiolase.

different from that of T2 deficiency. However, a case of MHBD deficiency mimicking T2 deficiency both clinically and in terms of the urinary organic acid profile (increased excretion of 2M3HB and TIG) has been reported.[2,29] Moreover, MHBD deficiency may produce the same abnormal results as T2 deficiency in a coupled assay.[1,30] Differentiation between T2 and MHBD deficiencies is based on the following: (1) MHBD deficiency is an X-linked disorder; (2) urinary excretion of 2MAA does not increase in MHBD deficiency, even after an oral isoleucine challenge (100 mg/kg body weight), although isoleucine challenge is usually not necessary[3]; and (3) the potassium-dependent AA-CoA thiolase assay gives a normal result in cases of MHBD deficiency.[28]

To overcome the aforementioned challenges, a number of procedures should be followed. Blood gases, electrolytes, glucose, ammonia, TKB (or 3HB if TKB is not available), and FFA are the most important initial investigations during acute attacks. Lactate and pyruvate concentrations should also be measured during the first crises of undiagnosed patients with T2 deficiency to exclude congenital lactic acidosis.[3] The collection of plasma or serum samples for acylcarnitine analysis and aminogram as well as urine samples for organic acid analysis is important at this stage. For accurate evaluation, samples for these analyses should be obtained before glucose infusion.[1,2,19] Enzymatic assays for both T2 and SCOT deficiencies should be performed in suspected cases even in the absence of typical biochemical abnormalities.[1,10]

It is worth emphasizing the importance of TKB levels in the diagnosis of T2 deficiency and other ketone body disorders. Total ketone body should be interpreted in light of clinical factors, such as fasting time and any ketogenic stresses, and biochemical factors, especially blood glucose and FFA. The FFA/TKB ratio is a useful tool; being lower than 0.3 in the early fasting stage in patients with T2 deficiency and other ketolytic disorders, it differentiates such conditions from physiological ketosis due to fasting.[31] In the case of associated hypoglycemia, the marked increase in TKB in relation to blood glucose differentiates T2 deficiency (and other ketolytic disorders) from ketotic hypoglycemia.[2] Figure 2 shows a diagnostic flow chart for T2 deficiency.

Molecular Analysis: Diagnostic Challenges

Molecular Analysis

The structure of the human T2 gene (gene symbol *ACAT1*) was determined in 1991. The gene is located on chromosome 11q22.3 to q23.1 is 27-kb in length and is composed of 12 exons and 11 introns.[32] Genetic mutations resulting in T2 deficiency are highly heterogeneous, with no clear genotype–phenotype correlation. To date, more than 50 different mutations have been discovered and at least 9 novel mutations have been reported in the last 6 years. To our knowledge, apart from the common R208X mutation that has been identified in

Vietnamese cases, no other common mutations have been determined.[1,4,7-15,17,20-25,28,29,33-59]

T2 deficiency can be confirmed if genomic DNA analysis reveals mutations in *ACAT1* gene that were previously identified as causative for T2 deficiency in a mutant complementary DNA (cDNA) expression assay. Screening of other family members for these mutations can identify asymptomatic patients without the need for other sophisticated biochemical or enzymatic assays. Unfortunately, because of the high heterogeneity of mutations in T2 deficiency, this is not the usual scenario.[19]

Diagnostic Challenges

DNA analysis of suspected patients with T2 deficiency may reveal novel variants in *ACAT1* gene that have never been reported or studied. This is usually enough for a justifiable diagnosis when such variants have not been reported as polymorphisms. However, confirmation of the diagnosis at the molecular level requires mutant cDNA expression assays to verify that these variants are responsible for T2 deficiency.[3] In the absence of any mutations in the coding regions (exons) of the genomic DNA, there are multiple possibilities that must be ruled out before T2 deficiency can be excluded. Although homozygous mutations involving nucleotide substitutions can usually be detected by traditional genomic DNA analysis, heterozygous mutations may be missed. Moreover, copy number variants, small or large heterozygous deletions, and heterozygous or homozygous whole exon duplications cannot be detected by this method.[55,58]

Multiplex ligation-dependent probe amplification is a semiquantitative technique by which the relative copy number of multiple DNA sequences can be determined in a single polymerase chain reaction (PCR). By this technique, heterozygous deletions and heterozygous or homozygous exon duplications can be detected.[60] Multiplex ligation-dependent probe amplification for the human *ACAT1* gene has already been achieved, and it helped in the detection of a heterozygous deletion including exons 3 to 4 in a patient with T2 deficiency.[58] Real-time PCR can also be used to determine the copy number of each exon. However, neither technique is widely applied.[60,61]

Aberrant splicing has been identified in 20% of mutations in the *ACAT1* gene.[57,58] Following analysis of genomic DNA, obvious exonic mutations may be reported as silent mutations or polymorphisms if we do not realize their impact on splicing. To discover the effects of mutations on splicing, we have to directly analyze messenger RNA structure.[57]

Enzymatic Assay: Diagnostic Challenges

Enzymatic Assay

Enzymatic assay, which is often required to confirm a diagnosis of T2 deficiency,[2] can be performed by different methods: (1) the potassium-dependent AA-CoA thiolase assay is based on the fact that T2 is the only thiolase that is activated in the presence of potassium ions[62]; (2) the use of 2MAA-CoA as a substrate provides a more sensitive and specific method for the study of residual T2 enzymatic activity[3]; and (3) the coupled assay for the detection of defects in isoleucine catabolism distal to enoyl-CoA hydratase, using tiglyl-CoA as a substrate, was described as a rapid, straightforward screening test for isoleucine catabolic pathway defects.[30] This procedure has been widely used in the United States and Europe for T2 enzymatic assay.[51]

Based on the enzymatic activity detected upon expression of mutant cDNAs, patients have been divided into 2 groups: patients with 2 null mutations and patients in whom at least one of the 2 mutations allows some residual T2 activity. The latter was designated as patients with mild mutations.[7] Patients with T2 deficiency with mild mutations develop ketoacidotic attacks as severe as those in patients with null mutations, but their blood acylcarnitine and urinary organic acid profiles may show only subtle abnormalities even during acute attacks.[1,2,19]

Diagnostic Challenges

The potassium-dependent AA-CoA thiolase assay using blood mononuclear cells is possible, but correct evaluation is difficult if the cell preparation includes a lot of erythrocytes. Thus, enzyme assays using fibroblasts are recommended for correct evaluation of T2 enzymatic activity.[3] 2MAA-CoA is, unfortunately, neither stable nor marketed.[3] The coupled assay test has 2 substantial flaws: (1) it cannot differentiate T2 deficiency from MHBD deficiency[30] and (2) cases involving mild mutations, where there is residual T2 enzymatic activity, may not be detected by this test. In fact, based on normal results obtained from this test, some patients with T2 deficiency were initially excluded as having the disorder but were later diagnosed with T2 deficiency based on results of the potassium-dependent AA-CoA thiolase assay.[51]

Because the coupled assay alone may give false-negative results in cases with residual enzymatic activity and 2MAA-CoA as a substrate is neither stable nor marketed, the potassium-dependent AA-CoA thiolase assay, either alone or combined with the coupled assay, remains the gold standard for T2 enzymatic assay.[3]

Screening: Diagnostic Challenges

Screening

Mass screening. Newborn screening programs are invaluable preventive health measures that enable early detection of serious and treatable disorders in the first few days of life before the appearance of any clinical manifestations.[63,64] However, some NBS programs in developing countries are very limited, including only a few disorders.[64,65]

Two cases of T2 deficiency were identified by NBS in North Carolina from 1997 to 2005 (by tandem mass spectrometry); however, a missed case (false negative) was identified later, at

15 months of age. That missed case showed an increased C5:1 level only during acute attacks.[13] In a similar NBS program in Minnesota, from January 2001 to November 2010, 1 case was identified, whereas 2 missed cases were discovered later.[10] In an expanded pilot NBS program (liquid chromatography–tandem mass spectrometry) in the Campania region, southern Italy, from 2007 to 2009, 1 case was identified, which led to a diagnosis of T2 deficiency in the patient's older sister as well.[14] In an interesting study in New South Wales (Australia), an NBS program (April 1998 to March 2002) resulted in a substantial increase in the detection of T2 deficiency to 7 cases compared with only 1 case in the period from April 1974 to March 1998.[66] In that study, there were also 3 missed cases that were discovered later.[67]

The results of previous NBS studies have some substantial implications: (1) NBS represents a valuable tool for the detection of T2 deficiency[10,13,14,66] and (2) NBS studies have shown a higher incidence of T2 deficiency than previously reported and provide strong evidence for the underestimation of T2 deficiency. The incidence of T2 deficiency in North Carolina from 1997 to 2005 was nearly 1 per 313 000 newborns, whereas that in Minnesota from January 2001 to November 2010 was 1 per 232 000 newborns.[10,13] Both figures are much higher than the previously estimated incidence of less than 1 per 1 million newborns.[5]

Selective screening. Selective screening provides a valuable alternative diagnostic method for the identification of inborn errors of metabolism in developing countries that lack NBS programs. The results may help in preventing further deterioration of the patient and in screening other family members.[65] For example, selective screening of high-risk neonates and children by tandem mass spectrometry in Oman (1998-2008) identified 2 cases of T2 deficiency.[68] In a similar Egyptian study (2008-2013), 6 cases were identified.[25]

Diagnostic Challenges

Newborn screening may yield false-negative results, and thus, exclusion of suspected T2 deficiency should not be based on normal NBS results.[2,10] In some countries, such as Japan, where most cases are of the mild genotypic type, the yield of NBS programs is expected to be low, with a high false-negative percentage.[1,28]

Selective screening has 2 major flaws. First, if tests are performed under stable clinical conditions, patients with T2 deficiency who lack biochemical abnormalities between attacks will be missed.[1,3] Second, screening may be based on the presence of clinical findings, and some of these findings, such as mental retardation, may be irreversible. In such cases, diagnosis through an NBS program might result in a better prognosis.[25,65,68]

Management

The management of T2 deficiency includes prevention of further ketoacidotic attacks, treatment of acute attacks, and screening of other family members.

General Measures for Prevention of Further Ketoacidotic Attacks

Avoidance of prolonged fasting is the cornerstone to prevent further ketoacidotic attacks of T2 deficiency. In case of fever and/or vomiting, increased carbohydrate intake is advised, and intravenous glucose infusion should be considered in such conditions. Monitoring of urinary ketone bodies is advised, and medical advice should be obtained in case of moderate or severe ketonuria. Mild protein restriction, avoidance of a fat-rich diet, and L-carnitine supplementation, particularly in cases with a low carnitine level, are also advised[1,3]; however, no evidence support the effectiveness of these measures.

Treatment of Acute Attacks

In the event of an acute ketoacidotic attack, administration of intravenous glucose should be started—even in cases with a normal blood glucose level—to keep blood glucose at the upper range of the normal level. This will help suppress ketogenesis. Second, appropriate intravenous fluids and electrolytes should be administered to maintain good urine output and keep serum electrolytes within normal limits. Third, if blood pH is < 7.1, a small bicarbonate bolus (1 mmol/kg over 10 minutes) can be given, followed by continuous infusion. This should be guided by frequent monitoring of blood gases and electrolytes to avoid hypernatremia or rapid correction of acidosis.[1] Finally, L-carnitine supplementation or other supportive measures, such as peritoneal dialysis or mechanical ventilation, may be required.[1,3]

Screening of Other Family Members

Screening of family members of a patient diagnosed with T2 deficiency can detect asymptomatic individuals before the development of any acute or chronic clinical manifestations.[3,8]

Summary and Conclusions

For 45 years, there have been many challenges in the diagnosis of T2 deficiency and underestimation of its incidence. Improvement in T2 diagnosis together with expansion of NBS programs to more countries will maximize the detection of previously undiagnosed cases. Early diagnosis and management of T2 deficiency enable prevention of its serious acute and chronic complications and remarkably improve the prognosis.

Acknowledgments

The authors thank the Cultural Affairs and Missions Sector, Egyptian Ministry of Higher Education, for their support. They also thank the reviewers for their invaluable comments and suggestions.

Declaration of Conflicting Interests

The author(s) declared no potential conflicts of interest with respect to the research, authorship, and/or publication of this article.

Funding

The author(s) disclosed receipt of the following financial support for the research, authorship, and/or publication of this article: The present study was supported in part by Grants in Aid for Scientific Research from the Ministry of Education, Culture, Sports, Science and Technology of Japan (grant numbers 26114708, 24591505); Health and Labor Science Research Grants for Research on Intractable Diseases from the Ministry of Health, Labour and Welfare of Japan; and the Practical Research Project for Rare/Intractable Diseases from the Japan Agency for Medical Research and Development to T.F. [grant number 15AeK0109050h002].

References

1. Hori T, Yamaguchi S, Shinkaku H, et al. Inborn errors of ketone body utilization. *Pediatr Int.* 2015;57(1):41-48.
2. Fukao T, Mitchell G, Sass JO, Hori T, Orii K, Aoyama Y. Ketone body metabolism and its defects. *J Inherit Metab Dis.* 2014;37(4):541-551.
3. Fukao T. Beta-ketothiolase deficiency. Orphanet encyclopedia, September 2004, Updated February, 2015. Web site. http://www.orpha.net/data/patho/GB/uk-T2.pdf. Accessed October 11, 2015.
4. Daum RS, Lamm PH, Mamer OA, Scriver CR. A "new" disorder of isoleucine catabolism. *Lancet.* 1971;2(7737):1289-1290.
5. US National Library of Medicine. Beta-ketothiolase deficiency. Genetics Home Reference [Internet]. Bethesda (MD): The Library; Updated August, 2015. Web site. http://ghr.nlm.nih.gov/condition/beta-ketothiolase-deficiency. Accessed September 14, 2015.
6. van Hasselt PM, Ferdinandusse S, Monroe GR, et al. Monocarboxylate transporter 1 deficiency and ketone utilization. *N Engl J Med.* 2014;371(20):1900-1907.
7. Fukao T, Scriver CR, Kondo N; T2 Collaborative Working Group. The clinical phenotype and outcome of mitochondrial acetoacetyl-CoA thiolase deficiency (beta-ketothiolase or T2 deficiency) in 26 enzymatically proved and mutation-defined patients. *Mol Genet Metab.* 2001;72(2):109-114.
8. Thümmler S, Dupont D, Acquaviva C, Fukao T, de Ricaud D. Different clinical presentation in siblings with mitochondrial acetoacetyl-CoA thiolase deficiency and identification of two novel mutations. *Tohoku J Exp Med.* 2010;220(1):27-31.
9. Buhaş D, Bernard G, Fukao T, Décarie JC, Chouinard S, Mitchell GA. A treatable new cause of chorea: beta-ketothiolase deficiency. *Mov Disord.* 2013;28(8):1054-1056.
10. Sarafoglou K, Matern D, Redlinger-Grosse K, et al. Siblings with mitochondrial acetoacetyl-CoA thiolase deficiency not identified by newborn screening. *Pediatrics.* 2011;128(1):246-250.
11. Schutgens RBH, Middleton B, van del Blij JF, et al. Beta-ketothiolase deficiency in a family confirmed by in vivo enzymatic assays in fibroblasts. *Eur J Pediatr.* 1982;139(1):39-42.
12. Merinero B, Pérez-Cerdá C, García MJ, et al. β-Ketothiolase deficiency: two siblings with different clinical conditions. *J Inherit Metab Dis.* 1987;10(2):276-278.
13. Frazier DM, Millington DS, McCandless SE, et al. The tandem mass spectrometry newborn screening experience in North Carolina: 1997-2005. *J Inherit Metab Dis.* 2006;29(1):76-85.
14. Catanzano F, Ombrone D, Di Stefano C, et al. The first case of mitochondrial acetoacetyl-CoA thiolase deficiency identified by expanded newborn metabolic screening in Italy: the importance of an integrated diagnostic approach. *J Inherit Metab Dis.* 2010;33(3):91-4.
15. Riudor E, Ribes A, Perez-Cerda C, et al. Metabolic coma with ketoacidosis and hyperglycaemia in 2-methylacetoacetyl-CoA thiolase deficiency. *J Inherit Metab Dis.* 1995;18(6):748-749.
16. Fukao T, Song XQ, Yamaguchi S, et al. Identification of three novel frameshift mutations (83delAT, 754insCT, and 435+IG to A) of mitochondrial acetoacetyl-coenzyme A thiolase gene in two Swiss patients with CRM-negative b-ketothiolase deficiency. *Hum Mutat.* 1997;9(3):277-279.
17. Weerasinghe WAG, Jasinge E, Sarathchandra JC, Chinthaka RAK. Intermittent episodes of metabolic ketoacidosis in a seven-year-old boy: mitochondrial beta-ketothiolase deficiency. *Gall Med J.* 2013;18(1):51-53.
18. Fontaine M, Briand G, Ser N, et al. Metabolic studies in twin brothers with 2-methylacetoacetyl-CoA thiolase deficiency. *Clin Chim Acta.* 1996;255(1):67-83.
19. Fukao T, Maruyama S, Ohura T, et al. Three Japanese patients with beta-ketothiolase deficiency who share a mutation, c. 431A>C (H144P) in ACAT1: subtle abnormality in urinary organic acid analysis and blood acylcarnitine analysis using tandem mass spectrometry. *JIMD Rep.* 2012;3:107-115.
20. Middleton B, Bartlett K, Romanos A, et al. 3-Ketothiolase deficiency. *Eur J Pediatr.* 1986;144(6):586-589.
21. Fukao T, Yamaguchi S, Scriver CR, et al. Molecular studies of mitochondrial acetoacetyl-coenzyme A thiolase deficiency in the two original families. *Hum Mutat.* 1993;2(3):214-220.
22. Gibson KM, Elpeleg ON, Bennett MJ. Beta-ketothiolase (2-methylacetoacetyl-coenzyme A thiolase) deficiency: identification of two patients in Israel. *J Inherit Metab Dis.* 1996;19(5):698-699.
23. Fukao T, Nguyen HT, Nguyen NT, et al. A common mutation, R208X, identified in Vietnamese patients with mitochondrial acetoacetyl-CoA thiolase (T2) deficiency. *Mol Genet Metab.* 2010;100(1):37-41.
24. Karam PE, Habbal MZ, Mikati MA, Zaatari GE, Cortas NK, Daher RT. Diagnostic challenges of aminoacidopathies and organic acidemias in a developing country: a twelve-year experience. *Clin Biochem.* 2013;46(18):1787-1792.
25. Selim LA, Hassan SA, Salem F, et al. Selective screening for inborn errors of metabolism by tandem mass spectrometry in Egyptian children: a 5 year report. *Clin Biochem.* 2014;47(9):823-828.
26. Saini N, Malhotra A, Chhabra S, Chhabra S. Methylmalonic acidemia mimicking diabetic ketoacidosis and septic shock in infants. *Indian J Crit Care Med.* 2015;19(3):183-185.
27. Ngu LH, Zabedah MY, Shanti B, Teh SH. Biochemical profiling in two siblings with mitochondrial 2-methylacetoacetyl-CoA thiolase deficiency. *Malays J Pathol.* 2008;30(2):109-114.
28. Fukao T, Zhang GX, Sakura N, et al. The mitochondrial acetoacetyl-CoA thiolase (T2) deficiency in Japanese patients: urinary organic acid and blood acylcarnitine profiles under stable conditions have subtle abnormalities in T2-deficient patients with

some residual T2 activity. *J Inherit Metab Dis*. 2003(5);26: 423-431.

29. Law CY, Lam CW, Ching CK, et al. NMR-based urinalysis for beta-ketothiolase deficiency. *Clin Chim Acta*. 2015;438:222-225.
30. Gibson KM, Lee CF, Kamali V, Søvik O. A coupled assay detecting defects in fibroblast isoleucine degradation distal to enoyl-CoA hydratase: application to 3-oxothiolase deficiency. *Clin Chim Acta*. 1992;205(1-2):127-135.
31. Bonnefont JP, Specola NB, Vassault A, et al. The fasting test in paediatrics: application to the diagnosis of pathological hypo- and hyperketotic states. *Eur J Pediatr*. 1990;150(2):80-85.
32. Kano M, Fukao T, Yamaguchi S, Orii T, Osumi T, Hashimoto T. Structure and expression of the human mitochondrial acetoacetyl-CoA thiolase-encoding gene. *Gene*. 1991;109(2): 285-290.
33. Daum RS, Scriver CR, Mamer OA, Delvin E, Lamm P, Goldman H. An inherited disorder of isoleucine catabolism causing accumulation of alpha-methylacetoacetate and alpha-methyl-beta-hydroxybutyrate, and intermittent metabolic acidosis. *Pediatr Res*. 1973;7(3):149-160.
34. Hiyama K, Sakura N, Matsumoto T, Kuhara T. Deficient beta-ketothiolase activity in leukocytes from a patient with 2-methylacetoacetic aciduria. *Clin Chim Acta*. 1986;155(2): 189-194.
35. Yamaguchi S, Orii T, Sakura N, Miyazawa S, Hashimoto T. Defect in biosynthesis of mitochondrial acetoacetyl-coenzyme A thiolase in cultured fibroblasts from a boy with 3-ketothiolase deficiency. *J Clin Invest*. 1988;81(3):813-817.
36. Fukao T, Yamaguchi S, Tomatsu S, et al. Evidence for structural mutation (347Ala to Thr) in a German family with 3-ketothiolase deficiency. *Biochem Biophys Res Commun*. 1991;179(1): 124-129.
37. Fukao T, Yamaguchi S, Orii T, Osumi T, Hashimoto T. Molecular basis of 3-ketothiolase deficiency: identification of an AG to AC substitution at the splice acceptor site of intron 10 causing exon 11 skipping. *Biochim Biophys Acta*. 1992;1139(3):184-188.
38. Fukao T, Yamaguchi S, Orii T, Schutgens RB, Osumi T, Hashimoto T. Identification of three mutant alleles of the gene for mitochondrial acetoacetyl-CoA thiolase: a complete analysis of two generations of a family with 3-ketothiolase deficiency. *J Clin Invest*. 1992;89(2):474-479.
39. Wajner M, Sanseverino MT, Giugliani R, et al. Biochemical investigation of a Brazilian patient with a defect in mitochondrial acetoacetylcoenzyme-A thiolase. *Clin Genet*. 1992;41(4): 202-205.
40. Yamaguchi S, Fukao T, Kano M, et al. Further analysis of mutant thiolase protein in fibroblasts from a Japanese boy with 3-ketothiolase deficiency. *Tohoku J Exp Med*. 1992;167(2): 143-153.
41. Fukao T, Yamaguchi S, Wakazono A, Orii T, Hoganson G, Hashimoto T. Identification of a novel exonic mutation at -13 from 5' splice site causing exon skipping in a girl with mitochondrial acetoacetyl-coenzyme A thiolase. *J Clin Invest*. 1994;93(3): 1035-1041.
42. Fukao T, Song XQ, Yamaguchi S, et al. Mitochondrial acetoacetyl-coenzyme A thiolase gene: a novel 68-bp deletion involving 3' splice site of intron 7, causing exon 8 skipping in a Caucasian patient with beta-ketothiolase deficiency. *Hum Mutat*. 1995;51(1):94-96.
43. Wakazono A, Fukao T, Yamaguchi S, et al. Molecular, biochemical, and clinical characterization of mitochondrial acetoacetyl-coenzyme A thiolase deficiency in two further patients. *Hum Mutat*. 1995;5(1):34-42.
44. Fukao T, Kodama A, Aoyanagi N, et al. Mild form of beta-ketothiolase deficiency (mitochondrial acetoacetyl-CoA thiolase deficiency) in two Japanese siblings: identification of detectable residual activity and cross-reactive material in EB-transformed lymphocytes. *Clin Genet*. 1996;50(4):263-266.
45. Gibson KM, Feigenbaum AS. Phenotypically mild presentation in a patient with 2-methylacetoacetyl-coenzyme A (beta-keto)thiolase deficiency. *J Inherit Metab Dis*. 1997;20(5):712-713.
46. Fukao T, Nakamura H, Song XQ, et al. Characterization of N93S, I312T, and A333P missense mutations in two Japanese families with mitochondrial acetoacetyl-CoA thiolase deficiency. *Hum Mutat*. 1998;12(4):245-254.
47. Sewell AC, Herwig J, Wiegratz W, et al. Mitochondrial acetoacetyl-CoA thiolase (β-ketothiolase) deficiency and pregnancy. *J Inherit Metab Dis*. 1998;21(4):441-442.
48. Nakamura K, Fukao T, Perez-Cerda C, et al. A novel single-base substitution (380C>T) that activates a 5-base downstream cryptic splice-acceptor site within exon 5 in almost all transcripts in the human mitochondrial acetoacetyl-CoA thiolase gene. *Mol Genet Metab*. 2001;72(2):115-121.
49. Fukao T, Nakamura H, Nakamura K, et al. Characterization of 6 mutations in 5 Spanish patients with mitochondrial acetoacetyl-CoA thiolase deficiency: effects of amino acid substitutions on tertiary structure. *Mol Genet Metab*. 2002;75(3):235-243.
50. Fukao T, Matsuo N, Zhang GX, et al. Single base substitutions at the initiator codon in the mitochondrial acetoacetyl-CoA thiolase (ACAT1/T2) gene result in production of varying amounts of wild-type T2 polypeptide. *Hum Mutat*. 2003;21(6):587-592.
51. Zhang GX, Fukao T, Rolland MO, et al. Mitochondrial acetoacetyl-CoA thiolase (T2) deficiency: T2-deficient patients with "mild" mutation(s) were previously misinterpreted as normal by the coupled assay with tiglyl-CoA. *Pediatr Res*. 2004; 56(1):60-64.
52. Mrázová L, Fukao T, Hálovd K, et al. Two novel mutations in mitochondrial acetoacetyl-CoA thiolase deficiency. *J Inherit Metab Dis*. 2005;28(2):235-236.
53. Zhang G, Fukao T, Sakurai S, Yamada K, Michael Gibson K, Kondo N. Identification of Alu-mediated, large deletion-spanning exons 2-4 in a patient with mitochondrial acetoacetyl-CoA thiolase deficiency. *Mol Genet Metab*. 2006;89(3):222-226.
54. Sakurai S, Fukao T, Haapalainen AM, et al. Kinetic and expression analyses of seven novel mutations in mitochondrial acetoacetyl-CoA thiolase (T2): identification of a Km mutant and an analysis of the mutational sites in the structure. *Mol Genet Metab*. 2007;90(4):370-378.
55. Fukao T, Zhang G, Rolland MO, et al. Identification of an Alu-mediated tandem duplication of exons 8 and 9 in a patient with mitochondrial acetoacetyl-CoA thiolase (T2) deficiency. *Mol Genet Metab*. 2007;92(4):375-378.

56. Fukao T, Boneh A, Aoki Y, Kondo N. A novel single-base substitution (c.1124A>G) that activates a 5-base upstream cryptic splice donor site within exon 11 in the human mitochondrial acetoacetyl-CoA thiolase gene. *Mol Genet Metab*. 2008;94(4):417-421.
57. Fukao T, Horikawa R, Naiki Y, et al. A novel mutation (c.951C>T) in an exonic splicing enhancer results in exon 10 skipping in the human mitochondrial acetoacetyl-CoA thiolase gene. *Mol Genet Metab*. 2010;100(4):339-344.
58. Fukao T, Aoyama Y, Murase K, et al. Development of MLPA for human ACAT1 gene and identification of a heterozygous Alu-mediated deletion of exons 3 and 4 in a patient with mitochondrial acetoacetyl-CoA thiolase (T2) deficiency. *Mol Genet Metab*. 2013;110(1-2):184-187.
59. Akella RR, Aoyama Y, Mori C, Lingappa L, Cariappa R, Fukao T. Metabolic encephalopathy in beta-ketothiolase deficiency: the first report from India. *Brain Dev*. 2014;36(3):537-540.
60. Stuppia L, Antonucci I, Palka G, Gatta V. Use of the MLPA assay in the molecular diagnosis of gene copy number alterations in human genetic diseases. *Int J Mol Sci*. 2012;13(3):3245-3276.
61. Dhanasekaran S, Doherty TM, Kenneth J, et al. Comparison of different standards for real-time PCR-based absolute quantification. *J Immunol Methods*. 2010;354(1-2):34-39.
62. Haapalainen AM, Meriläinen G, Pirilä PL, Kondo N, Fukao T, Wierenga RK. Crystallographic and kinetic studies of human mitochondrial acetoacetyl-CoA thiolase: the importance of potassium and chloride ions for its structure and function. *Biochemistry*. 2007;46(14):4305-4321.
63. La Marca G. Mass spectrometry in clinical chemistry: the case of newborn screening. *J Pharm Biomed Anal*. 2014;101:174-182.
64. Lim JS, Tan ES, John CM, et al. Inborn Error of Metabolism (IEM) screening in Singapore by electrospray ionization-tandem mass spectrometry (ESI/MS/MS): an 8 year journey from pilot to current program. *Mol Genet Metab*. 2014;113(1-2):53-61.
65. Golbahar J, Al-Jishi EA, Altayab DD, Carreon E, Bakhiet M, Alkhayyat H. Selective newborn screening of inborn errors of amino acids, organic acids and fatty acids metabolism in the Kingdom of Bahrain. *Mol Genet Metab*. 2013;110(1-2):98-101.
66. Wilcken B, Wiley V, Hammond J, Carpenter K. Screening newborns for inborn errors of metabolism by tandem mass spectrometry. *N Engl J Med*. 2003;348(23):2304-2312.
67. Estrella J, Wilcken B, Carpenter K, Bhattacharya K, Tchan M, Wiley V. Expanded newborn screening in New South Wales: missed cases. *J Inherit Metab Dis*. 2014;37(6):881-887.
68. Al Riyami S, Al Maney M, Joshi SN, Bayoumi R. Detection of inborn errors of metabolism using tandem mass spectrometry among high-risk Omani patients. *Oman Med J*. 2012;27(6):482-485.

2

Mitochondrial Disease and Anesthesia

Vincent C. Hsieh, MD[1], Elliot J. Krane, MD[2,3], and Philip G. Morgan, MD[1]

Abstract

It is increasingly common for children with mitochondrial disease to undergo surgery and anesthesia. Although many different anesthetics have been used successfully for these patients, serious, unexpected complications have occurred during and following anesthetic exposure. This has led to the widespread opinion among anesthesiologists that mitochondrial patients are at increased risk from the stress of surgery and anesthesia. Defects in function of the mitochondrial electron transport chain can lead to striking hypersensitivity to volatile anesthetics in children. Despite this striking finding, the connection between mitochondrial function and response to anesthetics is unknown. We review here the anesthetic considerations for patients with mitochondrial defects. In addition, we present an approach to anesthetic care of these patients at our institutions.

Keywords

anesthetics, genetics, biochemistry, mitochondria, perioperative

Introduction

Mitochondrial disease (MD) is recognized as an important cause of a wide range of physiologic changes that affect the perioperative period.[1-3] Organ systems with high metabolic requirements are uniquely dependent on the energy delivered by mitochondria, and therefore logically should have the lowest threshold for displaying symptoms of MD. Thus, mitochondrial dysfunction most commonly affects the function of the central nervous system, the heart, the gastrointestinal (GI) tract, and the muscular system.[3-5] These same systems are strongly affected by anesthetics.

As diagnosis and treatment improve for children with MDs, it has also become increasingly common for children with MD to undergo surgical procedures for their long-term care. One published case series of 122 patients with muscle biopsy–confirmed MD, and another smaller series of 38 pediatric patients show that patients with MD may undergo brief general anesthetics using volatile anesthetics or propofol without serious anesthesia-related adverse events.[6] Recently, an additional report of 26 patients with genetically confirmed MD found no correlation between anesthetic chosen and complication.[7] However, 4of 26 patients did have a hemodynamic complication in the perioperative period. In each report, the large diversity in molecular causes for MD limits the ability to generalize the results to all mitochondrial patients. Kinder Ross, in an editorial in *Pediatric Anesthesia*, pointed out that patients with myopathies and MD *usually* do well regardless of the specific anesthetic approach that is chosen,[8] a conclusion supported by more recent case reports.[9,10] However, on theoretical grounds and based upon several case reports in which adverse outcomes were observed,[11-16] many anesthesiologists believe that patients with MD are at an increased risk for perioperative complications including organ damage or death. Given the relatively small published experience of this vulnerable population, the following management principles are designed to minimize risk when a diagnosis of mitochondrial myopathy is known or suspected.

General Concerns

Surgical procedures for pediatric patients with MD usually require general anesthesia. Patients with advanced sequela

[1] Department of Anesthesiology and Perioperative Medicine, University of Washington, Seattle, WA, USA

[2] Department of Anesthesiology, Perioperative and Pain Medicine, Stanford University, Stanford, CA, USA

[3] Department of Pediatrics, Stanford University, Stanford, CA, USA

Corresponding Author:

Philip G. Morgan, Department of Anesthesiology and Perioperative Medicine, University of Washington, Seattle, WA, USA.

Email: pgm4@uw.edu

of MD may present with respiratory failure, cardiac depression, conduction defects, or dysphagia.[2,3] Several reports document that patients with MD may face an increased risk of perioperative complications such as respiratory depression, worsened cardiac function and arrhythmias, metabolic disturbances, or severe neurologic injury. Respiratory depression may occur simply from the combination of anesthetic drugs and preexisting muscle weakness seen in any myopathic state.

Since most of the medications used for general anesthesia are depressants of one or more of these systems, great care must be exercised in managing their use.[17] Mitochondrial patients often require smaller doses of general anesthetics, local anesthetics, sedatives, analgesics, and neuromuscular blockers (paralytics) to achieve the desired end points. Furthermore, it is important to avoid increasing the metabolic burden of patients with MD by not requiring prolonged fasting, and preventing hypoglycemia, postoperative nausea and vomiting, hypothermia (with resulting shivering), prolonged orthopedic tourniquet application, acidosis, and hypovolemia.[18,19] Obviously, anesthesiologists try to avoid these complications in all patients, but the consequences can be greater in patients with mitochondrial defects. Finally, some patients with MD do not metabolize lactate normally; therefore, lactate-containing intravenous fluids (eg, lactated Ringer's solution) should not be administered.[17]

It is worth reminding the reader that MD is not 1 disorder but represents hundreds of different enzymatic mitochondrial defects, both genetic and environmental in origin. And yet there are few reports of remarkably small numbers of mitochondrial patients that conclude that the use of anesthetics is uniformly safe.[11-13] It is therefore incorrect and inaccurate to generalize from limited case series. Furthermore, these few case series with limited observation periods do not rule out delayed postoperative complications or _metabolic decompensation that may indeed result from a biochemically stressed state exacerbated by a combination of anesthetics, preoperative fasting, catabolism, or prolonged exposure to pain.

Hypersensitivity to Anesthetics

Most MDs fall broadly into 2 categories: respiratory chain defects and fatty acid metabolism defects.[2] Of the 5 complexes of the respiratory chain, complex I is inhibited by all inhaled halogenated anesthetics (but not nitrous oxide) and many parenteral drugs as well.[20-22] In a small series of children with MD, several patients with complex I defects showed an exquisite hypersensitivity to the inhaled halogentated agent sevoflurane, observed when monitoring the depth of anesthesia using a processed electroenceohalogram (EEG), such as the bispectral index (BIS).[23]

But essentially, every general anesthetic and ancillary anesthetic drug studied depresses mitochondrial function in vitro, although some ancillary medications seem to be clinically well tolerated. Fatty acid metabolism defects do not appear to alter sensitivity to volatile anesthetics, but defects in acylcarnitine transferase may increase the cardiotoxicity of bupivacaine.[24] In addition, at least on theoretical grounds, defects in acylcarnitine transferase may increase the toxicity of propofol, which also inhibits this enzyme.[17,25,26] Defects in the tricarboxylic acid cycle, substrate transport, and many unknown defects can also lead to MD. The precise interaction of most of these other mitochondrial defects with anesthetics and surgical stress is not known at this time. We discuss specific interactions below.

Table 1. Listed below are Common Anesthetic Agents and the Sites Affected by Each. The References Match those in the Manuscript.

Medication	Mitochondrial Effects	References
Barbiturates	Complex I inhibition	33
Etomidate	Complex I inhibition, mild inhibition complex III	32
Propofol	Acylcarnitine transferase, complexes I/II/IV inhibition	25,37,38
Benzodiazepines	Complex I/II/III inhibition	34
Ketamine	Increase energy consumption +/− reports of complex I	35,36
Dexmedetomidine	None reported	None
Fentanyl/remifentanil	Minimal	39
Morphine	Mild complex I inhibition	39,40
Volatile Anesthetics	Complex I inhibition	20,21,27
Bupivacaine (Etidocaine)	Acylcarnitine translocase Mild complex I	24

Volatile Anesthetics

Volatile anesthetics (isoflurane, sevoflurane, and desflurane) suppress oxidative phosphorylation, particularly at complex I, coenzyme Q, and to a lesser extent complex V[20,21,27] (Table 1). Studies in model organisms (*Caenorhabditis elegans* and mice) with selective mutations in multiple mitochondrial proteins in complex I have shown markedly increased sensitivities to volatile anesthetics.[28-30] The increased sensitivities are well tolerated provided there is careful monitoring of the anesthetic depth of patients and the anesthetic dose is titrated to the appropriate anesthetic depth.[17] It is also worth noting that volatile anesthetics in common use today are minimally metabolized. They are predominantly excreted unchanged by the lungs within minutes of turning off the anesthetic vaporizer. Their rapid elimination allows return of mitochondrial function after their discontinuation, a benefit compared with most parenteral anesthetic agents, which undergo extensive hepatic metabolism and excretion for their offset.

Parenteral Anesthetics

Parenteral drugs commonly used during a general anesthetic (propofol, etomidate, ketamine, barbiturates, midazolam, etc.) exert the majority of their effects via ligand-gated ion channels in the central nervous system[31] (Table 1). However, all of these drugs also have an additional effect in mitochondria: either direct or indirect inhibition of oxidative phosphorylation. In the cases of midazolam, etomidate, and barbiturates, the effect is primarily an inhibition of complex I although each has minor effects at other sites.[32-34] Some reports indicate that ketamine may also have an effect on complex I, although the work is inconclusive at this time.[35,36] Propofol strongly inhibits complex I, other sites of oxidative phosphorylation and utilization of fatty acids.[37,38] Yet, each of these anesthetic drugs has been reported to have been used successfully in a small number of patients with MD by anesthesiologists familiar with the care of patients with myopathy.[6,8,17]

Propofol is unique among parenteral anesthetics in that it is known to affect mitochondrial metabolism by at least 4 separate mechanisms. In vitro, propofol has been shown to uncouple oxidative phosphorylation and inhibit complexes I, II, and IV.[25,37,38] The strongest effect of propofol is that it inhibits the transport of long-chain acylcarnitine esters via an inhibition of acylcarnitine transferase (specifically carnitine palmitoyl transferase 1).[25] The latter effect has been implicated as the mechanism behind propofol infusion syndrome, a potentially fatal complication of long-term propofol infusions used in intensive care. Given the multiple mitochondrial effect sites of propofol, it is prudent not to use propofol-based anesthetic techniques (ie, continuous infusions of propofol, or total intravenous anesthesia) to patients with known or suspected MD. As discussed later, however, limited boluses of propofol for anesthetic induction seem generally well tolerated.[6,17]

Local Anesthetics

Regional anesthetic techniques and wound infiltration with local anesthetics provide analgesia without the inhibitory effect of parenteral opioids on respiratory drive and upper airway tone. There is a single report of ventricular dysrhythmia after a patient with carnitine deficiency received a small dose of bupivacaine (an amide local anesthetic), which may have been caused by the inhibition of carnitine–acylcarnitine translocase that occurs with that particular local anesthetic in vitro. It should be noted that other clinically useful amide local anesthetics (ropivacaine and lidocaine) inhibit carnitine–acylcarnitine translocase to a lesser degree and therefore have less of a deleterious effect on carnitine-stimulated pyruvate oxidation than does bupivacaine.[24] They should therefore be chosen over bupivacaine when nerve blocks are performed in children with MD. Chlorprocaine and tetracaine (ester class local anesthetics) have not been studied to our knowledge.

Anesthetic Medications With Minimal Mitochondrial Effects

At present, several adjuvant drugs used with a general anesthetic have *not* been shown to affect mitochondrial function in vitro. These include most opioids with the exception of morphine (which has been reported to mildly inhibit complex I and alter the mitochondrial transmembrane potential).[39,40] Given that postoperative respiratory depression is a concern in this population, the use of remifentanil, an opioid with a fast offset because it is rapidly metabolized by serum cholinesterases, has proven extremely useful in many cases. Nonopioid analgesics such as nonsteroidal anti-inflammatory drugs (NSAIDs) have also been used safely; many neurologists advise against using repeated doses of acetaminophen due to the energy demands on the liver for metabolism. The sedative benzodiazepines as well as the central nervous system (CNS) alpha-adrenergic agonist dexmedetomidine have also proven useful, although their clearance may be slowed and effects prolonged. Finally, although the in vitro literature is not definitive, analgesic doses of ketamine have been well tolerated by the report.

Our Approach

The following represents the evidence-based approaches of the Seattle Children's Hospital and Stanford Children's Hospital. The first point of importance is to maintain the ongoing treatment for the patient's with MD for as long as possible in the preoperative period. Some patients with MD may be taking medications such as vitamins, coenzyme Q, L-Carnitine, EPI-743 (a novel medication presently in trial for MD therapy [41,42]) as well as other medications. As a rule, we continue these medications until nil per os (nothing by mouth) (NPO) requirements necessitate their discontinuation and often add L-Carnitine to their IV fluids in patients who have shown a strong clinical response to the drug.

Anesthetic management of patients with MD requires meticulous attention to cardiorespiratory physiology and specific attention to mitochondrial function. Patients with hypotonia and generalized myopathy may be prone to intra and postoperative upper airway obstruction, hypoventilation, hypercarbia, and therefore acidosis. They benefit therefore from opioid-sparing techniques such as the use of local anesthetics, regional anesthesia, NSAIDs as well as avoidance of nondepolarizing neuromuscular blocking drugs to which patients with MD may have exaggerated sensitivity. The depolarizing muscle relaxant succinylcholine should not be administered in any patient with myopathy out of concern for their upregulation of nicotinic acetylcholine receptors in skeletal muscle, resulting in potentially lethal acute hyperkalemia and acute myolysis after succinylcholine administration.

In the perioperative setting, several measures are taken to minimize physiologic changes and therefore stress on impaired mitochondrial function. A complete anesthetic assessment should be performed to establish baseline comorbidities and the degree of organ system involvement. In particular, the history and physical should seek signs and symptoms of MD including cardiomyopathy, the history or presence of cardiac arrhythmias, respiratory weakness or insufficiency, obstructive sleep apnea, seizures, and lactic acidosis. Classical patterns of maternal inheritance of undiagnosed symptoms should also alert the anesthetist to the possibility of MD. Preoperative fasting is minimized (limited to 2 hours if possible) in order to prevent hypovolemia, hypoglycemia, and increased reliance on fatty acid metabolism (in the setting of impaired β-oxidation of fatty acids that may be seen in MD), and dextrose-containing maintenance fluids should be initiated for all fasting inpatients with the following exception. Many patients with MD are managed with ketogenic diets for control of seizure.[43] A ketogenic diet contraindicates the administration of glucose and theoretically complicates the use of propofol due to its effect on fatty acid metabolism. When patients receive dextrose, they should be monitored to ensure that they do not develop either hyperglycemia or lactic acidosis.[44]

Outpatient surgery should be scheduled as the first case in the morning to minimize fasting intervals. Continuous temperature monitoring is used to prevent both hypo- and hyperthermia, with the use of active patient warming or cooling devices, and intravenous fluid warmers to maintain euthermia. Continuous intraoperative electrocardiogram, blood pressure, and end-tidal gas monitoring are routine for all patients undergoing anesthetics, of course. Application of surgical tourniquets should be minimized as much as possible to avoid tissue hypoperfusion and ischemia.

Maintenance anesthetics (volatile agents or intravenous drugs) should be titrated incrementally, slowly, and carefully, while monitoring anesthetic depth clinically or ideally with the BIS or other processed electroencephalography system if available. It is important to remember that some patients with MD, particularly those with disorders affecting complex I, have shown exquisite sensitivity to anesthetic agents.[23] Although induction of general anesthesia with either propofol bolus or volatile anesthetics has been used in patients with MD,[6,8] it is advised to not administer propofol by continuous infusion after induction of anesthesia out of concern for propofol infusion syndrome in this vulnerable population. However, both we and others[17,25] are of the opinion that boluses of propofol are generally well tolerated unless the patient is metabolically compromised.[16]

The following have been safely, but anecdotally, used to provide anesthesia without causing recognizable mitochondrial or physiologic decompensation:

- small intravenous boluses of propofol, benzodiazepines, or ketamine;
- continuous infusion of dexmedetomidine;
- inhalation of sevoflurane; and
- bolus dosing or continuous infusion of short- or ultrashort-acting opioids such as fentanyl, sufentanil, alfentanil, or remifentanil.

Volume resuscitation with a physiological electrolyte solution without lactate is preferable to lactated Ringer solution, since patients with MD may have impaired lactate metabolism, and serum lactate levels would be artifactually high if measured to determine the degree of metabolic decompensation, if it were suspected.

The question of how long to keep a patient with MD under observation postoperatively usually hinges on how long the patient is likely to remain in a catabolic state. Close postoperative monitoring is essential to ensure that patients return to their baseline level of function prior to discharge from the postanesthesia care unit.

Summary

Meticulous attention to the same parameters that are important for all children forms the foundation of care for patients with MD. In addition, the anesthesiologist must recognize that patients with MD have heightened sensitivity or even untoward responses to many medications routinely used in anesthesiology. Intravascular volume and hydration status require close attention, with no administration of lactate and, when appropriate, addition of intravenous glucose. Central nervous system monitoring with processed EEG has proven helpful in small case series, primarily to prevent excessive dosing of inhaled anesthetics.

Declaration of Conflicting Interests

The author(s) declared no potential conflicts of interest with respect to the research, authorship, and/or publication of this article.

Funding

The author(s) received no financial support for the research, authorship, and/or publication of this article.

References

1. Muravchick S, Levy RJ. Clinical implications of mitochondrial dysfunction. *Anesthesiology*. 2006;105(4):819-837.
2. Falk MJ, Sondheimer N. Mitochondrial genetic diseases. *Curr Opin Pediatr*. 2010;22(6):711-716.
3. Falk MJ. Neurodevelopmental manifestations of mitochondrial disease. *J Dev Behav Pediatr*. 2010;31(7):610-621.
4. Schaefer AM, Taylor RW, Turnbull DM, Chinnery PF. The epidemiology of mitochondrial disorders–past, present and future. *Biochim Biophys Acta*. 2004;1659(2-3):115-120.
5. Taylor RW, Schaefer AM, Barron MJ, McFarland R, Turnbull DM. The diagnosis of mitochondrial muscle disease. *Neuromuscul Disord*. 2004;14(4):237-245.
6. Driessen J, Willems S, Dercksen S, Giele J, van der Staak F, Smeitink J. Anesthesia-related morbidity and mortality after surgery for muscle biopsy in children with mitochondrial defects. *Paediatr Anaesth*. 2007;17(1):16-21.
7. Smith A, Dunne E, Mannion M, et al. A review of anaesthetic outcomes in patients with genetically confirmed mitochondrial disorders. *Eur J Pediatr*. 2017;176(1):83-88.
8. Allison KR. Muscular dystrophy versus mitochondrial myopathy: the dilemma of the undiagnosed hypotonic child. *Paediatr Anaesth*. 2007;17(1):1-6.
9. Miyamoto Y, Miyashita T, Takaki S, Goto T. Perioperative considerations in adult mitochondrial disease: a case series and a review of 111 cases. *Mitochondrion*. 2016;26:26-32.
10. Gurrieri C, Kivela JE, Bojanic K, et al. Anesthetic considerations in mitochondrial encephalomyopathy, lactic acidosis, and stroke-like episodes syndrome: a case series. *Can J Anaesth*. 2011;58(8): 751-763.

11. Kitoh T, Mizuno K, Otagiri T, Ichinose A, Sasao J, Goto H. Anesthetic management for a patient with Kearns-Sayre syndrome. *Anesth Analg*. 1995;80(6):1240-1242.
12. Cheam EW, Critchley LA. Anesthesia for a child with complex I respiratory chain enzyme deficiency. *J Clin Anesth*. 1998;10(6):524-527.
13. Footitt EJ, Sinha MD, Raiman JA, Dhawan A, Moganasundram S, Champion MP. Mitochondrial disorders and general anaesthesia: a case series and review. *Br J Anaesth*. 2008;100(4):436-441.
14. Thompson VA, Wahr JA. Anesthetic considerations in patients presenting with mitochondrial myopathy, encephalopathy, lactic acidosis, and stroke-like episodes (MELAS) syndrome. *Anesth Analg*. 1997;85(6):1404-1406.
15. Vanlander AV, Jorens PG, Smet J, et al. Inborn oxidative phosphorylation defect as risk factor for propofol infusion syndrome. *Acta Anaesthesiol Scand*. 2012;56(4):520-525.
16. Savard M, Dupre N, Turgeon AF, Desbiens R, Langevin S, Brunet D. Propofol-related infusion syndrome heralding a mitochondrial disease: case report. *Neurology*. 2013;81(8):770-771.
17. Niezgoda J, Morgan PG. Anesthetic considerations in patients with mitochondrial defects. *Paediatr Anaesth*. 2013;23(9):785-793.
18. Wallace JJ, Perndt H, Skinner M. Anaesthesia and mitochondrial disease. *Paediatr Anaesth*. 1998;8(3):249-254.
19. Lerman J. Perioperative management of the paediatric patient with coexisting neuromuscular disease. *Br J Anaesth*. 2011;107(suppl 1):i79-i89.
20. Harris RA, Munroe J, Farmer B, Kim KC, Jenkins P. Action of halothane upon mitochondrial respiration. *Arch Biochem Biophys*. 1971;142(2):435-444.
21. Cohen PJ. Effect of anesthetics on mitochondrial function. *Anesthesiology*. 1973;39(2):153-164.
22. Becker GL, Pelligrino DA, Miletich DJ, Albrecht RF. The effects of nitrous oxide on oxygen consumption by isolated cerebral cortex mitochondria. *Anesth Analg*. 1986;65(4):355-359.
23. Morgan PG, Hoppel CL, Sedensky MM. Mitochondrial defects and anesthetic sensitivity. *Anesthesiology*. 2002;96(5):1268-1270.
24. Weinberg GL, Palmer JW, VadeBoncouer TR, Zuechner MB, Edelman G, Hoppel CL. Bupivacaine inhibits acylcarnitine exchange in cardiac mitochondria. *Anesthesiology*. 2000;92(2):523-528.
25. Wolf A, Weir P, Segar P, Stone J, Shield J. Impaired fatty acid oxidation in propofol infusion syndrome. *Lancet*. 2001;357(9256):606-607.
26. Withington DE, Decell MK, Al Ayed T. A case of propofol toxicity: further evidence for a causal mechanism. *Paediatr Anaesth*. 2004;14(6):505-508.
27. Kayser EB, Sedensky MM, Morgan PG, Hoppel CL. Mitochondrial oxidative phosphorylation is defective in the long-lived mutant clk-1. *J Biol Chem*. 2004;279(52):54479-54486.
28. Kayser EB, Morgan PG, Hoppel CL, Sedensky MM. Mitochondrial expression and function of GAS-1 in Caenorhabditis elegans. *J Biol Chem*. 2001;276(23):20551-20558.
29. Falk MJ, Rosenjack JR, Polyak E, et al. Subcomplex Ilambda specifically controls integrated mitochondrial functions in Caenorhabditis elegans. *PLoS One*. 2009;4(8):e6607.
30. Falk MJ, Kayser EB, Morgan PG, Sedensky MM. Mitochondrial complex I function modulates volatile anesthetic sensitivity in C. elegans. *Curr Biol*. 2006;16(16):1641-1645.
31. Campagna JA, Miller KW, Forman SA. Mechanisms of actions of inhaled anesthetics. *N Engl J Med*. 2003;348(21):2110-2124.
32. Devin A, Nogueira V, Averet N, Leverve X, Rigoulet M. Profound effects of the general anesthetic etomidate on oxidative phosphorylation without effects on their yield. *J Bioenerg Biomembr*. 2006;38(2):137-142.
33. Chance B, Williams GR, Hollunger G. Inhibition of electron and energy transfer in mitochondria. I. Effects of Amytal, thiopental, rotenone, progesterone, and methylene glycol. *J Biol Chem*. 1963;238:418-431.
34. Colleoni M, Costa B, Gori E, Santagostino A. Biochemical characterization of the effects of the benzodiazepine, midazolam, on mitochondrial electron transfer. *Pharmacol Toxicol*. 1996;78(2):69-76.
35. Ito H, Uchida T, Makita K. Ketamine causes mitochondrial dysfunction in human induced pluripotent stem cell-derived neurons. *PLoS One*. 2015;10(5):e0128445.
36. Venancio C, Felix L, Almeida V, et al. Acute ketamine impairs mitochondrial function and promotes superoxide dismutase activity in the rat brain. *Anesth Analg*. 2015;120(2):320-328.
37. Bergamini C, Moruzzi N, Volta F, et al. Role of mitochondrial complex I and protective effect of CoQ10 supplementation in propofol induced cytotoxicity. *J Bioenerg Biomembr*. 2016;48(4):413-423.
38. Wu GJ, Tai YT, Chen TL, Lin LL, Ueng YF, Chen RM. Propofol specifically inhibits mitochondrial membrane potential but not complex I NADH dehydrogenase activity, thus reducing cellular ATP biosynthesis and migration of macrophages. *Ann N Y Acad Sci*. 2005;1042:168-176.
39. Mastronicola D, Arcuri E, Arese M, et al. Morphine but not fentanyl and methadone affects mitochondrial membrane potential by inducing nitric oxide release in glioma cells. *Cell Mol Life Sci*. 2004;61(23):2991-2997.
40. Cunha-Oliveira T, Silva L, Silva AM, Moreno AJ, Oliveira CR, Santos MS. Mitochondrial complex I dysfunction induced by cocaine and cocaine plus morphine in brain and liver mitochondria. *Toxicol Lett*. 2013;219(3):298-306.
41. Blankenberg FG, Kinsman SL, Cohen BH, et al. Brain uptake of Tc99m-HMPAO correlates with clinical response to the novel redox modulating agent EPI-743 in patients with mitochondrial disease. *Mol Genet Metab*. 2012;107(4):690-699.
42. Enns GM, Kinsman SL, Perlman SL, et al. Initial experience in the treatment of inherited mitochondrial disease with EPI-743. *Mol Genet Metab*. 2012;105(1):91-102.
43. Steriade C, Andrade DM, Faghfoury H, Tarnopolsky MA, Tai P. Mitochondrial encephalopathy with lactic acidosis and stroke-like episodes (MELAS) may respond to adjunctive ketogenic diet. *Pediatr Neurol*. 2014;50(5):498-502.
44. Haas RH, Parikh S, Falk MJ, et al; Mitochondrial Medicine Society's Committee on D. The in-depth evaluation of suspected mitochondrial disease. *Mol Genet Metab*. 2008;94(1):16-37.

3

The Central Nervous System Involvement in Fabry Disease

Alessandro Burlina, MD, PhD[1] and Juan Politei, MD[2]

Abstract

Fabry disease (FD) is an X-linked, lysosomal storage disorder caused by a mutation in the alpha galactosidase (GLA) gene leading to a deficiency in α-galactosidase A enzyme (α-Gal A) activity, which in turn results in accumulation of glycosphingolipids in different cells. The 2 major clinical phenotypes are the classic severe phenotype and the milder, later onset phenotype. In severe affected males with little or no α-Gal A activity, the onset of acroparesthesias, hypohidrosis, angiokeratomas, and corneal dystrophy is typically observed in childhood or adolescence. With advancing age, progressive multisystem microvasculopathic disease culminates in renal failure, cardiomyopathy, and/or cerebrovascular disease. Patients with later onset have residual enzyme activity and lack of vascular endothelial glycolipid accumulations; thus, they do not present with the early manifestations of the classic phenotype and typically present cardiac or renal disease in the fourth to seventh decade. Although the pathogenesis of cerebral vasculopathy in FD is poorly understood, it can be hypothesized that white matter changes may reflect the pathophysiology of the disease.

Keywords

pathophysiology, brain imaging findings, neuropsychiatry symptoms, cognitive dysfunction, treatment

Introduction

Fabry disease (FD) is a rare and highly debilitating storage disorder that results from a total lack of or deficiency in the lysosomal enzyme α-galactosidase A (α-Gal A) because of mutations in the *GLA* gene.[1] Fabry disease is inherited as an X-linked trait; many of the male patients develop a classic severe phenotype with early onset of symptoms, whereas heterozygous females exhibit phenotypes ranging from absence of symptoms to severe involvement of vital organs. Indeed, as recently demonstrated, the existence of skewed X chromosome inactivation in females with FD is the key molecular explanation of the wide range of severity in clinical manifestations.[2] The deficiency in α-Gal A causes accumulation of globotriaosylceramide (GL3), globotriaosylsphingosine (lyso-GL3) and related glycosphingolipids within the lysosomes of multiple cell types throughout the body.[1] Patients with later onset FD (also called type 2 phenotype, whereas the classic form is called type 1 phenotype) have residual α-Gal A activity and lack vascular endothelial GL3 accumulation; thus, they do not present with the early clinical manifestations of the severe phenotype. In the later onset phenotype, patients typically present with predominantly cardiac or renal disease in the fourth to seventh decade, indicating delayed onset and slower progression.[1]

Stroke is a common and serious clinical manifestation of FD. Recent evidence, from the literature on the natural history of FD and postmarketing surveillance databases of patients with FD treated with enzyme replacement therapy (ERT), has indicated that stroke may appear in young patients[3,4] and has been reported, in some patients, as the first disease's event.

The mechanisms underlying the stroke pathogenesis in FD have not been unraveled yet. Early pathophysiological changes are believed to predominantly involve microvasculature, but recently the compromise of large brain vessels has been reported even before the appearance of white matter lesions (WMLs) in brain magnetic resonance imaging (MRI).[5] Although ischemic strokes and transient ischemic attacks (TIAs) are the most prevalent types of overt cerebrovascular

[1] Neurological Unit, Department of Internal Medicine, St. Bassiano Hospital, Bassano del Grappa, Italy

[2] Fundación para el estudio de las enfermedades neurometabólicas (FESEN), Buenos Aires, Argentina

Corresponding Author:

Juan Politei, MD, Fundación para el estudio de las enfermedades neurometabólicas (FESEN), Buenos Aires, Argentina.

Email: jpolitei@hotmail.com

events in patients with FD, intracerebral hemorrhages, microbleeds, neurocognitive decline, and depression have also been reported.[6]

Prevalence

Silent WMLs are the most common findings in FD, before the onset of the "clinical" stroke, even though there are no reports on the frequency of other silent cerebrovascular events (ie, lacunar strokes and microbleeds). Several studies have estimated the incidence of stroke in various small cohorts of patients. Vedder et al[7] reported that 12 (48%) of 25 males and 13 (32%) of 41 females had experienced a cerebrovascular accident or lacunar stroke, at a median age of 46 and 52 years, respectively. Another group[8] reported that 4 (7%) of 54 female patients with Fabry had experienced strokes, at a median age of 51 years, and Mehta et al[4] found that 24 (11%) of 216 males and 27 (16%) of 172 females had experienced either a TIA or a stroke. Grewal et al reviewed various clinical and neuroradiological records and reported that 8 of 33 Fabry patients (24%) had experienced strokes at a median age as low as 26.5 years.[9] An analysis of a large cohort of 2446 patients in the Fabry Registry reported that stroke occurs in 6.9% of men and 4.3% of women.[3] Of these, 87% of first strokes were found to be ischemic, with hemorrhagic stroke reported in 13% of cases. Although the incidence of stroke increases with age in patients with FD, as in the general population, analysis of the Fabry Registry has indicated that the incidence of stroke among patients with FD is markedly higher than that observed in the general US population across all age categories.[3] From the Fabry Outcome Survey, the overall prevalence of ischemic stroke or TIAs was 13%.[4] Cerebrovascular events tending to occur at an earlier age with 12 times higher number of ischemic strokes in the male 25- to 44-year age-group compared to what could be expected in the general population.[6]

Fellgiebel et al reported that the frequency and severity of WMLs were similar for both sexes, with a prevalence of 31% in male and 36% in female patients.[10] In another study, the corresponding proportions were 27% (4 of 15) for women and 34% (11 of 32) for men.[11] Reisin et al described 36 adults with FD (14 men and 22 women) who were evaluated by MRI; 44% of them showed WMLs.[12] Among the 16 patients with abnormal MRI, 12 were women. The latter study is a further evidence confirming that women are not just carriers of FD and should be followed clinically and evaluated comprehensively to monitor for disease burden and progression.

In 2005, the first selective screening study in patients with cryptogenic stroke was published and reported a high number of presumed FD diagnoses: 4.9% of studied males and 2.4% of studied females.[13] However, other authors have failed to corroborate these relevant figures. Indeed, more recent studies indicate that the frequency of FD in cryptogenic stroke is likely less significant than initially suggested, probably below 1%.[14]

One possible explanation could be that in the study of 2005, there was the inclusion of intronic mutations, mutations of unknown clinical significance, or genetic variants/polymorphisms. It should be pointed out that the relationship between various types of *GLA* gene variants, the residual α-Gal A activity, and the clinical manifestations is complex and still under investigation. According to Schiffmann et al, we can classify *GLA* gene variants/mutations into 3 main groups: (1) *benign* genetic variants, not directly responsible for the clinical findings (eg, D313Y); (2) *risk factors*, genetic variants (eg, A143T) that concur with other risk factors for the clinical findings; (3) *causative mutations*, directly responsible for the disease.[15]

Pathophysiology

Historically, the cerebral pathology of FD has been considered a secondary manifestation of a primary endotheliopathy. Progressive accumulation of GL3 within the endothelium of intracranial blood vessels is thought to play a primary role in vasculopathy and risk of ischemic stroke. However, involvement of smooth muscle cells (SMCs) in the vessel wall has also been demonstrated, suggesting a more complex pathogenesis. The damage of SMCs in the medial vessel layer is the result of the storage of GL3 and derivatives, as a consequence of released hypertrophic factors such as Lyso-GL3 and sphingosine 1 phosphate.[16,17] This last mechanism has been confirmed by in vitro studies of cardiomyocytes and SMCs in culture.[18] A recent study showed that the removal of stored glycosphingolipid from the endothelial cells, as identified by conventional histological examination, does not prevent the progression of vascular disease.[19] Thus, the traditional concept that the storage in endothelial cells is the only mechanism responsible for the vascular dysfunction cannot be held. Indeed, other factors, such as the presence of a prothrombotic state,[20] abnormalities in cerebral blood flow velocity, autonomic dysfunction,[21] and increased production of reactive oxygen species, have also been identified to contribute to the development of stroke in patients with FD.[22] Another relevant mechanism contributing to stroke occurrence may be due to cardiac emboli and arrhythmias,[23] which are important and common cardiac manifestations in both genders of patients with Fabry.

The role of vascular or autonomic dysfunction as a pathogenic mechanism for stroke in patients with Fabry by compromising cerebral blood flow velocities and cerebral autoregulation has been studied by Hilz et al.[21] They investigated, by means of transcranial Doppler sonography, 22 patients with Fabry and 24 controls and assessed the resistance index, pulsatility index, cerebrovascular resistance, spectral powers of oscillations in electrocardiographic RR-intervals intervals, mean blood pressure, and mean cerebral blood flow velocities. The tested hypothesis was that the decreased cerebral blood flow velocities might result from downstream stenoses of resistance vessels and dilation of the insonated segment of the middle cerebral artery due to reduced sympathetic tone and vessel wall pathology with decreased elasticity. Furthermore, the augmented gain between blood pressure and cerebral blood flow velocity oscillations indicated an inability to dampen blood pressure fluctuations by cerebral

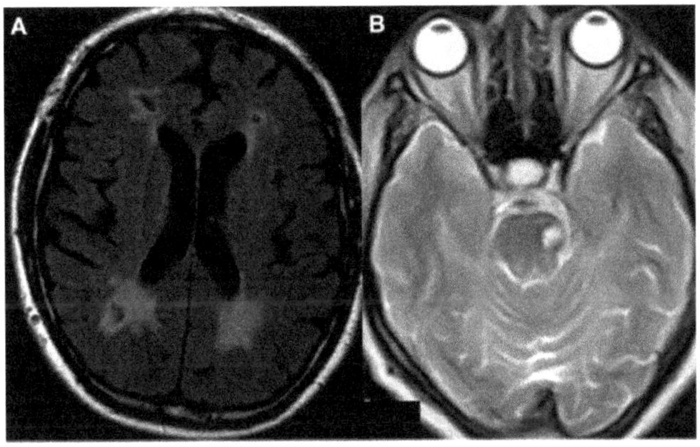

Figure 1. A, Periventricular white matter lesions in a 51-year-old male patient with Fabry disease. B, Ischemic lesion at the left pons level in a 42-year-old female patient with Fabry disease.

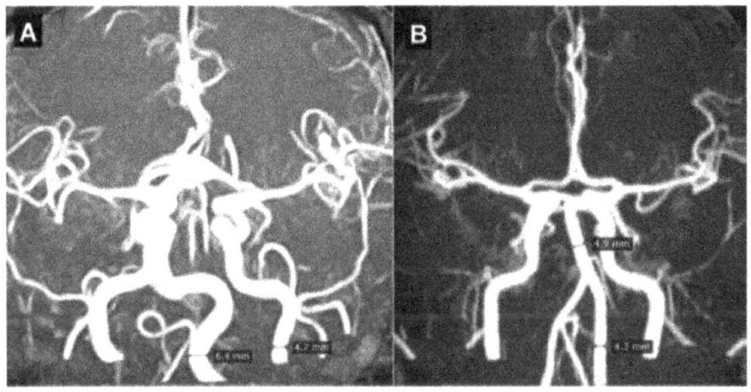

Figure 2. Vertebrobasilar dolichoectasia. A, 55-year-old male patient with Fabry disease, the diameter of the left vertebral artery is increased more than the homolateral internal carotid artery. B, 46-year-old female patient with Fabry disease; both diameters of the left vertebral artery and the basilar artery are increased.

autoregulation. The authors' conclusion was that, both reduced cerebral blood flow velocities and impaired cerebral autoregulation were likely to be involved in the increased risk of stroke in patients with FD.

Pathology studies regarding central nervous system (CNS) involvement in FD are rare. Nevertheless, a specific neuronal involvement has been reported.[24-27] The selective nature of the storage phenomenon is in accordance with the other disorders of the nervous system where accumulation of the substrate in nerve cells results from a metabolic disorder, as, for example, in gangliosidoses and metachromatic leucodystrophy.[28,29] Sites of selective storage in the CNS are amygdala, hypothalamus (supraoptic and paraventricular nuclei), substantia nigra, pontine reticular formation, the dorsal efferent nucleus of vagus, salivary nuclei, nucleus ambiguous, the mesencephalic nucleus of the fifth nerve, intermedial lateral columns, anterior horns, and dorsal root ganglia.[24-26] Numerous deposits of GL3 were visualized in the cytoplasm of the SMCs of the parenchymal and leptomeningeal vessels.[25,26] Other findings usually reported are the presence of segments of subarachnoidal medium-sized arteries with definite luminal stenosis due to intimal fibrosis, severe undulation of the internal elastic membrane, and stiffening due to subtotal or total replacement of medial SMCs by fibrosis.[26]

Brain Imaging Findings

The cerebrovascular involvement can be visualized on conventional MRI as (1) multiple lesions located in the deep white matter and in the subcortical gray matter of both hemispheres; (2) ischemic lesions, which can be silent lacunar strokes or clinically relevant strokes (Figure 1). The cerebral WML burden visible on brain MRI increases with age and can precede the onset of neurological symptoms.[30] The usual pattern of WMLs in FD shows a symmetric distribution, resembling a "vascular leukodystrophy." Nevertheless, the load of lesions and the pattern of distribution can be different according to aging, raising the question of differential diagnosis with multiple sclerosis. A recent study on a large cohort of patients with Fabry showed that the fourth decade of life is critical in the progression of WMLs.[31]

More recent studies, using proton emission tomography[32] and proton magnetic resonance spectroscopy,[33] have suggested that metabolic abnormalities can be found even in the absence of cerebral lesions in patients with FD.

Vertebrobasilar dolichoectasia (VBD) is a vascular condition that may cause severe morbidity due to ischemic or compressive dysfunction in the posterior fossa (ie, paroxysmal vertigo due to the compression of the VIII cranial nerve has been reported in a patient with FD).[34] Vertebrobasilar dolichoectasia may not be readily recognized by many neurologists or radiologists owing to the "normal" variation in the tortuosity or diameter of the vertebral and basilar arteries in healthy individuals. The study of dolichoectasia has been hampered by the lack of standardized diagnostic criteria. In 1996, Mitsias and Levine reviewed 53 cases and found elongated, ectatic, and tortuous vertebral and basilar arteries as the most common angiographic and pathologic features.[35] Recently, Politei et al reported that VBD was present in 55.5% of men and 34.8% of women (Figure 2) using Smoker's criteria.[5] The definitive prevalence and incidence of VBD is still unknown in the general population. According to the literature, the diagnostic frequency of VBD has been noted as 4.4% among 1440 magnetic resonance angiography records, 3.7% among 780 patients with posterior circulation ischemic stroke, 6% among 381 autopsies of fatal stroke, and 18.8% in 96 patients with isolated pontine infarction.[5] Pico et al reported that intracranial arterial dolichoectasia, including VBD, is found in 12% of patients with stroke.[36] It is important to emphasize that the median age in all the previous series is more than 50 years. The role of atherosclerosis in dolichoectasia is unknown, and whether atherosclerosis is the inciting event or an innocent bystander remains to be determined. The results from FD studies did not show a clear relationship between cardiovascular risk factors, cerebral ischemia, and the presence or absence of VBD or cerebral ischemia.[5] Currently, the different mechanisms involved in the cerebrovascular damage in FD have not indicated atherosclerosis as a major contributing risk factor. On the contrary, Doppler ultrasound studies showed an increase in the intima–media thickness without the presence of atherosclerotic plaques.[37,38] This finding has been reported in brain and coronary arteries in some autopsies.[39] The primary cause of dolichoectasia seems to be aberrant vascular remodeling. Dilation is associated with a large increase in the levels of early growth response factor 1 in endothelial cells, and the expression of this transcription factor is closely linked to the expression of matrix metalloproteinases (MMPs),[40] especially MMP-9.[41] Evidence indicates that MMPs break down the elastic lamina, and degradation of this component of the arterial wall is thought to aid the migration of SMCs, residing in the tunica intima, to the stressed medial layer.[38,42] Levels of MMP-9 were significantly higher in patients with FD than in controls and there was a positive correlation between MMP-9 levels and the Mainz Severity Score Index, a validated severity score for FD.[43] Dolichoectasia can affect both the anterior and the posterior circulations, but the posterior circulation and the basilar artery are most frequently affected in FD, one explanation could be that posterior circulation has less sympathetic innervation than the anterior circulation (Figure 2A).[5] Indeed, this asymmetry in trophic support that the sympathetic nerves confer on the vessel walls may render the posterior circulation more susceptible to deformity upon exposure to increases in blood flow. In 2009, Fellgiebel et al reported results of brain MR angiography of 25 patients with FD, in comparison with a control group.[44] The principal finding of this study was that the basilar artery diameter is clearly superior to the WML load for the differentiation of FD from controls. However, as recently reported by Üçeyler et al, the increased basilar artery of males with FD cannot distinguish patients with FD from patients with stroke.[45]

Moore et al[46] studied neuroradiologic images of 104 hemizygous patients with FD. Overall, 22 patients (23%) demonstrated pulvinar hyperintensity on T1-weighted images (the so-called *the pulvinar sign*). They concluded that hyperintensity in the pulvinar on T1-weighted images is a common, pathognomonic finding in FD, likely reflecting the presence of calcification, secondary to cerebral hyperperfusion and selective vulnerability of the pulvinar and adjacent thalamic nuclei. In the same issue of the *American Journal of Neuroradiology*, Takanashi et al reported the presence of T1 hyperintensity in 7 out of 9 male patients with Fabry.[47] This finding was later confirmed by Burlina et al[48] who investigated the pulvinar sign and its relationship with other clinical findings in a total of 36 patients from 14 families (Figure 3). The pulvinar sign was found in 5 severe affected male patients (with severe renal and cardiac involvement) but not in any of the investigated female patients. Furthermore, Burlina et al demonstrated that the pulvinar sign is not a pathognomonic neuroradiological sign of FD, being present under other pathological conditions.[48] Recently, the detection of a faint pulvinar sign in 2 female patients with no significant cardiac and renal involvement indicates that this sign is not restricted to advanced stages of FD.[49]

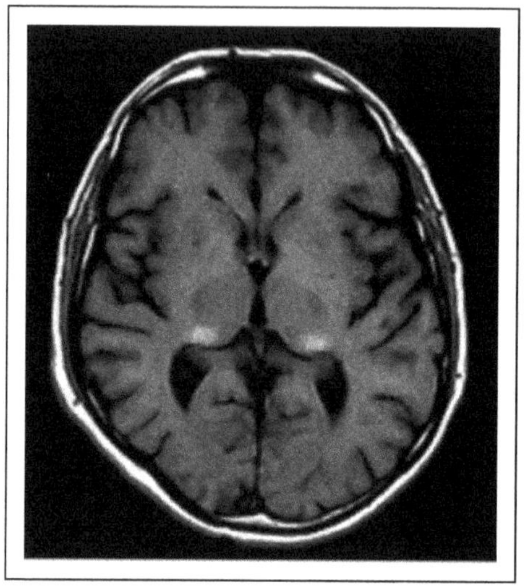

Figure 3. T1-axial image showing a well-defined symmetric hyperintensity of both pulvinar nuclei of a 46-year-old male patient with Fabry disease (Adapted from Burlina et al,[48] with permission from Springer).

Chiari type I malformation is a rare condition characterized by a herniation of the cerebellar tonsils, which extend more than 5 mm below the foramen magnum, often associated with syringomyelia. The prevalence has been reported to be lower than 0.24% in the literature.[50] In FD, the prevalence of this malformation was 10% and 12.7% in 2 different series patients, respectively.[51]

Neuropsychiatric Symptoms, Cognitive Dysfunction, and Sleep Disorders in FD

In FD, cognitive deficits have been described primarily in attention, executive functions, and psychomotor performance.[52,53] However, studies are inconclusive on the degree of these deficits and whether its development is a result of depressive symptoms or neurological alterations.

Schermuly et al could not find any relationship between depression and WML load in patients with FD.[53] In the same investigation, they found that 60% of the 25 patients with FD enrolled showed clinical depression compared to healthy controls. In fact, depression is by far the most frequently reported psychiatric complication of FD, ranging from 15% to 62.5% in all series.

Depression in FD has been reported to be directly associated with chronic pain. Cole et al[54] found 4 factors to be predictive of increased risk of depression in patients with FD. Two of these were factors related to depression in the general population (relationship status and financial status). The other 2 factors were more directly related to patients' illness. Firstly, having an additional chronic illness as well as FD increased the risk of depression. However, the strongest predictor of depression was the degree to which FD symptoms interfered with daily life, with both pain symptoms and inability to sweat (hypohidrosis/anhidrosis) being found to strongly predict depression. It is of note that cerebrovascular disease were not found to strongly predict depression.

Recently, 14 patients with Fabry (46.1 ± 10.8 years) participated in a neurocognitive investigation 8 years after the first assessment.[55] Patients were investigated by neuropsychiatric testing, brain MRI and MR angiography to determine WMLs, hippocampal volume, and the diameter of the larger intracranial arteries. While patients with Fabry did not differ in cognitive performance, they showed progressive and significant hippocampal volume loss over the 8-year observation period. None of the aforementioned brain imaging parameters were associated with the neuropsychiatric parameters. The depression frequency reduced from 50% at baseline to 21% at follow-up, but it did not reach significance. The authors concluded that patients with Fabry (10 patients were on ERT) have clinical stability in cognitive function, while pronounced hippocampal atrophy progressed throughout the 8 years.

A common finding in the clinical practice is the complain of excessive daytime sleepiness by patients with Fabry disease.[56,57] Indeed, as reported by Duning et al, excessive daytime sleepiness, with a frequency of 68%, can be considered one of the most common symptoms of FD.[56]

Treatment

Enzyme Replacement Therapy

There are 2 drugs available for ERT: agalsidase alfa (administered IV at a dosage of 0.2 mg/kg biweekly) and agalsidase beta (administered IV at a dosage of 1.0 mg/kg biweekly). Besides dosage and other different pharmacologic properties, both drugs share a common feature. They do not cross the blood–brain barrier. Short-term and long-term Fabry studies on ERT efficacy had focused on kidney and heart outcome.[58] There isn't any study designed to assess stroke prevention or recurrence. Nevertheless, data from the literature indicate that strokes can occur in patients on ERT.[59,60]

Recently, the WML burden and the effect of agalsidase beta 1 mg/kg biweekly on WML progression were assessed longitudinally in a phase 4 agalsidase beta placebo-controlled analysis of untreated and treated FD patients with mild to moderate renal involvement.[61] The primary end point was the difference in the number of patients with increased WML burden between the agalsidase beta and placebo groups at the end of treatment. Brain MRI scans from 41 patients with FD were analyzed. Patients with previous or recent strokes (n = 11, 39–68 years) showed an increase in the number of WMLs. A greater proportion of younger patients (≤50 years) on ERT had stable WML burden compared with younger patients in the placebo group (P = .014). Authors concluded that the WML burden in patients on ERT was more likely to remain stable, compared with patients on placebo. Thus, this study showed that agalsidase beta may reduce the progression of WML load, according to MRI analysis.

Concomitant/Supportive Therapy

Prevention of stroke is a critical issue in FD. Antiplatelet agents have been recommended for primary and secondary stroke prevention in FD, but their effectiveness has not been assessed with a specific study.[62] The same holds true for anticoagulants that are necessary if embolic events that stem from cardiac causes are a concern (warfarin is used in the clinical practice, while there are no reports on the use of the new oral anticoagulants). Blood pressure control is mandatory, and statin therapy should be considered.[63] Adequate intake of vitamins should be promoted, especially in cases of hyperhomocysteinemia.[64] Evaluation of comorbid prothrombotic risk factors may help to identify those with higher stroke risk (eg, patients with FD and the concurrent presence of factor V Leiden).[65] Although there are no evidence-based data, feasibility of thrombolysis in acute ischemic stroke in FD was recently demonstrated, as reported in 2 patients.[66,67]

Conclusions

The CNS is extensively involved in FD. Cerebrovascular findings include strokes, chronic WMLs, and brain vessel abnormalities. These clinical and neuroimaging findings are similar to those detected in other patients with cerebrovascular disease. Therefore, for diagnosing FD, an appropriate neurological workup that include detailed clinical history, neurological examination, and brain MRI investigations (search for WMLs, basilar artery dolichoectasia, and pulvinar sign) is necessary.

Until today, treatment studies did not address the specific issue of stroke prevention and recurrence. We hope that in the near future new studies on therapy will be designed, with the specific goal of neurological outcome for patients with FD.

Declaration of Conflicting Interests

The author(s) declared no potential conflicts of interest with respect to the research, authorship, and/or publication of this article.

Funding

The author(s) received no financial support for the research, authorship, and/or publication of this article.

References

1. Germain DP. Fabry disease. *Orphanet J Rare Dis*. 2010;5:30.
2. Echevarria L, Benistan K, Touissant A, et al. X-chromosome inactivation in female patients with Fabry disease. *Clin Genet*. 2016; 89(1): 44-54.
3. Sims K, Politei J, Banikazemi M, Lee P. Stroke in Fabry disease frequently occurs before diagnosis and in the absence of other clinical events: natural history data from the Fabry Registry. *Stroke*. 2009;40(3):788-794.
4. Mehta A, Ginsberg L; FOS Investigators. Natural history of the cerebrovascular complications of Fabry disease. *Acta Paediatr Suppl*. 2005;94(447):24-27.
5. Politei J, Schenone A, Burlina A, et al. Vertebrobasilar dolichoectasia in Fabry Disease: the earliest marker of neurovascular involvement? *J Inborn Err Metab Screening*. 2014;2:1-6.

6. Kolodny E, Fellgiebel A, Hilz M, et al. Cerebrovascular involvement in Fabry disease: current status of knowledge. *Stroke*. 2015; 46(1):302-313.
7. Vedder AC, Linthorst GE, van Breemen MJ, et al. The Dutch Fabry cohort: diversity of clinical manifestations and Gb3 levels. *J Inherit Metab Dis*. 2007;30(1):68-78.
8. Gupta S, Ries M, Kotsopoulos S, Schiffmann R. The relationship of vascular glycolipid storage to clinical manifestations of Fabry disease: a cross-sectional study of a large cohort of clinically affected heterozygous women. *Medicine (Baltimore)*. 2005; 84(5):261-268.
9. Grewal RP. Stroke in Fabry's disease. *J Neurol*. 1994;241(3): 153-156.
10. Fellgiebel A, Müller MJ, Mazanek M, Baron K, Beck M, Stoeter P. White matter lesion severity in male and female patients with Fabry disease. *Neurology*. 2005;65(4):600-602.
11. Ginsberg L, Manara R, Valentine AR, Kendall B, Burlina AP. Magnetic resonance imaging changes in Fabry disease. *Acta Paediatr Suppl*. 2006;95(451):57-62.
12. Reisin RC, Romero C, Marchesoni C, et al. Brain MRI findings in patients with Fabry disease. *J Neurol Sci*. 2011;305(1-2):41-44.
13. Rolfs A, Böttcher T, Zschiesche M, et al. Prevalence of Fabry disease in patients with cryptogenic stroke: a prospective study. *Lancet*. 2005;366(9499):1794-1796.
14. Linthorst GE, Ginsberg L.Prevalence of Fabry disease in TIA/ stroke cohorts. What define Fabry disease? *Eur J Neurol*. 2012; 19(11):1383-1384.
15. Schiffmann R, Fuller M, Clarke LA, Aerts JM. Is it Fabry disease? [published online May 19, 2016] *Genet Med*. 2016. doi:10.1038/ gim.2016.55.
16. Aerts JM, Groener JE, Kulper S, et al. Elevated globotriaosylsphingosine is a hallmark of Fabry disease. *Proc Natl Acad Sci U S A*. 2008;105(8):2812-2817.
17. Brakch N, Dormond O, Bekri S, et al. Evidence for a role of sphingosine-1 phosphate in cardiovascular remodelling in Fabry disease. *Eur Heart J*. 2010;31(1):67-76.
18. Barbey F, Brakch N, Linhart A, et al. Cardiac and vascular hypertrophy in Fabry disease: evidence for a new mechanism independent of blood pressure and glycosphingolipid deposition. *Arterioscler Thromb Vasc Biol*. 2006;26(4): 839-844.
19. Park JL, Whitesall SE, D'Alecy LG, Shu L, Shayman J. Vascular dysfunction in the alphagalactosidase A-knockout mouse is an endothelial cell-, plasma membrane-based defect. *Clin Exp Pharmacol Physiol*. 2008;35(10):1156-1163.
20. DeGraba T, Azhar S, Dignat-George F, et al. Profile of endothelial and leukocyte activation in Fabry patients. *Ann Neurol*. 2000; 47(2):229-233.
21. Hilz MJ, Kolodny EH, Brys M, Stemper B, Haendl T, Marthol H. Reduced cerebral blood flow velocity and impaired cerebral autoregulation in patients with Fabry disease. *J Neurol*. 2004;251(5): 564-570.
22. Shen JS, Meng XL, Moore DF, et al. Globotriaosylceramide induces oxidative stress and up-regulates cell adhesion molecule expression in Fabry disease endothelial cells. *Mol Genet Metab*. 2008;95(3):163-168.
23. Acharya D, Robertson P, Kay GN, et al. Arrhythmias in Fabry cardiomyopathy. *Clin Cardiol*. 2012;35(12):738-740.
24. Schiffmann R, Rapkiewicz A, Abu-Asab M, et al. Pathological findings in a patient with Fabry disease who died after 2.5 years of enzyme replacement. *Virchows Arch*. 2006;448(6):337-343.
25. Kaye EM, Kolodny EH, Logigian EL, Ullman MD. Nervous system involvement in Fabry's disease: clinicopathological and biochemical correlation. *Ann Neurol*. 1988;23(5):505-509.
26. Okeda R, Nisihara M. An autopsy case of Fabry disease with neuropathological investigation of the pathogenesis of associated dementia. *Neuropathology*. 2008;28(5):532-540.
27. Tagliavini F, Pietrini V, Gemignani F, Lechi A, Pallini R, Federico A. Anderson-Fabry's disease: neuropathological and neurochemical investigation. *Acta Neuropathol*. 1982;56(2):93-98.
28. Kornfeld M. Neuropathology of chronic GM2 gangliosidosis due to hexosaminidase A deficiency. *Clin Neuropathol*. 2008;27(5): 302-308.
29. Takashima S, Matsui A, Fujii Y, Nakamura H. Clinicopathological differences between juvenile and late infantile metachromatic leukodystrophy. *Brain Dev*. 1981;3(4):365-374.
30. Fellgiebel A, Müller MJ, Ginsberg L. CNS manifestations of Fabry's disease. *Lancet Neurol*. 2006;5(9):791-795.
31. Rost NS, Cloonan L, Kanakis AS, et al. Determinants of white matter hyperintensity burden in patients with Fabry disease. *Neurology*. 2016;86(20):1880-1886.
32. Moore DF, Altarescu G, Herscovitch P, Schiffmann R. Enzyme replacement reverses abnormal cerebrovascular responses in Fabry disease. *BMC Neurol*. 2002;18(2):4.
33. Politei JM, Capizzano AA. Magnetic resonance image findings in 5 young patients with Fabry disease. *Neurologist*. 2006;12(2): 103-105.
34. Prüss H, Bohner G, Zschenderlein R. Paroxysmal vertigo as the presenting symptom of Fabry disease. *Neurology*. 2006;66(2): 249.
35. Mitsias P, Levine SR. Cerebrovascular complications of Fabry's disease. *Ann Neurol*. 1996;40(1):8-17.
36. Pico F, Labreuche J, Touboul PJ, Leys D, Amarenco P. Intracranial arterial dolichoectasia and small-vessel disease in stroke patients. *Ann Neurol*. 2005;57(4):472-479.
37. Boutouyrie P, Laurent S, Laloux B, Lidove O, Grunfeld JP, Germain DP. Arterial remodelling in Fabry disease. *Acta Paediatr Suppl*. 2002;91(439):62-66.
38. Barbey F, Brakch N, Linhart A, et al. Increased carotid intimamedia thickness in the absence of atherosclerotic plaques in an adult population with Fabry disease. *Acta Paediatr Suppl*. 2006; 95(451):63-68.
39. Suzuki O, Abe M. An autopsy case of Fabry's disease with cardiac manifestations. *J Clin Exp Hematop*. 2009;49(2):121-123.
40. Sho E, Sho M, Singh TM, et al. Arterial enlargement in response to high flow requires early expression of matrix metalloproteinases to degrade extracellular matrix. *Exp Mol Pathol*. 2002; 73(2):142-153.
41. Tronc F, Mallat Z, Lehoux S, Wassef M, Esposito B, Tedgui A. Role of matrix metalloproteinases in blood flow-induced arterial enlargement: interaction with NO. *Arterioscler Thromb Vasc Biol*. 2000;20(12):E120-E126.

42. Lehoux S, Castier Y, Tedgui A. Molecular mechanisms of the vascular responses to haemodynamic forces. *J Intern Med.* 2006;259(4):381-392.
43. Shah JS, Hughes DA, Tayebjee MH, MacFadyen RJ, Mehta AB, Elliott PM. Extracellular matrix turnover and disease severity in Anderson-Fabry disease. *J Inherit Metab Dis.* 2007;30(1):88-95.
44. Fellgiebel A, Keller I, Marin D, et al. Diagnostic utility of different MRI and MR angiography measures in Fabry disease. *Neurology.* 2009;72(1):63-68.
45. Üçeyler N, Homola GA, Guerrero Gonzalez H, et al. Increased arterial diameters in the posterior cerebral circulation in men with Fabry disease. *PLoS One.* 2014;9(1):e87054.
46. Moore DF, Ye F, Schiffmann R, Butman JA. Increased signal intensity in the pulvinar on T1-weighted images: a pathognomonic MR imaging sign of Fabry disease. *Am J Neuroradiol.* 2003;24(6):1096-1101.
47. Takanashi JI, Barkovich J, Dillon WP, Sherr EH, Hart KA, Packman S. T1 hyperintensity in the pulvinar: key imaging feature for diagnosis of Fabry disease. *Am J Neuroradiol.* 2003;24(6):916-921.
48. Burlina AP, Manara R, Caillaud C, et al. The pulvinar sign: frequency and clinical correlations in Fabry disease. *J Neurol.* 2008;255(5):738-744.
49. Burlina AP, Politei J, Cinque S, et al. The pulvinar sign in Fabry patients: the first report in female patients. *J Neurol.* 2012;259(6):1227-1228.
50. Milhorat TH, Chou MW, Trinidad EM, et al. Chiari I malformation redefined: clinical and radiographic findings for 364 symptomatic patients. *Neurosurgery.* 1999;44(5):1005-1017.
51. Germain DP, Benistan K, Halimi P. Chiari type I malformation in four unrelated patients affected with Fabry disease. *Eur J Med Genet.* 2006;49(5):419-425.
52. Bolsover FE, Murphy E, Cipolotti L, Werring DJ, Lachmann RH. Cognitive dysfunction and depression in Fabry disease: a systematic review. *J Inherit Metab Dis.* 2014;37(2):177-187.
53. Schermuly I, Muller MJ, Muller KM, et al. Neuropsychiatric symptoms and brain structural alterations in Fabry disease. *Eur J Neurol.* 2011;18(2):347-353.
54. Cole AL, Lee PJ, Hughes DA, Deegan PB, Waldek S, Lachmann RH. Depression in adults with Fabry disease: a common and underdiagnosed problem. *J Inherit Metab Dis.* 2007;30(6):943-951.
55. Lelieveld IM, Böttcher A, Hennermann JB, Beck M, Fellgiebel A. Eight-Year follow-up of neuropsychiatric symptoms and brain structural changes in Fabry disease. *PLoS One.* 2015;10(9):e0137603.
56. Duning T, Deppe M, Keller S, et al. Excessive daytime sleepiness is a common symptom in Fabry disease. *Case Rep Neurol.* 2009;1(1):33-40.
57. Löhle M, Hughes D, Milligan A, et al. Clinical prodromes of neurodegeneration in Anderson-Fabry disease. *Neurology.* 2015;84(14):1454-1464.
58. Germain DP, Charrow J, Desnick RJ, et al. Ten-year outcome of enzyme replacement therapy with agalsidase beta in patients with Fabry disease. *J Med Genet.* 2015;52(5):353-358.
59. Jardim L, Vedolin L, Schwartz IV, et al. CNS involvement in Fabry disease: clinical and imaging studies before and after 12 months of enzyme replacement therapy. *J Inherit Metab Dis.* 2004;27(2):229-240.
60. Buechner S, Moretti M, Burlina AP, et al. Central nervous system involvement in Anderson-Fabry disease: a clinical and MRI retrospective study. *J Neurol Neurosurg Psychiatry.* 2008;79(11):1249-1254.
61. Fellgiebel A, Gartenschläger M, Wildberger K, Scheurich A, Desnick RJ, Sims K. Enzyme replacement therapy stabilized white matter lesion progression in Fabry disease. *Cerebrovasc Dis.* 2014;38(6):448-456.
62. Eng CM, Germain DP, Banikazemi M, et al. Fabry disease: guidelines for the evaluation and management of multiorgan system involvement. *Genet Med.* 2006;8(9):539-548.
63. Politei JM. Can we use statins to prevent stroke in Fabry disease? *J Inherit Metab Dis.* 2009;32(4):481-487.
64. Demuth K, Germain DP. Endothelial markers and homocysteine in patients with classic Fabry disease. *Acta Paediatr Suppl.* 2002;91(439):57-61.
65. Lenders M, Karabul N, Duning T, et al. Thromboembolic events in Fabry disease and the impact of factor V Leiden. *Neurology.* 2015;84(10):1009-1016.
66. Zenone T, Chan V. Young woman with recurrent ischemic strokes diagnosed as Fabry disease: lessons learned from a case report. *Clin Neurol Neurosurg.* 2011;113(7):586-588.
67. Saarinen JT, Sillanpää N, Kantola I. A male Fabry disease patient treated with intravenous thrombolysis for acute ischemic stroke. *J Clin Neurosci.* 2015;22(2):423-425.

4

The Link Between Lysosomal Storage Disorders and More Common Diseases

Michael Beck, MD[1]

Abstract

In the last decades, it has become more and more evident that lysosomal storage disorders and common neurodegenerative diseases such as Alzheimer and Parkinson diseases have clinical, neuropathological, and genetic features in common, including lysosomal dysfunction and impaired autophagy. Patients with Gaucher and even carriers of Gaucher disease have an increased risk to develop Parkinson disease. Likewise, individuals who are heterozygous for a mutation of a gene that causes an adult form of neuronal ceroid lipofuscinosis are more likely to be affected by a form of frontotemporal dementia in their later life. A further example is the gene *NAGLU* encoding the enzyme α-*N*-acetylglucosaminidase, which is deficient in patients with mucopolysaccharidosis type IIIB. Mutations of the *NAGLU* gene have been observed in patients affected by an axonal neuropathy. An interesting unexpected finding was the link between stuttering and genes that are essential for the function of all lysosomal enzymes. This review will present some example of the association of lysosomal storage disorders and neurodegenerative disease and discuss possible pathogenic mechanisms that are common to both conditions. The understanding of the pathophysiology of the endosomal–lysosomal–autophagic system may help to develop drugs, which might provide benefit not only for patients with rare lysosomal storage disorders but also for individuals affected by more common diseases.

Keywords

lysosomal storage disorders, Parkinson disease, Alzheimer disease, endosomal–lysosomal network, stuttering, frontotemporal dementia, neuropathy, ceroid lipofuscinosis, mucopolysaccharidosis

Introduction

Lysosomes cannot be regarded anymore as simple waste bags that have the singular task of degrading high-molecular-weight compounds but must now be recognized as the central regulator of cell homeostasis, with a functional role in many cellular processes. Lysosomes continuously fuse or interact transiently with other compartments in the autophagic and endocytic pathways and even with the plasma membrane, thereby forming a complex cellular system, the endosomal–lysosomal–autophagic pathway, which plays an essential role in signaling, growth, cell dynamics, defense, and regulation of metabolic homeostasis.[1-3]

It has been shown that in lysosomal storage disorders, the primary storage material can impair also the clearance of other cellular cargo, for example, amyloid β and α synuclein, processed through the endocytic and autophagic routes.

From the other side, a dysfunction of the endosomal–lysosomal (E/L) network plays an essential role in the pathogenesis of secondary storage disorders such as Alzheimer and Huntington diseases, as these conditions are caused by mutations of genes whose function directly or indirectly regulates part of the autophagic pathway, even though they do not encode lysosomal enzymes.

All storage disorders are characterized by the accumulation of material such as gangliosides or undegraded proteins within the endosomal–lysosomal–autophagic system. At the end, the accumulations of these compounds trigger degenerative processes. Postmitotic neurons are particularly vulnerable to the effect of toxic substances because they are unable to dilute the

[1] Institute of Human Genetics, University Medical Center, Mainz, Germany

Corresponding Author:
Michael Beck, MD, Institute of Human Genetics, University Medical Center, Langenbeckstrasse 1, Mainz 55131, Germany.
Email: dr.m.beck@t-online.de

storage material, unlike mitotic cells, which can remove their accumulated cargo through cell division.

In this review, clinical, pathophysiological, genetic, and therapeutic aspects of the association between lysosomal storage disorders and common neurodegenerative diseases will be discussed.

Common Neurodegenerative Diseases in the Context of Lysosomal Storage Disorders

Alzheimer Disease

Alzheimer, Parkinson, and Huntington diseases are neurodegenerative disorders, called proteinopathies, that are characterized by the presence of insoluble protein aggregates in the brain. A typical neuropathological feature of these conditions is the accumulation of cellular substances in neuronal cells that become toxic aggregates. In Parkinson disease, the aggregates consist of α-synuclein; in Huntington disease, Huntingtin is the accumulating compound; and Alzheimer disease is characterized by the deposition of neurofibrillary tangles (NFTs) and amyloid β (Aβ). The major component of the NFTs is hyperphosphorylated tau, a microtubule-stabilizing protein.

From pathological and genetic studies, it has become more and more clear that dysfunction of the E/L network plays an essential role in the pathogenesis of Alzheimer disease. It was first recognized 20 years ago that the E/L system is upregulated in this neurodegenerative disorder.[4] Alterations of the E/L system are evident in familiar forms of Alzheimer disease: The most common cause of early-onset familial Alzheimer disease is mutations of presenilin 1 (*PS1*), a transmembrane protein (TMEM) that is involved in the autophagic turnover of proteins. The PS1 has been shown to be essential for lysosomal acidification and proteolysis during autophagy, and defective lysosomal proteolysis is apparently responsible for pathogenic protein accumulations and neuronal cell death in Alzheimer disease.[5]

In some families, the duplication of the amyloid precursor protein (*APP*) gene is the cause of early-onset Alzheimer disease, and in an animal model of Down syndrome, it was shown that the triplication of the *APP* gene leads to the dysfunction of the endocytic pathway, resulting in defective neurotrophic signaling and neurodegeneration.[6] The epsilon4 allele of ApoE polymorphism represents the strongest genetic risk factor for late-onset Alzheimer disease, and Cataldo et al were able to demonstrate that inheritance of this polymorphism accelerates the abnormal endocytic upregulation seen in early Alzheimer disease.[7]

Studies in patients and mouse models have demonstrated that the disruption of the E/L system is an essential component in the pathophysiology of Alzheimer disease; conversely, a dysfunction of the E/L network results in the formation of tau insoluble aggregates, which leads to neurodegeneration, as seen in human neuroblastoma cells.[8] And Ohmi et al have detected hyperphosphorylated tau in a mouse model of Sanfilippo syndrome type B (mucopolysaccharidosis type IIIB [MPS IIIB]), and based on these findings, the author speculated that this lysosomal storage disorder should be regarded as a tauopathy.[9] Pathological abnormalities characteristic of Alzheimer disease, such as fragments of Aβ within enlarged neurons, have been demonstrated in the brain of patients affected by Niemann-Pick type C, thus reinforcing the close link between lysosomal storage disorders and more common neurodegenerative diseases.[10]

Parkinson Disease

In Parkinson disease, the main symptoms are rest tremor, rigidity, bradykinesia, postural instability, and nonmotor impairments such as autonomic dysfunction, depression, and cognitive deficits. Characteristic neuropathological changes are marked degeneration of dopamonergic neurons in the substantia nigra and the presence of Lewy body (LB) inclusions. Lewy bodies consist mainly of α-synuclein that is abnormally phosphorylated and tends to form insoluble fibrils.

For a long time, Parkinson disease was assumed to be a single, non-genetic disorder, but genetic analysis in a great number of affected individuals and their families has revealed a great number of genes associated with this condition.[11]

Clinical features similar to that of Parkinson disease are also observed in some lysosomal storage disorders, for example, bradykinesia and cognitive decline in Gaucher disease (defect of β-glucocerebrosidase). In 1996, Neudorfer et al reported that the incidence of Parkinson disease in patients with type I Gaucher was higher than expected.[12] Based on this and other observations, Tayebi et al studied the association of mutations of the β-glucocerebrosidase gene and Parkinson disease in 17 patients who, in addition to type I Gaucher disease, had symptoms of this neurodegenerative disorder such as rigidity, bradykinesia, and tremor. Genotyping in 14 patients revealed the common "non-neuronopathic" N370S mutation.[13] Using data from the International Gaucher Registry, it was calculated that patients with type I Gaucher have a 9% to 12% probability of developing Parkinson disease before the eighth decade of life,[14] as compared to a probability of 2.6% in the general population.[15] A study performed by Goker-Alpan et al in relatives of patients with Gaucher revealed that also heterozygotes of this lysosomal storage disorder have an increased risk for developing Parkinson disease.[16]

Aharon-Peretz investigated 99 Ashkenazi patients with idiopathic Parkinson disease and 1543 healthy Ashkenazi Jews for the occurrence of the 6 most common mutations of the *GBA* gene. Her results showed that 31 (31.3%) patients with Parkinson disease had 1 or 2 mutant *GBA* alleles, but only 6.2% (95 of 1543) of control participants carried a *GBA* mutation (92 were heterozygous for the mutation N370S and 3 were heterozygous for the mutation 84GG).[17] The suggestion that heterozygosity for a *GBA* mutation predisposes to Parkinson disease was confirmed in an international study in which 5691 patients with Parkinson disease (780 Ashkenazi Jews) and 4898 controls (387 Ashkenazi Jews) from 16 centers were enrolled. In both Jewish and non-Jewish patients with Parkinson disease, the frequency of a *GBA* mutation was significantly higher than in the control group. Furthermore, individuals who carried a *GBA* mutation had an earlier onset of symptoms and more often demonstrated atypical clinical manifestations compared to patients who were not carriers.[18]

The concept of an association of *GBA* mutations and Parkinson disease is based not only on clinical observations but also on neuropathology findings. In the brain of 4 patients who had symptoms of Parkinson disease in addition to type I Gaucher disease, LBs were detected. The level of the storage compound glucosylsphingosine, however, was not elevated.[13] When neuropathological, genetic, and immunofluorescence studies were performed in brain samples from 7 patients with Parkinson disease who had Gaucher disease or were heterozygous for a *GBA* mutation, immunofluorescence showed the presence of glucocerebrosidase in 75% of LBs. In samples from 7 participants without a GBA mutation, however, less than 10% of LBs were glucocerebrosidase positive.[19] These results demonstrate again that β-glucocerebrosidase represents an important component of pathological α-synuclein-positive inclusions.

Although the role of *GBA* mutations in the pathogenesis of Parkinson disease is not yet fully understood, several possible mechanisms have been proposed. It has been shown, for example, that α-synuclein is predominantly degraded by lysosomes, in part by chaperone-mediated autophagy.[20] In mouse models of lysosomal storage disorders that are associated with severe neurodegeneration (MPS type IIIA and multiple sulfatase deficiency), an impairment of the autophagic pathway was observed, leading to insufficient degradation of proteins such as α-synuclein or huntingtin.[21] Conversely, abnormalities of α-synuclein have an influence on the lysosomal function, as demonstrated by the studies of Cuervo et al who have shown that the pathogenic A53T and A30P α-synuclein mutants, bound to the lysosomal membrane via the receptor LAMP2A, inhibit both their own degradation and that of other proteins.[20] This observation, however, cannot explain why in the cerebrospinal fluid of patients with Parkinson disease a significant decrease in the activity of several lysosomal enzymes (including β-glucocerebrosidase) was observed.[22]

A direct physical interaction between β-glucocerebrosidase and α-synuclein at acidic pH has been detected by the use of fluorescence and nuclear magnetic resonance spectroscopy. This interaction apparently enables lysosomal degradation or prevents aggregation of α-synuclein, whereas the N370S mutant form of β-glucocerebrosidase has shown a reduced affinity for α-synuclein, possibly impairing its degradation.[23] In mice, elevated α-synuclein levels were observed within nigral cell bodies as well as in astroglia after the inhibition of β-glucocerebrosidase with conduritol B epoxide.[24]

Based on a comprehensive literature search, Shachar et al found that not only patients with Gaucher disease but also individuals affected by another neurodegenerative lysosomal storage disorder might develop symptoms of Parkinson disease and show pathological abnormalities such as α-synuclein aggregation in the brain and substantia nigra pathology.[25] An association with Parkinson disease has been described in GM1- and GM2-gangliosidosis, Niemann-Pick disease type C, neuronal ceroid lipofuscinoses (NCLs), and mucopolysaccharidoses, for example.

It has already been reported that mechanisms that might be implicated in the link between a rare lysosomal storage disorder and a more common neurodegenerative disease include impairment of autophagy, disturbance of calcium homeostasis, oxidative stress, and dysfunction of the ubiquitin–proteasome system.[26] All in all, one has to state that the present theories that try to explain the link between a group of lysosomal storage disorders and a synucleinopathy still have their limitations.

Frontotemporal Dementia and NCL

Frontotemporal dementia (FTD), the second most common form of young-onset dementia, is characterized by atrophy of the frontal and temporal lobes and is clinically, neuropathologically, and genetically heterogeneous.[27] The clinicopathological spectrum named frontotemporal lobar degeneration (FTLD) can be divided into 3 clinical syndromes: frontal variant (fvFTD) with predominant behavioral disorders, semantic dementia, and progressive nonfluent aphasia, in which language disturbances predominate. Two major pathological categories of FTLD can be distinguished. There are FTLD with tau-positive (FTLD-tau) inclusions and FTLD with ubiquitin and TAR DNA-binding protein of 43 kDa (TDP-43) positive, but tau-negative inclusions (FTLD-TDP). In only a small number of cases, immunoreactivity with the fused in sarcoma (FUS) antibody (FTLD-FUS) has been detected, and FUS-positive inclusions were additionally found in patients with neuronal filament inclusion disease. About a half of the familial FTD cases are caused by mutations in the microtubule associated protein tau (*MAPT*) and *GRN* (progranulin) genes, whereas mutations valosin-containing protein (*VCP*), charged multivesicular body protein 2B (*CHMP2B*), *TDP-43*, and *FUS* genes are found in less than 5% of cases.[27]

The assumption that dysfunction of the E/L pathway contributes to the pathogenesis of not only Alzheimer and Parkinson diseases but also of frontal lobar dementia was supported by many morphological and biochemical studies in the brains and cell culture models of affected patients. In fibroblasts of patients with FTD who carried a *CHMP2B* mutation, a malfunction of endosomal trafficking, namely the disruption of the fusion of endosomes with lysosomes, was detected.[28] Tresse et al have demonstrated an accumulation of large autophagic vesicles with cathepsin B activity in cells (myoblasts) from patients with FTD having a mutation of the *VCP* gene, indicating an autophagy defect. From this finding, the authors concluded that *VCP* is essential for maturation of ubiquitin-containing autophagosomes and that a defect in this function may contribute to FTD pathogenesis.[29]

The assumption that FTD and lysosomal storage disorders share common pathophysiological mechanisms was confirmed by the observation of a co-occurrence of NCL and FTD in 1 family[30]: In this family, the index cases were 2 adult siblings who had typical features of NGL, but in whom no mutation in known NCL genes could be found. Using linkage analysis and exome sequencing in the siblings, the homozygous deletion c.813_816del (p.Thr272Serfs *10) in the progranulin (*GRN*) gene was detected, and a similar 4 base pair (bp) deletion in exon 7 (c.811–814delCTCA) was already known as a pathogenic mutation, causing FTD when present in heterozygosity.[31] Later on, the ceroid lipofuscinosis, caused by a progranulin mutation, has been designated as CLN11.[32]

Neither parent of the siblings described by Smith et al had symptoms of dementia at the time of their clinical evaluation, although they were heterozygous for the 4 bp deletion, but one has to take into account that they were still in their 50s. There was, however, a history of dementia in several ancestors of both families.[30]

Additionally, studies in several animal models of FTD and NCL showed an overlap of morphological and biochemical abnormalities. In Grn$^{(-/-)}$ mice, in which the progranulin gene is completely absent, not only increased levels of TMEM 106B (a known risk factor for FTLD-TDP) but also an accumulation of lipofuscin and other components characteristic of NCL were detected.[33] Vice versa, in the brain of mice deficient in cathepsin D, which are a model for the most severe form of ceroid lipofuscinosis (congenital NCL10), an accumulation not only of saposin D, the typical storage material of patients with NCL10, but also increased levels of the FTLD-associated proteins progranulin and TMEM106B have been found.[33] The observation that in the brain of several patients with NCL, phosphorylated TDP-43 was detected in addition to the characteristic accumulation of saposin D, again implicates that lysosomal storage disorders and FTD share common features. This applies not only for *GRN*-associated frontal lobar dementia but also for FTLD cases caused by *CHMP2B* and *VCP* mutations that apparently also impair lysosomal function.[28,29] However, the mechanisms that lead to a malfunction of the lysosomal–endosomal–autophagic pathway in mutations of several genes of frontal lobar dementia are still unclear.

Axonal Neuropathy and MPS Type IIIB (Sanfilippo Disease IIIB)

Genetic sensory neuropathies, which are often accompanied by varying degrees of autonomic dysfunction, are usually painless and have an early onset.[34] Late-onset painful polyneuropathies, however, rarely have a genetic basis. Most are associated with other systemic disorders such as diabetes or alcohol abuse.[35] Little is known about genetically determined adult-onset forms of sensory neuropathy, but the identification of the underlying genetic defects may become possible by the application of new molecular techniques such as next generation sequencing. Whole exome sequencing was used by Tetreault et al to discover the mutated gene in a large family with many members affected by a dominant late-onset painful neuropathy.[36] Of 45 individuals of this French Canadian family, 21 had symptoms. Pedigree analysis suggested a dominant mode of inheritance, whereby a significant intrafamilial variability in age of onset and severity could be observed. All patients complained of painful sensations, and the diagnosis of a peripheral neuropathy was based upon the finding of decreased vibration sense and/or a loss of some deep tendon reflexes. Whole exome sequencing analysis in 4 affected individuals did not reveal a mutation in the genes for the types 1 to 5 of hereditary sensory and autonomic neuropathy, for Fabry disease, or for GM2-gangliosidosis. The great number of variants that was found by exome sequencing analysis was filtered against several databases in order to eliminate common polymorphisms. After the last step of filtering, 4 candidate variants were left, and only the missense mutation c.1208T>C (p.Ile403Thr) in exon 6 of the α-*N*-acetylglucosaminidase (*NAGLU*) gene was predicted to be pathogenic by the bioinformatics programs. This result was validated by Sanger sequencing, and segregation analysis in the whole family demonstrated that only the *NAGLU* mutation p.Ile403Thr segregated with the disease. This variant was not found in any available databases, but its location on the protein structure suggests an impact on the activity of α-*N*-acetyl-glucosaminidase. The activity of α-*N*-acetyl-glucosaminidase was measured in 42 individuals of this family and showed a reduction of about 50% of normal control, confirming the biological effect of the p.Ile403Thr mutation. No second *NAGLU* variant could be detected in any of the affected patients. In order to find additional patients affected by a neuropathy who might carry a *NAGLU* mutation, the authors searched a database of the University of Miami, the Genomes Management Application. In this database, a patient with Charcot-Marie-Tooth (CMT) was detected, who carried the nonsense p.Glu123X variant of the α-*N*-acetyl-glucosaminidase gene, that undoubtedly has a biological effect, as it leads to a truncation of the protein in the *N*-terminal domain before the catalytic domain. Many family members of the patient with CMT had diminished reflexes, reduced sense of vibration, and complained of pain. Segregation analysis, performed in 3 affected members from whom DNA was available, confirmed the presence of the NAGLU p.Glu123X variant.[36]

The lysosomal enzyme α-*N*-acetyl-glucosaminidase is involved in the degradation of the glycosaminoglycan heparan sulfate. A deficiency of this enzyme, caused by *NAGLU* mutations, leads to the neurodegenerative disorder Sanfilippo disease IIIB (MPS type IIIB), which is inherited in an autosomal recessive manner and characterized by a broad clinical heterogeneity.[37] Very mildly affected patients, described by Selmer et al, presented with sensory ataxia but had hyperactive tendon reflexes.[38] From the observation that *NAGLU* knockout mice develop significantly reduced response to painful stimuli by the age of about 4 months,[39] Tetreault and coworkers speculated that involvement of the peripheral nervous system could also be present in patients with MPS IIIB but that they are masked by the severe neurodegenerative symptoms.[36] Furthermore, it could be possible that the late-onset phenotype in heterozygotes of a *NAGLU* mutation is caused by the neurotoxic effects of slowly accumulating glycosaminoglycans, as in the brain of *NAGLU* knockout mice, an increased level of not only glycosaminoglycans but also of GM3 ganglioside and P-tau has been detected.[9] However, it is obvious that the association of peripheral neuropathy and *NAGLU* mutations cannot be fully explained at the present time.

Stuttering and Mucolipidosis

Stuttering is a speech disorder characterized by excessive repetitions of sounds and syllables as well as blockages of the vocal tract. The disorder typically arises in childhood but generally stops spontaneously. Only in a minority of cases, stuttering persist into adulthood. The cause of stuttering is unknown. From twin and family studies, however, it has become clear that genetic factors also play role in the etiology of this condition. Genetic studies in large families have uncovered linkage with several loci across the genome, for example, linkage with chromosome 3,13, and 15.[40] Riaz et al have performed a linkage analysis in a group of 44 consanguineous Pakistani families, each of them containing numerous individuals affected by stuttering. In these families, a very strong linkage with a locus on the chromosome 12q, giving a LOD score above 3, was detected.[41] Kang et al analyzed this region in more detail in Pakistani and North American families who had affected members, as well as in control participants.[42] They found a high incidence of mutations of genes that are required for the generation of the mannose-6-phosphate residue, a signal that directs lysosomal enzymes to the lysosome. These genes are the *N*-acetylglucosamine-1-phosphate transferase gene *GNPTAB*, which encodes the α and β subunits of GlcNAc-phosphotransferase (GNPT), the *GNPTG* gene, which encodes the γ subunit of GNPT, and the gene *NAGPA*, which encodes the so-called uncovering enzyme (UCE) that is responsible for removing 1 *N*-acetylglucosamine group, thereby exposing the targeting signal mannose-6-phosphate.

Mutations of the *GNTAB* gene, localized in chromosome 12q.23.3, and of the *GNPTG* gene, localized in chromosome 16p13.3, are known to cause the lysosomal storage disorders such as mucolipidosis type II and type III, which are multisystemic diseases in which also the central nervous system is often involved.[43] However, the mutations that have been observed in stuttering cases are totally different from those found in mucolipidosis. To date, there are no known disorders caused by mutations the *NAGPA* gene (localization: chromosome 16p13.3).

Kang et al reported a high incidence of mutations of the *GNPTAB*, *GNTPG*, and *NAGPA* genes in patients who had stuttering.[42] In order to confirm these preliminary results, the frequency of rare mutations in these genes was reexamined in a larger number of patients.[44] In this study, 1013 individuals with persistent stuttering from the United States, England, Pakistan, and Brazil were included. And 164 (16%) of the patients were found to carry a rare, non-synonymous coding variant in 1 of these 3 genes, this frequency being significantly higher in comparison to population-matched controls. In total, 81 different variants were detected in the stuttering participants. Almost all coding variants were missense amino acid substitutions. Only 1 mutation, a 3-bp in-frame deletion in the *GNPTAB* gene, has been previously described in a mildly affected patient with mucolipidosis type III.[45] In summary, Raza et al demonstrated that rare non-synonymous coding variants of the genes *GNPTAB*, *GNTPG*, or *NAGPA* account for as much 16% of persistent stuttering cases.[44]

The question arises, however, whether the variants of these genes in a heterozygous status even have an impact on the activity of the enzymes they are encoding. In order to answer this question, Lee et al analyzed the consequences of 3 mutations in the *NAGPA* gene, detected in individuals with persistent stuttering, on the function of the UCE.[46] These mutations (2 missense and 1 deletion/frameshift) resulted in impaired folding and rapid degradation, respectively, of the synthesized protein and finally in a reduction of cellular enzyme activity.

It was even demonstrated in an animal model, that mutations in genes essential for the function of lysosomal enzymes can significantly contribute to stuttering: Barnes reported on experiments he performed in a mouse that carried a missense mutation in the *GNTPAB* gene. This mouse was shown to produce fewer vocalizations per unit time and had longer pauses between vocalizations in comparison with controls, speech abnormalities that are comparable to those exhibited by stutterers.[47]

Taking together all findings from genetic investigations in large families, biochemical analyses, and the animal model, there is no doubt anymore that mutations of the *GNTPAB*, *GNPTGG*, and *NAGPA* genes, which function sequentially in the metabolic pathway of lysosomal enzymes, play an important role in the pathogenesis of stuttering. However, the functional mechanism behind the association of mutations in these genes and stuttering remains unknown, and to be able to find an explanation for this association, a better understanding of the pathophysiology of stuttering and the identification of neurons that are crucial for this process will be required.

Therapeutic Aspects

As many common neurodegenerative disorders are associated with a dysfunction of the E/L system, therapeutic interventions that aim to restore lysosomal function may also be useful for the treatment of conditions such as Alzheimer or Parkinson disease. A positive lysosomal modulation can be achieved in different ways. One possibility is to increase the activity of lysosomal enzymes, since it is known that in neuronal cells the accumulation of toxic agents leads to upregulation of catabolic enzymes, as this is apparent in the brain of patients with Alzheimer and in related transgenic mouse models. The compensatory mechanism, however, which should increase the degradation of the accumulating material, is not sufficient to prevent damage to the neuronal cells. Therefore, a further increase in the level of catabolic enzymes could be a therapeutic target. One way to increase the activity of lysosomal enzymes is to use small molecules that act as specific chaperones. In Alzheimer disease, Aβ forms complexes with the gangliosides GM2 and GM3. Assuming that a reduction in

Aβ could be achieved by lowering the GM2 level, Knight et al used the iminosugar OT1001, a chaperone for β-hexosaminidase, in an in vivo model of Alzheimer disease (Dutch APP^{E693Q} mouse). These transgenic mice, which overexpress APP and show intraneuronal accumulation of Aβ, also display significant learning deficits.[48] Treatment of the mice with OT1001 for 3 months led to a significant increase in brain β-hexosaminidase and a substantial reduction in Aβ in the perirhinal cortex. Additionally, an improvement in learning behavior could be demonstrated.[49]

The increased risk of Parkinson disease in patients and carriers of Gaucher disease is explained by the fact that deficient β-glucocerebrosidase activity leads to increased accumulation of α-synuclein in the central nervous system. It could be shown that, on the other hand, the formation of the membrane-bound α-synuclein complex with glucocerebrosidase inhibits enzyme function,[50] suggesting that β-glucocerebrosidase deficiency may also play a role in sporadic Parkinson disease. In order to investigate whether an increase in wild-type β-glucocerebrosidase activity by the use of a chaperone could be a therapeutic strategy for sporadic Parkinson disease in the absence of a *GBA* mutation, Richter et al performed an experiment in transgenic mice overexpressing human wild-type α-synuclein (Thy1-aSyn mice).[51] These animals were treated with AT2101 (afegostat-tartrate, isofagomine) that has been demonstrated to be a potential pharmacological chaperone of β-glucocerebrosidase.[52] Thy1-aSyn mice that received AT2101 for 4 months showed a reduction in α-synuclein immunoreactivity in dopaminergic neurons and an improvement in mobility and non-motor function, namely of olfactory deficits.[51]

A positive effect of enzyme enhancement on the level of α-synuclein, which is believed to be the major neurotoxic agent in the neurodegenerative process of Parkinson disease and other synucleinopathies, could be demonstrated not only in mouse models but also in patients affected by Gaucher disease. In these individuals, increased plasma levels of α-synuclein oligomers have been observed. Patients with Gaucher, however, who received enzyme replacement therapy for more than 5 years, showed much lower α-synuclein levels than untreated individuals.[53] From these results, it can be concluded that mutations in the *GBA* gene apparently are associated with an increase in plasma α-synuclein, and enzyme replacement therapy used for treatment of Gaucher disease might decrease the formation of this toxic compound.

Another way to improve lysosomal function, and thereby reverse abnormal aggregation of proteins, is the use of substances that have a direct effect on autophagic clearance. And in the last years, several non-toxic small molecules have been identified that are able to restore autophagy in neurons. Rapamycin, for example, is known to block mTOR, the master regulator of growth that is also an inhibitor of autophagy. Rapamycin has also been demonstrated to be able to ameliorate Aβ and tau pathology and rescue cognitive deficits in an animal model of Alzheimer disease.[54]

Latrepirdine, a Russian antihistaminic compound also known as Dimebon, has been assessed for its ability to regulate mTOR-dependent autophagy. In cultured cells, latrepirdine led to enhanced autophagy, and in a mouse model of Alzheimer disease, latrepirdine treatment was associated with a reduction in accumulation of Aβ- and α-synuclein.[55] In Russia, a randomized, placebo-controlled phase 2 clinical trial was performed in 134 patients with Alzheimer disease. Patients who were treated with Dimebon for 26 weeks showed a significant improvement in the Alzheimer disease assessment scale (ADAS-cog) in comparison to the placebo group.[56] The molecular mechanisms underlying the putative positive effects of latrepirdine in patients with Alzheimer are hardly understood. In a phase 3 clinical trial, however, Dimebon failed to show any significant effect in 2 coprimary and several secondary outcome measures.[57]

Many other autophagy-enhancing molecules have been studied in cell culture systems and mouse models that in the future may serve as therapeutics in neurodegenerative disorders.

Conclusion

Clinical, histological, biochemical, and genetic investigations in patients and animal models have clearly demonstrated that rare lysosomal storage disorders and more frequent neurodegenerative diseases share a common underlying feature, namely an impaired clearance of cellular cargo through the E/L network. However, the exact pathophysiological mechanisms tying together the various factors involved are not yet fully understood. In Alzheimer and Parkinson diseases, aggregates of undegraded proteins (Aβ, tau protein, α-synuclein) may impede the endosomal transport of not only these compounds but also of gangliosides and other possibly toxic macromolecules. On the other hand, a reduced activity of a lysosomal enzyme, as seen in heterozygous carriers of a lysosomal storage disorder causing mutation, might be insufficient to remove protein aggregates that should be degraded by the E/L. Examples of this possible mechanism are the link between frontotemporal lobar dementia and heterozygosity for *CLN11* mutations and the link between axonal neuropathy and heterozygosity for MPS IIIB mutations.

Up to now, there is no explanation for the association between stuttering and mutations of the genes sharing a role in the pathway of mannose-6-phosphate formation (an essential signaling marker for lysosomal enzymes). Patients who have stuttering and carry a mutation in one of these genes do not show any symptoms associated with mucolipidosis, and patients affected by mucolipidosis II or III do not stutter. Furthermore, the mutations in *GNPTAB* and *GNPTG* causing stuttering are completely different from those observed in ML II or ML III. One may hypothesize that the products of these gene have several functions and that different mutations have an influence on this function in different ways, leading to mucolipidosis II or III on one side and to stuttering on the other side.

The finding that there is a close link between neurodegenerative disorders and lysosomal storage disorders offers the opportunity for new therapeutic strategies. Compounds that induce autophagy, such as rapamycin, may have a beneficial effect in Alzheimer disease. In animal models and even in humans, it has been shown that drugs used for the treatment of Gaucher disease, such as enzyme replacement therapy and the chaperone isofagomine, are able to reduce levels of α-synuclein and therefore may be helpful in treating patients with Parkinson disease. It can be expected that in the future, drugs will be developed that are able to efficiently enhance protein clearance and slow down the progression of proteinopathies. Perhaps those drugs may provide a benefit for patients with a lysosomal storage disorder as well.

Declaration of Conflicting Interests

The author(s) declared no potential conflicts of interest with respect to the research, authorship, and/or publication of this article.

Funding

The author(s) received no financial support for the research and/or authorship of this article.

References

1. Luzio JP, Pryor PR, Bright NA. Lysosomes: fusion and function. *Nat Rev Mol Cell Biol*. 2007;8(8):622-632.
2. Saftig P, Klumperman J. Lysosome biogenesis and lysosomal membrane proteins: trafficking meets function. *Nat Rev Mol Cell Biol*. 2009;10(9):623-635.
3. Huotari J, Helenius A. Endosome maturation. *EMBO J*. 2011; 30(17):3481-3500.
4. Cataldo AM, Barnett JL, Berman SA, et al. Gene expression and cellular content of cathepsin D in Alzheimer's disease brain: evidence for early up-regulation of the endosomal-lysosomal system. *Neuron*. 1995;14(3):671-680.
5. Lee JH, Yu WH, Kumar A, et al. Lysosomal proteolysis and autophagy require presenilin 1 and are disrupted by Alzheimer-related PS1 mutations. *Cell*. 2010;141(7):1146-1158.
6. Cataldo AM, Petanceska S, Peterhoff CM, et al. App gene dosage modulates endosomal abnormalities of Alzheimer's disease in a segmental trisomy 16 mouse model of down syndrome. *J Neurosci*. 2003;23(17):6788-6792.
7. Cataldo AM, Peterhoff CM, Troncoso JC, et al. Endocytic pathway abnormalities precede amyloid beta deposition in sporadic Alzheimer's disease and Down syndrome: differential effects of APOE genotype and presenilin mutations. *Am J Pathol*. 2000; 157(1):277-286.
8. Hamano T, Gendron TF, Causevic E, et al. Autophagic-lysosomal perturbation enhances tau aggregation in transfectants with induced wild-type tau expression. *Eur J Neurosci*. 2008;27(5): 1119-1130.
9. Ohmi K, Kudo LC, Ryazantsev S, et al. Sanfilippo syndrome type B, a lysosomal storage disease, is also a tauopathy. *Proc Natl Acad Sci U S A*. 2009;106(20):8332-8337.
10. Jin LW, Shie FS, Maezawa I, et al. Intracellular accumulation of amyloidogenic fragments of amyloid-beta precursor protein in neurons with Niemann-Pick type C defects is associated with endosomal abnormalities. *Am J Pathol*. 2004;164(3):975-985.
11. Hardy J, Lewis P, Revesz T, et al. The genetics of Parkinson's syndromes: a critical review. *Curr Opin Genet Dev*. 2009;19(3): 254-265.
12. Neudorfer O, Giladi N, Elstein D, et al. Occurrence of Parkinson's syndrome in type I Gaucher disease. *QJM*. 1996;89(9):691-694.
13. Tayebi N, Walker J, Stubblefield B, et al. Gaucher disease with Parkinsonian manifestations: does glucocerebrosidase deficiency contribute to a vulnerability to parkinsonism? *Mol Genet Metab*. 2003;79(2):104-109.
14. Rosenbloom B, Balwani M, Bronstein JM, et al. The incidence of parkinsonism in patients with type 1 Gaucher disease: data from the ICGG Gaucher Registry. *Blood Cells Mol Dis*. 2011;46(1):95-102.
15. Elbaz A, Bower JH, Maraganore DM, et al. Risk tables for parkinsonism and Parkinson's disease. *J Clin Epidemiol*. 2002;55(1): 25-31.
16. Goker-Alpan O, Schiffmann R, LaMarca ME, et al. Parkinsonism among Gaucher disease carriers. *J Med Genet*. 2004;41(12): 937-940.
17. Aharon-Peretz J, Rosenbaum H, Gershoni-Baruch R. Mutations in the glucocerebrosidase gene and Parkinson's disease in Ashkenazi Jews. *N Engl J Med*. 2004;351(19):1972-1977.
18. Sidransky E, Nalls MA, Aasly JO, et al. Multicenter analysis of glucocerebrosidase mutations in Parkinson's disease. *N Engl J Med*. 2009;361(17):1651-1661.
19. Goker-Alpan O, Stubblefield BK, Giasson BI, et al. Glucocerebrosidase is present in alpha-synuclein inclusions in Lewy body disorders. *Acta Neuropathol*. 2010;120(5):641-649.
20. Cuervo AM, Stefanis L, Fredenburg R, et al. Impaired degradation of mutant alpha-synuclein by chaperone-mediated autophagy. *Science*. 2004;305(5688):1292-1295.
21. Settembre C, Fraldi A, Jahreiss L, et al. A block of autophagy in lysosomal storage disorders. *Hum Mol Genet*. 2008;17(1):119-129.
22. Balducci C, Pierguidi L, Persichetti E, et al. Lysosomal hydrolases in cerebrospinal fluid from subjects with Parkinson's disease. *Mov Disord*. 2007;22(10):1481-1484.
23. Yap TL, Gruschus JM, Velayati A, et al. Alpha-synuclein interacts with Glucocerebrosidase providing a molecular link between Parkinson and Gaucher diseases. *J Biol Chem*. 2011;286(32): 28080-28088.
24. Manning-Bog AB, Schule B, Langston JW. Alpha-synuclein-glucocerebrosidase interactions in pharmacological Gaucher models: a biological link between Gaucher disease and parkinsonism. *Neurotoxicology*. 2009;30(6):1127-1132.
25. Shachar T, Lo Bianco C, Recchia A, et al. Lysosomal storage disorders and Parkinson's disease: Gaucher disease and beyond. *Mov Disord*. 2011;26(9):1593-1604.
26. Vitner EB, Platt FM, Futerman AH. Common and uncommon pathogenic cascades in lysosomal storage diseases. *J Biol Chem*. 2010;285(27):20423-20427.
27. Seelaar H, Rohrer JD, Pijnenburg YA, Fox NC, van Swieten JC. Clinical, genetic and pathological heterogeneity of frontotemporal dementia: a review. *J Neurol Neurosurg Psychiatry*. 2011; 82(5):476-486.
28. Urwin H, Authier A, Nielsen JE, et al. Disruption of endocytic trafficking in frontotemporal dementia with CHMP2B mutations. *Hum Mol Genet*. 2010;19(11):2228-2238.

29. Tresse E, Salomons FA, Vesa J, et al. VCP/p97 is essential for maturation of ubiquitin-containing autophagosomes and this function is impaired by mutations that cause IBMPFD. *Autophagy*. 2010;6(2):217-227.
30. Smith KR, Damiano J, Franceschetti S, et al. Strikingly different clinicopathological phenotypes determined by progranulin-mutation dosage. *Am J Hum Genet*. 2012;90(6):1102-1107.
31. Benussi L, Binetti G, Sina E, et al. A novel deletion in progranulin gene is associated with FTDP-17 and CBS. *Neurobiol Aging*. 2008;29(3):427-435.
32. Warrier V, Vieira M, Mole SE. Genetic basis and phenotypic correlations of the neuronal ceroid lipofusinoses. *Biochim Biophys Acta*. 2013;1832(11):1827-1830.
33. Gotzl JK, Mori K, Damme M, et al. Common pathobiochemical hallmarks of progranulin-associated frontotemporal lobar degeneration and neuronal ceroid lipofuscinosis. *Acta Neuropathol*. 2014;127(6):845-860.
34. Axelrod FB, Gold-von Simson G. Hereditary sensory and autonomic neuropathies: types II, III, and IV. *Orphanet J Rare Dis*. 2007;2:39.
35. Hoeijmakers JG, Faber CG, Lauria G, Merkies IS, Waxman SG. Small-fibre neuropathies–advances in diagnosis, pathophysiology and management. *Nat Rev Neurol*. 2012;8(7):369-379.
36. Tetreault M, Gonzalez M, Dicaire MJ, et al. Adult-onset painful axonal polyneuropathy caused by a dominant NAGLU mutation. *Brain*. 2015;138(pt 6):1477-1483.
37. Valstar MJ, Bruggenwirth HT, Olmer R, et al. Mucopolysaccharidosis type IIIB may predominantly present with an attenuated clinical phenotype. *J Inherit Metab Dis*. 2010;33(6):759-767.
38. Selmer KK, Gilfillan GD, Stromme P, et al. A mild form of mucopolysaccharidosis IIIB diagnosed with targeted next-generation sequencing of linked genomic regions. *Eur J Hum Genet*. 2012;20(1):58-63.
39. Fu H, Bartz JD, Stephens RL Jr. et al. Peripheral nervous system neuropathology and progressive sensory impairments in a mouse model of mucopolysaccharidosis IIIB. *PLoS One*. 2012;7(9):e45992.
40. Wittke-Thompson JK, Ambrose N, Yairi E, et al. Genetic studies of stuttering in a founder population. *J Fluency Disord*. 2007;32(1):33-50.
41. Riaz N, Steinberg S, Ahmad J, et al. Genomewide significant linkage to stuttering on chromosome 12. *Am J Hum Genet*. 2005;76(4):647-651.
42. Kang C, Riazuddin S, Mundorff J, et al. Mutations in the lysosomal enzyme-targeting pathway and persistent stuttering. *N Engl J Med*. 2010;362(8):677-685.
43. Kollmann K, Pohl S, Marschner K, et al. Mannose phosphorylation in health and disease. *Eur J Cell Biol*. 2010;89(1):117-123.
44. Raza MH, Domingues CE, Webster R, et al. Mucolipidosis types II and III and non-syndromic stuttering are associated with different variants in the same genes. *Eur J Hum Genet*. 2016;24(4):529-534.
45. Cathey SS, Leroy JG, Wood T, et al. Phenotype and genotype in mucolipidoses II and III alpha/beta: a study of 61 probands. *J Med Genet*. 2010;47(1):38-48.
46. Lee WS, Kang C, Drayna D, Kornfeld S. Analysis of mannose 6-phosphate uncovering enzyme mutations associated with persistent stuttering. *J Biol Chem*. 2011;286(46):39786-39793.
47. Barnes TD, Wozniak DF, Gutierrez J, Han TU, Drayna D, Holy TE. A mutation associated with stuttering alters mouse pup ultrasonic vocalizations [published online April 13, 2016]. *Curr Biol*. doi:10.1016/j.cub.2016.02.068.
48. Gandy S, Simon AJ, Steele JW, et al. Days to criterion as an indicator of toxicity associated with human Alzheimer amyloid-beta oligomers. *Ann Neurol*. 2010;68(2):220-230.
49. Knight EM, Williams HN, Stevens AC, et al. Evidence that small molecule enhancement of beta-hexosaminidase activity corrects the behavioral phenotype in Dutch APP (E693Q) mice through reduction of ganglioside-bound Aβ. *Mol Psychiatry*. 2015;20(1):109-117.
50. Yap TL, Velayati A, Sidransky E, Lee JC. Membrane-bound alpha-synuclein interacts with glucocerebrosidase and inhibits enzyme activity. *Mol Genet Metab*. 2013;108(1):56-64.
51. Richter F, Fleming SM, Watson M, et al. A GCase chaperone improves motor function in a mouse model of synucleinopathy. *Neurotherapeutics*. 2014;11(4):840-856.
52. Kornhaber GJ, Tropak MB, Maegawa GH, et al. Isofagomine induced stabilization of glucocerebrosidase. *Chembiochem*. 2008;9(16):2643-2649.
53. Pchelina SN, Nuzhnyi EP, Emelyanov AK, et al. Increased plasma oligomeric alpha-synuclein in patients with lysosomal storage diseases. *Neurosci Lett*. 2014;583:188-193.
54. Caccamo A, Majumder S, Richardson A, Strong R, Oddo S. Molecular interplay between mammalian target of rapamycin (mTOR), amyloid-beta, and tau: effects on cognitive impairments. *J Biol Chem*. 2010;285(17):13107-13120.
55. Steele JW, Lachenmayer ML, Ju S, et al. Latrepirdine improves cognition and arrests progression of neuropathology in an Alzheimer's mouse model. *Mol Psychiatry*. 2013;18(8):889-897.
56. Doody RS, Gavrilova SI, Sano M, et al. Effect of dimebon on cognition, activities of daily living, behaviour, and global function in patients with mild-to-moderate Alzheimer's disease: a randomised, double-blind, placebo-controlled study. *Lancet*. 2008;372(9634):207-215.
57. Alzforum: Dimebon Disappoints in Phase 3 Trial. 2010. http://www.alzforum.org/news/research-news/dimebon-disappoints-phase-3-trial. Accessed November 29, 2016.

Validation of a Multiplex Tandem Mass Spectrometry Method for the Detection of Selected Lysosomal Storage Diseases in Dried Blood Spots

Graziela Schmitt Ribas, PhD[1], Jurema Fátima De Mari[1], Gabriel Civallero, PhD[1], Heryk Motta de Souza[2], Maira Graeff Burin, PhD[1], Carmen Regla Vargas, PhD[1,3], and Roberto Giugliani, PhD[1,4,5]

Abstract

Background: Interest in screening methods for lysosomal storage diseases (LSDs) has increased in recent years, since early diagnosis and treatment are essential to prevent or attenuate the onset of symptoms and the complications of these diseases. In the current work, we evaluated the performance of tandem mass spectrometry (MS/MS) for the detection of some LSDs, aiming the future use of this methodology for the screening of these disorders. **Methods:** Standard curves and quality control dried blood spots were assayed to evaluate the precision, linearity, and accuracy. A total of 150 controls were grouped according to age and subjected to measurement of lysosomal enzymes deficient in Niemann-Pick A/B, Krabbe, Gaucher, Fabry, Pompe, and Mucopolysaccharidosis type I diseases. Samples from 59 affected patients with a diagnosis of LSDs previously confirmed by fluorimetric methods were analyzed. **Results:** Data from standard calibration demonstrated good linearity and accuracy and the intra- and interassay precisions varied from 1.17% to 11.60% and 5.39% to 31.24%, respectively. Except for galactocerebrosidase and α-L-iduronidase, enzyme activities were significantly higher in newborns compared to children and adult controls. Affected patients presented enzymatic activities significantly lower compared to all control participants. **Conclusion:** Our results show that MS/MS is a promising methodology, suitable for the screening of LSDs, but accurate diagnoses will depend on its correlation with other biochemical and/or molecular analyses.

Keywords

lysosomal storage diseases, multiplex enzyme assay, tandem mass spectrometry

Introduction

Lysosomal storage diseases (LSDs) comprise a heterogeneous group of more than 50 genetic disorders, which result in the accumulation of macromolecular substrates that would normally be degraded/processed by proteins/enzymes involved in lysosomal metabolism.[1,2] Although individual LSDs are rare, their combined incidence has been estimated at 1 per 7700 live births.[1] The progressive accumulation of these molecules leads to cellular dysfunction, which may affect both somatic organs and the central nervous system. Clinical features suggestive of LSDs include developmental delay, progressive regression after a period of normal development, ataxia, seizures, weakness, and dementia.[2,3]

Since substrate accumulation and its tissue distribution can be variable even among patients with identical genotypes, the

[1] Medical Genetics Service, HCPA, and WHO Collaborating Center for the Development of Medical Genetic Services in Latin America, Porto Alegre, Rio Grande do Sul, Brazil
[2] Faculdade de Farmácia, UFRGS, Porto Alegre, Rio Grande do Sul, Brazil
[3] Departamento de Análises, Faculdade de Farmácia, UFRGS, Porto Alegre, Rio Grande do Sul, Brazil
[4] Department of Genetics and Postgraduate Program in Genetics and Molecular Biology, UFRGS, Porto Alegre, Rio Grande do Sul, Brazil
[5] Instituto Nacional de Genética Médica Populacional—INAGEMP, Porto Alegre, Rio Grande do Sul, Brazil

Corresponding Author:
Roberto Giugliani, Medical Genetics Service, Hospital de Clinicas de Porto Alegre, Rua Ramiro Barcelos 2350, Porto Alegre, RS 90035-903, Brazil.
Email: rgiugliani@hcpa.edu.br

symptoms of LSDs are not always recognized early in life.[4] Lysosomal storage diseases are usually diagnosed through biochemical assays for the enzyme of interest by using an artificial substrate with a fluorescent tag such as 4-methylumbelliferone.[5] However, the availability of suitable treatments for some of these disorders has resulted in increased efforts to develop new, reliable, and robust methods to perform high-throughput population screening. Thus, there is a growing consensus for the development of methods to detect these disorders before the onset of clinical symptoms, then allowing the early begin of therapeutic interventions.[6,7]

In 2006, Gelb and colleagues[8] designed a method to directly analyze the activity of lysosomal enzymes by using electrospray ionization tandem mass spectrometry (MS/MS). The method was first tested to detect galactocerebrosidase (GALC) activity, which is deficient in Krabbe disease, in human cell lysates. Later, this technique was adapted for dried blood spot (DBS) samples and new substrates (S) and internal standards (IS) were developed for Gaucher, Fabry, Pompe, and Niemann-Pick diseases, and more recently, for Mucopolysaccharidosis type I (MPS-I).[9] Since then, screening for LSDs by MS/MS has been implemented in North America and European countries as pilot projects.[10-12]

The present study addresses the implementation of the detection of 6 LSDs by MS/MS (Fabry, Niemann-Pick A/B, Pompe, Gaucher, Krabbe, and MPS-I diseases) by measuring the activities of α-galactosidase (GLA), acid sphingomyelinase (ASM), α-glucosidase (GAA), β-glucocerebrosidase (ABG), GALC, and α-L-iduronidase (IDUA), respectively, in DBS samples from affected and control individuals with different ages. Analyses were performed at Medical Genetic Service of Hospital de Clínicas de Porto Alegre (SGM/HCPA), Brazil, which is a reference center for the diagnosis of inborn errors of metabolism in Latin America.

Materials and Methods

Reagents

Reagents were purchased from Sigma Chemical Co (St Louis, Missouri). Cocktails containing the enzyme substrates and ISs were kindly donated by the Newborn Screening Translation Research Initiative at the North American Center for Disease Control and Prevention (CDC, Atlanta, Georgia). For the instrument calibration, standards with known ratios between the product of the reaction and the IS for each enzyme of interest were injected, which were also provided by CDC.

Patients and Controls

All participants of this study were recruited from SGM/HCPA, Brazil. A total of 150 control individuals were divided into 3 groups according to age: 50 newborns (mean age: 7.12 days), 42 children (mean age: 4.15 years), and 58 adults (mean age: 37.0 years).

Sixty-two DBSs from affected patients diagnosed at our institution by classic fluorimetric or radioisotopic methods (8 with Niemann-Pick A/B, 18 with MPS-I, 7 with Krabbe disease, 10 with Gaucher disease, 6 with Pompe disease, 10 with Fabry disease, and 3 heterozygous women for Fabry disease) were used as positive controls. Informed consent was obtained from all patients. For method validation, DBSs of the CDC Quality Assurance Program were used as positive controls.[13] This research was approved by the institutional ethics committee of HCPA, Brazil (project 13-0239).

Assay Cocktails Preparation

For preparing the GAA assay cocktail, 1.8 mL of a 100 g/L solution of CHAPS in water, 15.9 mL of a buffer 0.34 M sodium phosphate + 0.17 M sodium citrate, pH 4.0, and 0.3 mL of a 8 mM solution of acarbose in water were added to a vial containing GAA-S/IS. The GLA assay cocktail was prepared by adding 0.45 mL of a 120 g/L solution of sodium taurocholate in water, 14.67 mL of 0.174 M sodium acetate buffer pH 4.6, and 2.88 mL of 1 M solution of *N*-acetylgalactosamine in water to a vial containing GLA-S/IS. The ABG assay cocktail consisted of 2.4 mL of a 120 g/L solution of sodium taurocholate in water and 15.6 mL of 0.72 M phosphate–0.36 M citrate buffer, pH 5.1, in a vial containing ABG-S/IS. For preparing the ASM assay cocktail, 0.15 mL of a 120 g/L solution of sodium taurocholate in water and 17.85 mL of 0.93 M sodium acetate plus 0.604 mM zinc chloride buffer, pH 5.7, were added to a vial containing ASM-S/IS. The GALC assay cocktail was prepared by adding 1.8 mL of a solution containing 96 g/L sodium taurocholate with 12 g/L oleic acid in water and 16.2 mL of 0.2 M phosphate–0.1 M citrate buffer, pH 4.4, to a vial containing GALC-S/IS. Finally, for preparing the IDUA assay cocktail, 0.5 mL of inhibitor solution (3.0 mM D-saccharic acid 1,4 lactone monohydrate in water) and 17.5 mL of 0.11 M sodium formate–0.16 M formic acid buffer, pH 3.6, were added to a vial containing IDUA-S/IS.

Sample Preparation

All the procedures were conducted based on the methods described by Zhang et al[14] and Duffey et al.[15] We punched out 2 DBS disks of 3.2-mm diameter from each card. One disk was placed in a 96-well plate for the GALC assay, and the other disk was placed on a plate containing 70 μL of sodium phosphate elution buffer and then mixed on an orbital shaker for 1 hour at 250 rpm at 37°C. Each enzyme cocktail (15 μL), except the GALC assay cocktail, was added to a separate plate, and 10 μL of this DBS extract was added to it. The GALC assay cocktail (30 μL) was added to the GALC assay plate. All the plates were incubated at 37°C for 22 hours. After the reactions were complete, they were quenched with 100 μL of ethyl acetate–methanol (1:1) solution. Then, the 6 enzyme assays were mixed and the samples were extracted by adding 400 μL of both ethyl acetate and water to the plate. Then, 300 μL of the top organic layer was transferred to a deep-well plate, which was dried under N_2 gas. The dried extract was resuspended in a 100 μL of ethyl acetate–methanol (19:1) solution. Next, a solid-phase extraction was conducted by adding 100 μL of the resuspended extract into a multi-well filter plate (AcroPrep 96 Filter Plate 0.45 μm polytetrafluoroethylene) containing 100 mg of silica gel. This plate was washed 4 times with 400 μL of ethyl acetate–methanol (19:1) solution by using a microplate vacuum filtration apparatus. After drying the plate under N_2 gas, the extract was resuspended in 100 μL of the mobile phase (80% acetonitrile, 20% water containing 0.2% formic acid) for injection in the MS/MS equipment.

Tandem Mass Spectrometry Analysis

Electrospray ionization MS/MS was performed using a Waters Quattro Micro API tandem mass spectrometer (Waters, Massachusetts) in a positive-ion, multiple-reaction monitoring mode. A volume of 20 μL for each resuspended sample was injected into a Binary HPLC Pump using a Waters 2777C Sample Manager via a flow injection of 0.1 mL/min for 0.10 minutes, then decreasing to 0.05 mL/min until 1.5 minutes and backing to 0.1 mL/min until 2 minutes. The mobile phase consisted of 80/20 acetonitrile/water with 0.2% formic acid. The amount of product was calculated by multiplying the ratio of ion abundance of the product to that of the IS with the amount of the added IS and then dividing the value by the ratio of the response factor for each enzyme, which was calculated from the calibration curves obtained for the standards containing known ratios of product and IS. The enzyme activities were expressed in μmol/h/L and were calculated from the amount of product by assuming that a 3.2-mm DBS disk contained 3.2 μL of blood.

Evaluation of Precision, Accuracy, and Linearity

Intra-assay precisions (intra-assay coefficients of variation [CVs]) were determined by performing 3 replicated assays for the CDC QC samples at concentrations that showed medium and high activity. To evaluate the interassay CVs, enzyme activities of the same CDC samples were measured on 7 consecutive assays. Linearity was evaluated by analyzing the slopes and the correlation coefficients R^2 obtained from calibration curves constructed by injection of 6 calibration solutions containing the substrate and IS for each enzyme in predefined ratios (P/IS: 0, 0.10, 0.50, 1.0, 2.0, and 5.0). The accuracy was evaluated by comparing the enzymatic activities obtained in quality control DBSs with the results predetermined by the CDC.

Statistical Analysis

Comparison between enzyme activities from different individuals was performed using the nonparametric Mann-Whitney *U* test. A *P* value lower than .05 was considered significant. For the determination of the intra-assay and interassay CVs, results were expressed as mean (standard deviation). All analyses were performed using Statistical Package for the Social Sciences (SPSS) software, version 19.0, on a PC-compatible computer.

Table 1. Conditions for Tandem Mass Spectrometry and Multiple Reaction Monitoring (MRM) Transitions of the Products and Internal Standards.

	Cone Voltage, V	Collision Energy, eV	MRM Transition, m/z
ASM-P	28	25	398.4-264.4
ASM-IS	25	19	370.4-264.4
ABG-P	20	28	482.4-264.4
ABG-IS	28	27	510.4-264.4
GAA-P	20	20	498.4-398.4
GAA-IS	20	18	503.4-403.4
GLA-P	20	15	484.4-384.4
GLA-IS	18	15	489.4-389.4
GALC-P	20	20	426.4-264.4
GALC-IS	30	28	454.4-264.4
IDUA-P	12	15	391.1-291.20
IDUA-IS	19	12	377.10-277.20

Abbreviations: ABG, β-glucocerebrosidase; ASM, acid sphingomyelinase; GAA, α-glucosidase; GALC, galactocerebrosidase; GLA, α-galactosidase; IDUA, α-L-iduronidase; IS, internal standards; P, products.

Results

Parameters of MS/MS analysis and data for the calibration standards are listed in Tables 1 and 2, respectively. Data demonstrated good linearity, with correlation coefficient R^2 ranged from 0.975 to 0.9991. In order to evaluate the precision and accuracy of the technique, quality control materials provided by the CDC were assayed. These materials correspond to a pool of inactivated cord blood supplemented with 5% (low), 50% (medium), and 100% (high) unprocessed cord blood.[13] As demonstrated in Table 3, the mean of the enzyme activities measured in 7 consecutive assays was comparable to those reported by the CDC. The intra-assay CVs for GAA were 11.60% and 4.97%, for GLA were 5.96% and 4.91%, for ABG were 4.15% and 5.19%, for ASM were 1.42% and 6.67%, for IDUA were 11.33% and 6.08%, and for GALC were 7.86% and 1.17%, in medium and high QC samples, respectively. Interassay CVs were higher compared to intra-assay CVs; the interassay CVs for GAA were 5.8% and 11.25%, for GLA were 30.08% and 31.24%, for ABG were 8.37% and 5.39%, for ASM were 13.70% and 14.22%, for IDUA were 17.20% and 13.07%, and for GALC were 18.22% and 19.91%, at medium and high levels of enzyme activity, respectively.

The enzyme activities in the DBS samples from normal participants (newborns, infants, and adults) and nonnewborn patients are shown in Figures 1-6. As expected, the enzyme activities in the DBSs of patients were consistently lower than those obtained for the controls. Interestingly, the median activities of the enzymes GAA, GLA, ABG, and ASM were higher in newborns in relation to older controls. α-L-Iduronidase activity in control infants was higher in relation to newborns and adults. However, GALC activity did not present significant

Table 2. Calibration Results and Linearity Parameters.

Ratio P/IS	GAA, Observed Ratio	GLA, Observed Ratio	ABG, Observed Ratio	ASM, Observed Ratio	IDUA, Observed Ratio	GALC, Observed Ratio
0.00	0.03	0.003	0.019	0.022	0.03	0.02
0.10	0.11	0.12	0.094	0.11	0.12	0.11
0.50	0.57	0.54	0.45	0.47	0.47	0.49
1.00	1.09	0.99	0.90	1.11	0.96	0.99
2.00	1.93	2.11	2.07	1.96	1.91	1.96
5.00	3.54	5.06	4.17	4.6	4.63	4.8
R^2	0.975	0.99	0.99	0.99	0.99	0.99
Slope	0.70	0.99	0.84	0.92	0.92	0.97

Abbreviations: ABG, β-glucocerebrosidase; ASM, acid sphingomyelinase; GAA, α-glucosidase; GALC, galactocerebrosidase; GLA, α-galactosidase; IDUA, α-L-iduronidase; IS, internal standards; P, products.

Table 3. Comparison Between the Enzyme Activities Measurements (μmol/h/L) in Quality Control DBS Samples Determined in SGM/HCPA and by the CDC.

	ASM	GALC	ABG	GAA	GLA	IDUA
Reference values determined in QC DBS samples by the CDC						
Base pool	(0.0-0.33)	(0.03-0.12)	(0.0-0.45)	(0.0-0.60)	(0.0-0.90)	(0.0-0.41)
Low	(0.10-0.40)	(0.26-0.43)	(0.19-0.90)	(0.47-1.02)	(0.19-1.23)	(0.0-0.99)
Medium	(1.25-1.96)	(2.36-3.48)	(3.93-6.29)	(5.42-7.83)	(4.60-6.88)	(3.54-5.46)
High	(2.33-3.70)	(4.95-6.83)	(7.03-12.35)	(10.14-15.63)	(8.01-14.09)	(7.04-12.42)
Enzyme activities obtained from 7 consecutive assays in SGM/HCPA. Results were expressed as mean ± SD						
Base pool	0.18 ± 0.07	0.07 ± 0.02	0.28 ± 0.14	0.48 ± 0.21	0.79 ± 0.45	0.44 ± 0.12
Low	0.39 ± 0.17	0.33 ± 0.08	0.75 ± 0.24	0.98 ± 0.16	1.16 ± 0.33	0.82 ± 0.27
Medium	2.20 ± 0.30	2.82 ± 0.51	5.61 ± 0.47	5.30 ± 0.30	6.16 ± 1.85	5.53 ± 0.95
High	4.48 ± 0.63	5.54 ± 1.10	11.30 ± 0.60	10.37 ± 1.16	12.62 ± 3.94	11.59 ± 1.51

Abbreviations: ABG, β-glucocerebrosidase; ASM, acid sphingomyelinase; CDC, Centers for Diseases Control and Prevention; DBS, dried blood spots; GAA, α-glucosidase; GALC, galactocerebrosidase; GLA, α-galactosidase; IDUA, α-L-iduronidase; SGM/HCPA, Medical Genetic Service of Hospital de Clínicas de Porto Alegre; SD, standard deviation.

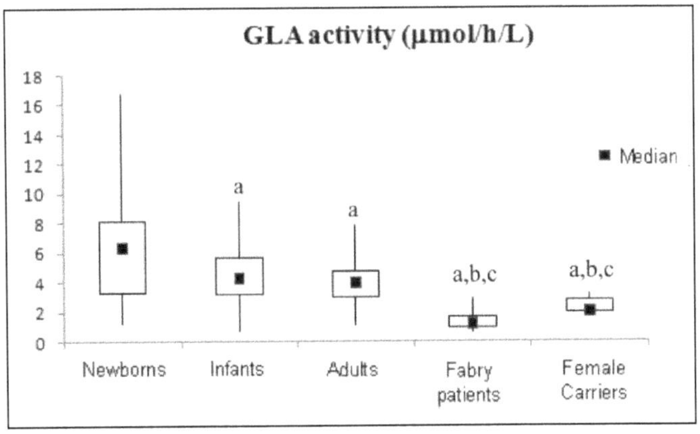

Figure 1. α-Galactosidase (GLA) activity in dried blood spot (DBS) samples from controls grouped according to age and from patients with Fabry disease. The error bars show the range of enzyme activity, the box represents those results within the 95th percentile, and the "■" symbol represents the median (Mann-Whitney *U* test, $P < .05$). [a]Different from newborns. [b]Different from infants. [c]Different from adult controls.

alterations between the different groups of controls. Using cutoff points of 30% of the median activity observed (0.51 μmol/h/L for Krabbe disease, 4.0 μmol/h/L for Gaucher disease, 1.91 μmol/h/L for Fabry disease, 3.0 μmol/ h/L for Pompe disease, 2.15 μmol/h/L for MPS-I, and 2.5 μmol/h/L for Niemann-Pick A/B), we did not observe overlaps between the enzyme activities of the affected patients and healthy controls of any age group for the enzymes GALC, ASM, GAA, and ABG. For MPS-I, 3 patients presented IDUA activity higher than those observed in newborn controls but lower in relation to nonnewborn normal participants. For Fabry disease, some patients presented GLA activity similar to the values of normal individuals, which could be associated with the enzyme replacement therapy.

Discussion and Conclusion

The availability of therapies for many LSDs, the relatively high combined incidence, the delay between the onset of symptoms

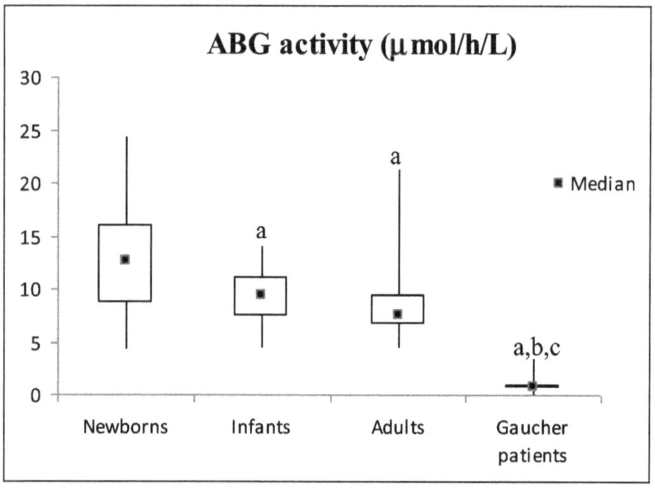

Figure 2. β-Glucocerebrosidase (ABG) activity in dried blood spot (DBS) samples from controls grouped according to age and from patients with Gaucher disease. The error bars show the range of enzyme activity, the box represents those results within the 95th percentile, and the "■" symbol represents the median (Mann-Whitney *U* test, $P < .05$). [a]Different from newborns. [b]Different from infants. [c]Different from adult controls.

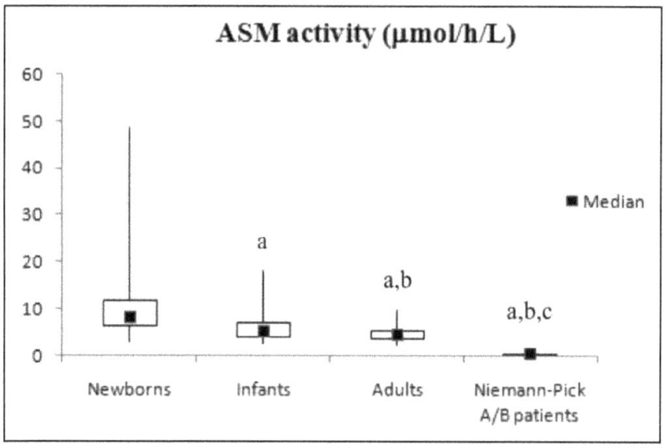

Figure 3. Acid sphingomyelinase (ASM) activity in dried blood spot (DBS) samples from controls grouped according to age and from patients with Niemann-Pick A/B disease. The error bars show the range of enzyme activity, the box represents those results within the 95th percentile, and the "■" symbol represents the median (Mann-Whitney *U* test, $P < .05$). [a]Different from newborns. [b]Different from infants. [c]Different from adult controls.

and diagnosis, and the benefits of early start of treatment justify the implementation of LSDs into routine newborn screening protocols.[6] Studies carried out in Brazil indicated an average delay of 4.8 years between the onset of symptoms in patients with MPS and conclusive laboratory diagnosis,[16] which may also occur for other LSDs. In Brazil, a study demonstrated that the median time between the onset of first symptoms of Fabry disease and diagnosis was 20.3 years in males and 14.3 years in females.[17] This delay in diagnosis does not allow early initiation of appropriate treatment that could prevent many complications of the disease.

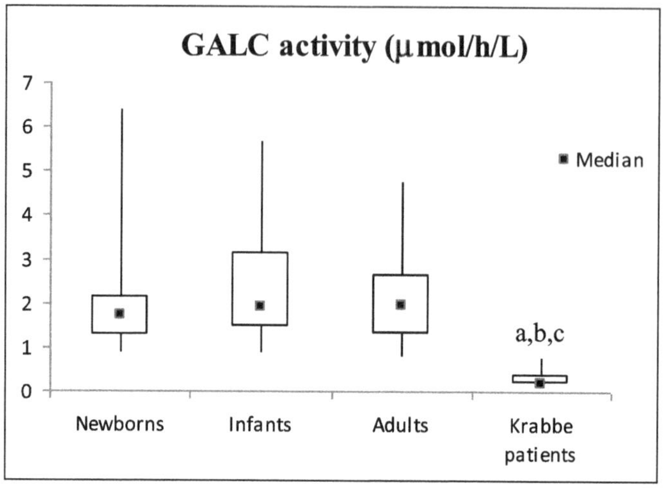

Figure 4. Galactocerebrosidase (GALC) activity in dried blood spot (DBS) samples from controls grouped according to age and from patients with Krabbe disease. The error bars show the range of enzyme activity, the box represents those results within the 95th percentile, and the "■" symbol represents the median (Mann-Whitney *U* test, $P < .05$). [a]Different from newborns. [b]Different from infants. [c]Different from adult controls.

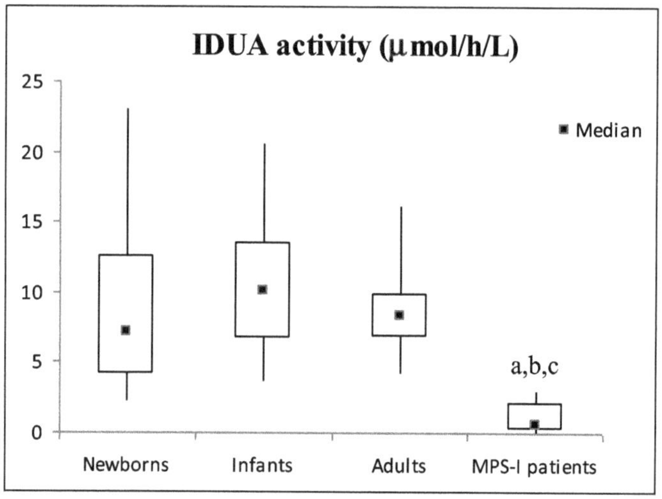

Figure 5. α-L-Iduronidase (IDUA) activity in dried blood spot (DBS) samples from controls grouped according to age and from patients with mucopolysaccharidosis type I (MPS-I). The error bars show the range of enzyme activity, the box represents those results within the 95th percentile, and the "■" symbol represents the median (Mann-Whitney *U* test, $P < .05$). [a]Different from newborns. [b]Different from infants. [c]Different from adult controls.

In 2001, Chamoles and colleagues[18] reported the possibility of diagnosing lysosomal enzymes using DBSs, opening the door for the screening of LSDs. Considering that conventional methods of quantifying enzymatic activity, such as spectrophotometry and fluorometry, have the technical limitations of non-specificity and limited capacity for multiplexing, MS/MS has become an excellent option for this purpose, enabling the investigation of different LSDs simultaneously in a single patient's sample, with high specificity and sensitivity.[7]

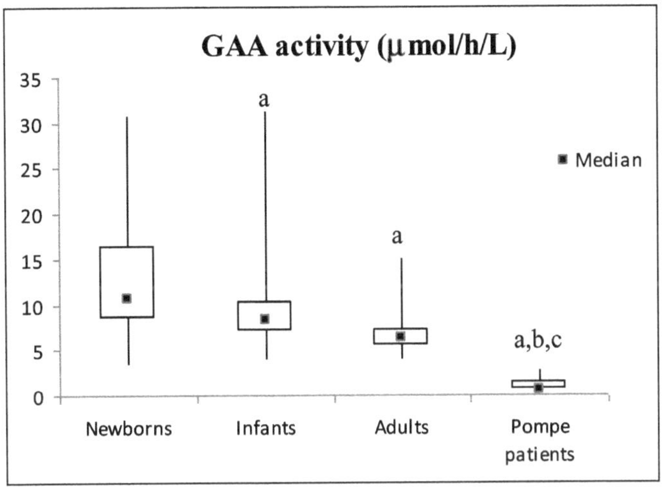

Figure 6. α-Glucosidase (GAA) activity in dried blood spot (DBS) samples from controls grouped according to age and from patients with Pompe disease. The error bars show the range of enzyme activity, the box represents those results within the 95th percentile, and the "■" symbol represents the median (Mann-Whitney *U* test, $P < .05$). [a]Different from newborns. [b]Different from infants. [c]Different from adult controls.

Although pilot projects for LSD screening by MS/MS are being reported since 2006 in North America, Europe, and Asia,[9] there are few laboratories in Brazil investing in this area. Lysosomal storage diseases seem to be relatively frequent in Brazil. In 1997, a study published by Coelho et al[19] demonstrated a higher proportion of LSDs (59.8%) diagnosed by selective screening at Medical Genetic Service of Hospital de Clínicas de Porto Alegre, Brazil, during the period from 1982 to 1995, compared to other groups of inborn errors of metabolism, such as aminoacidopathies and organic acidemias.

Therefore, aiming the future use of the MS/MS methodology for the screening of LSDs in our laboratory, in this work we validated the methodology for analysis of 6 lysosomal enzymes, GAA, GLA, ABG, ASM, IDUA and GALC, in DBS samples, evaluating the precision and accuracy of the method, as well as the ability in discriminating between positive and negative cases.

Results obtained from the calibration curves for method validation demonstrated linearity with the expected P/IS ratios and the enzyme activities determined in QC DBS samples correlated well with those reported by the CDC, demonstrating a good accuracy. Besides, CDC quality control specimens showed a good distinction between high and low activity levels for all analytes. In relation to the precision, the intra- and interassay CVs were comparable to those reported by other authors,[20,21] except for GLA which showed higher rates of variation.

When analyzing the activities of GAA, GLA, ABG, ASM, IDUA, and GALC in DBS samples from healthy controls, a wide variation in the reference values has been reported by different laboratories, which can be explained by analytical and instrumental modifications used in the analysis. Although the number of normal samples analyzed in this work is small, our preliminary results showed that the median activities of these 6 enzymes for newborns and nonnewborn controls were comparable to those reported in the literature[22,23] and the assays enabled unambiguous differentiation between samples obtained from healthy individuals and patients, suggesting that the method was effective in detecting Pompe, Fabry, Gaucher, Niemann-Pick A/B, MPS-I, and Krabbe diseases. Corroborating with findings published by Brand et al,[24] our results also demonstrated that some lysosomal enzymes present a higher activity in newborns when compared to older individuals.

In this study, GLA was the enzyme that showed less discrimination between samples from affected patients and healthy individuals, especially when compared with the activities found in adults. The median GLA activity in patients with Fabry disease was 71.36% lower than those observed in adult controls; however, the medians for GAA, ABG, ASM, IDUA, and GALC were 90%, 89.02%, 90.2%, 93%, and 89.44%, respectively, lower than those obtained for normal adult individuals. It is also important to emphasize that 5 patients with Fabry disease were under enzyme replacement therapy, which probably contributed to higher levels of enzyme activity. Only through the screening of a higher number of samples from untreated patients will be possible to accurately determine the difference in GLA activity in Fabry disease compared to normal participants. Even so, other biochemical assays may be interesting for Fabry disease investigation to confirm the diagnosis. Our results also agree with those obtained by other authors, showing that women heterozygous for Fabry disease present GLA activity close to normality.[7,25]

In the current work, we were able to detect precision in patients with Pompe, Fabry, Gaucher, Niemann-Pick A/B, MPS-I, and Krabbe diseases by MS/MS. However, additional analyses with a larger number of DBS samples are in progress in order to better determine the normal range of these enzyme activities, as well as the specificity of the method by analyzing false-negative or false-positive cases. It should also be mentioned that for all cases of abnormal or nondiscriminative results, leukocytes isolation or a fibroblast skin culture should be requested for confirmation of the enzyme deficiency. It is also important to correlate the results of biochemical assays with clinical data of patients aiming to achieve an accurate diagnosis.

In conclusion, we evaluated the performance of MS/MS in detecting 6 LSDs, and the preliminary results of this study suggest that this methodology can be successfully employed in the screening of LSDs, which will allow faster diagnosis and treatment of patients, reducing the morbidity of the diseases and improving patient survival and quality of life.

Acknowledgments

The authors thank CDC (Centers for Disease Control and Preventions) and Genzyme for supplying part of the reagents and standards needed for the study.

Declaration of Conflicting Interests

The author(s) declared no potential conflicts of interest with respect to the research, authorship, and/or publication of this article.

Funding

The author(s) disclosed receipt of the following financial support for the research, authorship, and/or publication of this article: This work was supported in part by grants from CAPES, CNPq, FAPERGS and FIPE/HCPA-Brazil.

References

1. Meikle PJ, Hopwood JJ, Clague AE, Carey WF. Prevalence of lysosomal storage diseases. *JAMA*. 1999;281(3):249-254.
2. Wenger DA, Coppola S, Liu SL. Insights into the diagnosis and treatment of lysosomal storage diseases. *Arch Neurol*. 2003;60(3):322-328.
3. Marsden D, Levy H. Newborn screening of lysosomal storage disorders. *Clin Chem*. 2010;56(7):1071-1079.
4. Wilcox WR. Lysosomal storage disorders: the need for better pediatric recognition and comprehensive care. *J Pediatr*. 2004;144(5 suppl):S3-S14.
5. Parkinson-Lawrence E, Fuller M, Hopwood JJ, Meikle PJ, Brooks DA. Immunochemistry of lysosomal storage disorders. *Clin Chem*. 2006;52(9):1660-1668.
6. Giugliani R. Newborn screening for lysosomal diseases: current status and potential interface with population medical genetics in Latin America. *J Inherit Metab Dis*. 2012;35(5):871-877.
7. Li Y, Scott CR, Chamoles NA, et al. Direct multiplex assay of lysosomal enzymes in dried blood spots for newborn screening. *Clin Chem*. 2004;50(10):1785-1796.
8. Gelb MH, Turecek F, Scott CR, Chamoles NA. Direct multiplex assay of enzymes in dried blood spots by tandem mass spectrometry for the newborn screening of lysosomal storage disorders. *J Inherit Metab Dis*. 2006;29(2-3):397-404.
9. Zhou H, Fernhoff P, Vogt RF. Newborn bloodspot screening for lysosomal storage disorders. *J Pediatr*. 2011;159(1):7-13.e1.
10. Orsini JJ, Morrissey NA, Slavin LN, et al. Implementation of newborn screening for Krabbe disease: population study and cut off determination. *Clin Biochem*. 2009;42(9):877-884.
11. Orsini JJ, Martin MM, Showers AL, et al. Lysosomal storage disorder 4 + 1 multiplex assay for newborn screening using tandem mass spectrometry: application to a small-scale population study for five lysosomal storage disorders. *Clin Chim Acta*. 2012;413(15-16):1270-1273.
12. Mechtler TP, Stary S, Metz TF, et al. Neonatal screening for lysosomal storage disorders: feasibility and incidence from a nationwide study in Austria. *Lancet*. 2012;379(9813):335-341.
13. De Jesus VR, Zhang XK, Keutzer J, et al. Development and evaluation of quality control dried blood spot materials in newborn screening for lysosomal storage disorders. *Clin Chem*. 2009;55(1):158-164.
14. Zhang XK, Elbin CS, Chuang WL, et al. Multiplex enzyme assay screening of dried blood spots for lysosomal storage disorders by using tandem mass spectrometry. *Clin Chem*. 2008;54(10):1725-1728.
15. Duffey TA, Bellamy G, Elliott S, et al. A tandem mass spectrometry triplex assay for the detection of Fabry, Pompe, and mucopolysaccharidosis-I (Hurler). *Clin Chem*. 2010;56(12):1854-1861.
16. Vieira T, Schwartz I, Muñoz V, et al. Mucopolysaccharidoses in Brazil: what happens from birth to biochemical diagnosis? *Am J Med Genet A*. 2008;146A(13):1741-1747.
17. Martins AM, Kyosen SO, Garrote J, et al. Demographic characterization of Brazilian patients enrolled in the Fabry Registry. *Genet Mol Res*. 2013;12(1):136-142.
18. Chamoles NA, Blanco M, Gaggioli D. Diagnosis of α-L-iduronidase deficiency in dried blood spots on filter paper: the possibility of newborn diagnosis. *Clin Chem*. 2001;47(4):780-781.
19. Coelho JC, Wajner M, Burin MG, Vargas CR, Giugliani R. Selective screening of 10,000 high-risk Brazilian patients for the detection of inborn errors of metabolism. *Eur J Pediatr*. 1997;156(8):650-654.
20. Liao HC, Chiang CC, Niu DM, et al. Detecting multiple lysosomal storage diseases by tandem mass spectrometry—a national newborn screening program in Taiwan. *Clin Chim Acta*. 2014;431:80-86.
21. Han M, Jun SH, Song SH, Park KU, Kim JQ, Song J. Use of tandem mass spectrometry for newborn screening of 6 lysosomal storage disorders in a Korean population. *Korean J Lab Med*. 2011;31(4):250-256.
22. Metz TF, Mechtler TP, Orsini JJ, et al. Simplified newborn screening protocol for lysosomal storage disorders. *Clin Chem*. 2011;57(9):1286-1294.
23. Kasper DC, Herman J, De Jesus VR, Mechtler TP, Metz TF, Shushan B. The application of multiplexed, multi-dimensional ultra-high-performance liquid chromatography/tandem mass spectrometry to the high-throughput screening of lysosomal storage disorders in newborn dried bloodspots. *Rapid Commun Mass Spectrom*. 2010;24(7):986-994.
24. Brand GD, de Matos HC, da Cruz GC, Fontes Ndo C, Buzzi M, Brum JM. Diagnosing lysosomal storage diseases in a Brazilian non-newborn population by tandem mass spectrometry. *Clinics (Sao Paulo)*. 2013;68(11):1469-1473.
25. Dajnoki A, Fekete G, Keutzer J, et al. Newborn screening for Fabry disease by measuring GLA activity using tandem mass spectrometry. *Clin Chim Acta*. 2010;411(19-20):1428-1431.

6

Reducing the False-Positive Rate for Isovalerylcarnitine in Expanded Newborn Screening: The Application of a Second-Tier Test

Sara Poggiali, BSc, MT[1], Daniela Ombrone, BSc[1], Giulia Forni, BSc[1], Sabrina Malvagia, BSc[1], Silvia Funghini, BSc, PhD[1], Massimo Mura, Pharm Sc[1], Elisabetta Pasquini, MD[2], Laura Santoro, BSc[3], Vincenzo Bellavia, BSc[3], Orazia Maria Granata, BSc[3], Cinzia Castana, MD[4], Kathleen S. McGreevy, PhD[5], Tommaso Silvano Aronica, MD[3], and Giancarlo la Marca, Pharm Sc[1,6]

Abstract

The isodecyl neopentanoate is an ingredient used in the cosmetic industry to prepare a nipple fissure balm. We report on 12 newborns that showed elevated C5-acylcarnitine levels upon newborn screening following treatment with balm. The first 3 neonates were immediately recalled for confirmatory tests and resulted negative for both isovaleric acidemia and short/branched chain acyl-CoA dehydrogenase deficiency. In the other 9 cases, the immediate recall was avoided by applying a new second-tier test able to confirm the presence of pivaloylcarnitine. The concentration of C5-acylcarnitine was measured in the days following the suspension of balm application. Abnormal concentrations of C5-acylcarnitine did not seem to be associated with free carnitine deficiency, probably due to the short time of exposure. A direct correlation between balm ingestion and the elevation in pivaloylcarnitine has been demonstrated in 10 adult volunteers. The commercial balm containing a pivalic acid derivative is causal of false-positive results during newborn screening, and it could have the potential to cause secondary carnitine deficiency when used chronically.

Keywords

newborn screening, tandem mass spectrometry, false positive, pivalic acid, second-tier test

Introduction

Acylcarnitine profile analysis using the flow injection analysis–tandem mass spectrometry (MS/MS) method is commonly used in newborn screening programs for the biochemical screening of fatty acid oxidation and organic acid metabolism disorders.

The profile is analyzed in positive-ion mode, usually using a precursor ion scan experiment or a multiple reaction monitoring (MRM) experiment. A common fragment (85 *m/z*) containing the quaternary ammonium function could be detected with high sensitivity and specificity. Flow injection analysis–MS/MS methods cannot distinguish between isobaric compounds, making chromatographic separation essential when the separation of isomers is required for the differential diagnosis of some inborn errors of metabolism.[1,2]

Several authors have developed methods for the determination of C4-acylcarnitine and C5-acylcarnitine isomers in plasma and dried blood spots (DBSs) by ultra-performance

[1] Newborn Screening, Biochemistry and Pharmacology Laboratory, Pediatric Neurology Clinic and Laboratories, Meyer Children's University Hospital, Florence, Italy

[2] Metabolic and Muscular Unit, Pediatric Neurology Clinic, Meyer Children's University Hospital, Florence, Italy

[3] UOS Newborn Screening Center, UOC Pediatric Clinical Pathology, P.O.G. Di Cristina, Palermo, Italy

[4] UOC Pediatric Clinic, P.O.G. Di Cristina, Palermo, Italy

[5] Research, Innovation and International Relations Office, Meyer Children's University Hospital, Florence, Italy

[6] Department of Experimental and Clinical Biomedical Sciences, University of Florence, Florence, Italy.

Corresponding Author:

Giancarlo la Marca, Pharm Sc, Newborn Screening, Biochemistry and Pharmacology Laboratory, Pediatric Neurology Clinic and Department of Experimental and Clinical Biomedical Sciences, University of Florence; Laboratories, Meyer Children's University Hospital, Viale Pieraccini 24, 50139 Florence, Italy. Emails: g.lamarca@meyer.it; giancarlo.lamarca@unifi.it

Table 1. Free Carnitine and C5-Acylcarnitine Concentrations Detected During Expanded Newborn Screening Program in 12 Infants Whose Mothers Used the Nipple Fissure Balm.

	C5 (nv 0-0.56) Concentration Expressed in µmol/L			C0 (nv 5.5-45) Concentration Expressed in µmol/L		
Case	Newborn Screening	Retesting (Without Suspension)	Retesting (Days After Suspension)	Newborn Screening	Retesting (Without Suspension)	Retesting (Days After Suspension)
1[a]	1.18	3.63	0.29 (7)	24.4	24.1	26.9 (7)
2[a]	0.82	0.85	0.11 (10)	13.02	12.02	23.6 (10)
3[a]	1.13	1.32	0.30 (4)	20.38	18.11	29.5 (4)
4	0.86	-	0.44 (3)	22.33	-	29.4 (3)
5	0.62	-	0.22 (2)	25.62	-	26.7 (2)
6	0.91	-	0.64 (3)	20.74	-	29.1 (3)
7	1.02	-	0.34 (4)	22.9	-	21.2 (4)
8	0.66	-	0.19 (4)	31.9	-	31.6 (4)
9	0.89	-	0.22 (2)	33.37	-	26.5 (2)
10	0.73	-	0.15 (10)	20.51	-	20.5 (10)
11	1.8	-	0.29 (5)	29	-	27.5 (5)
12	1.1	-	0.17 (4)	10.7		15.0 (4)

Abbreviation: nv, normal value.
[a]Newborns immediately recalled for clinical evaluation.

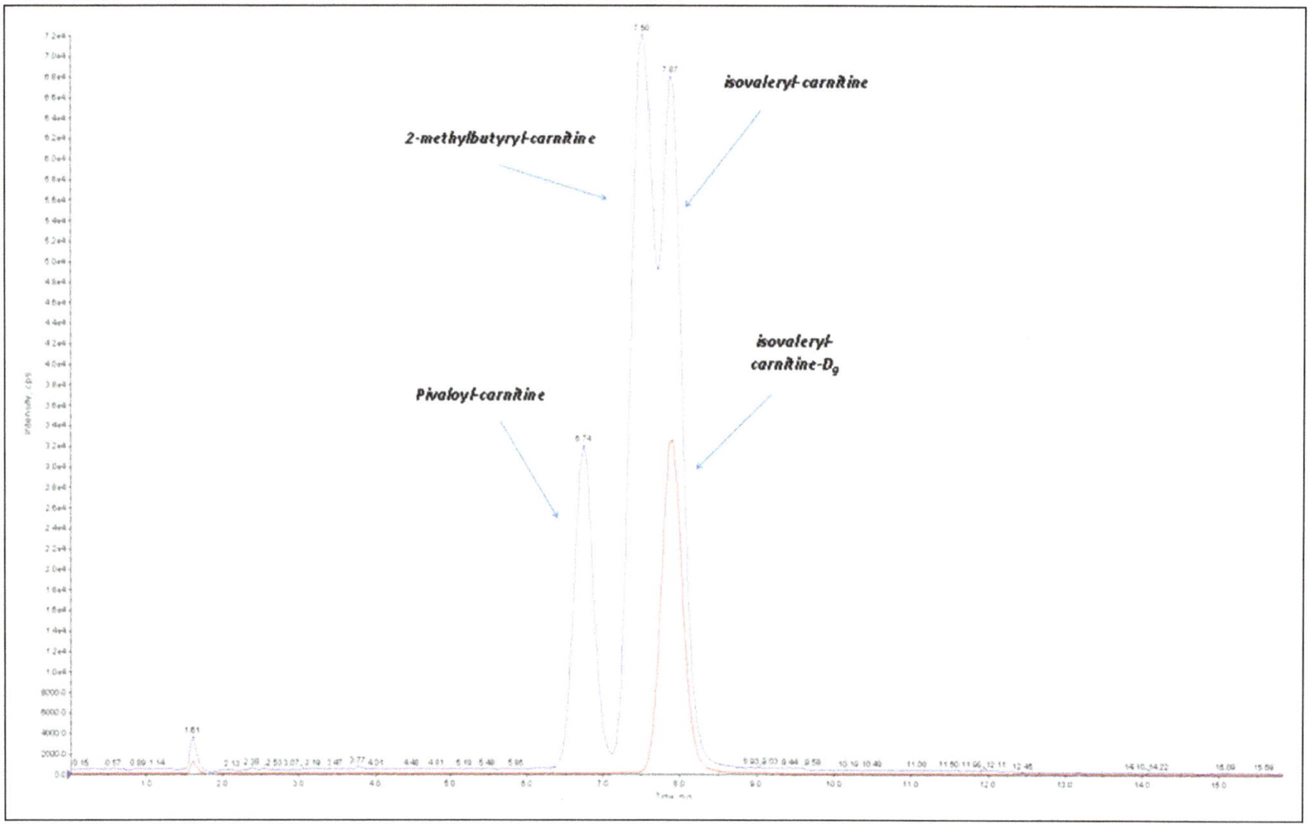

Figure 1. Chromatographic separation of the selected transition 302 → 85.0 m/z. The chromatogram corresponds to a solution spiked with 0.05 µmol/L of pivaloylcarnitine, 0.1 µmol/L of 2-methylbutyrylcarnitine, and 0.1 µmol/L of isovalerylcarnitine in the presence of D_9-isovalerylcarnitine (311 → 85.0 m/z). The separate peaks show enough chromatographic resolution of C5-acylcarnitine isomers.

liquid chromatography (LC)–MS/MS as a second-tier test following flow injection–MS/MS acylcarnitine profile analysis.[3] In particular, an increase in C5-acylcarnitine in a newborn screening profile indicates a possible isovaleric acidemia (IVA) with elevated isovalerylcarnitine (IC) or a possible short/branched chain acyl-CoA dehydrogenase deficiency (SBCADD) with elevated 2-methylbutyrylcarnitine (2MBC).

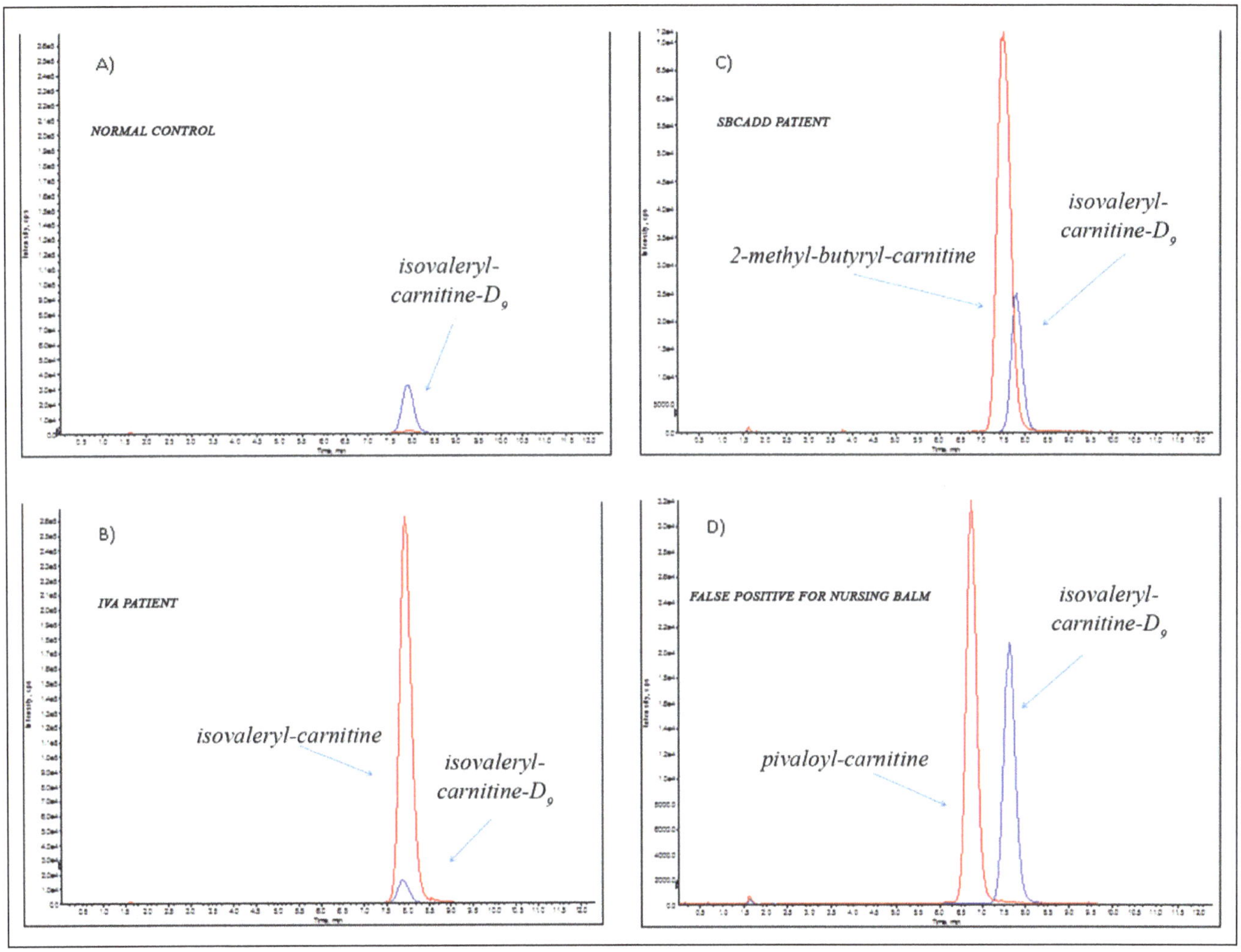

Figure 2. Extracted ion chromatogram of the monitored mass transitions 302→85 m/z and 311→85 m/z (used as internal standard) in a normal newborn (A), in a patient with isovaleric acidemia (IVA; B), in a patient with short-branched chain acyl-CoA dehydrogenase deficiency (SBCADD; C), and in a breast-fed neonate whose mother was using nipple cream (D).

Moreover, an increase in C5-acylcarnitine due to the presence of pivaloylcarnitine (PC) originating from pivalic acid in some antibiotic preparations and generating many false-positive results in newborn screening programs has been reported in the literature.[4,5] More recently, Boemer and collaborators described a pivalic acid derivative "neopentanoate" used in the cosmetic industry to formulate a nipple fissure unguent that leads to false-positive increases in C5-acylcarnitine.[6] In 2015, Yamada and colleagues reported on 2 cases that developed elevated C5-acylcarnitine levels following treatment with sivelestat, a neutrophil elastase inhibitor used to treat acute respiratory distress syndrome.[7]

Patients with SBCADD are generally asymptomatic, and its clinical consequences are not yet known.[8,9] On the contrary, IVA is a branched-chain amino acid metabolism disorder characterized by severe episodes of ketoacidosis, vomiting, and lethargy, progressing to coma.[10]

It is therefore very important to differentiate between IVA, SBCADD, and increased levels of C5 due to PC. In 2014, an increased false-positivity rate due to elevated C5-acylcarnitine was observed in the newborn screening programs of Tuscany and Northern Sicily.

Here, we report 12 cases presenting elevated C5-acylcarnitine due to nipple fissure balm, and we describe the second-tier method developed to identify specific isobars on DBS from newborns. Moreover, a direct correlation between the ingestion of nipple fissure balm and growing values of C5-carnitine has been demonstrated in 10 adult volunteers.

Materials and Methods

Standards and Solvents

D_9-isovalerylcarnitine (D_9-IC) was purchased from Cambridge Isotope Laboratories (Andover, Massachusetts) to be used as an internal standard. The PC, 2MBC, and IC standard solutions were a gift from the Department of Chemistry of the University of Florence. Stock solutions of chemical and labeled standards at 100 mmol/L were prepared in methanol and stored at −20°C. Other reagents such as LC/MS-grade water, formic acid (purity

98%-100%), and LC/MS grade acetonitrile were purchased from Panreac (Barcelona, Spain). *N*-butanol containing 3N HCl, used as a derivatizing agent for the second-tier test, was purchased from Regis Chemical (Morton Grove, Illinois).

Sample Preparation and Chromatography

For the sample extraction, 200 μL of methanol solution containing D_9-IC as an internal standard at a concentration of 40 nmol/L was added to a DBS punch (3.2-mm diameter, about 3.3-3.5 μL) and kept at 37°C for 25 minutes in an orbital shaker. The extracted samples were completely dried under nitrogen flow at room temperature (Evaporator Porvair Micro-DS 96; Stepbio, Bologna, Italy) and were then derivatized using 75 μL of 3N HCl in n-butanol and kept at 65°C for 20 minutes. The derivatized samples were completely dried under nitrogen flow at 40°C and finally reconstituted with 200 μL of water/acetonitrile 30:70 (vol/vol) + 0.1% of formic acid to prepare them for analysis.

The chromatographic separations were performed on an Agilent 1260 Quaternary Capillary Pump with a Synergi Polar-RP 80A, 4 μm 150 × 2 mm high-performance liquid chromatography column (Phenomenex, Anzola, Bologna, Italy) and 4 × 2 mm precolumn cartridge (Phenomenex) for separation.

The mobile phase was composed of water (eluent A) and methanol (eluent B) with a flow rate of 200 μL/min. Gradient elution was achieved using a program with mobile phase A and mobile phase B as follows: 5% B to 50% B in 3 minutes and maintained for 0.1 minute, then from 50% B to 80% in 0.1 minute and maintained for 4.5 minutes, then back to 5% B in 0.1 minute and reequilibration for 4.2 minutes. The total analysis run time was 12 minutes. One microliter of the extracted sample was injected for the LC–MS/MS experiments.

An API 4000 Triple-Quad Mass Spectrometer equipped with the Turbo V-spray source with the turbo gas temperature set at 400°C was used for the MS/MS tests. The source operates in positive ionization polarity at a potential of +5500 V. The transitions for the MRM experiments were 302.2 → 85 m/z for C5 isomers and 311.2 → 85 m/z for the labeled internal standard D_9-IC. Optimal Collision Energy (CE), Cell exit Potential (CXP) and Declustering Potential (DP) were found at 25, 7, and 40 V, respectively, for both transitions.

Experimental Design and Sample Collection

About 300 mg of a nipple fissure balm containing neopentanoate as a cosmetic ingredient was added to 50 mL of commercial fresh pasteurized cow milk and administered to 3 males and 5 females, all volunteers from the NBS laboratory of Meyer Children's Hospital.

Additionally, 2 volunteers, 1 male and 1 female, drank only 50 mL of commercial fresh pasteurized cow milk (vehicle) without balm. Dried blood spot samples from each volunteer were obtained by finger prick before and after balm ingestion (T0, T1, T2, T4, T8, T24 hours). A fully automated finger incision device for blood sampling was used (Tenderfoot Preemie; ITC, Edison, New Jersey). Dried blood spots were prepared by spotting whole blood onto filter paper cards (903; Whatman GmbH, Dassel, Germany), which were then left to dry and stored at −20°C in a sealed plastic bag containing desiccant until analysis. Samples were prepared in triplicate for routine screening tests, as previously described.[11]

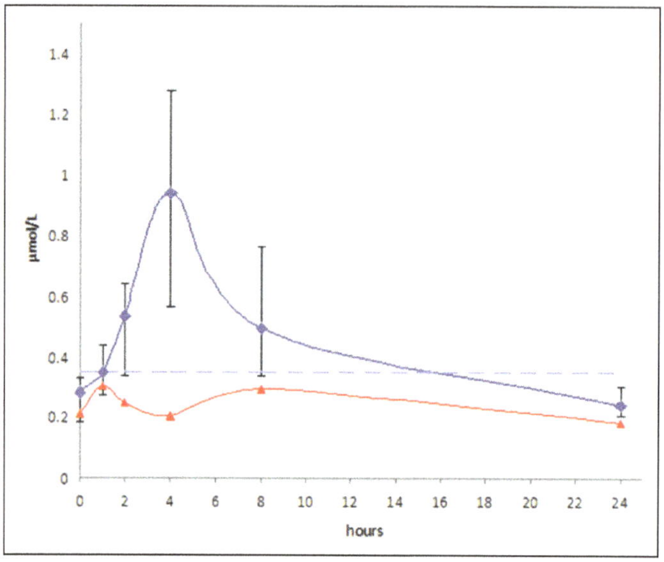

Figure 3. Graphic representation of the effect of balm ingestion on blood C5-carnitine levels. Blood samples were collected sequentially over a 24-hour period from 10 healthy volunteers, 8 who received an oral dose of nursing balm (purple line) and 2 monitored as controls (red line). The horizontal dashed line represents the higher cutoff of C5 (0.35 μmol/L) on blood for normal adults.

Results

Between January and December 2014, the newborn screening programs of Tuscany (n = 37111) and Northern Sicily (n = 16020), limited to LC–MS/MS testing, had a detection rate of 1:2062 and 1:2620, respectively. Of 91 total recalls in Tuscany, 5 (5.5%) were for abnormal values of isolated C5-acylcarnitine (normal values ≤0.56 μmol/L). Of 529 total recalls in Sicily, 27 (5.1%) were for abnormal values of isolated C5 (normal values ≤ 0.56 μmol/L). Only 2 of the 32 were true IVA positives—1 from Tuscany and 1 from Sicily.

Twelve of the 32 neonates showed abnormal C5-acylcarnitine concentrations due to indirect absorption of isodecyl neopentanoate originating from a nipple fissure balm used by nursing mothers to prevent rhagades. Three of them were from the Tuscany Newborn Screening Center and 9 were from the Northern Sicily Newborn Screening Center. The remaining 18 false positives from newborn screening resulted negative upon the second-tier test. The C5-acylcarnitine and free carnitine concentrations of the 12 false-positive newborns for balm are reported in Table 1.

As IVA can lead to acute metabolic decompensation, in the period preceding the setup of the second-tier test, newborns 1

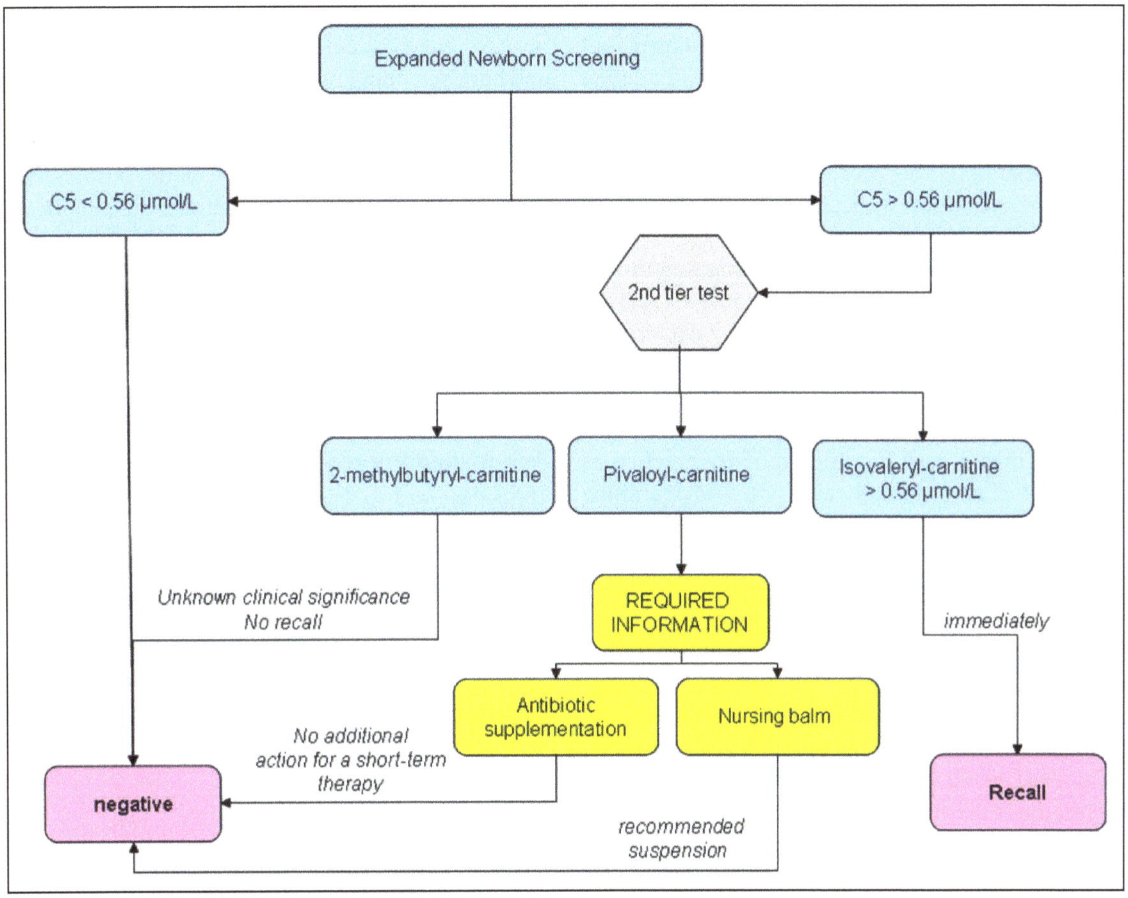

Figure 4. Flow diagram for the C5-carnitine evaluation in the newborn screening.

(from Tuscany), 2, and 3 (from Sicily) were immediately recalled following the newborn screening results for clinical evaluation and second-level confirmatory testing according to internal protocol. However, IVA was considered to be unlikely because isovalerylglycine and 3-OH-isovaleric acid were not detected by urinary organic acid analysis. Moreover, no abnormal findings such as body smell or hypoglycemia, which are typical symptoms of IVA, were noted in these patients. During the anamnestic evaluation, their mothers referred to the use of the same nipple fissure balm (to prevent rhagades) at the time that blood was drawn (as preventive of rhagades) without concomitant drug supplementation. After these first 3 cases, we decided to develop a second-tier test able to separate C5-acylcarnitine isomers.

Figure 1 shows the chromatographic separation of butylated C5 isomers at 0.05 µmol/L (D_9-IC and PC) and at 0.1 µmol/L (2MBC and IC) in acetonitrile/water 70:30 + 0.1% formic acid. The corresponding retention times were 7.83, 6.74, 7.50, and 7.87 minutes, respectively.

To assess whether second-tier testing could be effective, we applied it to 100 blood spots reported as normal during newborn screening by LC–MS/MS, and 32 spots recalled for abnormal values of C5 (newborns 1, 2, and 3 were retrospectively analyzed). In addition, we tested 4 truly positive newborn screening blood spots (2 IVA and 2 SBCADD). No quantifiable signal corresponding to IC or 2MBC was detected for controls or false positives. Figure 2 shows the extracted ion chromatogram from a normal neonatal DBS (panel A), patient with IVA (panel B), patient with SBCADD (panel C), and false positive due to PC (panel D).

In the period of April to December 2014, the application of the second-tier test allowed the identification of 9 additional cases of false positives due to balm application during breastfeeding. For all of them, we decided to ask for a new DBS after the suspension of balm application to control the C5-acylcarnitine normalization (Table 1).

A new experiment was performed in 10 adult volunteers to demonstrate the direct correlation between balm ingestion and the increase in C5-acylcarnitine blood levels. Eight of them (3 males and 5 females, age 25-46 years) received 50 mL of commercially available fresh cow milk containing about 300 mg of the balm. One male (42 years old) and 1 female (46 years old) drank only 50 mL of commercially available fresh cow milk (vehicle) without balm. Dried blood spot samples were obtained from each volunteer by finger prick over 24 hours.

Figure 3 shows the C5-acylcarnitine trend. The reported C5 acylcarnitine values are the average of 3 replicates for all volunteers at each time point. The maximum C5-acylcarnitine blood concentration was reached 4 hours after balm ingestion in all volunteers.

Considering that the pivalic acid derivative neopentanoic acid conjugates the free carnitine[4-6] and that the breast-feeding period could be quite long (generally some months), we cannot exclude a potentially dangerous secondary carnitine deficiency due to a long-term nipple fissure balm application. Exogenous unusual long-term pivalate exposure from pivalic esters of antibiotics to mothers or newborns had previously been reported as responsible for carnitine depletion and hypoglycemic convulsions.[12]

Moreover, Ito and collaborators reported that serum-free and total carnitine levels decreased by about 50% even after short-term administration of these drugs.[4] In our experience, the free carnitine levels in the 12 false-positive newborns and in adult volunteers were within the normal ranges (Table 1 and Figure 3), probably due to short-term exposure.

The NBS protocol has been modified in daily practice as reported in Figure 4. If an abnormal value of C5-acylcarnitine is present during a routine newborn screening procedure, the second-tier test is immediately performed. If PC is present, we contact the mother by phone and ask if she has been using some antibiotics or the balm. In the first case, no further action is required if a short-term therapy has been recommended by a physician; in the latter, we recommend the suspension of balm application and/or possibly replacement with other creams. If IC is present and the concentration in blood is higher than 0.56 μmol/L, we proceed to the immediate recall of the baby for clinical evaluation and second-level confirmatory testing.

Considering that patients with SBCADD are generally asymptomatic,[8,9] SBCADD is not included in the NBS panel because of its unknown clinical significance; therefore, if 2MBC is present, the newborn is not recalled.

Conclusion

The aim of this work is to declare that the use of the nipple fissure cream containing neopentanoate esters as an ingredient causes false-positive results during newborn screening. Warning nurseries, pediatric facilities, and manufacturing companies about the effects of these compounds is very important in order to decrease diagnostic errors and consequent recalls. Recalls induce stress in the families of newborns and may also cause the loss of milk in mothers or influence the child-parent relationship.[13]

In the experiences of Tuscany and Sicily, the biomarker C5-acylcarnitine is not causative of many recalls during newborn screening (about 5%-6% of total recalls); however, the positive predictive value of the biomarker is not good (2 IVA of the 32 positives corresponding to 6.25%). Based on the conviction that the combination of first- and second-tier testing for many metabolic disorders must be considered the best working practice to achieve the most benefit out of newborn screening programs, in our opinion, the new second-tier test for C5-acylcarnitine can reduce the false-positive rate, improve the positive predictive value, and above all avoid superfluous urgent recalls with a consequent reduction in laboratory analyses, personnel costs for repeat tests, and considerable anxiety for parents. The use of pivalic acid derivatives in drugs or cosmetics is still widespread worldwide, in spite of important reports. During the preparation of this article, a new false positive for C5-acylcarnitine was identified by the Tuscan newborn screening program because of a newborn's exposure to an antibiotic named "cefditoren pivoxil," a semisynthetic cephalosporin used in pediatric patients with laryngopharyngitis and tonsillitis. New and better strategies should be developed to provide testing options that, applied to newborn screening programs, reduce recall rate, overall expenses, and parental anxiety.

Authors' Note

Sara Poggiali and Daniela Ombrone are contributed equally to this work.

Acknowledgments

The authors wish to thank Drs Fabio Villanelli, Sara Peli, Paola Meloni, Rodolfo Tonin, and Patrizia Porcina, who served as volunteers for some experiments; moreover, the authors would like to thank Dr Cristiano Rizzo from Bambino Gesù Children's Hospital for the constructive discussion regarding chromatography separation.

Declaration of Conflicting Interests

The author(s) declared no potential conflicts of interest with respect to the research, authorship, and/or publication of this article.

Funding

The author(s) received no financial support for the research, authorship, and/or publication of this article.

References

1. la Marca G, Malvagia S, Pasquini E, et al. Hyperhydroxyprolinaemia: a new case diagnosed during neonatal screening with tandem mass spectrometry. *Rapid Commun Mass Spectrom.* 2005;19(6):863-864.
2. Alodaib A, Carpenter K, Wiley V, et al. An improved ultra performance liquid chromatography-tandem mass spectrometry method for the determination of alloisoleucine and branched chain amino acids in dried blood samples. *Ann Clin Biochem.* 2011;48(pt 5):468-470.
3. Forni S, Fu X, Palmer SE, et al. Rapid determination of C4-acylcarnitine and C5-acylcarnitine isomers in plasma and dried blood spots by UPLC-MS/MS as a second tier test following flow-injection MS/MS acylcarnitine profile analysis. *Mol Genet Metab.* 2010;101(1):25-32.
4. Ito T, Sugiyama N, Kobayashi M, et al. Alteration of ammonia and carnitine levels in short-term treatment with pivalic acid-containing prodrug. *Tohoku J. Exp. Med.* 1995;175(1):43-53.
5. Cloppenborg T, Janzen N, Wagner H, et al. Application of a second-tier newborn screening assay for C5 isoforms. *JIMD Rep.* 2014;13:23-26.
6. Boemer F, Schoos R, de Halleux V, Kalenga M, Debray FG. Surprising causes of C5-carnitine false positive results in newborn screening. *Mol Genet Metab.* 2014;111(1):52-54.
7. Yamada K, Kobayashi H, Bo R, et al. Elevation of pivaloylcarnitine by sivelestat sodium in two children. *Mol Genet Metab.* 2015;116(3):192-194.

8. van Calcar SC, Baker MW, Williams P, et al. Prevalence and mutation analysis of short/branched chain acyl-CoA dehydrogenase deficiency (SBCADD) detected on newborn screening in Wisconsin. *Mol Genet Metab.* 2013;110(1-2):111-115.
9. van Calcar SC, Gleason LA, Lindh H, et al. 2-methylbutyryl-CoA dehydrogenase deficiency in Hmong infants identified by expanded newborn screen. *Wisconsin Medical Journal.* 2007; 106(1):12-15.
10. Vockley J, Ensenauer R. Isovaleric acidemia: new aspects of genetic and phenotypic heterogeneity. *Am J Med Genet C Semin Med Genet.* 2006;142C(2):95-103.
11. la Marca G, Canessa C, Giocaliere E, et al. Diagnosis of immunodeficiency caused by a purine nucleoside phosphorylase defect by using tandem mass spectrometry on dried blood spots. *J Allergy Clin Immunol.* 2014;134(1):155-159.
12. Nakajima Y, Ito T, Maeda Y, et al. Detection of pivaloylcarnitine in pediatric patients with hypocarnitinemia after long-term administration of pivalate-containing antibiotics. *Tohoku J Exp Med.* 2010;221(4):309-313.
13. Gurian EA, Kinnamon DD, Henry JJ, Waisbren SE. Expanded newborn screening for biochemical disorders: the effect of a false-positive result. *Pediatrics.* 2006;117(6):1915-1921.

7

Coenzyme Q_{10} in the Treatment of Mitochondrial Disease

Viruna Neergheen, MSc[1], Annapurna Chalasani, MSc[1], Luke Wainwright, MSci, MRes[2], Delia Yubero, PhD[3], Raquel Montero, PhD[3], Rafael Artuch, MD, PhD[3], and Iain Hargreaves , PhD[1,4]

Abstract

Currently, there is a paucity of available treatment strategies for oxidative phosphorylation disorders. Coenzyme Q_{10} (CoQ_{10}) and related synthetic quinones are the only agents to date that have proven to be beneficial in the treatment of these heterogeneous disorders. The therapeutic efficacy of CoQ_{10} is not restricted to patients with an underlying CoQ_{10} deficiency and is thought to result from its ability to restore electron flow in the mitochondrial respiratory chain (MRC) as well as to increase the cellular antioxidant capacity. At present, however, there is no consensus on the appropriate dosage or therapeutic plasma level of CoQ_{10}, and this information will be required before CoQ_{10} can be utilized effectively in the treatment of mitochondrial disease. The following review will outline our current knowledge on the use of CoQ_{10} in the treatment of MRC disorders and primary CoQ_{10} deficiencies.

Keywords

coenzyme Q_{10}, mitochondrial respiratory chain (MRC), oxidative stress, antioxidant

Introduction

The mitochondrial respiratory chain (MRC; Figure 1) is located in the inner mitochondrial membrane and consists of 4 enzyme complexes: complex I (NADH: ubiquinone reductase; EC 1.6.5.3), complex II (succinate: ubiquinone reductase; EC 1.3.5.1), complex III (ubiquinol: cytochrome c reductase; EC 1.10.2.2), and complex IV (cytochrome c oxidase; EC 1.9.3.1;).[1,2] The MRC together with complex V (adenosine triphosphate [ATP] synthase; EC 3.6.3.14) synthesizes ATP, the energy currency of the cell by the process of oxidative phosphorylation.[1,2] In addition to existing as discrete entities, recent studies have indicated that the MRC enzymes can also exist as supercomplexes within the inner mitochondrial membrane consisting of aggregates of complexes I, III, and IV; complexes I and III; and complexes III and IV.[3]

The MRC disorders are a heterogeneous group of multisystemic diseases that develop as the result of mutations in either nuclear or mitochondrial DNA.[2] Once believed to be rare, inherited disorders of the MRC are now thought to represent one of the more commoner groups of inborn errors of metabolism with a birth prevalence of 1 in 5000.[4] The treatment of MRC disorders is extremely difficult and in general woefully inadequate with no overall consensus on appropriate therapeutic strategies.[5] To date, coenzyme Q_{10} (CoQ_{10}) and its analogues are among a small group of agents that have been reported to offer some therapeutic potential in the treatment of MRC disorders.

[1] Neurometabolic Unit, The National Hospital for Neurology and Neurosurgery, Queen Square, London, UK
[2] Department of Molecular Neuroscience, Institute of Neurology, University College London, London, UK
[3] Clinical Biochemistry department, Institut de Recerca Sant Joan de Déu and CIBERER, Barcelona, Spain
[4] School of Pharmacy and Biomolecular Science, Liverpool John Moores University, Liverpool, UK

Corresponding Author:
Viruna Neergheen, Neurometabolic Unit, The National Hospital for Neurology and Neurosurgery, Queen Square, London, UK.
Email: viruna.neergheen@uclh.nhs.uk

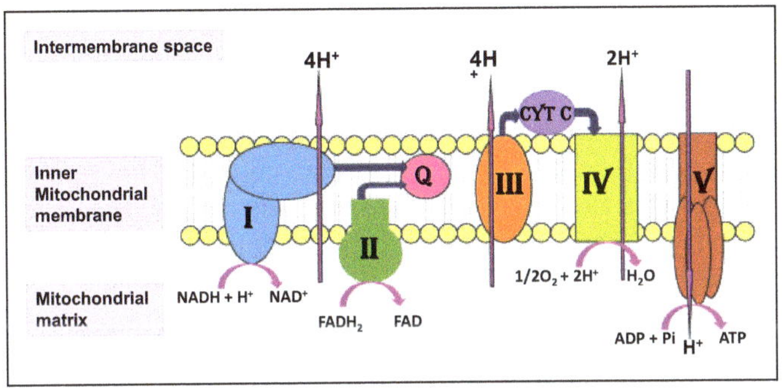

Figure 1. Mitochondrial respiratory chain (MRC).

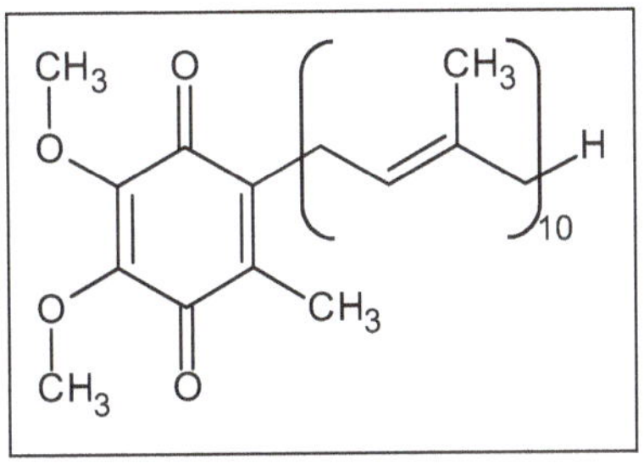

Figure 2. Structure of coenzyme Q_{10} (CoQ_{10}).

Coenzyme Q_{10}

Coenzyme Q_{10} is a small lipophilic molecule consisting of a benzoquinone nucleus and an isoprenoid side chain (Figure 2), which is synthesized by all cells apart from red blood cells, and shares a common biosynthetic pathway with cholesterol.[6] Coenzyme Q_{10} serves as an essential electron carrier within the MRC, transferring electrons derived from complexes I and II to complex III and therefore allowing a continuous passage of electrons within the chain, which is essential for the process of oxidative phosphorylation. In addition to its role as an electron carrier, CoQ_{10} functions as a lipid-soluble antioxidant, protecting cellular membranes and plasma lipoproteins against free radical–induced oxidation.[7] The antioxidant function of CoQ_{10} is attributed to its fully reduced ubiquinol form.[7] Other functions of CoQ_{10} include membrane stabilization and modulation of gene expression.[8,9] In view of all these functions, a deficiency in CoQ_{10} status could conceivably contribute to disease pathophysiology by causing a failure in mitochondrial energy metabolism, compromising cellular antioxidant capacity as well as adversely affecting membrane stability and gene expression. A deficiency in CoQ_{10} status can result from either a genetic defect in the CoQ_{10} biosynthetic pathway, known as a primary deficiency, or as the result of a mutation in a gene not directly involved in CoQ_{10} biosynthesis, known as a secondary deficiency.[10]

Primary CoQ_{10} Deficiencies

The first reported cases of CoQ_{10} deficiency in the literature described 2 sisters born to unrelated parents who presented with recurrent rhabdomyolysis, seizures, and mental retardation.[11] On assessment, the muscle CoQ_{10} status of these patients was found to be approximately 3.7% of mean control values indicating the evidence of a primary defect in CoQ_{10} biosynthesis, as yet however, the genetic cause of this defect has yet to be elucidated. Since this time, well over 150 patients have been reported with CoQ_{10} deficiency, although there are no precise epidemiological data for the overall incidence of this condition.[12] Coenzyme Q_{10} deficiency appears to have a particularly heterogeneous clinical presentation, although it can be divided into 5 distinct clinical phenotypes: encephalomyopathy, severe infantile multisystemic disease, nephropathy, cerebellar ataxia, and isolated myopathy.[12] In most cases, the family history indicates an autosomal recessive mode of inheritance; and to date, mutations in 9 genes involved in the human CoQ_{10} biosynthetic pathway have been reported (*PDSS1*, *PDSS2*, *COQ2*, *COQ4*, *COQ6*, *COQ7*, *ADCK3*, *ADCK4*, and *COQ9*).[13,14]

Secondary CoQ_{10} Deficiencies

Overall, the incidence of secondary CoQ_{10} deficiencies appears to be more common than that of primary CoQ_{10} deficiencies,[10] being a common feature among diseases, such as MRC disorders.[10,12,15,16] Furthermore, it has been suggested that a deficit in CoQ_{10} status may be a good predictor of an MRC deficiency.[17] Indeed, a CoQ_{10} deficiency has been reported in patients with a range of MRC disorders originating from mutations either in mitochondrial DNA such as Kearns Sayre Syndrome or nuclear DNA such as mitochondrial DNA depletion syndrome.[16,18,19,20] A CoQ_{10} deficiency has been detected in plasma/serum[18,19,21] as well as in muscle[15,17] in these patient groups. The cause of the CoQ_{10} deficiency in MRC disorders has yet to be fully elucidated, but it may result from the oxidative degradation of CoQ_{10} as a consequence of the increase in oxidative stress that is associated with MRC dysfunction[22] or just be a reflection of generalized mitochondrial impairment.[16] The decrease of plasma/serum CoQ_{10} levels in patients may also reflect an increased utilization or requirement by the MRC defective tissue(s)/organ(s) as well as liver impairment, as this is the major site of synthesis for circulatory CoQ_{10}.[23] Furthermore, since the enzymes involved in CoQ_{10} synthesis are thought to exist in a superenzyme complex closely associated with the MRC in the inner mitochondrial membrane, an incomplete or abnormal MRC may adversely impact on the structural formation of the CoQ_{10} superenzyme complex resulting in impaired CoQ_{10} biosynthesis.[24]

Treatment of Primary CoQ_{10} Deficiency

A primary CoQ_{10} deficiency is unique among MRC disorders in that it is potentially treatable if oral supplementation is commenced with high-dose CoQ_{10} during the early stages of the disease with clinical improvement being reported in all forms of this condition.[25] However, treatment protocols for CoQ_{10}-deficient patients have not yet been standardized, and results have varied between studies.[25] Although muscle symptoms associated with CoQ_{10} deficiency appear to improve in most cases upon CoQ_{10} supplementation, cerebral symptoms are generally less responsive to treatment.[12] This is illustrated in patients with the ataxic presentation of CoQ_{10} deficiency who show a variable response to CoQ_{10} supplementation. Four patients with mutations in the *ADCK3* gene have been reported to show improvement following CoQ_{10} supplementation with stabilization of the cerebellar ataxic features, reduction in myoclonus, improvement in speech, and ataxic symptoms.[12,26] In contrast, no improvement in symptoms have been reported in 7 patients carrying mutations in the same gene.[27,28] Furthermore, 11 patients with cerebellar ataxia and CoQ_{10} deficiency of undefined molecular cause also failed to show any sign of clinical improvement following CoQ_{10} supplementation.[29,30] In addition, despite almost complete amelioration of muscle symptoms, cerebral symptoms in patients with the encephalomyopathic phenotype again showed a variable response to CoQ_{10} treatment.[11,31,32] The reasons for the refractory nature of the neurological sequelae associated with a CoQ_{10} deficiency are as yet unknown and may be a consequence of irreversible damage prior to supplementation, the retention of CoQ_{10} in the blood-brain barrier (BBB) itself or simply reflect poor transport across the BBB. Animal studies have indicated that CoQ_{10} can be transported across the BBB following high-dose supplementation.[33,34] However, it is uncertain whether the degree of CoQ_{10} uptake demonstrated in these animal studies would be sufficient to replenish the cerebral levels of this quinone in a deficiency state.

Patients who develop renal dysfunction as the result of a CoQ_{10} deficiency appear to respond well to high-dose CoQ_{10} supplementation if treatment is initiated early in the course of diseases, with progressive recovery of renal function and decreased proteinuria being reported.[35,36] In contrast, CoQ_{10} supplementation was reported to be unsuccessful in inducing the recovery of renal function once chronic renal failure had developed.[37] In order to exploit the "window of opportunity" whereby organ dysfunction may be amenable to CoQ_{10} treatment, supplementation at birth has been suggested for siblings of CoQ_{10}-deficient patients.[38]

In vitro studies have indicated that the use of modified precursors of the quinone ring of CoQ_{10} to bypass the enzymatic defect may be effective in treating specific mutations of the *COQ6* and *COQ7* genes.[39] Studies in yeast harboring the mutant *COQ6* gene revealed that treatment with vanillic acid as well as 3-4-hydroxybenzoic acid could restore respiratory growth.[13,14] These compounds may therefore prove efficacious in the treatment of patients with *COQ6* mutations and are now being evaluated in mammalian cells.[40] The CoQ_{10} analogue, 2,4-dihydroxybenzoic acid, also demonstrated some therapeutic potential by its ability to restore CoQ_{10} biosynthesis in *COQ7* mutant human fibroblasts.[42]

Treatment of MRC Disorders

At present, there are no standardized therapeutic protocols for the treatment of patients with oxidative phosphorylation disorders, and treatment can vary between specialist centers. An extensive review about the current status of small molecule treatments and clinical trials in mitochondrial patients has recently been published.[41] However, once diagnosed, patients generally receive a "mitochondrial cocktail" containing antioxidants and cofactors for the various constituents of the MRC. The "cocktail" can consist of antioxidants such as vitamin E and C, the flavoprotein precursor riboflavin, and creatine monohydrate to assist in ATP generation.[43,44] Coenzyme Q_{10} is often a constituent of this "cocktail" because in addition to serving as an antioxidant it can serve to restore electron flow in the MRC.[45] Unfortunately, it has been suggested that patients with complex V deficiencies such as those with the clinical syndrome Neuropathy, ataxia, and retinitis pigmentosa (NARP), which has been associated with increased oxidative stress, may not benefit from CoQ_{10} therapy.[46] This is because the general blockage of electron flow in the MRC as the result of a complex V deficiency may impede the redox recycling of ubiquinol from CoQ_{10}, which is facilitated by redox exchange with the MRC. A number of small studies have assessed the therapeutic potential of CoQ_{10} in the treatment of MRC disorders with variable outcomes,[15,18,19,47,48] although evidence of clinical improvement has been documented in a number of these studies with reports of increased strength,[49] accelerated postexercise recovery,[50] and improvement in oxygen consumption.[51] Coenzyme Q_{10} therapy was also reported to correct pancreatic β-cell dysfunction in patients with mitochondrial encephalomyopathy and lactic acidosis and diabetes mellitus.[52] However, the most consistent finding appears to be at the biochemical level with a decrease in plasma/serum lactate and pyruvate levels being widely reported following exercise[48,51,53,54,55,56,57,58]. In contrast, some studies have shown no evidence of clinical or biochemical improvement in patients following CoQ_{10} supplementation[59,60]. The failure to elicit a therapeutic effect in these studies may in part be attributable to the dosage or duration of the CoQ_{10} supplementation employed. However, it has been suggested that patients who show some form of biochemical or clinical improvement (responders) following CoQ_{10} supplementation may be those patients who harbor an underlying CoQ_{10} deficiency[19,61]. This is demonstrated in the study by Sacconi et al[15] who reported the evidence of clinical improvement in 7 out of 8 patients with MRC disorder having an underlying CoQ_{10} deficiency following CoQ_{10} supplementation, as opposed to clinical benefit being reported in only 1 out of 15 patients with MRC disorder having no evidence of a muscle CoQ_{10} deficiency. This illustrates the importance of determining CoQ_{10} status prior to commencing CoQ_{10} supplementation in order to identify this subgroup of patients who may respond to treatment. An in vitro study by Chan and colleagues[62] reported that CoQ_{10} supplementation of hepatocytes with a pharmacologically induced MRC complex I deficiency was able to restore both mitochondrial membrane potential (MMP) and cellular antioxidant status. This indicated the potential of CoQ_{10} to be reduced by cytosolic DT-diaphorase (NQO1 or NAD(P)H: quinone oxidoreductase) and then bypass the deficiency at complex I, feeding electrons directly into complex III of the MRC to restore MMP. The short-chain synthetic quinone analogue of CoQ_{10}, idebenone, is also thought to display a similar mechanism of action in the treatment of the mitochondrial disorder, Lebers hereditary optic neuropathy, which in general results from an MRC complex I deficiency.[45] However, in vitro studies have demonstrated the potential of idebenone to inhibit complex I activity and therefore, the therapeutic efficacy of this quinone in vivo may be attributable to a metabolite of this drug formed following the administration.[45] Another synthetic quinone, EPI-743, which is also reduced by NQO1 activity has shown some beneficial effects in the treatment of patients with MRC disorders.[63] Although its precise mechanism of cellular action has yet to be fully elucidated, EPI-743 treatment has been shown to replenish the level of the antioxidant, reduced glutathione (GSH), possibly resulting from its ability to facilitate the transfer of electrons between NOQ1 and GSH reductase.[64] In addition to its ability to restore cellular GSH status, the beneficial effects of EPI-743 in the treatment of mitochondrial disease may result from its possible interaction with the transcription factor, nuclear factor E2-related factor 2 (Nrf2), which regulates both the expression of antioxidant proteins and cellular energy metabolism.[63,65]

Although a number of small studies and case reports have illustrated the potential benefits of CoQ_{10} in the treatment of patients with MRC disorder,[25] few controlled clinical trials have been conducted to evaluate its effectiveness. The trials that have been undertaken to date generally included patients with MRC disorder having variable genotypes and clinical phenotypes making it difficult to draw any firm conclusions to the responsiveness of particular groups of patients to CoQ_{10} therapy[21,48,66,67]. Although 2 trials demonstrated no benefit in any of the outcomes,[61] evidence of improvement in muscle strength[21] and a decrease in plasma lactate levels following exercise[48] was reported. It has been suggested that both the dose of CoQ_{10} administered and the duration of the study are factors that may compromise the therapeutic efficacy of CoQ_{10} in clinical trials[21,58]. The paucity of controlled clinical trials that have evaluated CoQ_{10} in the treatment of mitochondrial disease can be attributed to the difficulties encountered in recruiting sufficient patients and the relatively large expense of conducting such trials. However, phase 3 of a large-scale, double-blind, randomized clinical trial evaluating CoQ_{10} in the treatment of children with primary MRC disease has been completed, although the results are yet to be published.[42]

Absorption and Bioavailability of CoQ_{10} Formulations

Although all cells of the body apart from red blood cells are capable of synthesizing CoQ_{10}, the body also receives CoQ_{10} from dietary sources such as meat, fish, and some vegetables, with an estimated intake of 3 to 5 mg per day.[68] In view of its similar physicochemical properties to that of vitamin E, CoQ_{10} appears to follow an analogous pattern of digestive uptake. Gastric digestion releases dietary CoQ_{10} from the food matrix, secretions from the pancreas, and bile and then facilitates micelle formation leading to absorption of the solubilized lipid in the small intestine. Coenzyme Q_{10} is then incorporated into chylomicrons and transported via the lymphatic system into the circulation.[69] Following absorption from the gastrointestinal (GI) tract, CoQ_{10} is reduced into its ubiquinol form which is thought to occur in the enterocytes of intestine prior to its entry into the lymphatic system.[70] After release into the circulation, chylomicron remnants are readily taken up by the liver, where ubiquinol is repackaged into lipoproteins, primarily, low-density lipoproteins, and then rereleased into the circulation.[71] In general, tissues with a high-metabolic turnover or energy demand, such as the heart, kidney, liver, and muscle, contain relatively high concentrations of CoQ_{10}, and it is thought that most of this CoQ_{10} pool is synthesized in such tissues. Approximately 95% of plasma and 61% to 95% of tissue CoQ_{10} are present in the reduced, ubiquinol form.[71,72] The brain and lungs are exceptions with ≤25% of total CoQ_{10} being found as ubiquinol.[72] This may reflect the higher degree of oxidative stress in these 2 tissues.

In cases of primary and secondary CoQ_{10} deficiency, acquisition of CoQ_{10} from the diet may be insufficient to meet cellular requirements as intestinal absorption of CoQ_{10} is very limited[71] and supplementation may be a consideration. An important factor to consider which may influence the clinical response to CoQ_{10} supplementation is the type of CoQ_{10} formulation employed, as this will have an important bearing on absorption and bioavailability.[40,73]

In view of their superior absorption, the use of gel and oil-based formulations of CoQ_{10} has been recommended in preference to tablets[74] in the treatment of patients with mitochondrial disorders. Recently, a study by Martinefski et al[75] reported that liquid emulsion improved the bioavailability of CoQ_{10} with respect to solid formulations. Following administration, CoQ_{10} takes approximately 6 hours to reach its maximal plasma concentration. Subsequently, a second plasma CoQ_{10} peak is often observed at about 24 hours, which has been attributed to enterohepatic recycling as well as redistribution to the circulation.[76,77] Once administered, the circulatory half-life of CoQ_{10} has been reported to be approximately 36 hours requiring a 2-week period of cessation of treatment before it returns to its baseline level following 4 weeks of supplementation.[78] There is a lot of debate at present as to whether formulations of ubiquinol have a better absorption from the GI tract than those of CoQ_{10}. It has been estimated that the GI absorption of ubiquinol is 3 to 4 times greater than that of CoQ_{10}.[74,79] However, since upon absorption from the GI tract, CoQ_{10} undergoes reduction to ubiquinol, the purported superior bioavailability of ubiquinol formulations to that of CoQ_{10} may in part be attributable to the matrix in which the quinol is encapsulated. Furthermore, there is limited data available from patient studies and no clear indications of dosage compatibility.[40] Interestingly, ubiquinol treatment, in contrast to an equivalent dosage of CoQ_{10}, was reported to increase the CoQ_{10} status of mitochondria from the cerebrum of a mouse model of CoQ_{10} deficiency due to a *COQ9* mutation.[79] The results of this study may therefore have important implications for the treatment of the cerebral presentations of CoQ_{10} deficiency.

The efficiency of absorption of CoQ_{10} formulations has been reported to decrease as the dosage increases with a suggested block of GI absorption above 2400 mg,[74] and split doses have been recommended in preference to a single dose.[80] Dietary fat together with grapefruit juice consumption have been reported to improve the absorption of CoQ_{10}.[74,81] In contrast, ingestion of high-dose vitamin E together with CoQ_{10} may impede the absorption of CoQ_{10} resulting in lower plasma levels of the quinone,[82] possibly as a result of competition during the GI absorption process.

Coenzyme Q_{10} Monitoring and Dosage

In view of its relative accessibility, clinical monitoring of CoQ_{10} status is generally based on plasma determinations with an established reference interval ranging from 0.5 to 1.7 μM. However, this will vary between centers.[83] Although the level of plasma CoQ_{10} is influenced by both diet and circulatory lipoprotein status, it may have utility in identifying both evidence of cellular CoQ_{10} deficiency[19] and increased tissue utilization and demand.[18] However, in view of the questionable reliability of plasma CoQ_{10} status to reflect that of cells, blood mononuclear cells[84] and urine epithelial cells[85] may be more appropriate surrogates to determine endogenous CoQ_{10} status. However, the "gold standard" for the assessment of tissue CoQ_{10} status is skeletal muscle, and this is commonly used to identify evidence of an underlying CoQ_{10} deficiency.[86]

Currently, there is no consensus on the dosage of CoQ_{10} or the plasma level required that may prove efficacious in the treatment of patients with a primary CoQ_{10} deficiency and/or MRC disorders. Coenzyme Q_{10} supplementation is safe and well tolerated, exhibiting an excellent safety profile with doses as high as 2400 mg/d being used in the treatment of Parkinson disease.[87] Typically, doses in the range 5 to 30 mg/kg/d have been administered to patients with documented low levels of tissue CoQ_{10} as well as those with a primary CoQ_{10} deficiency.[25,88,89] In the absence of a demonstrable CoQ_{10} deficiency, doses of 5 to 30 mg/kg/d may also be used in the treatment of cases of known and suspected mitochondrial disease.[25,78] In Parkinson disease, a plasma CoQ_{10} level of 4.6 μmol/L was reported to be the most effective in slowing functional decline in patients.[90] An in vitro study using CoQ_{10}-deficient human fibroblasts has shown evidence of an improvement in bioenergetics status/normalization of cellular antioxidant status following 7 days of treatment with 5 μM CoQ_{10}.[91] Furthermore, a recent study by Duberley et al[92] indicated that supplementation with >10 μM CoQ_{10} may be required to restore MRC enzyme activities to control levels in CoQ_{10}-deficient human neuroblastoma cells. To date, the highest plasma CoQ_{10} concentration reported is 10.7 μmol/L, using a solubilized ubiquinol formulation[74,83] that may have the potential to show some therapeutic efficacy in the treatment of the neurological presentation of CoQ_{10} deficiency. These latter in vitro studies indicate that the dosage/plasma level of CoQ_{10} required to elicit biochemical or clinical improvement may be dependent on the organ of disease presentation.

Discussion/Conclusion

The ability of CoQ_{10} to demonstrate some beneficial effect in the treatment of mitochondrial disease is thought to rely mainly on its ability to restore electron flow in the MRC and replenish cellular antioxidant capacity. As would be expected, patients with an underlying deficit in CoQ_{10} status may be more responsive to such therapy. However, factors such as the time of diagnosis, the dosage, and duration of CoQ_{10} therapy may influence the efficacy of this treatment. Although a number of case reports and small studies have indicated some therapeutic potential of CoQ_{10} in the treatment of patients with MRC disorders and primary CoQ_{10} deficiencies, there is as yet no consensus of the dosage or plasma level of CoQ_{10} required to achieve some clinical benefit and whether this is influenced by the organ of disease presentation. Determination of CoQ_{10} status in other biological specimens beyond plasma/serum may also be advisable. In this sense, CoQ_{10} monitoring in blood mononuclear cells[84] or in urine samples[85] may better reflect the cellular uptake of exogenous CoQ_{10}. Furthermore, in view of the purported impermeability of the BBB to CoQ_{10}, monitoring of cerebral spinal fluid CoQ_{10} levels in preference to those of plasma may be more appropriate in patients with cerebral disease presentations.[93] The possibility arises that the underlying cause of a particular oxidative phosphorylation disorder may dictate the appropriate quinone therapy to implement, whether utilizing CoQ_{10}, a synthetic quinone, or a combination of the 2 in the treatment regime. At present however, this information is not available, and studies aimed at establishing these treatment protocols may improve the therapeutic efficacy of quinone supplementation.

Authors' Note

The Centro de Investigación Biomédica en Red de Enfermedades Raras (CIBERER) is an initiative of the Instituto de Salud Carlos III.

Declaration of Conflicting Interests

The author(s) declared no potential conflicts of interest with respect to the research, authorship, and/or publication of this article.

Funding

The author(s) disclosed receipt of the following financial support for the research and/or authorship of this article: This work was supported by grant from the Spanish Ministerio de Economia y Competitividad PI14/00028 and FEDER Funding Program from the European Union.

References

1. Land JM, Morgan-Hughes JA, Hargreaves I, Heales SJ. Mitochondrial disease: a historical, biochemical, and London perspective. *Neurochem Res*. 2004;29(3):488-491.
2. Rahman S, Hanna MG. Mitochondrial disorders: diagnosis and new treatments in mitochondrial disease. *J Neurol Neurosurg Psychiatry*. 2009;80(9):943-953.

3. Lapuente-Brun E, Moreno-Loshuertos R, Acin-Perez R, et al. Super-complex assembly determines electron flux in the mitochondrial electron transport chain. *Science*. 2013;340(6140): 1567-1570.
4. Haas RH, Parikh S, Falk MJ, et al. Mitochondrial disease: a practical approach for primary care physicians. *Pediatrics*. 2007; 120(6):1326-1333.
5. Dimauro S, Mancuso M, Naini A. Mitochondrial encephalomyopathies: therapeutic approach. *Ann N Y Acad Sci*. 2004;1011:232-245.
6. Hargreaves IP. Ubiquinone: cholesterol's reclusive cousin. *Ann Clin Biochem*. 2003;40(pt 3):207-218.
7. Bentinger M, Brismar K, Dallner G. The antioxidant role of coenzyme Q. *Mitochondrion*. 2007;7(suppl);S41-S51.
8. Turunen M, Olsson J, Dallner G. Metabolism and function of coenzyme Q. *Biochem Biophys Acta*. 2004;1660(1-2):171-199.
9. Groneberg DA, Kindermann B, Althammer M, et al. Coenzyme Q10 affects expression of genes involved in cell signalling, metabolism and transport in human CaCo-2 cells. *Int J Biochem Cell Biol*. 2005;37(6):1208-1218.
10. Yubero D, Montero R, Martin MA, et al. Secondary coenzyme Q10 deficiencies in oxidative phosphorylation (OXPHOS) and non –OXPHOS disorders. *Mitochondrion*. 2016;30:51-58.
11. Ogasahara S, Engel AG, Frens D, Mack D. Muscle coenzyme Q deficiency in familial mitochondrial encephalomyopathy. *Proc Natl Acad Sci USA*. 1989;86(7):2379-2382.
12. Emmanuele V, Lopez LC, Berardo A, et al. Heterogeneity of coenzyme Q10 deficiency: patient study and literature review. *Arch Neurol*. 2012;69(8):979-983.
13. Doimo M, Desbats MA, Cerqua C, Cassina M, Trevisson E, Salviati L. Genetics of coenzyme Q10 deficiencies. *Mol Syndromol*. 2014;5(3-4):156-162.
14. Doimo M, Trevisson E, Airik R, et al. Effect of vanillic acid on CoQ6 mutants identified in patients with coenzyme Q10 deficiency. *Biochim Biophys Acta*. 2014;1842(1):1-6.
15. Sacconi S, Trevisson E, Salviati L, et al. Coenzyme Q10 is frequently reduced in muscle of patients with mitochondrial myopathy. *Neuromuscul Disord*. 2010;20(1):44-48.
16. Montero R, Grazina M, Lopez-Gallardo E, et al. Coenzyme Q10 deficiency in mitochondrial DNA depletion syndromes. *Mitochondrion*. 2013;13(4):337-341.
17. Miles MV, Miles L, Tang LM, et al. Systemic evaluation of muscle coenzyme Q10 content in children with mitochondrial respiratory chain enzyme deficiencies. *Mitochondrion*. 2008; 8(2):170-180.
18. Bresolin N, Bet L, Binda A, et al. Clinical and biochemical correlations in mitochondrial myopathies treated with coenzyme Q10. *Neurology*. 1988;38(6):892-899.
19. Zierz S, Jahns G, Jerusalem F. Coenzyme Q in serum and muscle of 5 patients with Kearns-Sayre syndrome and 12 patients with ophthalmoplegia plus. *J Neurol*. 1989;236(2):97-101.
20. Matsuoka M, Nagawa F, Okazaki K, et al. Detection of somatic DNA recombination in transgenic mouse brain. *Science*. 1991; 254(5028):81-86.
21. Chen RS, Huang CC, Chu NS. Coenzyme Q10 treatment in mitochondrial encephalomyopathies. Short-term double-blind, crossover study. *Eur Neurol*. 1997;37(4):212-218.
22. Miranda S, Foncea R, Guerrero J, Leighton F. Oxidative stress and upregulation of mitochondrial biogenesis genes in mitochondrial DNA-depleted HeLa cells. *Biochem Biophys Res Commun*. 1999;258(1):44-49.
23. Hargreaves IP, Duncan AJ, Heales SJR, Land JM. The effect of HMG-CoA reductase inhibitors on coenzyme Q10: possible biochemical/clinical implications. *Drug Saf*. 2005;28(8):659-676.
24. He CH, Xie LX, Allan CM, Tran UC, Clarke CF. Coenzyme Q supplementation or over-expression of the yeast Coq8 putative kinase stabilizes multi-subunit coq polypeptide complexes in yeast coq null mutants. *Biochim Biophys Acta*. 2014;1841(4):630-644.
25. Marin SE, Haas RH. Coenzyme Q10 and the treatment of mitochondrial disease. In: Hargreaves IP, Hargreaves AK, eds. *Coenzyme Q_{10}: From fact to fiction*. New York: Nova Science Publishers, Inc. 2015;85–107.
26. Liu YT, Hersheson J, Plagnol V, et al. Autosomal-recessive cerebellar ataxia caused by a novel ADCK3 mutation that elongates the protein: clinical, genetic and biochemical characterisation. *J Neurol Neurosurg Psychiatry*. 2014;85(5):493-498.
27. Mollet J, Delahodde A, Serre V, et al. CABC1 gene mutations cause ubiquinone deficiency with cerebellar ataxia and seizures. *Am J Hum Genet*. 2008;82(3):623-630.
28. Horvath R, Czermin B, Gulati S, et al. Adult-onset cerebellar ataxia due to mutations in CABC1/ADCK3. *J Neurol Neurosurg Psychiatry*. 2012;83(2):174-178.
29. Lamperti C, Naini A, Hirano M, et al. Cerebellar ataxia and coenzyme Q10 deficiency. *Neurology*. 2003;60(7):1206-1208.
30. Terracciano A, Renaldo F, Zanni G, et al. The use of muscle biopsy in the diagnosis of undefined ataxia with cerebellar atrophy in children. *Eur J Paediatr Neurol*. 2012;16(3):248-256.
31. Sobreira C, Hirano M, Shanske S, et al. Mitochondrial encephalomyopathy with coenzyme Q10 deficiency. *Neurology*. 1997; 48(5):1238-1243.
32. Di Giovanni S, Mirabella M, Spinazzola A, et al. Coenzyme Q10 reverses pathological phenotype and reduces apoptosis in familial CoQ10 deficiency. *Neurology*. 2001;57(3):515-518.
33. Smith KM, Matson S, Matson WR, et al. Dose ranging and efficacy study of high dose coenzyme Q10 formulations in Huntington's disease. *Biochim Biophys Acta*. 2006;1762(6):616-626.
34. Mathews RT, Yang L, Browne S, Baik M, Beal F. Coenzyme Q10 administration increases brain mitochondrial concentrations and exerts neuroprotective effects. *Proc Natl Acad Sci USA*. 1998; 95(15):8892-8897.
35. Diomedi-Camassei F, Di Giandomenico S, Santorelli FM, et al. COQ2 nephropathy: a newly described inherited mitochondriopathy with primary renal involvement. *J Am Soc Nephrol*. 2007; 18(10):2773-2780.
36. Heeringa SF, Chernin G, Chaki M, et al. COQ6 mutations in human patients produce nephrotic syndrome with sensorineural deafness. *J Clin Invest*. 2011;121(5):2013-2024.
37. Montini G, Malaventura C, Salviat L. Early coenzyme Q10 supplementation in primary coenzyme Q10 deficiency. *N Eng J Med*. 2008;358(26):2849-2850.
38. Desbats MA, Vetro A, Limongeli I, et al. Primary coenzyme Q10 deficiency presenting as fatal neonatal multiorgan failure. *Eur J Hum Genet*. 2015b;23(9):1254-1258.

39. Ozeir M, Muhlenhoff U, Webert R, et al. Coenzyme Q biosynthesis: CoQ6 deficiency. *Chem Biol*. 2011;18(9):1134-1142.
40. Desbats MA, Lunardi G, Doimo M, Trevisson E, Salviati L. Genetic bases and clinical manifestations of coenzyme Q10 (CoQ10) deficiency. *J Inherit Metab Dis*. 2015;38(1):145-56.
41. Freyer C, Stranneheim H, Naess K, et al. Rescue of primary ubiquinone deficiency due to a novel COQ7 defect using 2,4-dihydroxybensoic acid. *J Med Genet*. 2015;52(11):779-783.
42. Koopman WJH, Beyrath J, Fung CW, et al. Mitochondrial disorders in children: toward development of small-molecule treatment strategies. *EMBO Mol Med*. 2016;8(4):311-327.
43. Chinnery P, Majamaa K, Turnbull D, Thorburn D. Treatment for mitochondria disorders. *Cochrane Database Syst Rev*. 2006; 25(1):CD004426.
44. Kerr DS. Treatment of mitochondrial electron transport chain disorders: a review of clinical trials over the past decade. *Mol Genet Metab*. 2010;99(3):246-255.
45. Hargreaves IP. Coenzyme Q10 as a therapy for mitochondrial disease. *Int J Biochem Cell Biol*. 2014;49:105-111.
46. Geromel V, Darin N, Chretien D, et al. Coenzyme Q10 and idebenone in the therapy of respiratory chain diseases: rational and comparative benefits. *Mol Genet Metab*. 2002;77(1-2):21-30.
47. Nishikawa Y, Takahashi M, Yorifuji S, et al. Long-term coenzyme Q10 therapy for a mitochondrial encephalomyopathy with cytochrome c oxidase deficiency: a 31P NMR study. *Neurology*. 1989;39(3):399-403.
48. Glover EI, Martin J, Maher A, Thornhill RE, Moran GR, Tarnopolsky MA. A randomized trial of coenzyme Q10 in mitochondrial disorders. *Muscle Nerve* 2010;42(5):739-748.
49. Ogasahara S, Yorifuji S, Nishikawa Y, et al. Improvement of abnormal pyruvate metabolism and cardiac conduction defect with coenzyme Q10 in Kearns-Sayre syndrome. *Neurology*. 1985;35(3):372-377.
50. Ihara Y, Namba R, Kuroda S, Sato T, Shirabe T. Mitochondrial encephalopmyopathy (MELAS): pathological study and successful therapy with coenzyme Q10 and idebenone. *J Neurol Sci*. 1989;90(3):263-271.
51. Abe K, Matsuo Y, Kadekawa J, Inoue S, Yanagihara T. Effect of coenzyme Q10 in patients with mitochondrial myopathy, encephalopathy, lactic acidosis, and stroke-like episodes (MELAS): evaluation by noninvasive tissue oximetry. *J Neurol Sci*. 1999; 162(1):65-68.
52. Liou CW, Huang CC, Lin TK, Tsai JL, Wei YH. Correction of pancreatic beta-cell dysfunction with coenzyme Q(10) in a patient with mitochondrial encephalomyopathy, lactic acidosis and stroke like episodes syndrome and diabetes mellitus. *Eur Neurol*. 2000;43(1):54-55.
53. Ogasahara S, Nishikawa Y, Yorifuli S, et al. Treatment of Kearns-Sayre syndrome with coenzyme Q10. *Neurology*. 1986;36(1): 45-53.
54. Goda S, Hamada T, Ishimoto S, Kobayashi T, Goto I, Kuroiwa Y. Clinical improvement after administration of coenzyme Q10 in a patient with mitochondrial encephalomyopathy. *J Neurol*. 1987; 234(1):62-63.
55. Bendahan D, Desnuelle C, Vanuxem D, , et al. 31P NMR spectroscopy and ergometer exercise test as evidence for muscle oxidative performance improvement with coenzyme Q in mitochondrial myopathies. *Neurology*. 1992;42(6):1203-1208.
56. Fadic R, Johns DR. Clinical spectrum of mitochondrial diseases. *Semin Neurol*. 1996;16(1):11-20.
57. Chan A, Reichmann H, Kogel A, et al. Metabolic changes in patients with mitochondrial myopathies and effects of coenzyme Q10 therapy. *J Neurol*. 1998;245(10):681-685.
58. Bresolin N, Doriguzzi C, Ponzetto C, et al. Ubidecarenone in the treatment of mitochondrial myopathies: a multi-center double-blind trial. *J Neurol Sci*. 1990;100(1-2):70-78.
59. Matthews PM, Ford B, Dandurand RJ, et al. Coenzyme Q10 with multiple vitamins is generally ineffective in treatment of mitochondrial disease. *Neurology*. 1993;43(5):884-890.
60. Zierz S, von Wersebe O, Bleistein J, Jerusalem F. Exogenous Coenzyme Q (Coq) Fails to Increase Coq in Skeletal Muscle of Two Patients With Mitochondrial Myopathies. *J Neurol Sci*. 1990;95(3):283-290.
61. Chan A, Reichmann H, Kögel A, Beck A, Gold R. Metabolic changes in patients with mitochondrial myopathies and effects of coenzyme Q10 therapy. *J Neurol*. 1989;245(10):681-685.
62. Chan T, Teng S, Wilson J, Galati G, Khan S, O'Brien PJ. Coenzyme Q cytoprotective mechanisms for mitochondrial complex I cytopathies involves NAD(P)H Quinone oxidoreductase 1 (NQO1). *J Free Radic Res*. 2002;36(4):421-427
63. Enns GM, Kinsma SL, Perlman SL, et al. Initial experience in the treatment of inherited mitochondrial disease with EPI-743. *Mol Genet Metab*. 2012;105(1):91-102.
64. Martinelli D, Catteruccia M, Piemonte F, et al. EPI-743 reverses the progression of the pediatric mitochondrial disease. *Mol Genet Metab*. 2012;107(3):383-388.
65. Homstrom KH, Baird L, Zhang Y, et al. NrF2 impacts cellular bioenergetics by controlling substrate availability for mitochondrial respiration. *Biol Open*. 2013;2(8):761-770.
66. Muller W, Reimers CD, Berninger T, et al. Coenzyme Q10 in ophthalmoplegia plus—a double blind, cross over therapeutic trial. *J Neurol Sci*. 1990;98(suppl):442.
67. Rodriguez MC, MacDonald JR, Mahoney DJ, Parise G, Beal MF, Tarnopolsky MA. Beneficial effects of creatine, CoQ10 and lipoic acid in mitochondrial disorders. *Muscle Nerve*. 2007;35(2): 235-242.
68. Garrido-Maraver J, Cordero MD, Oropesa-Avila M, et al. Clinical applications of coenzyme Q10. *Front Biosci*. 2014; 19:619-633.
69. Katayama K, Fujita T. Studies on lymphatic absorption of 1', 2'-(3 H)-coenzyme Q10 in rats. *Chem Pharm Bull*. 1972;20(12): 2585-2592.
70. Bhagavan HN, Chopra RK, Craft NE, Chitchumroonchokchai C, Failla ML. Assessment of coenzyme Q10 absorption using an in vitro digestion-Caco-2 cell model. *Int J Pharm*. 2007;333(1-2): 112-117.
71. Bhagavan HN, Chopra RK. Coenzyme Q10: absorption, tissue uptake, metabolism and pharmacokinetics. *Free Radic Res*. 2006;40(5):445-453.
72. Aberg F, Appelkvist EL, Dallner G, Ernster L. Distribution and redox state of ubiquinones in rat and human tissues. *Arch Biochem Biophys*. 1992;295(2):230-234.

73. Trevisson E, Dimauro S, Nava P, et al. Coenzyme Q10 deficiency in muscle. *Curr Opin Neurol*. 2011;24(5):449-456.
74. Bhagavan HN, Chopra RK. Plasma coenzyme Q10 response to oral ingestion of coenzyme 10 formulations. *Mitochondrion*. 2007;7(suppl):S78-S88.
75. Martinefski M, Samassa P, Buontempo F, Höcht C, Lucangioli S, Tripodi V. Relative bioavailability of coenzyme Q10 formulation for paediatric individualized therapy. *J Pharm Pharmacol*. 2017; 69(5):567-573. doi:10.1111/jphp.12613.
76. Miles MV, Horn P, Miles L. Bioequivalence of coenzyme Q10 from over-the counter supplements. *Nutr Res*. 2002;22(8): 919-929.
77. Weis M, Mortensen SA, Rassing MR, Møller-Sonnergaard J, Poulsen G, Rasmussen SN. Bioavailability of four oral coenzyme Q10 formulations in healthy volunteers. *Mol Aspects Med*. 1994; 15(suppl): s273-s280.
78. Parikh S, Saneto R, Falk MJ, et al. A modern approach to the treatment of mitochondrial disease. *Curr Treat Options Neurol*. 2009;11(6):414-430.
79. Garcia-Corzo L, Luna-Sanchez M, Doerrier C, et al. Ubiquinol-10 ameliorates mitochondrial encephalopathy associated with CoQ10 deficiency. *Biochim Biophys Acta*. 2014;1842(7): 893-901.
80. Miles MV, Patterson BJ, Schapiro MB, et al. Coenzyme Q10 absorption and tolerance in children with Down syndrome: a dose ranging trial. *Pediatr Neurol*. 2006;35(1):30-37.
81. Itagaki S, Ochiai A, Kobayash M, Sugawara M, Hirano T, Iseki K. Grapefruit juice enhance the uptake of coenzyme Q10 in the human intestinal cell-line Caco-2. *Food Chem*. 2010;120(2): 552-555.
82. Kaikkonen J, Nyyssonen K, Tomasi A, et al. Antioxidative efficacy of parallel and combined supplementation with coenzyme Q10 d-alpha-tocopherol in mildly hypercholesterolemic subjects: a randomized placebo-controlled clinical study. *Free Radic Res*. 2000;33(3):329-340.
83. Molyneux SL, Young JM, Florkowski CM, et al. Coenzyme Q10: is there a clinical role and a case for measurement? *Clin Biochem Rev*. 2008;29(2):71-81.
84. Duncan AJ, Heales SJ, Mills K, Eaton S, Land JM, Hargreaves IP. Determination of coenzyme Q10 status in blood mononuclear cells, skeletal muscle and plasma by HPLC with a di-propoxy-coenzyme Q10 as an internal standard. *Clin Chem*. 2005;51(12): 2380-2382.
85. Yubero D, Montero R, Ramos M, et al. Determination of urinary coenzyme Q10 by HPLC with electrochemical detection: reference values for a paediatric population. *Biofactors*. 2015;41(6): 424-430.
86. Yubero D, Montero R, Artuch R, Land JM, Heales SJ, Hargreaves IP. Biochemical diagnosis of coenzyme Q10 deficiency. *Mol Syndromol*. 2014;5(3-4):147-155.
87. Shults CW, Beal F, Song D, Fontaine D. Pilot trial of high dosages of coenzyme Q10 in patients with Parkinson's disease. *Exp Neurol*. 2004;188(2):491-494.
88. Rotig A, Appelkvist EL, Geromel V, et al. Quinone-responsive multiple respiratory chain dysfunction due to widespread coenzyme Q10 deficiency. *Lancet*. 2000;356(9227):391-395.
89. Pineda M, Montero R, Aracil A, et al. Coenzyme Q(10)-responsive ataxia: 2-year-treatment follow-up. *Mov Disord*. 2010;25(9): 1262-1268.
90. Shults CW, Oakes D, Kieburtz K, et al. Effects of coenzyme Q10 in early Parkinson disease: evidence of slowing of the functional decline. *Arch Neurol*. 2002;59(10):1541-1550.
91. Lopez LC, Quinzii CM, Area E, et al. Treatment of CoQ10 deficient fibroblasts with ubiquinone, CoQ analogs, and vitamin C: time- and compound-dependent effects. *PloS One*. 2010;5(7): e11897.
92. Duberley KE, Heales SJ, Abramov AY, et al. Effect of Coenzyme Q10 supplementation on mitochondrial electron transport chain activity and mitochondrial oxidative stress in Coenzyme Q10 deficient human neuronal cells. *Int J Biochem Cell Biol*. 2014; 50:60-63.
93. Duberley KE, Hargreaves IP, Chaiwatanasirikul KA, et al. Coenzyme Q10 quantification in muscle, fibroblasts and cerebrospinal fluid by liquid chromatography/tandem mass spectrometry using a novel deuterated internal standard. *Rapid Commun Mass Spectrom*. 2013;27(9):924-930.

8

Chilean Nutrition Management Protocol for Patients With Phenylketonuria

Gabriela Castro[1]**, Valerie Hamilton**[1]**, and Verónica Cornejo**[1]

Abstract

Since neonatal screening and early nutritional treatment began, it has been possible to reverse the neurological damage that phenylketonuria (PKU) causes. Scientific evidence gathered over more than 50 years on the monitoring of individuals with PKU indicates that a phenylalanine level of about 6 mg/dL (360 μmol/L) is ideal and points to the necessity of starting a long-term phenylalanine-restricted diet in which blood phenylalanine level should stay between 2 and 6 mg/dL (120-360 μmol/L). This article aims to establish the general basis for proper monitoring of people with PKU and provide a useful tool for clinicians overseeing treatment. We hope to establish similar criteria throughout Latin America and create a uniform protocol in order to have comparative monitoring results for the region.

Keywords

phenylketonuria, blood phenylalanine level, PHE levels in follow-up.

Introduction

Phenylketonuria (PKU; OMIM 261600) is caused by a defect in the enzyme phenylalanine (PHE) hydroxylase, which is responsible for transforming PHE to tyrosine (TYR). Inheritance is autosomal recessive and recurrence is 25% in each pregnancy. Starting at neonatal diagnosis, PHE restriction is used as a treatment for PKU in order to prevent the neurological sequelae that this disease causes. The Medical Research Council has established that any child with a PHE level of 6 mg/dL (360 μmol/L), normal or decreased TYR, and receiving a normal diet should start a PHE-restricted diet in combination with protein-free PHE substitutes, minerals and essential fatty acids supplementation, and special foods low in protein. Optimal treatment requires diagnosis to be done as soon as possible, ideally in the second week of life (before 1 month of life), strict monitoring throughout life and maintaining a PHE-restricted diet. Additionally, dietary intake must be adjusted to the PHE value that is considered safe for maintaining normal growth and development. Good metabolic control means maintaining blood levels between 2 and 6 mg/dL (120-360 μmol/L) throughout life.[1-7]

The diet prohibits all foods of animal origin because of the high PHE content. Foods such as cereals and most fruits and vegetables should be carefully monitored, and the exact PHE content of each should be known. To provide energy, protein, and TYR, the diet must include PHE-free protein substitutes. Nutritional therapy should be monitored periodically for clinical, biochemical, and nutritional status methods, mainly by observing physiological and pathophysiological changes that lead to increases or decreases in PHE level.

This article aims to establish the general basis for proper monitoring of people with PKU and provide a useful tool for clinicians responsible for treatment. The article is meant to be used as educational material to facilitate clinical monitoring and encourage similar criteria be used across Latin America. In this way, a single protocol could facilitate treatment-monitoring comparisons in the region.

Objectives of Diet Therapy Treatment

The objective is to maintain optimal growth and development and plasma PHE levels within ranges that prevent mental retardation, normal plasma TYR level, and promote anabolism.[8]

[1] Instituto de Nutrición y Tecnología de los Alimentos, Universidad de Chile, Santiago, Chile

Corresponding Author:

Verónica Cornejo, Instituto de Nutrición y Tecnología de los Alimentos, Universidad de Chile, Santiago, Chile.

Email: vcornejo@inta.uchile.cl

Table 1. Allowed Levels of Phenylalanine for Patients With Phenylketonuria (PKU) by Age.

Age Group	Phenylalanine Level (mg/dL)
Newborn to 2 years old	2-4
>2 years old	2-6
Pregnant patients with PKU	2-6

Metabolic Control Goals

Plasma PHE level keeps blood values between 2 and 6 mg/dL (120-360 μmol/L), which vary according to age (Table 1).[1,6] Plasma TYR level maintains levels between 1.0 and 1.8 mg/dL (55-100 μmol/L). If levels fall below 0.8 mg/dL (<44 μmol/L), TYR intake should be evaluated and, if necessary, PHE-free protein substitutes should be increased or free form supplementation (600-1200 mg/d) should be considered depending on availability and following up 1 month later with acylcarnitines to adjust dose.[9,10]

Plasma PHE Level, Intake Tolerance, and Mutation Type

Classic PKU has plasma PHE above 20 mg/dL (1200 μmol/L) at the time of diagnosis. The plasma PHE level for neonatal screening is greater than 7 mg/dL, with a ratio of PHE/TYR greater than 5. The PHE dietary tolerance until 1 year is between 25 and 45 mg/kg/d (130-330 mg/d). Between 2 and 5 years, the recommended level is below 20 mg/kg/d, maintaining a plasma PHE value less than 5 mg/dL (300 μmol/L). After 5 years of age, less than 12 mg/kg/d of PHE is tolerated, with the goal being to maintain plasma PHE level between 2 and 6 mg/dL (120-360 μmol/L).

Moderate PKU has a plasma PHE level between 15 and 20 mg/dL (900-1200 μmol/L) at diagnosis. The ratio of PHE/TYR is greater than 3. Dietary PHE tolerance until 1 year of life is between 45 and 50 mg/kg/d. Between 2 and 5 years, the recommended level is between 20 and 25 mg/kg/d (350-400 mg/d), maintaining a plasma PHE value less than 5 mg/dL (300 μmol/L). Over 5 years, patients have a PHE dietary tolerance between 12 and 18 mg/kg/d, maintaining plasma PHE level between 2 and 6 mg/dL (120-360 μmol/L).

Mild PKU has PHE plasma level 10 to 15 mg/dL (600-900 μmol/L), with a ratio of PHE/TYR greater than 3. The phenylalanine dietary tolerance up to 1 year is 55 mg/kg/d. Between 2 and 5 years, it is 25 to 50 mg/kg/d (400-600 mg/d), maintaining PHE plasma less than 5 mg/dL (300 μmol/L). Over 5 years, the PHE dietary tolerance is greater than 18 mg/kg/d, maintaining PHE plasma level between 2 and 6 mg/dL (120-360 μmol/L).

Moderate hyperphenylalaninemia or gray area has PHE plasma level between 6 and 10 mg/dL (360-600 μmol/L). The PHE/TYR ratio is greater than 3. Dietary tolerance of PHE in the first year is 70 mg/kg/d. Between 2 and 5 years, it is greater than 50 mg/kg/d, maintaining a plasma PHE value of less than 5 mg/dL (300 μmol/L).

Moderate hyperphenylalaninemia not requiring nutritional treatment has plasma PHE level between 2 and 6 mg/dL (120-360 μmol/L). The PHE level for neonatal screening between 2.5 and 6 mg/dL (151-360 μmol/L). An average PHE/TYR ratio is 3.3 (between 0.8 and 8.25). Normal dietary PHE intake and normal PHE value.

Tetrahydropterin deficiencies have normal or elevated plasma PHE levels. The PHE blood level of neonatal screening between 2 and 35 mg/dL (120-2120 μmol/L). Patients tolerate PHE intake and have variable PHE values. A specific genotype has not been determined. Many of protein deficiencies require BH4 supplementation and neurotransmitter precursors.[6]

Nutritional Therapy at Diagnosis by PHE Level

Nutritional therapy should be started as early as possible, preferably during the second week of life, considering that diagnostic confirmation will take place during the first week of life. Depending on the initial value, PHE intake should be excluded until PHE values attain ranges that do not cause neurological damage. It is important to note that beginning treatment in a timely manner requires coordination between the neonatal screening laboratory, a search of the suspect cases, and a short confirmation period to establish a correct case.[11] On this basis, we recommend:

- If, at diagnosis, the newborn has a PHE value less than 6 mg/dL (360 μmol/L), patient should maintain exclusive breast-feeding, with PHE blood levels checked weekly. If value is greater than 6 mg/dL, patient should begin nutritional treatment, controlling PHE intake.
- When PHE value is between 6 and 10 mg/dL (360-600 μmol/L), treatment should begin in the form of a PHE-restricted diet. As PHE value is not extremely high, 50% of the total volume should be PHE-free formula and 50% breast milk or infant formula. This requires estimating the total volume of liquids, considering the recommendation of 150 mL/kg/d *(recommended dietary intake [RDI])*. Blood PHE value should be measured weekly, and according to the results obtained, PHE intake should be adjusted. If values remain high, the contribution of breast-feeding should be reduced and the volume of PHE-free formula increased. The recommendation is always to provide PHE-free formula first and then place the baby to the breast.
- When initial value of PHE is over 10 mg/dL (600 μmol/L), breast-feeding and/or infant formula should be discontinued immediately. First, determine the total fluid volume (150 mL/kg/d); 100% of the daily volume should be PHE-free formula, which provides all the nutrient necessities for this age group. After 5 to 7 days, if PHE value has dropped below 10 mg/dL, PHE intake is reintroduced through combined breast milk with special formula, providing the lower amount of PHE recommendations (Table 2). It is important to note that

Table 2. Recommended Intake of Phenylalanine (PHE), Tyrosine (TYR), and Protein for Individuals With Phenylketonuria (PKU).

	PHE, mg/d	TYR, mg/d	Protein RDI + 30%, g/kg
Age, months			
0-3	130-430	1000-1300	2.1
3-6	135-400	1400-2100	1.7
6-9	145-370	2500-3000	1.7
9-12	135-330	2500-3000	1.7
Age, years			
1-4	200-320	2800-3500	1.1-1.2
4 to adult	200-1100	4000-6000	1.2-1.5

Abbreviation: RDI, recommended dietary intake.

PHE-free formula is always given before breast milk. The PHE values are tested weekly until PHE is able to stabilize between 2 and 4 mg/dL (120-240 μmol/L).

Calorie intake provides recommendations based on age and sex, keeping a ratio of 150 kcal/g of nonprotein nitrogen. Maltodextrin and vegetable oil, preferably with oils containing essential fatty acids precursors (eg, α-linolenic acid and docosahexaenoic acid [DHA]), can be used to complete 120 to 150 kcal/kg/d and promote anabolism.

Long-Term Nutritional and Metabolic Monitoring

Phenylalanine prescription according to blood PHE levels.

- The PHE levels measured every 7 days, making sure that there is adequate physical growth.
- If plasma PHE level is less than 2 mg/dL (120 μmol/L), the supply of PHE should be increased to 50 mg/d. If PHE is more than 6 mg/dL (360 μmol/L), PHE intake should decrease 30 to 100 mg/d depending on the detected plasma level.
- Each change in diet is followed by an assessment of PHE value every 7 days after a change, and necessary adjustments should be made to the diet in order to maintain PHE values between 2 and 4 mg/dL (120-240 μmol/L) in infants and between 2 and 6 (120-360 μmol/L) in older children.
- For actual PHE intake measurement, a 24-hour dietary recall close to PHE measurement date should be completed by parents or caregivers in order to evaluate PHE requirements according to the metabolic status of the child.
- Between the third and fifth month of life, there is a slowdown in growth, thus PHE contribution should be discreetly decreased and adjusted in each case if PHE value increased without apparent cause. If the child spontaneously stops taking formula during the night, total volume must be distributing during the day.
- At 5 months, pureed fruit (50-150 mL/d) is introduced. It should be noted that delivery time is midmorning and this contribution of PHE not be quantified due to its low PHE level. Fruits low in PHE, such as pears or apples, are suggested.
- At 6 months, solid meals of vegetables begin with PHE contributions between 100 and 120 mg. This amount of PHE should be considered within the total PHE estimated for each child. It is important to teach parents or caregiver how to calculate the daily PHE. Written explanation and examples should be provided if possible, together with a table of the PHE contents of different foods.[12]
- At 8 months, the second solid food meal begins, increasing the contribution of PHE from natural foods such as vegetables, grains, and fruits to about 200 mg/d. The volume of each meal will vary according to gastric tolerance of the child (200-250 mL in average). At least 3 doses of phenylalanine-free protein substitutes should be kept, if possible, these should be divided in more takes in order to promote anabolism. Increasing intake of solid foods involves a reduction in breast milk and/or infant formula. At this age, in addition to the formula indicated, the child must consume 2 meals and 1 snack (preferably midmorning and consisting of natural fruit).
- At 1 year, PHE intake recommendations are set according to plasma level of previously maintained PHE. First, pureed or semipureed foods are introduced. At 15 months, children have molars, thus chopped foods can be provided, and by 18 months, whole foods are offered. The use of low-protein foods, specially formulated for aminoacidopathies, is an excellent tool to increase volume, providing satiety, and promoting diet adherence.

Recommended PHE level during times of physiological stress.

- Vaccines should be applied when PHE value is low or equal to 2 mg/dL (<120 μmol/L), as these induce increased plasma level for protein catabolism. If the value of PHE is above 2 mg/dL, PHE intake should be reduced between 10% and 25% (depending on plasma value) and reevaluated after 1 week. If, after 1 week, PHE values have dropped below 2 mg/dL, vaccination should proceed. Regular intake of PHE must be reset 72 hours postvaccination, as long as the child is without fever, if not wait until the fever is gone.
- In the presence of infectious conditions or surgeries, a reduction in the intake of PHE by 15% to 25% is suggested since PHE level tends to increase regardless of diet. Energy intake should increase by 10% over normal intake (from maltose dextrin, vegetable oil, etc.) to prevent catabolism. An adequate level of hydration and electrolyte balance should be maintained. Oral rehydration salts can be used where appropriate.
- Keep recommended intake of PHE-free formula at all times; if there is less tolerance, reduce volumes no greater than 50 to 100 mL/h.

Protein recommendations. Natural protein intake is inadequate to maintain PHE values between 2 and 6 mg/dL, and foods of animal origin are prohibited, thus it is not possible to maintain adequate growth through natural foods only. Thus, it is mandatory to provide a PHE-free formula, which provides the necessary amounts of amino acids to maintain normal growth, and supplies the appropriate intake of vitamins and minerals. We recommend:

- The special PHE-free formula is the only source of protein of high biological value for children with classic PKU. To determine the amount of PHE-free formula to be delivered each the day, calculate the amount of protein according to the 2007 World Health Organization recommendations by age, sex, and weight and by adding 30% extra for a synthetic diet (Table 2).[13,14]
- At the beginning of treatment, less than 50% of total protein can come from PHE-free formula. The nutritional needs of this period, which is characterized by rapid growth, require that patients also receive breast milk or infant formula. Subsequently, protein intake from PHE-free formulas increases to 70% or 80%, becoming the only source of protein of high biological value. There is a wide variety of PHE-free products that differ in protein levels and can be consumed in amounts according to the age and PKU physiological stage. Products have different forms—powders, "ready-to-drink" liquids, and bars in order to improve intake adherence throughout life.[2]
- Currently, various products have been developed such as glycomacropeptide, a product that delivers intact natural proteins from whey, has excellent biological value and contains small amounts of PHE. Its use is recommended to improve both diet adherence and protein quality[15]; nevertheless, more evidence related to its effectiveness is needed.
- The PHE-free formula should be distributed evenly throughout the day and in similar quantities to ensure better absorption and stability of PHE plasma level. At the start of treatment, frequency will be every 3 hours (8 servings/day) and, subsequently, decreasing in the preschool stage 3 to 4 times a day and 3 servings/day in the adolescent stage. The recommendation is to keep as many servings as possible.
- Protein requirements increase during periods of rapid growth and physiological stress, needs that are satisfied by increasing the volume of PHE-free special formula.[1,2,6]

Calorie recommendations. Energy needs are set according to RDI, by sex and nutritional status, in order to maintain growth and development within normal ranges. Due to natural food restrictions and the contribution of PHE-free formula, we recommend the following:

- In children less than 12 months of age, 100 to 120 kcal/kg/d should be provided. If complete energy supply is not achieved with PHE-free formula, a caloric supplement (maltose dextrin) and/or vegetable oils (canola = α-linolenic acid or fish oil = eicosapentaenoic acid [EPA]/DHA) are recommended. Starting at 1 year, energy recommendations should be based on RDI, adjusted for nutritional status. At least 150 nonprotein kcal/g of nitrogen is recommended.
- Inadequate intake of energy can produce stunted growth and weight loss, among other complications. Weight loss is a catabolic process thus may induce an endogenous increase in plasma levels of PHE.

Low-protein food or low-protein–modified food products have been created, which are an excellent source of energy and provide satiety, but care must be taken in the quantities consumed daily, as they may increase risk of overweight or obesity if intake is not controlled. These products that include bread and pasta are prepared with wheat starch and other grains, are very low in PHE, and have allowed the diet of PKU children to resemble that of a child without PKU.

Liquid recommendations.

- In the first months of life, 150 mL/kg/d is recommended, corresponding to 1.5 mL by ingested calorie. In children and adults, 1 mL per calorie ingested is calculated.
- When there is an increase in body temperature, vomiting, or diarrhea, fluid requirements are increased according to the degree of temperature change.

Vitamin and mineral supplementation. Starting at the first month, in countries or regions at latitudes below 35° (southern Chile and Argentina), should include mandatory supplementation with 400 IU/d of vitamin D. If a daily dose is not consumed, give 2 to 3 doses of 100 000 IU during the first year of life.[16]

- Premature and/or low-birth-weight children should be supplemented with iron (2 mg/kg/d).[17]
- In the fourth month of life for breast-fed children, iron supplementation should start providing 1 mg/kg/d to prevent iron deficiency anemia.
- Supplementing with 5 mg/d of zinc between the fourth month and the first year and up to 3 years with 10 mg/d and then 15 to 20 mg/d.
- At 12 months, if calcium intake is low, 400 mg/d of calcium is recommended. At 10 years, between 800 and 1000 mg/d is suggested, as at this stage one-third of adult bone mass is deposited. Individuals with PKU have been observed to have lower bone densitometry compared to controls. Measurement of bone mineral density can be used as a complement to suggested supplementation.[18]
- From treatment start, supplementation with omega 3 fatty acids is recommended, as it is important in retina and central nervous system structure formation, which favors the development of visual, motor, and cognitive skills.

Table 3. Phenylalanine (PHE) Monitoring Frequency for Patients With Phenylketonuria (PKU).

Age	PHE Monitoring Frequency
<12 months or breast-feeding	Every 7 days
1 to 2 years	Every 15 days
> 2 years	Monthly, depending on adherence

Between 1% and 3% of total calories, soybean oil, canola (α-linolenic acid, the precursor of DHA fatty acids), or fish oil containing EPA and DHA is recommended.[19]

Monitoring PHE and TYR Values

Dietary manipulation requires frequent monitoring of blood PHE, with the aim of keeping levels in safe ranges and preventing neurological damage but also enough to achieve growth with PHE in normal ranges. Together, PHE intake and PHE blood value must be adapted based on growth, physiological state, disease, and comorbidity. It is also important to monitor TYR value. We recommend:

- The Weekly PHE blood level checking in the first year of life is highly recommended with values between 2 and 4 mg/dL (120-240 μmol/L). In this period, many factors interfere with PHE level, such as physiological (growth, teething, breast-feeding, etc) and pathophysiological (infections and frequent vaccinations). A value less than 0.5 mg/dL (30 μmol/L) is considered as levels risky for affecting growth. If a child has values between 1 and 2 mg/dL (60-120 μmol/L) and has high PHE intake, they are considered low risk.[6,20] Between 1 and 2 years, testing PHE level every 15 days is recommended. After 2 years, frequency depends on adherence to the monthly diet (Table 3).
- The TYR value during the first year should be measured every 3 months in conjunction with PHE level, then semiannually or once a year, depending on child development. If there is growth arrest, TYR should be evaluated independent of age. Values between 1.0 and 1.8 mg/dL (55-100 μmol/L) are recommended.
- A profile of amino acids, transferrin, complete blood count, albumin, ferritin, 25-OH vitamin D, essential fatty acids, trace minerals (zinc, copper, and selenium), vitamin A, and folic acid. Between 6 and 8 years, a dual energy X-ray absorptiometry is recommended to evaluate bone health.

Education. Diet for PKU children is based on vegetables and fruits and small portions of cereals. Thus, nutrition education focuses on establishing good habits early in life and providing a varied diet, with different flavors and textures. We recommend creating written material to support education and improve adherence to nutritional therapy. Families should be taught to select foods with a low PHE contribution and avoid bad eating habits that, in the future, could affect adherence to nutritional therapy. It is important to note that starting at 10 years of age, education should include the concept of self-control, that is, learning to prepare the special formula, knowing how to calculate the PHE content of foods, to choose foods low in PHE, and maintain healthy habits as physical exercises.

Discussion

This work represents an effort to share the experience developed by a Chilean group with more than 25 years of experience in the treatment of more than 300 patients with PKU. There are similar criteria published by Singh and colleagues[21] regarding nutrition management guidelines for PKU, specifically in relation to metabolic control goals, critical nutrients intake, and parameters to start treatment.

The management guidelines for PKU recommend maintaining PHE levels between 2 and 6 mg/dL throughout life.[21] In Chile, we maintain the same level, except in the first 2 years of life, where we recommend a maximum level of 4 mg/dL. A lower level allows greater control over catabolism increases in PHE associated with vaccinations and intercurrent infections, both frequent occurrences during this period.

In our country, special formula intake represents 80% of the protein intake in children over 1 year of age. Through various efforts of our working group, PHE-free formula is now distributed by the ministry of health, up to 25 years of age. Certain special formulas generate high rejection in patients, due to low palatability. This has the consequence that patients do not consume 100% of the nutritional indication given as a special formula. Therefore, unlike the guidelines published by Singh and colleagues, we supplement children with calcium, iron, and zinc, to comply with micronutrient recommendations.[21]

In recent years, it has been shown that PKU treatment should be for life, and new nutrition management guidelines, emphasize this, exposing the neurological changes that occur in older children and adults without treatment.[21] Therefore in Chile, we have developed various strategies to promote self-care and educate patients and families to achieve compliance with lifelong treatment; this includes the creation of educational workshops for adolescents and adults, developing applications for patients and parents to access PHE levels and for calculating daily PHE. In addition, with the extension of the national program of special formulas provided by the ministry of health, it was possible to reengage the majority of patients older than 18 years who had left treatment.

Conclusion

A PHE-restricted diet, plus the use of special PHE-free formula and micronutrient supplementation, is effective in preventing the nerve damage caused by high levels of PHE in persons living with PKU. To achieve good metabolic control and prevent neurological disorders, PHE levels should be kept between 2 and 6 mg/dL throughout life.

Our goal was to present nutritional management guidelines based on our 25 years of experience in Chile and the current literature. Our guidelines can be used as educational materials to facilitate clinical monitoring. We encourage similar criteria to be used across Latin America.

Declaration of Conflicting Interests

The author(s) declared no potential conflicts of interest with respect to the research, authorship, and/or publication of this article.

Funding

The author(s) received no financial support for the research, authorship, and/or publication of this article.

References

1. Camp KM, Parisi MA, Acosta PB, et al. Phenylketonuria Scientific Review Conference: state of the science and future research needs. *Mol Genet Metab.* 2014;112(2):87-122.
2. MacDonald A, Rocha JC, van Rijn M, Feillet F. Nutrition in phenylketonuria. *Mol Genet Metab.* 2011;(104 suppl):S10-S18.
3. Okano Y, Nagasaka H. Optimal serum phenylalanine for adult patients with phenylketonuria. *Mol Genet Metab.* 2013;110(4): 424-430.
4. Robert M, Rocha JC, van Rijn M, et al. Micronutrient status in phenylketonuria. *Mol Genet Metab.* 2013;(110 suppl):S6-S17.
5. Strisciuglio P, Concolino D. New Strategies for the Treatment of Phenylketonuria (PKU). *Metabolites* 2014;4(4):1007-17.
6. Vockley J, Andersson H, Antshel K, et al; American College of Medical Genetics and Genomics, Therapeutics Committee. Phenylalanine hydroxylase deficiency: diagnosis and management guideline. *Genet Med.* 2014;16(2):88-200.
7. Report of Medical Research Council Working Party on Phenylketonuria, Recommendations on the dietary management of phenylketonuria. *Arch Dis Child.* 1993;68(3):426-427.
8. National Institutes of Health Consensus Development Panel. National Institutes of Health Consensus Development Conference Statement: Phenylketonuria: Screening and Management, October 16-18, 2000. *Pediatrics.* 2001;108(4):972-982.
9. van Spronsen FJ, van Rijn M, Bekhof J, Koch R, Smit PG. Phenylketonuria: tyrosine supplementation in phenylalanine-restricted diets. *Am J Clin Nutr.* 2001;73(2):153-157.
10. Webster D, Wildgoose J. Tyrosine supplementation for phenylketonuria. *Cochrane Database Syst Rev.* 2013;(6):CD001507. doi:10.1002/14651858.
11. Cornejo V, Raimann E. Errores innatos del metabolismo de los aminoácidos. En: Colombo M, Cornejo V, Raimann E. eds. *Errores innatos en el metabolismo del niño.* Santiago: Editorial Universitaria; 2010:65-132. Capítulo 3.
12. Gobierno de Chile MdS. Guía de alimentación del niño(a) menor de 2 años hasta la adolescencia. en: *Departamento de nutrición y ciclo vital.* Santiago: Gobierno de Chile; 2005:25-27.
13. Joint WHO/FAO/UNU Expert Consultation. Protein and amino acid requirements in human nutrition. *World Health Organ Tech Rep Ser.* 2007;(935):1-265.
14. Aguiar A, Ahring K, Almeida MF, et al. Practices in prescribing protein substitutes for PKU in Europe: no uniformity of approach. *Mol Genet Metab.* 2015;115(1):17-22.
15. van Calcar S, Ney D. Food products made with glycomacropeptide, a low-phenylalanine whey protein, provide a new alternative to amino acid-based medical foods for nutrition management of phenylketonuria. *J Acad Nutr Diet.* 2012; 112(8):1201-1210.
16. Rebollo G. Suplementos nutricionales en pediatría. *Rev Chil Nut.* 2002;29:294-299.
17. Olivares G M. Suplementación con hierro. *Rev Chil Nut.* 2004; 31(3):272-275.
18. de Groot M, Hoeksma M, van Rijn M, Slart R, van Spronsen F. Relationships between lumbar bone mineral density and biochemical parameters in phenylketonuria patients. *Mol Genet Metab.* 2012;105(4):566-570.
19. Giovannini M, Verduci E, Salvatici E, Paci S, Riva E. Phenylketonuria: nutritional advances and challenges. *Nutr Metab (Lond).* 2012;9(1):1-7.
20. Cornejo V, Castro G, Fernández E, et al. Modelo chileno de seguimiento a largo plazo para fenilcetonuria (PKU). *Acta Pediatr Mex.* 2012;33(6):301-307.
21. Singh RH, Cunningham AC, Mofidi S, et al. Updated, web-based nutrition management guideline for PKU: an evidence and consensus based approach. *Mol Genet Metab.* 2016;118(2):72-83. doi:10.1016/j.ymgme.2016.04.008.

9

Pulmonary Arterial Hypertension in Glycogen Storage Disease Type I

Rachel D. Torok, MD[1], Stephanie L. Austin, MS[2], Lisa K. Britt, RDCS[1], Jose E. Abdenur, MD[3,4], Priya S. Kishnani, MD[2], and Stephanie B. Wechsler, MD[1,2]

Abstract

Pulmonary arterial hypertension (PAH) is a rare and highly fatal disease that has been reported in 8 patients with glycogen storage disease type I (GSDI). We describe an additional case of an acute presentation of PAH in a 14-year-old patient with GSDI, which was successfully treated with inhaled nitric oxide and sildenafil. We investigated the incidence of PAH in 28 patients with GSDI on routine echocardiography and found no evidence of PAH and no significant cardiac abnormalities. This study highlights that PAH is a rare disease overall, but our case report and those previously described suggest an increased incidence in patients with GSDI. Should cardiopulmonary symptoms develop, clinicians caring for patients with GSDI should have a high degree of suspicion for acute PAH and recognize that prompt intervention can lead to survival in this otherwise highly fatal disease.

Keywords

glycogen storage disease type I, pulmonary arterial hypertension, echocardiography, sildenafil

Introduction

Glycogen storage disease type I (GSDI) is an autosomal recessive disease with an incidence of approximately 1 in 100 000 newborns. Two main subtypes exist, with type Ia (von Gierke disease) caused by a deficiency of glucose-6-phosphatase and type Ib caused by defects in glucose-6-phosphate translocase. Abnormal accumulation of glycogen and fat and inadequate glucose production lead to hypoglycemia, growth retardation, hepatomegaly, lactic acidosis, hyperlipidemia, and hyperuricemia.[1] Prognosis has improved with continuous gastric feeding and the use of uncooked cornstarch to maintain euglycemia, but short stature, gout, renal dysfunction, osteoporosis, and hepatic adenomas are known complications.[1,2] Eight cases of pulmonary arterial hypertension (PAH) in patients with GSDI have been described,[3-9] but the incidence and etiology of PAH in patients with GSDI remain unknown.

Pulmonary arterial hypertension is a rare disease with an incidence of 2.4 to 7.6 cases/million cases. Pulmonary arterial vascular changes lead to increased pulmonary vascular resistance and right heart failure, and the typical annual mortality rate is 15%.[10] Transthoracic echocardiography serves as a noninvasive, accurate, sensitive, and specific screening tool for PAH.[11,12] An estimate of pulmonary arterial pressure is obtained from the tricuspid regurgitation (TR) jet velocity, with a peak velocity >2.8 to 2.9 m/s used as the cutoff for PAH.[13,14]

Here, we present the case of acute PAH in a 14-year-old boy with GSDI who acutely responded to treatment with inhaled nitric oxide and sildenafil. Additionally, the echocardiographic data from a cohort of 28 patients with GSDI followed at Duke University Medical Center were reviewed to investigate the incidence of PAH in these patients.

[1] Divisions of Pediatric Cardiology, Department of Pediatrics, Duke University Medical Center, Durham, NC, USA
[2] Divisions of Medical Genetics, Department of Pediatrics, Duke University Medical Center, Durham, NC, USA
[3] Division of Metabolic Disorders, Children's Hospital of Orange County, Orange, CA, USA
[4] Department of Pediatrics, University of California Irvine School of Medicine, Orange, CA, USA

Corresponding Author:
Stephanie B. Wechsler, MD, Divisions of Pediatric Cardiology and Medical Genetics, Department of Pediatrics, Duke University Medical Center Box 3090, Durham, NC 27710, USA.
Email: stephanie.wechsler@dm.duke.edu

Table 1. Case Report Laboratory Values Over Time.

	2 Months Prior to Acute PAH	Acute PAH Presentation	9 Years After Acute PAH
Glucose (60-115 mg/dL)	65	105	84
Bicarbonate (22-28 mg/dL)	27	22	28
AST (15-41 U/L)	18	39	32
ALT (3-35 U/L)	12	5	37
Lactic acid (0.7-2.2 mmol/L)	2.5	36	1.9
Cholesterol (100-200 mg/dL)	164	ND	178
Triglycerides (40-160 mg/dL)	274	ND	508

Abbreviations: ALT, alanine aminotransferase; AST, aspartate aminotransferase; ND, not done; PAH, pulmonary arterial hypertension.

Case Report

A 14-year-old Pacific Islander male with GSDI diagnosed in infancy had shown normal growth and several years of excellent metabolic control (Table 1) on frequent cornstarch feedings. Baseline echocardiogram and electrocardiogram at 12 years of age were normal. He initially presented to the emergency department for emesis, leading to hypoglycemia, which was successfully treated with intravenous glucose prior to discharge home. However, 2 weeks later, he presented to the emergency department again with a 2-day history of breathing difficulty and palpitations. His evaluation showed sinus tachycardia at 148 beats/min, tachypnea with normal oxygen saturations, no fever, and a normal chest X-ray. Initial blood work was notable for a significantly elevated brain natriuretic peptide level of 877 pg/mL, mildly elevated creatinine of 1.1 mg/dL, and slightly elevated troponin at 0.07 μg/L (normal <0.04 μg/L). All other laboratory values were normal, and there was no significant leukocytosis, hypoglycemia, or evidence of liver dysfunction. He was admitted to the pediatric intensive care unit and quickly developed hypotension, bradycardia, and severe metabolic acidosis, requiring intubation, fluid resuscitation, and pressors. An emergent echocardiogram demonstrated an elevated TR jet velocity of 3.2 m/s, and he was started on inhaled nitric oxide at 20 parts per million and sildenafil 20 mg twice daily for suspected acute PAH. Infection was initially considered as a cause for his acute presentation, and an extensive infectious disease workup was performed for bacterial, fungal, and viral infections in blood, urine, respiratory, and cerebrospinal fluid (CSF) cultures. All infectious disease testing was negative, and antibiotics were discontinued shortly after admission. He remained afebrile without a significant leukocytosis throughout his stay, and infection was felt to be an unlikely etiology of his presentation. Instead, his rapid cardiopulmonary collapse, significantly elevated right heart pressures on echocardiogram, and clinical response to pulmonary vasodilators all suggested an acute onset of PAH. He was followed with serial echocardiograms, with a peak TR jet velocity of 3.4 m/s on hospital day 2. He clinically improved, and the inhaled nitric oxide was weaned off over 4 days. He was extubated on hospital day 8, and his echocardiogram on hospital day 15 showed a peak TR jet velocity of 2.9 m/s. Given his clinical improvement and declining TR jet velocity indicating normalizing pulmonary arterial pressures, a sildenafil wean was started, and sildenafil was discontinued on hospital day 20. He had developed renal failure initially requiring 6 days of dialysis and associated systemic hypertension, both of which normalized. He remained hospitalized for 1 month and required several subsequent months of outpatient rehabilitation for generalized weakness. He recovered fully over time, and echocardiogram obtained 1 year after his episode of acute PAH showed a high normal TR jet velocity of 2.8 m/s with no septal flattening.

Most recent follow-up at 23 years of age shows no recurrent evidence of PAH, with a normal echocardiogram and TR jet velocity of 2.0 m/s. He has no evidence of liver or kidney dysfunction (Table 1). He was recently diagnosed with systemic hypertension, for which he was started on low-dose lisinopril. He otherwise maintains good glucose control with cornstarch feedings five times per day.

Materials and Methods

Patients with GSDI who attend the Metabolic Diseases Clinic at Duke University Medical Center consented for participation in a GSDI natural history study, which was approved by the Duke Institutional Review Board. Of the 57 patients who consented for the GSDI natural history study, 29 had echocardiograms available for review. One patient's echocardiogram was eliminated for poor image quality, leaving a total of 28 patients for review. This cohort included follow-up data of 6 patients from a previous study by Kishnani et al at Duke University Medical Center examining PAH in GSDI.[7] All echocardiograms were reviewed in their entirety by 2 of the authors (R.D.T. and S.B.W.). Two echocardiograms were performed at outside institutions and reviewed by digital recording, and the rest were performed at Duke University Medical Center. Several specific features were documented for each echocardiogram: peak TR jet velocity (if present) in the parasternal and apical views, the presence of right ventricular hypertrophy, dilation, or dysfunction, the presence of septal flattening, increased right ventricular outflow gradient, and any additional structural abnormalities of the heart. These findings were then compared to the documented final report. In the event of significant discrepancies between the final clinical report and findings of research review, an independent assessment by a third reviewer was planned.

Results

Patient demographics are summarized in Table 2. Of the 28 patients in this review, 24 patients were diagnosed with GSDIa and 4 carried a diagnosis of GSDIb. The gender distribution was equal, with 14 males and 14 females. The median patient age at the time of echocardiogram was 24 years, with a range of

Table 2. Patient Demographics.

	GSD Type Ia	GSD Type Ib	Total
Age range (years)	3-51	4-28	3-51
Median age (years)	26	17.5	24
Males	13	1	14
Females	11	3	14
Echos reviewed			
Single echo	10	1	11
>1 echo	14	3	17

Abbreviation: GSD, Glycogen storage disease.

3 to 51 years. A total of 51 echocardiograms were reviewed, with 17 patients having multiple echocardiograms reviewed. The median time interval between echocardiograms was 35.9 months, with a range of 12 months to 12 years. The longest duration of follow-up over time by echocardiography was 18 years.

None of the echocardiograms reviewed showed evidence of PAH. Of the 6 patients in our review described previously by Kishnani et al,[7] 2 had been noted to have estimated systolic pulmonary artery pressures >20 mm Hg (TR jet velocity >2.2 m/s). However, on follow-up, none of the patients showed abnormalities or progression to PAH on echocardiogram. The maximum TR jet velocity in the entire cohort was 2.5 m/s, and none of the echocardiograms showed septal flattening. There was no right ventricular dilation, hypertrophy, or dysfunction. One patient had moderate aortic insufficiency and severe mitral insufficiency, and 2 patients had mild aortic insufficiency. Finally, 1 patient had a slightly elevated right ventricular outflow gradient ranging between 1.9 and 2.1 m/s on serial echocardiograms, but there was no evidence of obstruction or pulmonary hypertension. There were no other significant structural abnormalities among our patient cohort, and there were no major discrepancies between the results of our review and the final documented echocardiogram reports.

Discussion

None of the patients with GSDI in our cohort showed evidence of PAH. Given the low incidence of PAH in general, this result is not surprising. However, we add another case report to the previously described 8 cases of PAH in patients with GSDI, further strengthening the well-described association between these two rare diseases.[3-9] The complex pathogenesis of PAH is largely unknown, but recent progress has been made in identifying some genetic causes for familial PAH, and clinical testing for mutations in *BMPR2*, *ALK1*, *ENG*, *SMAD8*, and *CAV1* genes are now available. PAH is associated with congenital heart disease in the setting of a systemic to pulmonary shunt, connective tissue diseases, human immunodeficiency virus, portal hypertension, toxins and drugs, hemoglobinopathies, and several other conditions.[15,16] Pediatric PAH is associated with several genetic syndromes, including GSDI and III, but the etiology of PAH in GSD remains unclear.[15-17] Given the common association of

Table 3. Reported Cases of Pulmonary Arterial Hypertension in Patients With GSDI.

Author	Age at PAH Diagnosis (years)	Sex	Shunt[a]	Survival	Pathology (Pulmonary Arteries)
Pizzo[3]	16	F	Yes	No	Intimal fibrosis, medial hypertrophy, plexiform lesions
Hamaoka et al[4]	12	F	No	No	Fibrous occlusion, plexiform lesions
Hamaoka et al[4]	16	M	Yes	No	ND
Ohura et al[5]	21	F	No	No	ND
Bolz et al[6]	4	F	No	No[b]	Intimal fibrosis
Kishnani et al[7]	24	F	No	No	ND
Humbert et al[8]	25	M	Yes	Yes	ND
Ueno et al[9]	17	M	No	Yes	NA
Torok et al	14	M	No	Yes	NA

Abbreviations: GSDI, glycogen storage disease type I; NA, not applicable; ND, not done; PAH, pulmonary arterial hypertension.
[a]Portal vein or intestinal vein surgical shunt to inferior vena cava.
[b]Patient had an atrial septal defect and died 4 years after PAH diagnosis.

PAH in both GSDI and GSDIII, it is possible that a common mechanism leads to PAH in both diseases.

Characteristics of the 9 current case reports of PAH in patients with GSDI, including our case, are listed in Table 3. Patients with GSDI were typically diagnosed with PAH in the second to third decade of life, except 1 patient described by Bolz et al, who was diagnosed with PAH at 4 years of age and died 4 years later. This patient had an atrial septal defect, which typically does not lead to PAH until adulthood. However, the combination of an intracardiac shunt and GSDI was felt to accelerate PAH progression.[6] PAH is more common among females, with a 1.6- to 1.7-fold increase in idiopathic PAH and a 2- to 2.7-fold increase in incidence compared to males in familial PAH.[18] For PAH-associated diseases, the gender distribution is thought to be more heavily influenced by the epidemiology of the underlying condition,[19] and in the reported cases of PAH in patients with GSDI, 5 were females, and 4 were males. Three patients underwent surgical shunt placement from the portal or intestinal vein to the inferior vena cava, which was previously performed to promote growth in patients with GSDI. Some have questioned if blood returning directly to the lungs without passing through the hepatic circulation increases the risk of PAH. As previously mentioned, portal hypertension is associated with PAH, but none of the reported patients showed evidence of portal hypertension. Regarding survival, only the 3 most recent patients with GSDI and PAH survived, with the rest succumbing typically months after being diagnosed with PAH.

In the search for the mechanism of PAH in GSDI, increased levels of pulmonary vasoconstrictors such as serotonin, purine, histamine, and catacholamines have been proposed.[4] The most focus has been placed on serotonin, which is a vasoconstrictor produced by the enterochromaffin cells of the intestine and rapidly metabolized by endothelial monoamine oxidase in the liver and lung.[8] Genetic variation in the serotonin transporter and a serotonin receptor have been noted in the platelets and lung tissue of patients with PAH, and transgenic mice overexpressing the serotonin transporter develop PAH.[15] Humbert et al demonstrated elevated plasma serotonin levels in both patients with severe PAH and patients with GSDI, and plasma serotonin was significantly elevated in 1 patient with both PAH and GSDI. However, the level of serotonin alone did not predict the development of PAH, as only 1 of the patients with GSDI with elevated serotonin had PAH.[8] Also, selective serotonin-reuptake inhibitors are widely used clinically and have not been correlated with development of PAH.[11] Perhaps instead of causing PAH, an elevated serotonin level may serve as a marker of diseased tissue or altered signaling in the lungs and/or liver, as these are the sites of serotonin metabolism.

Considering the multiple genetic mutations which may lead to GSDI, we hypothesize that these variations could lead to different alterations in cell signaling, which may or may not lead to PAH. Perhaps some mutations leading to GSDI affect the glucose metabolism in the liver and also affect the pulmonary vasculature, making these patients more likely to develop PAH. Additionally, it is quite possible that the development of PAH is multifactorial, and triggers such as systemic illness, poor metabolic control, or decreased hepatic circulation contribute to the development of PAH in some patients with GSDI. In our patient, baseline echocardiogram was normal without evidence of PAH, but he had an episode of hypoglycemia 2 weeks prior to his acute presentation with pulmonary hypertension, which perhaps served as a trigger for his acute presentation.

While the etiology of PAH in GSDI remains unclear and the prognosis typically grim, in our case report and 2 of the previously reported cases, medical management of PAH led to survival. In the previous reports, 1 patient was treated with exercise limitation, warfarin, and diuretics,[8] and 1 was treated with the prostacyclin analog beraprost sodium, with subsequent transition to sildenafil.[9] In our case report, the patient was managed transiently on inhaled nitric oxide and sildenafil. Inhaled nitric oxide was weaned off within the first week of admission, and sildenafil was weaned off within 3 weeks of his admission, suggesting a transient pulmonary hypertensive crisis. It is quite possible that PAH is acute and transient in these patients due to acute triggers such as poor metabolic control. Many acute therapies were not available for pulmonary hypertension in the past, and it is not surprising that earlier, patients with GSDI and PAH succumbed.[3-7] The use of new agents such as inhaled oxide, prostacyclin analogs, and phosphodiesterase type 5 inhibitors such as sildenafil may enable stabilization and recovery without the need for lifelong therapy.

Given the available treatment options for PAH in patients with GSDI, clinicians must have a high index of suspicion for this diagnosis when patients with GSDI complain of shortness of breath, tachypnea, fatigue, chest pain, syncope, or edema, especially in the second decade of life. Chest X-ray, electrocardiogram, and echocardiogram should be ordered promptly in addition to basic laboratory chemistries to assess for signs of PAH.[16] Early detection and treatment of PAH in these patients could prevent progressive worsening or a sudden, severe pulmonary hypertensive crisis and can lead to improved outcomes.

In conclusion, PAH is a rare but highly fatal disease that has been associated with GSDI. Given the rarity of both GSDI and PAH, the exact incidence of PAH in patients with GSDI is difficult to quantify, and clinical collaboration among institutions will be required to further address this question. Additionally, further work is needed to explore the causes of PAH in patients with GSDI, which is likely multifactorial and could be related to genetic variations within GSDI and overall metabolic control. Finally, clinicians caring for patients with GSDI should have a high degree of suspicion for PAH, should cardiopulmonary symptoms develop, as prompt intervention can lead to survival in this otherwise highly fatal disease.

Authors' Note

All authors were involved in the concept and design and/or the interpretation of data for the manuscript, were involved in drafting or critical revision of the manuscript, and approved the version to be published.

Acknowledgments

We thank the patients and their families for their participation in the GSDI natural history study at Duke University Medical Center. We thank the Division of Metabolic disorders at Children's Hospital of Orange County for contributing the presented case report.

Declaration of Conflicting Interests

The author(s) declared no potential conflicts of interest with respect to the research, authorship, and/or publication of this article.

Funding

The author(s) received no financial support for the research, authorship, and/or publication of this article.

References

1. Rake JP, Visser G, Labrune P, Leonard JV, Ullrich K, Smit GP; European Study on Glycogen Storage Disease Type I (ESGSD I). Guidelines for management of glycogen storage disease type I—European Study on Glycogen Storage Disease Type I (ESGSD I). *Eur J Pediatr*. 2002;161(suppl 1):S112-S119.
2. Wang DQ, Carreras CT, Fiske LM, et al. Characterization and pathogenesis of anemia in glycogen storage disease type Ia and Ib. *Genet Med*. 2012;14(9):795-799.
3. Pizzo CJ. Type I glycogen storage disease with focal nodular hyperplasia of the liver and vasoconstrictive pulmonary hypertension. *Pediatrics*. 1980;65(2):341-343.

4. Hamaoka K, Nakagawa M, Furukawa N, Sawada T. Pulmonary hypertension in type I glycogen storage disease. *Pediatr Cardiol.* 1990;11(1):54-56.
5. Ohura T, Inoue CN, Abukawa D, et al. Progressive pulmonary hypertension: a fatal complication of type I glycogen storage disease. *J Inherit Metab Dis.* 1995;18(3):361-362.
6. Bolz D, Stocker F, Zimmermann A. Pulmonary vascular disease in a child with atrial septal defect of the secundum type and type I glycogen storage disease. *Pediatr Cardiol.* 1996;17(4):265-267.
7. Kishnani P, Bengur AR, Chen YT. Pulmonary hypertension in glycogen storage disease type I. *J Inherit Metab Dis.* 1996;19(2):213-216.
8. Humbert M, Labrune P, Sitbon O, et al. Pulmonary arterial hypertension and type-I glycogen-storage disease: the serotonin hypothesis. *Eur Respir J.* 2002;20(1):59-65.
9. Ueno M, Murakami T, Takeda A, Kubota M. Efficacy of oral sildenafil in a beraprost-treated patient with severe pulmonary hypertension secondary to type I glycogen storage disease. *Circ J.* 2009;73(10):1965-1968.
10. Archer SL, Weir EK, Wilkins MR. Basic science of pulmonary arterial hypertension for clinicians: new concepts and experimental therapies. *Circulation.* 2010;121(18):2045-2066.
11. McLaughlin VV, Archer SL, Badesch DB, et al; American College of Cardiology Foundation Task Force on Expert Consensus Documents; American Heart Association; American College of Chest Physicians; American Thoracic Society, Inc; Pulmonary Hypertension Association. ACCF/AHA 2009 expert consensus document on pulmonary hypertension a report of the American College of Cardiology Foundation Task Force on Expert Consensus Documents and the American Heart Association developed in collaboration with the American College of Chest Physicians; American Thoracic Society, Inc.; and the Pulmonary Hypertension Association. *J Am Coll Cardiol.* 2009;53(17):1573-1619.
12. Lafitte S, Pillois X, Reant P, et al. Estimation of pulmonary pressures and diagnosis of pulmonary hypertension by Doppler echocardiography: a retrospective comparison of routine echocardiography and invasive hemodynamics. *J Am Soc Echocardiogr.* 2013;26(5):457-463.
13. Galie N, Hoeper MM, Humbert M, et al; ESC Committee for Practice Guidelines (CPG). Guidelines for the diagnosis and treatment of pulmonary hypertension: the Task Force for the Diagnosis and Treatment of Pulmonary Hypertension of the European Society of Cardiology (ESC) and the European Respiratory Society (ERS), endorsed by the International Society of Heart and Lung Transplantation (ISHLT). *Eur Heart J.* 2009;30(20): 2493-2537.
14. Rudski LG, Lai WW, Afilalo J, et al. Guidelines for the echocardiographic assessment of the right heart in adults: a report from the American Society of Echocardiography endorsed by the European Association of Echocardiography, a registered branch of the European Society of Cardiology, and the Canadian Society of Echocardiography. *J Am Soc Echocardiogr.* 2010;23(7):685-713; quiz 786-688.
15. Ma L, Chung WK. The genetic basis of pulmonary arterial hypertension. *Hum Genet.* 2014;133(5):471-479.
16. Abman SH, Hansmann G, Archer SL, et al; American Heart Association Council on Cardiopulmonary, Critical Care, Perioperative and Resuscitation; Council on Clinical Cardiology; Council on Cardiovascular Disease in the Young; Council on Cardiovascular Radiology and Intervention; Council on Cardiovascular Surgery and Anesthesia; and the American Thoracic Society. Pediatric Pulmonary Hypertension: Guidelines From the American Heart Association and American Thoracic Society. *Circulation.* 2015;132(21): 2037-2099.
17. Lee TM, Berman-Rosenzweig ES, Slonim AE, Chung WK. Two cases of pulmonary hypertension associated with type III glycogen storage disease. *JIMD Rep.* 2011;1:79-82.
18. Sanchez O, Marie E, Lerolle U, Wermert D, Israel-Biet D, Meyer G. Pulmonary arterial hypertension in women [in French]. *Rev Mal Respir.* 2008;25(4):451-460.
19. Manes A, Palazzini M, Dardi F, D'Adamo A, Rinaldi A, Galie N. Female gender and pulmonary arterial hypertension: a complex relationship [in Italian]. *G Ital Cardiol(Rome).* 2012;13(6): 448-460.

10

Small Molecules: Substrate Inhibitors, Chaperones, Stop-Codon Read Through, and Beyond

Saida Ortolano, PhD[1]

Abstract

Lysosomal storage disorders are rare genetic disorders due to deficient lysosomal activity, which leads to progressive accumulation of nonmetabolized substrates. Patient's clinical outcomes have significantly improved since the advent of enzyme replacement therapy, even though this therapeutic approach presents important limitations, such as immune reactions, low bioavailability of recombinant enzymes, and incapability to reach the central nervous system. New strategies based on gene therapy or small molecules have been proposed and tested as an alternative to enzyme replacement therapy or to complement it. Small molecules are orally administrated, no antigenic compound that can diffuse across cell membranes and distribute in steady-state concentrations, also reaching the central nervous system. Substrate reduction therapy, pharmacological chaperones, and stop-codon read-through enhancers are small molecules currently available for the treatment of lysosomal storage disorders. This article describes the characteristics of this class of compounds and the possible strategies to improve their efficiency in future development.

Keywords

lysosomal storage disorders, substrate reduction therapy, pharmacological chaperones, stop-codon read through, cotreatment with enzyme replacement therapy

Introduction

Lysosomal storage disorders (LSDs) are a group of more than 50 different diseases due to a functional deficiency of a lysosomal protein (ie, acidic hydrolases, activator transporters, or nonlysosomal proteins necessary for lysosomal function), which leads to the accumulation of a variety of substrates, such as glycosaminoglycans (GAGs), glycosphingolipids, glycogen, oligosaccharides, cholesterol, peptides, and glycoproteins.[1] A broad clinical presentation is associated with LSDs, which includes visceral, ocular, hematological, skeletal, and neurological manifestations. These outcomes eventually affect lifespan, as well as physical and intellectual performance of the patients, determining an important challenge in terms of public health, social rights, and economic costs for the society. Even if LSDs are considered singularly as rare diseases (incidence ranging between 1:7000 and 1:1 000 000), collectively these pathologies are as frequent as 1:5000 to 1:7000 live births.[2]

Nowadays, the most frequent LSDs (ie, Gaucher disease [GD], Fabry disease [FD], Pompe disease [PD], mucopolysaccharidosis [MPS], type I, II, IV, VI, and acid lipase deficiency) are treated by enzyme replacement therapy (ERT) or substrate reduction therapy (SRT).[3]

The ERT consists of periodic intravenous administration of the recombinant form of the human wild-type enzyme, which can be internalized by the cells with deficient lysosomal activity, through the mannose 6-phosphate receptor (MP6). The ERT has been used in the clinic for around 15 years with relevant benefits in patients' quality of life, allowing, as an example, the normalization of hematologic parameters and organ volumes in GD or the decrease in neuropathic pain crisis

[1] Group of Neonatal Pathology, Pediatrics and Rare Diseases, Instituto de Investigación Sanitaria Galicia Sur, Vigo, Spain

Corresponding Author:
Saida Ortolano, Hospital Alvaro Cunqueiro, bloque tecnico, pl 2, zona A, Estrada Clara Campoamor 341, 36312 Vigo, Pontevedra, Spain.
Email: saida.ortolano@sergas.es

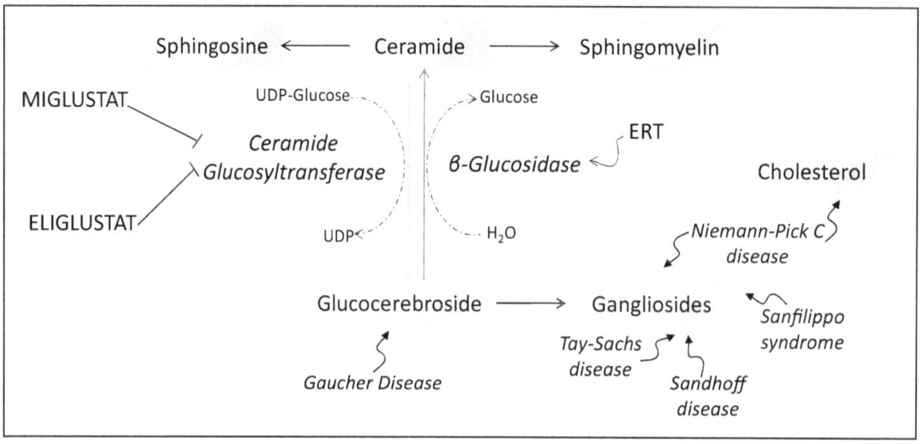

Figure 1. Mechanism of action of SRT drugs for GD and other LSDs. The SRT drugs like miglustat and eliglustat are competitive inhibitors of ceramide glucosyltransferase. By reducing glucocerebroside concentration, these drugs facilitate the degradation of the substrate by the β-glucosidase, the enzyme affected in GD. Glucocerebroside is a precursor of gangliosides accumulated in TSD, MPS III, SD, and Niemann-Pick C diseases. ERT enhances the activity of β-glucosidase. GD indicates Gaucher disease; LSD, lysosomal storage disorder; SRT, substrate reduction therapy; TSD, Tay-Sachs disorder; MPS III, mucopolysaccharidosis type III; SD, Sandhoff disorder; ERT, enzyme replacement therapy.

in patients with FD.[4,5] Nevertheless, ERT still presents important limitations, such as the low bioavailability and half-life of the drugs, the possibility to induce immunologic intolerance, and the incapability to cross the blood–brain barrier (BBB).[6]

Alternative therapeutic approaches, based on both in vivo or ex vivo gene therapy, are being tested to meliorate enzyme biodistribution and thus increase the therapeutic window for treatment administration and the possibilities of delivering into the central nervous system (CNS). The LSDs are particularly prone to be cured through gene therapy for the possibility of cross-correction of the enzyme defect,[7] and positive results have already been reported for metachromatic leukodystrophy.[8] Nevertheless, gene therapy still needs to be optimized for clinical applications, especially in terms of immunogenicity and control of viral genome integration sites.

A second alternative to ERT is represented by the use of orally administrated, no antigenic small molecules that can diffuse across multiple cell membranes and distribute in steady-state concentration through different tissues including the CNS. In this article, we will describe the characteristic of the different class of small molecules in use or in development for the treatment of LSDs.

Substrate Reduction Therapy

Small molecules can be used in LSDs to reduce accumulated substrate concentration by inhibiting the enzyme that synthesizes these substrates or one of their precursors. In this way, accumulation rate is lowered, facilitating the clearance of the storage by the defective, but yet partially functional, enzyme (Figure 1).[9]

The SRT-based drugs are now available for the treatment of GD type I (Table 1), an LSD in which patients usually present with anemia, thrombocytopenia, hepatosplenomegaly, and skeletal deformations. However, in the most severe manifestations of the disease (GD type III), these symptoms are associated with neurological involvement. The GD is characterized by a deficit of β-glucosidase (also called glucocerebrosidase), which removes glucose moieties from glucosylceramide, causing the accumulation of the substrate, predominately in macrophages.[10]

Miglustat (*N*-butyldeoxynojirimycin), a competitive inhibitor of glucosylceramide synthetase, was the first SRT medicament to be approved with a therapeutic indication for patients with GD who cannot be treated by ERT (ie, for immunological reaction or low compliance).[11] Around 800 patients worldwide[9] currently use this drug, which is an oral agent with good gastrointestinal adsorption and wide tissue distribution, including the CNS. It seems that naive patients may respond later and with less efficiency to miglustat compared to ERT in terms of hematological and visceral values normalization[12]; however, patients who achieved therapeutic response through ERT may be switched to miglustat without compromising previous benefits.[13,14]

Miglustat causes nonsevere sides effects such as diarrhea, flatulence, abdominal pain, or weight loss, which are due to intestinal α-disaccharides malabsorption, probably related to the inhibition of α-glucosidase isomers.[15] Nevertheless, this effects can be minimized with continued treatment, dose escalation, and/or by implementing a low sucrose–maltose diet.[16] Tremor was also reported in 30% of the patients during trials and in postapproval treated patients,[17,18] since miglustat is a potent agonist of the human glucose sensor SGLT3, which is expressed at the neuromuscular junction.[19] However, tremor is generally mild and may be reverted with dose adjustment. Paresthesia and burning sensations were also reported, although it is not known whether they are drug dependent. The potential neurotoxicity of miglustat compromises its possible use in patients with GD type III with neurological involvement, who did not show any improvement during the clinical trials that were performed.[20]

Since miglustat can retard biosynthesis of glucosylceramide-based compounds, its efficacy was also tested for the treatment

Table 1. SRT for GD Type I.[a]

Properties	Miglustat	Eliglustat
Structure	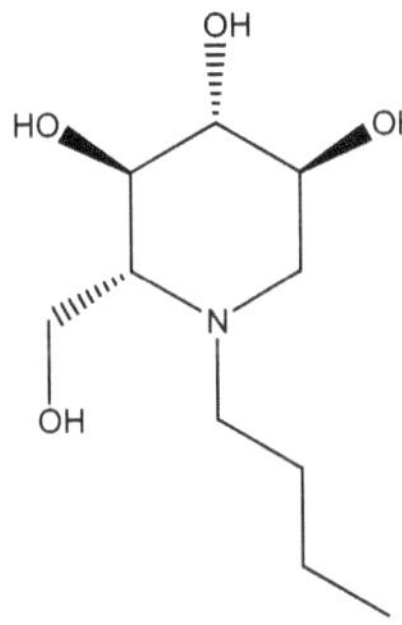	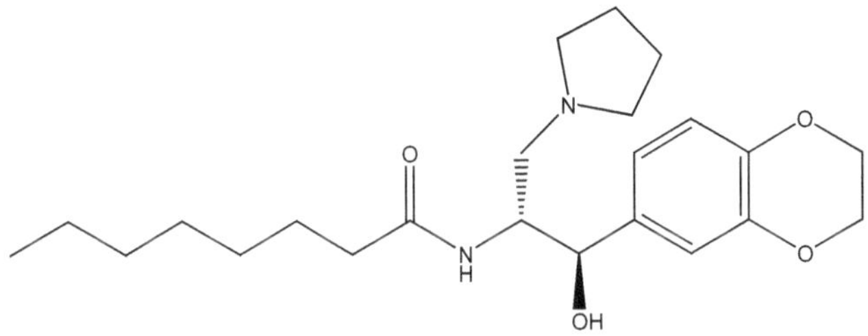
Targeted enzyme	Glucocerebrosidase	Glucocerebrosidase
Diffusion in CNS	Yes	No
Approved for other LSDs	NPC GD type I	GD type I
Comparison with ERT	Slower rate of substrate degradation	No inferior to imiglucerase
Administration form	Oral capsules	Oral capsule
Frequency	Three times per day	Extensive metabolizer: twice per day, poor metabolizer: once daily
Dose	100 mg	84 mg
Metabolization in human	No evidence	Yes (cytochrome P450)
Known interactions with drugs	Not known	Antiarrhythmics and other drugs metabolized by CP450
Agonist for	Glucose sensor SGLT3	P-glycoprotein transporter
Disaccharide absorption	Inhibits α-glucosidase isomers	No significant

Abbreviations: CNS, central nervous system; ERT, enzyme replacement therapy; GD, Gaucher disease; LSDs, lysosomal storage disorders; NPC, Niemann-Pick disease type C; SRT, substrate reduction therapy.
[a]Comparative description of the 2 small molecules used in clinical practice for GD type I treatment, which are based on SRT.

of Niemann-Pick disease type C (NPC), gangliosidosis, and MPS III (Sanfilippo syndrome).

The NPC1 and NPC2 are lipid storage disorders caused by mutations of genes involved in endosomal–lysosomal transport of lipids.[21] Cells, predominantly in the brain, accumulate unesterified cholesterol and other lipids with structural similarity to glycosphingolipids. Progressive accumulation determines that the disease manifestations may appear either at birth or later in life course, until the sixth decade of life. Onset in infants presents a more severe phenotype and may cause sudden failure, whereas late-onset patients develop neuropsychiatric manifestations and other neurological conditions, such as cerebellar ataxia, dystonia, dysarthria, seizure, cognitive problems, and progressive dementia.[22]

Treatment with miglustat managed to correct abnormal lipid trafficking in lymphocytes of patients with NPC-1 and to slow progression of neurological manifestations in animal models (mouse and cat) of the disease.[23,24] When used in clinical trial, miglustat improved saccadic eye movement and swallowing capacity of the patients, with better evidence in patients with later onset.[25,26] These results were confirmed in extended clinical trials, through assessments of cognitive functions and disability, and lead to the approval of miglustat for the treatment of NPC-1.[27]

Preclinical studies also showed positive results for the potential use of miglustat in the treatment of Tay-Sachs disorder (TSD) and Sandhoff disorder (SD). Both SD and TSD are gangliosidoses caused by the deficiency of β-hexosaminidase (β-Hex). β-Hexosaminidase is a dimeric enzyme (α and/or β subunits) that is required for the removal of the terminal *N*-acetylgalactosamine from several glycosphingolipids, as well as from some glycoproteins and oligosaccharides. Genetic mutations in the β-subunit result in compromised activity of both β-HexA and β-HexB leading to the accumulation of glycosphingolipids, GAGs, acetylgalactosamine, and *N*-acetylglucosamine, which are responsible for SD. On the other end, TSD results from mutations in the α-subunit, leading to β-HexA deficiency and the accumulation of ganglioside GM-2 as major storage product.[28] In TSD, GM-2 accumulation is confined to CNS, whereas in SD, there are multisystemic manifestations.

In mouse model of SD, miglustat was able to reverse neuronal pathophysiological and biochemical abnormalities, as well as to delay symptom of onset and to increase life expectancy. Moreover, treatment with the same drug prevented accumulation of GM-2 in the brain of the TSD model.[29,30]

Unfortunately, these results were not confirmed in a trial performed in 5 teenagers with GM-2 gangliosidosis observed over 2 years, failing to prevent neurological deterioration,[31] nor it did with patients with TSD,[32] in spite of previously reported positive data of an isolated study performed with patients with SD.[33]

Treatment with miglustat also failed to show any improvement or stabilization in patients with Sanfilippo syndrome, either in terms of clinical condition or of ganglioside concentration in the brain.[34] Genistain, another SRT-based compound, was also reported to improve cognitive and behavioral functions in MPS III,[35] although a more extended trial did not confirm the initial results.[36]

The second SRT-based treatment for GD type I to be approved was eliglustat, a highly specific oral glucosylceramide synthase inhibitor structurally different from miglustat.[37] In a double-blind 9-month phase III multinational clinical trial (ENGAGE, Phase III, randomized double-blind, placebo controlled, multicentre study confirming the efficacy and safety of Genz-112638 in patients with Gaucher disease Type I, NCT00891202), the drug significantly improved hematological parameters, bone marrow burden score, and also reduced organomegaly in naive patients with GD type I.[38] Moreover, in a second clinical trial, comparing eliglustat to ERT (a study of Eliglustat tartrate (Genz-112638) in patients with Gaucher disease, who have reached therapeutic goals with enzyme replacement therapy, NCT00943111), the end points that were reached proved that this drug is not inferior to imiglucerase after 12 months of treatment.[39] Eliglustat does not inhibit intestinal glucosidases and had no neurotoxic effect, since it is a substrate for P-glycoprotein transporter and is extruded from the CNS.[40] On the other end, other P-glycoprotein substrates such as digoxin, phenytoin, and colchicine can compete with eliglustat, affecting its pharmacokinetics. This active compound is metabolized through the cytochrome P450 complex, therefore, it can potentially interact with other drugs that are degraded through the same pathway. Pharmacokinetics of eliglustat can also be affected by the genetic heterogeneity of the patients with respect to the CYP2D6 enzyme of the cytochrome P450 complex. Prior to initiating eliglustat therapy, patients should be genotyped for CYP2D6 to determine their CYP2D6 metabolizer status and to find the adequate individual dosage. For this reason, the medicament obtained therapeutic indication for patients with GD type I, who are CYP2D6 extensive metabolizers, intermediate metabolizers, or poor metabolizers.[41,42]

The SRT is also used for the treatment of infantile nephropathic cystinosis, a rare genetic disease due to dysfunction of cystinosine transporter expressed in lysosomal membrane. Cysteamine converts accumulated cystine into cysteine and cysteine–cysteamine mixed disulfide, both of which can pass through the lysosomal membrane of patients with cystinosis.[43] Cysteamine bitartrate has been approved by the Food and Drug Administration since 1994, and in 2013, a delayed release formulation, no inferior to the previous one, was also approved.[44,45] In spite of its use in clinical practice, long-term studies indicate that cysteamine treatment even when started early (before 5) is not curative and 30% of the patients require renal transplant before 16 years.[46] The same active compound was also tested for the treatment of neuronal ceroid lipofuscinosis caused by *PPT1*, which is involved in lysosomal degradation of S-fatty acylated proteins.[47]

Pharmacological Chaperones

In several LSDs, substrate accumulation that determines clinical manifestations occurs when residual enzyme activity decays below a certain threshold. It was determined that an activity >10% significantly prevents storage in many LSDs and even values between 3% and 5% could be sufficient to slow down the disease progression.[48,49] In terms of treatment, this means that even a low improvement in enzyme activity could be effective to meliorate clinical evidence. A pharmacological chaperone (PC) is a small molecule that stabilizes the tertiary structure of a mutant enzyme, avoiding its degradation by the quality control mechanisms of the endoplasmic reticulum (ER) and allowing its trafficking to the lysosome through the secretory pathway (Figure 2).[50] Once the complex has reached the target organelle, the PC is released from the enzyme upon acid hydrolysis and the protein can, at least partially, catalyze substrate degradation, still in the presence of the mutation. Even though lysosomal enzymes are active at acid pH, their synthesis normally occurs at neutral pH; therefore, these proteins may be thermodynamically less stable during synthesis process, especially in the presence of a mutation. The PCs stabilize protein conformation, inhibit premature misfolding, and prevent aggregation.

Several PCs were designed and synthesized based on the structure of the natural substrate (iminosugars, azasugars, carbasugars, etc) or alternatively identified by high-throughput screening (HTS) studies. These compounds, potentially active for LSDs therapy, showed encouraging results in preclinical studies for the treatment of FD, GD, PD, or gangliosidosis 1 and 2 (Table 2).

In 2016, the first PC-based therapy (Galafold, Amicus Therapeutics) obtained marketing approval by the European Medicines Agency for the treatment of patients with FD with specific missense mutations. The active compound of this drug is 1-deoxygalactonojirimycin (DGJ), an iminosugar mimicking the structure of D-galactose, which is also denominated migalastat.[57] The FD is an X-linked LSD, caused by the impairment of α-galactosidase A (α-GalA), which leads to the progressive accumulation of glycosphingolipids such as globotriaosylceramide (GL-3) and Lyso-GL3 in vascular endothelium, smooth muscle, kidney, dorsal ganglia, brain, gastrointestinal tract, and so on.[58]

The chaperoning action of DGJ depends on the interaction of its amino group with the carboxylate of the aspartic acid 170 in the active site of the enzyme, as shown by crystallography.[59] Exposure to DGJ (0.2-20 μmol/L) of primary lymphoblast cultures from patients with FD caused a concentration-dependent increase in α-Gal A activity, which was maintained for 5 days.[57] In vivo studies with DGJ on FD transgenic mouse models showed significant increase in α-Gal A activity in heart, kidney, spleen, and liver of the treated animals, as well as decreased levels of GL-3 in the affected tissues.[59] A phase 2 clinical trial performed with migalastat hydrochloride as monotherapy showed increased α-Gal A activity and decreased GL-3 concentration in skin, urine, and kidneys. Reduction in renal peritubular capillary inclusions was also found in heterozygous women.[60] In phase 3 studies, stabilization of renal function, reduction in left ventricular mass, and improvement in gastrointestinal symptoms were demonstrated, as well as a generally good tolerability.[61] Long-term effects of the drugs as well as its possible synergistic effect in the cotreatment with ERT are currently being evaluated.

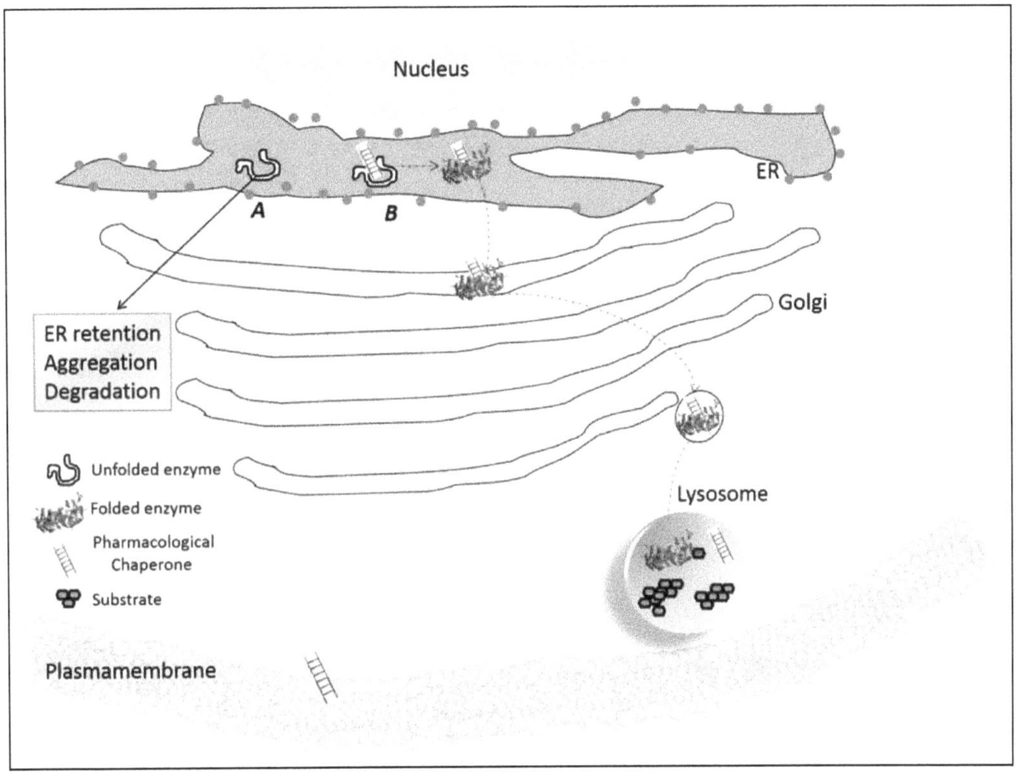

Figure 2. Pharmacological chaperones: mechanism of action. A, Mutated lysosomal enzyme that does not fold correctly is degraded at ER level. B, Pharmacological chaperone diffuses through the plasma membrane into the cell and binds to the mutated enzyme, allowing proper folding of the protein. The complex traffics through the secretory pathway and enters the lysosome, where the PC is released and the enzyme can catalyze substrate degradation. ER indicates endoplasmic reticulum; PC, pharmacological chaperone.

Two potential PCs for GD, isofagamin and ambroxol, were identified through HTS.[62,63] Isofagamin increased β-glucosidase activity in cells derived from p.N370S- and p.L444P-affected patients.[64] These results were confirmed in transgenic mice with different mutations including the p.L444P[65,66] and put the basis for phase 1 and 2 clinical trials, which unfortunately were discontinued, failing to show a clinically meaningful end point in most of the involved patients (NCT00446550 and NTC00875160). Ambroxol was also able to stabilize p.N370S-mutated β-glucosidase in patient's derived cells and animal models.[67,68] In clinical trials, ambroxol showed reduction of 15% to 40% in spleen volume and increased platelet counts after more than 6 months therapy in 1 patient.[53]

The PCs have been proposed to complement ERT also for PD. The PD is an LSD caused due to mutations in *GAA* gene, which encodes acid α-glucosidase. The enzymatic deficit produces accumulation of glycogen predominantly in heart and skeletal muscles.[69] Both 1-deoxynojirimycin (DNJ, duvoglu stat) and miglustat can increase acid α-glucosidase activity in cells expressing different mutant forms of the enzyme and in animal models, since these iminosugars are 10- to 250-fold more selective for α-glucosidase compared to β-glucosidase.[70,71] In particular, DNJ administration to PD mouse model showed daily important reduction of substrate in heart, diaphragm, gastrocnemius, soleus, and brain.[72] In spite of the positive tolerability results of phase 1 studies, duvoglustat showed severe adverse events in 2 patients during phase 2 clinical trial.[55] A follow-up study, showing the pharmacokinetic profile of the drug in the muscle, demonstrated that the dose selected for phase 2 study was excessive (>Half Maximal Inhibitory Concentration $[IC]_{50}$ for inhibition of the enzyme), and therefore, appropriate balance between chaperoning and inhibition was not achieved, causing the adverse events.[56]

On the other end, miglustat was tested as a combination therapy for PD to enhance the effects of ERT in patients with infantile and late onsets in a phase 2 trial. In the whole population (13 patients), acid α-glucosidase activity was significantly increased with the cotreatment.[73]

Since PCs can diffuse to the CNS, they are a potential good treatment for LSDs with important neurological manifestation such as SD and TSD, since ERT drugs do not cross the BBB. Among the tested compounds for SD and TSD, pyrimethamine, an approved antimalarial agent, significantly increased enzymatic activity in all the β-subunit mutants evaluated, however, it determined an insufficient increase in enzymatic activity of the α-subunit mutants.[54] In spite of this limitation, a clinical trial phase 1/2 was initiated in patients with SD or TSD. The 8 treated patients showed significant enzymatic activity increase; however, severe side effects, such as ataxia or blurred vision, among others, appeared during the trial, causing the suspension of the study.[74] Likewise, in the case of duvoglustat trial in

Table 2. Clinical Trials of PCs.[a]

Compound	Structure	Diseases	Clinical Trial	Phase	References
Migalastat	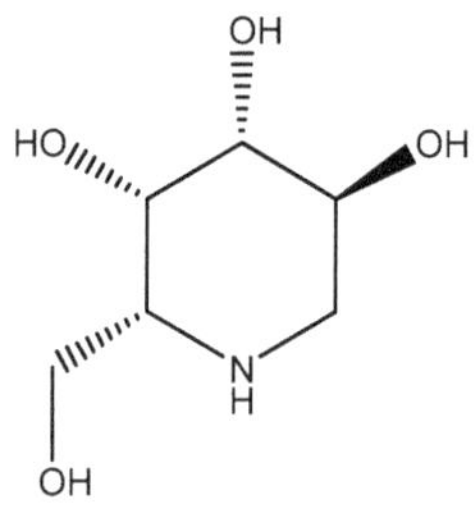	FD FD (long-term study)	NCT01458119 NCT02194985	Approved	51
Migalastat + ERT		FD	NCT01196871	II	52
Isofagomine	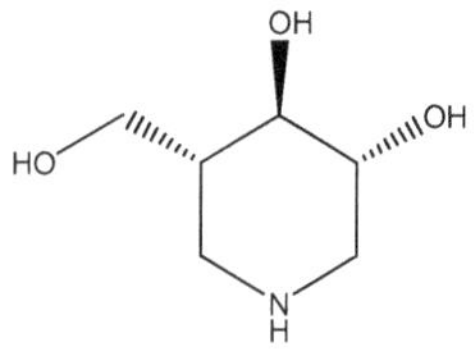	GD	NCT00875160	II	
Ambroxol	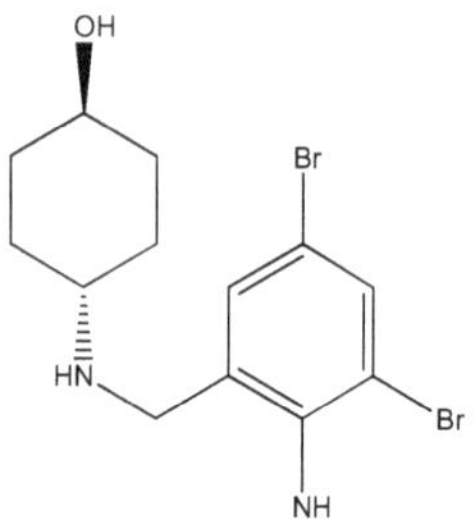	GD	NCT01463215	I/II	53
Pyrimethamine	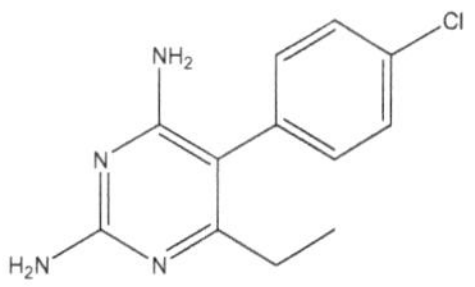	SD and TSD	NCT01102686	I/II	54
Miglustat + ERT	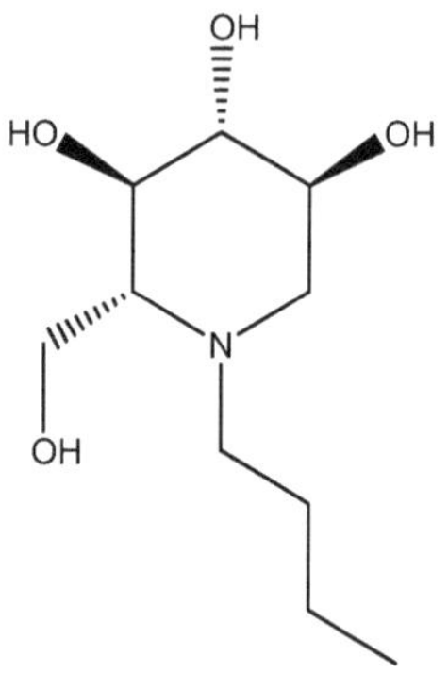	PD	NCT02185651	I	55
Duvoglustat Duvoglustat + ERT	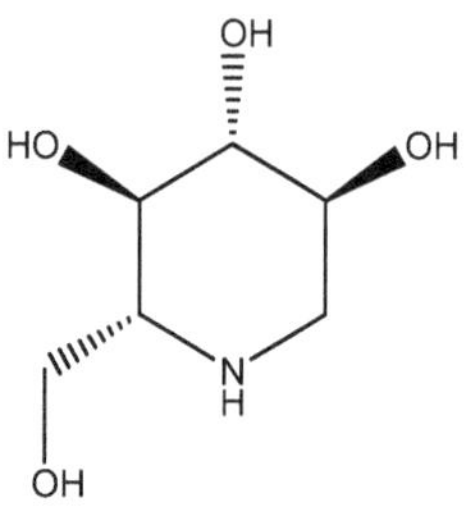	PD PD	NTC00688597 NCT01380743	II II	56

Abbreviations: ERT, enzyme replacement therapy; FD, Fabry disease; GD, Gaucher disease; PCs, pharmacological chaperones; SD, Sandhoff disorder; TSD, Tay-Sachs disorder; PD, Pompe disease.

[a]PC has been or is being tested in clinical trials, either in monotherapy or in combination with ERT. The identification number of the clinical trials corresponds to the database clinicaltrial.gov (https://clinicaltrials.gov).

patients with PD, it is possible that the dose of pyrimethamine selected for the study was too elevated for appropriate balance between chaperoning and inhibitory activity of the molecule. The majority of PCs that have been proposed binds to the active center of the target enzyme, therefore, they may act as inhibitors if the affinity is too high. This represents a major limitation for PC therapies for which the concentration has to be finely tuned to determine a net gain in chaperoning activity. Turnover is favored by high substrate concentration and by binders that present shorter half-life than the enzyme, as well as reduced binding affinity at lysosomal pH.

The increase in activity, however, depends on the disease and on the affected enzyme maturation process and its lysosomal trafficking. Moreover, the efficacy of PC-based drugs is mutation dependent, and a single compound may have different effects on patients with the same LSD, but different mutations. The PCs are more prone to stabilize proteins with missense mutations (either inside or outside the active site), which affect protein folding, thermodynamic stability, or lysosomal trafficking, while they are not suitable for large deletions, insertions, splice variants, or frameshift mutations.

Stop-Codon Read-Through Enhancement

Many patients with LSD present nonsense mutations in one or both alleles of the gene encoding for the lysosomal enzyme, which generate a premature stop codon. As an example, mucopolysaccharidosis type I (Hurler and Scheie syndromes), an LSD caused by the deficit of α-L-iduronidase, is often due to the frequent mutations p.Q70X and p.W402X in the *IDUA* gene.[75] In this disease, as well as in neuronal ceroid lipofuscinosis type I, over 50% of the patients carry a nonsense mutation.[76,77] Premature stop-codon mutations are usually associated with more severe clinical phenotypes, since truncated messenger RNA (mRNA) or protein is generally eliminated with resulting null or minimal net enzyme activity in the cells. Most mRNA transcripts containing stop-codon mutations are preferentially targeted for degradation by a cellular quality control system called nonsense-mediated decay, which limits the synthesis of potentially toxic or unwanted protein fragments that might interfere with normal cellular function.[78] Normally, during the splicing process, an exon–exon junction complex is recruited to mRNA and binds 20 to 24 nucleotides upstream of the exon–exon junction. A premature stop codon, upstream of this junction can elicit nonsense-mediated decay.[79] If a protein escapes this degradation mechanism, a truncated polypeptide is produced and often degraded by the control mechanisms of the ER. However, the read-through process may originate normal or mutated full-length proteins by incorporating an amino acid instead of terminating the synthesis at the premature stop codon. These products can be enough stable to bypass the ER degradation system and perform its function within the cell (Figure 3).

The read-through process can also be induced by drugs, such as gentamicin or other aminoglycosides, which bind to ribosomal RNA and affect the stop-codon transfer RNA recognition process.[80,81] The degree of read-through process will depend on the amounts of available RNA, the kind of stop codon of the nonsense mutation (UAA has high fidelity and little read-through potential, the UAG has intermediate fidelity, and the UGA sequence has the lowest fidelity and higher potential), the surrounding sequence (ie, nucleotide plus 4 is determinant), and correlates with the efficacy of nonsense-mediated decay.

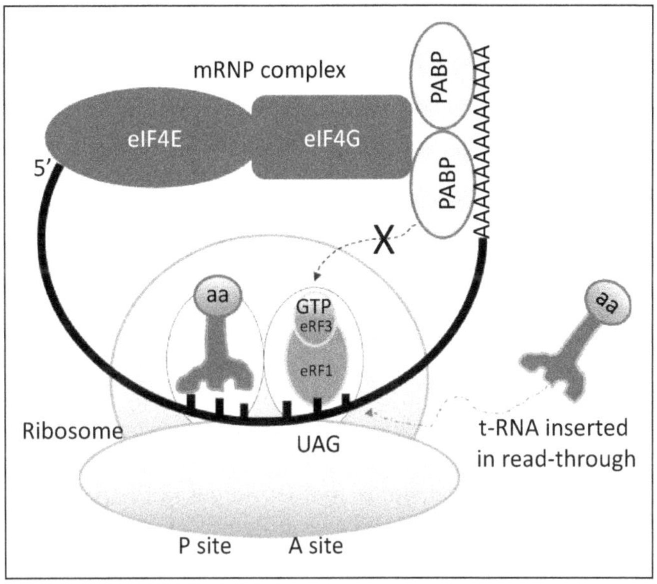

Figure 3. Stop-codon read-through process. The association of 3 proteins at the messenger ribonucleoprotein (mRNP) complex leads to a circular messenger RNA (mRNA) structure. The cap-binding protein eukaryotic initiation factor 4E (eIF4E) binds the 5′ extremity of mRNA; the poly(A)-binding protein (PABP) binds the 3′ end of mRNA; and the eIF4G protein binds both eIF4E and PABP. In mRNAs with wild-type stop codons, PABP is close to the termination complex and can interact with termination factor eukaryotic release factor 3 (eRF3) to stimulate polypeptide chain release. In the presence of a premature stop codon, PABP is at a larger distance and PABP interaction with eRF3 is more difficult, which increases the possibility of activate aminoacyl-transfer RNA to reach the complex and follow the translation (read-through process). Termination factor eRF1 directly recognize any of the 3 stop codons.

The amino acid that is inserted in read-through process is not always the correct one, but the protein that is produced may still be stable. The amino acids that are inserted with the highest probability during read through are the glutamine and the tryptophan, which is an advantage in the case of patients with MPS I carrying p.Q70X or p.W402X mutations.[82] Gentamicin gave promising results when tested in vitro for cystic fibrosis or Duchenne muscular dystrophy and also for MPS I, among the LSDs.[81,83,84]

The principal limitations for the use of gentamicin as read-through inducer are its low cell permeability and its toxic side effects, including kidney damage and hearing loss. For this reason, different analogues of this compound have been proposed. It has been shown that the C1a-subunit of gentamicin (amikacin) preserves efficacy but has reduced side effects.[85] Another stop-codon read-through active compound, which was identified during HTS, is PTC124. This active molecule, which inhibits nonsense-mediated decay and allows read through without affecting normal termination codons, presents high permeability and no toxic side effects.[86]

PTC124 proved to be more efficient than gentamicin in cystic fibrosis and Duchenne muscular dystrophy in preclinical studies. Phase 3 clinical trials were performed in patients with cystic fibrosis and Duchenne muscular dystrophy (NCT00803205 and NCT0182647), leading to the conditional approval of the compound for Duchenne muscular dystrophy.[87,88]

PTC124 was also tested in cells derived from patients with MPS VI (Maroteaux-Lamy). The MPS VI is an LSD without CNS involvement, which is caused by arylsulfatase B (*ARSB*, gene) deficiency. It is characterized by dysostosis multiplex, corneal clouding, heart valve defects, and urinary excretion of GAGs. A subgroup of patients with MPS VI carries nonsense mutations (p.R315X, p.R327X, p.Q456X, and p.Q503X) and therefore is eligible for enhancing of stop-codon read through, using small molecules. PTC124, but not gentamicin, showed to significantly increase the level of arylsulfatase B activity, resulting in a significant reduction in lysosomal size.[89]

In a second study, gentamicin, geneticin, PTC124, and 4 no aminoglycosidic compounds (RTC13, RTC14, BZ6, and Bz16) were tested in fibroblast derived from patients with MPS VI and MPS III B or C (Sanfilippo) with premature stop-codon mutations. Cells from 1 patient with Maroteaux-Lamy carrying the p.W322X mutation responded to treatment with gentamicin (2- to 3-fold increase in enzyme activity); however, the effects of the other compounds were not tested.

In Sanfilippo B and C patients' cells, an increase in mRNA levels of *NAGLU* and *HGSNAT* was found after treatment with, respectively, geneticin and RTC14 or PTC124, although no enzyme activity was recovered.[90]

Conclusions and Future Perspectives

The use of small molecules, comprising SRT, PCs, and read-through enhancer, could represent a great advantage in the treatment of LSDs compared to ERT, since they can be administrated orally, achieve homogenous steady-state concentrations, and possibly lower production costs. Nevertheless, important challenges have still to be faced to advance in the development of these drugs.

Small molecules can potentially diffuse in the CNS; however, up to date, the only commercialized treatment for LSDs with neurological involvement is miglustat, which has a therapeutic indication for NPC, and there is still no available treatment for a considerable number of LSDs. Indeed, the clinical trials performed in GD type III with miglustat or in gangliosidoses with pyrimethamine did not give the expected results due to toxic side effects, which were probably related to unoptimized doses.

Reviewing patents databases[6] (https://worldwide.espacenet.com/), many registered molecules claim PC activity for LSDs, nevertheless, at the moment the only PC to be commercialized is migalastat. The delay in the translation to the clinic could be related to the difficulty to select an appropriate dose of administration for PC-based treatment, which should allow maximal substrate turnover without inhibitory effect. An option to reach this goal is to administer the PC in alternative intervals, since the turnover of the small molecule is generally faster than that of the defective enzyme. In hR301Q α-GalA transgenic mice, oral administration of migalastat in cycle of 4 days during a week resulted in greater substrate clearance, compared to daily administration.[90]

Alternatively, next-generation PC should be directed to the domains of the lysosomal enzyme, which do not include the active site but have a crucial role in the stabilization of the protein (allosteric sites). This will preserve PC scaffolding function without affecting its catalytic action. Potential PCs binding to allosteric sites have already been identified for acid α-glucosidase[52,91] and glucocerebrosidase.[92,93]

Finally, a therapeutic option that is being explored for the treatment of LSDs is the coadministration of ERT with small molecules. Among the limitations of ERT, low half-life and uneven distribution of the recombinant enzyme are crucial in lowering the efficacy of the treatment. As an example, ERT for PD has to be administered at higher frequency and dose compared to other enzyme, due to the low expression of MP6 receptors in the muscle and the higher adaptive immune system activation in these patients. Nevertheless, it has been shown that wild-type lysosomal enzymes like the ones affected in FD, PD, and GD respond to PCs, increasing the rate of substrate degradation. Interestingly, only some of the wild-type enzymes related to LSDs respond to chaperons, depending on the folding efficiency of the enzyme, which may also be different across cell types and species. As mentioned previously, cotreatment was tested in patients with PD, achieving significant increase in blood α-glucosidase activity by administering miglustat or eliglustat prior to ERT.[55,56] Similar results were obtained in patients with FD treated with migalastat before ERT infusion, increasing α-Gal A activity in the blood and the skin of all the patients.[94,95]

For their action mechanism, SRT and read-through enhancer can also potentially contribute to higher storage metabolization, when used in combination with ERT. Therefore, cotreatment could be the key to achieve clinical improvement in patients with LSDs.

Due to the heterogeneity of LSDs and the variability of the expressed phenotypes, the ideal treatment for all affected patients has not been developed up to date. Nevertheless, thanks to the recent advances exposed in this review, crucial problems and possible solutions have been identified and will allow to design new tools and specific management protocols based on the association of different therapeutic agents to face individual diversity.

Declaration of Conflicting Interests

The author(s) declared the following potential conflicts of interest with respect to the research, authorship, and/or publication of this article: Saida Ortolano has collaborated in projects sponsored by the pharmaceutical company Shire Iberica Human Genetic Therapies.

She also has been invited to attend or give a conference by Shire Iberica Human Genetic Therapies.

Funding

The author(s) received no financial support for the research, authorship, and/or publication of this article.

References

1. Kingma SD, Bodamer OA, Wijburg FA. Epidemiology and diagnosis of lysosomal storage disorders; challenges of screening. *Best Pract Res Clin Endocrinol Metab*. 2015;29(2):145-157.
2. Fuller M, Meikle PJ, Hopwood JJ. Epidemiology of lysosomal storage diseases: an overview. In: Metha A, Beck M, Sunder-Plassmann G, eds. *Fabry Diseases: Perspectives From 5 Years of FOS*. Oxford, UK: Oxford Pharmagenesis; 2006.
3. Beck M. New therapeutic options for lysosomal storage disorders: enzyme replacement, small molecule and gene therapy. *Hum Genet*. 2007;121(1):1-22.
4. Charrow J, Scott CR. Long-term treatment outcomes in Gaucher disease. *Am J Hematol*. 2015;90(suppl 1):S19-S24.
5. Arends M, Hollak CE, Biegstraaten M. Quality of life in patients with Fabry disease: a systematic review of the literature. *Orphanet J Rare Dis*. 2015;10:77.
6. Ortolano S, Vieitez I, Navarro C, Spuch C. Treatment of lysosomal storage disease: recent patents and future strategies. *Rec Pat Endocr Metab Immune Drug Discov*. 2014;8(1):9-25.
7. Rastal DP, Amalfitano A. Recent advances in gene therapy for lysosomal storage disorders. *Appl Clin Genet*. 2015;8:157-169.
8. Biffi A, Montini E, Lorioli L, et al. Lentiviral hematopoietic stem cell gene therapy benefits metachromatic leukodystrophy. *Science*. 2013;341(6148):1233158.
9. Weinreb NJ. Oral small molecule therapy for lysosomal storage diseases. *Pediatr Endocr Rev*. 2013;11(supp 1):77-90.
10. Linari S, Castaman G. Clinical manifestation and management of Gaucher disease. *Clin Cases Miner Bone Metab*. 2015;12(2): 157-164.
11. McCormack PL, Goa KL. Miglustat. *Drugs*. 2003;63(22): 2427-2434.
12. Pastores GM, Giraldo P, Cherin P, Mehta A. Goal-oriented therapy with miglustat in Gaucher disease. *Curr Med Res Opin*. 2009; 25(1):23-37.
13. Elstein D, Dweck A, Attias D, et al. Oral maintenance clinical trial with miglustat for type I Gaucher disease: switch from or combination with intravenous enzyme replacement. *Blood*. 2007; 110(7):2296-2301.
14. Giraldo P, Alfonso P, Atutxa K, et al. Real world clinical experience with long-term miglustat maintenance therapy in type I Gaucher disease: the ZAGAL project. *Haematologica*. 2009; 94(12):1771-1775.
15. Amiri M, Naim HY. Miglustat-induced intestinal carbohydrate malabsorption is due to the inhibition of α-glucosidases, but not β-galactosidase. *J Inherit Metab Dis*. 2012;35(6):949-954.
16. Champion H, Ramaswami U, Imrie J, et al. Dietary modifications in patients receiving miglustat. *J Inher Metab Dis*. 2010;33(suppl 3):S379-S383.
17. Pastores GM, Barnett NL, Kolodny EH. An open-label noncomparative study of miglustat in Type I Gaucher disease: efficacy and tolerability over 24 months of treatment. *Clin Ther*. 2005; 27(8):1215-1227.
18. Hollak CE, Hughes D, van Schaik IN, Schwierin B, Bembi B. Miglustat (Zavesca) in type I Gaucher disease: 5-year results of a post-authorization safety surveillance program. *Pharmacoepidemiol Drug Saf*. 2009;18(9):770-777.
19. Voss AA, Diez-Sampedro A, Hirayama BA, Loo DD, Wright EM. Iminosugars are potent agonists of the human glucose sensor SGLT3. *Mol Pharmacol*. 2007;71(2):628-634.
20. Schiffmann R, Fitzgibbon EJ, Harris C, et al. Randomized controlled trial of miglustat in Gaucher's type 3. *Ann Neurol*. 2008; 64(5):514-522.
21. Vanier MT. Complex lipid trafficking in Niemann-Pick disease type C. *J Inherit Metab Dis*. 2015;38(1):187-199.
22. Santos-Lozano A, Vilamandos-Garcia D, Sanchis-Gomar F, et al. Niemann-Pick disease treatment: a systematic review of clinical trials. *Ann Trasl Med*. 2015;3(22):360.
23. Lachmann RH, te Vruchte D, Lloyd-Evans E, et al. Treatment with miglustat reverses the lipid-trafficking defect in Niemann-Pick disease type C. *Neurobiol Dis*. 2004;16(3):654-658.
24. Stein VM, Crooks A, Ding W, et al. Miglustat improves Purkinje cell survival and alters microglial phenotype in feline Niemann-Pick disease type C. *J Neuropathol Exp Neurol*. 2012;71(5): 434-448.
25. Patterson MC, Vecchio D, Jacklin E, et al. Long-term miglustat therapy in children with Niemann-Pick disease type C. *J Child Neurol*. 2010;25(3):300-305.
26. Wraith JE, Vecchio D, Jacklin E, et al. Miglustat in adult and juvenile patients with Niemann-Pick disease type C: long-term data from a clinical trail. *Mol Genet Metab*. 2010;99(4): 351-357.
27. Chien YH, Peng SF, Yang CC, et al. Long-term efficacy of miglustat in pediatric patients with Niemann-Pick disease type C. *J Inherit Metab Dis*. 2013;36(1):129-137.
28. Mahuran DJ. The biochemistry of HEXA and HEXB gene mutations causing GM2 gangliosidosis. *Biochim Biophys Acta*. 1991; 1096(2):87-94.
29. Pelled D, Lloyd-Evans E, Riebeling C, Jeyakumar M, Platt FM, Futerman AH. Inhibition of calcium uptake via the sarco/endoplasmic reticulum Ca^{2+}-ATPase in a mouse model of Sandhoff disease and prevention by treatment with N-butyldeoxnojirimycin. *J Biol Chem*. 2003;278(32):29496-29501.
30. Platt FM, Neises GR, Reinkensmeir G, et al. Prevention of lysosomal storage in Tay-Sachs mice treated with N-butyldeoxynojirimycin. *Science*. 1997;276(5311):428-431.
31. Maegawa GH, Banwell BL, Blaser S, et al. Substrate reduction therapy in juvenile GM2 gangliosidosis. *Mol Genet Metab*. 2009; 98(1-2):215-224.
32. Shapiro BE, Pastores GM, Gianutsos J, Luzy C, Kolodny EH. Miglustat in late onset Tay-Sachs disease: a 12-month, randomized, controlled clinical study with 24 months of extended treatment. *Genet Med*. 2009;11(6):425-433.
33. Wortmann SB, Lefeber DJ, Dekomien G, Willemsen MA, Wevers RA, Morava E. Substrate deprivation therapy in juvenile

Sandhoff disease. *J Inherit Metab Dis*. 2009;32(suppl 1): S307-S311.
34. Guffon N, Bin-Dorel S, Decullier EP, Paillet C, Guitton J, Fouilhoux A. Evaluation of miglustat treatment in patients with type III mucopolysaccharidoses: a randomized double-blind placebo-controlled study. *J Pediatr*. 2011;159(5): 838-844.
35. Piotrowska E, Jakobkiewicz-Banecka J, Maryniak A, et al. Two-year follow-up of Sanfilippo disease patients treated with a genistein-rich isoflavone extract: assessment of effects on cognitive functions and general status of patients. *Med Sci Monit*. 2011; 17(4):CR196-CR202.
36. de Ruijter J, Valstar MJ, Narajczyc M, et al. Genistain in Sanfilippo disease: a randomized controlled crossover trial. *Ann Neurol*. 2012;71(1):110-120.
37. Scott LJ. Eliglustat: a review in Gaucher disease Type I. *Drugs*. 2015;75(14):1669-1678.
38. Mistry P, Amato DJ, Dasouki M, et al. ENGAGE—a phase III randomized, double-blind, placebo controlled, multi-center study to investigate the efficacy and safety of eliglustat in adults with Gaucher disease type I: results after 11 months. *Mol Genet Metab*. 2015;114(2):S81-S82.
39. Cox TM, Drelichman GI, Cravo R, et al. ENCORE a randomized controlled, open-label no inferiority study comparing eliglustat to imiglucerase in Gaucher disease type I patients stabilized on enzyme replacement therapy: 24 months results. *Mol Genet Metab*. 2015;114(2):S33-S34.
40. Shayman JA. Eliglustat tartrate: glucosyl ceramide synthase inhibitor treatment of type 1 Gaucher disease. *Drugs Future*. 2010; 35(8):613-620.
41. European Medicine Agency. Cerdelga: summary of product characteristics. 2015. http://www.ema.europa.eu. Accessed August 22, 2016.
42. Genzyme Ireland Ltd. Cerdelga (eliglustat) capsules for oral use: US prescribing information. 2014. http://www.cerdelga.com/ Accessed August 22, 2016.
43. Tsilou ET, Rubin BI, Reed G, et al. Nephropathic cystinosis: posterior segment manifestations and effects of cysteamine therapy. *Ophtalmology*. 2006;113(6):1002-1009.
44. Cerqui S. Cysteamine therapy: a treatment for cystinosis, not a cure. *Kidney Int*. 2012;81(2):127-129.
45. Langman C, Greenbaum LA, Sarwal M, et al. A randomized controlled crossover trial with delayed release cysteamine bitartrate in nephropathic cystinosis: effectiveness on white blood cell cystine levels and comparison of safety. *Clin J Am Soc Nephrol*. 2012;7(7):1112-1120.
46. Brodin-Sartorius A, Tete MJ, Niaudet P, et al. Cysteamine therapy delays the progression of nephropatic cystinosis in late adolescent and adults. *Kidney Int*. 2012;81(2):179-189.
47. Gavin M, Wen GY, Messing J, et al. Substrate reduction therapy in four patients with milder CLN1 mutations and juvenile-onset Batten disease using cysteamine bitartrate. *JIMD Rep*. 2013;11:87-92.
48. Hopwood JJ, Muller V. Biochemical discrimination of Hurler and Schie syndromes. *Clin Sci*. 1979;57(3):265-272.
49. Leinekugel P, Michel S, Conzelmann E, Sandhoff K. Quantitative correlation between the residual activity of beta-hexosaminidase A and arylsulphatase A and the severity of the resulting lysosomal storage disease. *Hum Genet*. 1992;88(5):513-523.
50. Parenti G, Andria G, Valenzano KJ. Pharmacological chaperone therapy: preclinical development, clinical translation and prospects for the treatment of lysosomal storage disorders. *Mol Ther*. 2015;23(7):1138-1148.
51. Khanna R, Soska R, Lun Y, et al. The pharmacological chaperone 1-deoxygalactonojirimycin reduces tissue globotriaosylceramide levels in a mouse model of Fabry disease. *Mol Ther*. 2010;18(1): 23-33.
52. Porto C, Ferrara MC, Meli M, et al. Pharmacological enhancement of α-glucosidase by allosteric chaperone *N*-acetylcysteine. *Mol Ther*. 2012;20(12):2201-2211.
53. Zimran A, Altarescu G, Elstein D. Pilot study using ambroxol as a pharmacological chaperone in type I Gaucher disease blood cell. *Mol Dis*. 2013;50(2):134-137.
54. Tropak MB, Blanchard JE, Withers SG, Brown ED, Mahuran D. High-throughput screening for human lysosomal beta-*N*-acetyl hexosaminidase inhibitors acting as pharmacological chaperones. *Chem Biol*. 2007;14(2):153-164.
55. Web site: https://clinicaltrials.gov/Reference:NCT01380743, Accessed August 22, 2016.
56. Kishnani P, Tarnopolski M, Sivakumar K, et al. A phase 2a study to investigate drug–drug interactions between escalating doses of AT2220 (duvoglustat hydrochloride) and acid alpha-glucosidase in subjects with Pompe disease. *Mol Genet Metab*. 2013;108(2):S54.
57. Fan JQ, Ishii S, Asano N, Suzuki Y. Accelerated transport and maturation of lysosomal alpha-galactosidase A in Fabry lymphoblasts by an enzyme inhibitor. *Nat Med*. 1999;5(1): 112-115.
58. El-Abassi R, Singhal D, England JD. Fabry's disease. *J Neurol Sci*. 2014;344(1-2):5-19.
59. Guce AI, Clark NE, Rogich JJ, Garman SC. The molecular basis of pharmacological chaperoning in human alpha-galactosidase. *Chem Biol*. 2011;18(12):1521-1526.
60. Giugliani R, Waldek S, Germain DP, et al. A phase 2 study of migalastat hydrochloride in female with Fabry disease: selection of population, safety and pharmacodynamic effects. *Mol Gen Metab*. 2013;109(1):86-92.
61. Nicholls K, Germain DP, Feliciani C, et al. Phase III study of migalastat HCl for Fabry disease: stage 1 results [abstract 168]. *Mol Genet Metab*. 2013;108:S70.
62. Chang HH, Asano N, Ishii S, Ichikawa Y, Fan JQ. Hydrophilic iminosugar active site-specific chaperones increase residual glucocerebrosidase activity in fibroblasts from Gaucher patients. *FEBS J*. 2006;273(17):4082-4092.
63. Maegawa GH, Tropak MB, Buttner JD, et al. Identification and characterization of ambroxol as an enzyme enhancement agent for Gaucher disease. *J Biol Chem*. 2009;284(35): 23502-23516.
64. Sun Y, Liou B, Xu YH, et al. Ex vivo and in vivo effects of isofagomine on acid β-glucosidase variants and substrate levels in Gaucher disease. *J Biol Chem*. 2012;287(6):4275-4287.
65. Khanna R, Benjiamin ER, pellegrino L, et al. The pharmacological chaperone isofagomine increases the activity of the Gaucher

disease L444P mutant form of beta-glucosidase. *FEBS J*. 2010; 277(7):1618-1638.
66. Sanders A, Hemmelgarn H, Melrose HL, Hein L, Fuller M, Clarke LA. Transgenic mice expressing human glucocerebrosidase variants, utility for the study of Gaucher disease. *Blood Cell Mol Dis*. 2013;51(2):109-115.
67. Bendikov-Bar I, Maor G, Filocamo M, Horowitz M. Ambroxol as a pharmacological chaperone for mutant glucocerebrosidase. *Blood Cell Mol Dis*. 2013;50(2):141-155.
68. Luan Z, Li L, Higaki K, Nanba E, Suzuki Y, Ohno K. The chaperone activity and toxicity of ambroxol on Gaucher cells and normal mice. *Brain Dev*. 2013;35(4):317-322.
69. van der Ploeg AT, Rauser AJ. Pompe's disease. *Lancet*. 2008; 372(9646):1342-1353.
70. Parenti G, Zuppaldi A, Pittis GM, et al. Pharmacological enhancement of mutated alpha-glucosidase activity in fibroblasts from patients with Fabry disease. *Mol Ther*. 2007;15(3):508-514.
71. Tajima Y, Saito S, Ohno K, Tsukimura T, Tsujino S, Sakuraba H. Biochemical and structural study on a S529V mutant acid alpha-glucosidase responsive to pharmacological chaperones. *J Hum Genet*. 2011;56(6):440-446.
72. Khanna R, Flanagan JJ, Feng J, et al. The pharmacological chaperone AT2220 increases recombinant human alpha-glucosidase uptake and glycogen reduction in a mouse model of Pompe disease. *PLoS One*. 2012;7(7):e40776.
73. Parenti G, Fecarotta S, La Marca G, et al. A chaperone enhance blood alpha-glucosidase activity in Pompe disease patients treated with enzyme replacement therapy. *Mol Ther*. 2014;22(11):2004-2012.
74. Clarke JT, Mahuran DJ, Sathe S, et al. An open-label Phase I/II clinical trial of pyrimethamine for the treatment of patients affected with chronic GM2 gangliosidosis (Tay-Sachs or Sandhoff variants). *Mol Genet Metab*. 2011;102(1):6-12.
75. Wraith JE, Jones S. Mucopolysaccharidosis type I. *Pediatr Endocrinol Rev*. 2014;12(suppl 1):102-106.
76. Hein LK, Bawden M, Muller VJ, Sillence D, Hopwood JJ, Brooks DA. alpha-L-iduronidase premature stop codons and potential read-through in mucopolysaccharidosis type I patients. *J Mol Biol*. 2004;338(3):453-462.
77. Brooks DA, Muller VJ, Hopwood JJ. Stop-codon read-through for patients affected by a lysosomal storage disorder. *Trends Mol Med*. 2006;12(8):367-373.
78. Maquat LE. Nonsense mediated mRNA decay, in mammals. *J Cell Sci*. 2005;118(pt 9):1773-1776.
79. Dreyfuss G, Kim VN, Kataoka N. Messenger-RNA-binding protein and the message they carry. *Nat Rev Mol Cell Biol*. 2002;3(3): 195-205.
80. Francois B, Russell RJ, Murray JB, et al. Crystal structures of complexes between aminoglycosides and decoding A site oligonucleotides: role of the number of rings and positive charges in the specific binding leading to miscoding. *Nucleic Acids Res*. 2005;33(17):5677-5690.
81. Howard MT, Shirts Bh, Petros LM, Flanigan KM, Gesteland RF, Atkins JF. Sequence specificity of aminoglycoside-induced stop codon read-through: potential implications for treatment of Duchenne muscular dystrophy. *Ann Neurol*. 2000;48(2):164-169.
82. Harrell L, Melker U, Atkins JF. Predominance of six different hexanucleotide recording signals 3' of read-through stop codons. *Nucleic Acid Res*. 2002;30(9):2011-2017.
83. Wilschanski M, Yahav Y, Yaacov Y, et al. Gentamicin-induced correction of *CFTR* functions in patients with cystic fibrosis and *CFTR* stop mutations. *N Engl J Med*. 2003;349(15):1433-1441.
84. Keeling KM, Brooks DA, Hopwood JJ, Li P, Thompson JN, Bedwell DM. Gentamicin mediated suppression of Hurler syndrome stop mutations restores a low level of α-L-iduronidase activity and reduces lysosomal glycosaminoglycan accumulation. *Hum Mol Genet*. 2001;10(3):291-299.
85. Du M, Keeling KM, Fan L, et al. Clinical doses of amikacin provide more effective suppression of the human CFTR-G542X stop mutation than gentamicin in a transgenic CF mouse model. *J Mol Med*. 2006;84(7):573-582.
86. Welch EM, Barton ER, Zhuo J, et al. PTC124 targets genetic disorders caused by nonsense mutations. *Nature*. 2007; 447(7140):87-91.
87. Konstan M, Accurso F, De Boeck K, et al. Targeting class 1 mutations: update on ataluren as a promising treatment for nonsense mutation cystic fibrosis. *Pediatr Pulmonol*. 2012;47(S35): 108-109.
88. Bushby K, Finkel R, Wong B, et al; PTC124-GD-007-DMD STUDY GROUP. Ataluren treatment of patients with nonsense mutation dystrophinopathy. *Muscle Nerve*. 2014;50(4):477-487.
89. Bartolomeo R, Polishchuk EV, Volpi N, Polishchuk RS, Auricchio A. Pharmacological read-through of nonsense *ARSB* mutations as a potential therapeutic approach for mucopolysaccharidosis VI. *J Inherit Metab Dis*. 2013;36(2):363-371.
90. Gomez-Grau M, Garrido E, Cozar M, et al. Evaluation of aminoglycoside and non-aminoglycoside compound for stop-codon read-through therapy in four lysosomal storage diseases. *PLoS One*. 2015;10(8):e0135873.
91. Marugan JJ, Zheng W, Ferrer M, et al. Discovery, SAR and biological evaluation of a non-inhibitory chaperone for acid alpha-glucosidase. Probe reports from the NIH Molecular libraries program. MD, USA: National Center for Biotechnology Information Bethesda. http://www.ncbi.nlm.nih.gov/books/NBK153221.
92. Zheng W, Padia J, Urban DJ, et al. Three classes of glucocerebrosidase inhibitors identified by quantitative high-throughput screening are chaperone leads for GD. *Proc Nat Acad Sci U S A*. 2007;104(32):13192-13197.
93. Landon MR, Lieberman RL, Hoang QQW, et al. Detection of ligand binding hot spots on protein surfaces via fragment-based methods: application to DJ-1 and glucocerebrosidase. *J Comput Aided Mol Des*. 2009;23(8):491-500.
94. Warnock D, Bichet D, Holida M, et al. A phase 2A study to investigate the effect of a single dose of migalastat HCl, a pharmacological chaperone, on agalsidase activity in subjects with Fabry disease [abstract 248]. *Mol Genet Metab*. 2013;108:S96.
95. Hugues D, Adera M, Castelli J, et al. Preliminary long-term safety, tolerability and assessments of renal function of adult Fabry patients receiving treatment with AT1001 (migalastat, hydrochloride), a pharmacological chaperone, for up to 3 years [abstract 473-O]. *J Inher Metab Dis*. 2010;33(suppl 1):S148.

11

Cardiac Manifestation of Fabry Disease: From Hypertrophic Cardiomyopathy to Early Diagnosis and Treatment in Patients Without Left Ventricular Hypertrophy

Adrián Fernández, MD[1] and Juan Politei, MD[2]

Abstract

Although Fabry disease was identified a century ago, it is still a challenging condition to diagnose and treat. Registries data suggest that at least 10% of patients may first present with a cardiac event and that cardiac disease is 1 of the 3 major causes of morbidity and mortality in affected males and females. Cardiac involvement in Fabry disease may be expressed as left ventricular hypertrophy (LVH), coronary disease, atrioventricular conduction disturbances, arrhythmias, and valvular involvement. The exact mechanism by which hypertrophy and fibrosis in the heart occur is not fully understood. Lysosomal globotriaosylceramide accumulation in the myocardium is responsible for only 3% of the mass in the hypertrophic heart, indicating that the LVH is not a direct result of substrate infiltration. One of the most important contributions that cardiologists can make is to consider the diagnosis of Fabry disease in patients with cardiac manifestations preceding the development of LVH and conduct family screening to identify patients with early cardiac involvement which will benefit more from enzyme replacement therapy (ERT). Fabry patients without cardiac manifestations of the disease should be evaluated annually by a cardiologist specialized in Fabry disease, regardless of the indication for ERT.

Keywords

Fabry disease, hypertrophic cardiomyopathy, enzyme replacement therapy, lysosomal GL-3 accumulation, cardiac involvement

Introduction

Hypertrophic cardiomyopathy (HCM) is defined by the presence of a thickening of the left ventricular wall not accounted for by abnormal loading conditions only.[1-3] It is the most common genetic disease (1 of 500 births) caused by mutations in different genes encoding proteins of the cardiac sarcomere, and a low percentage is a result of other genetic disorders including metabolic diseases, genetic syndromes, and hereditary neuromuscular diseases, and in approximately 25% to 30% of patients no mutation can be identified despite a complete genetic study.[3,4] Therefore, there are diseases in which genetic and metabolic causes interact and have similar phenotypic manifestations (phenocopies) as in the case of Fabry disease (FD).[1-6] Although FD was originally considered as an X-linked recessive disorder, we now know that heterozygous females may be severely affected, is a relatively common cause of HCM, and is associated with significant morbidity and premature death due to heart failure or sudden cardiac death (SCD).[7-10] Although the prevalence of FD in patients with HCM is estimated between 0% and 6%, recent studies including more patients showed a prevalence of 0.5% to 1%.[11-17] However, given that the development of left ventricular hypertrophy (LVH) in FD is progressive, we must find cardiac manifestation of FD even in patients who do not still have LVH.

Pathophysiology

Fabry disease is caused by reduced or absent activity of the hydrolase α-galactosidase A (αGAL) enzyme due to mutations in the gene encoding the αGAL protein (GAL).[7-10] Patients with FD are not able to catabolize the membrane neutral

[1] Favaloro Foundation University Hospital, Buenos Aires, Argentina
[2] Division of Neurometabolism, Department of Neurology, Foundation for Study of Neurometabolic Diseases (FESEN), Buenos Aires, Argentina

Corresponding Author:
Adrián Fernández, MD, Favaloro Foundation University Hospital, 1746, Belgrano Avenue, C1093AAS Buenos Aires, Argentina.
Email: afernandez@ffavaloro.org; afernan@intramed.net

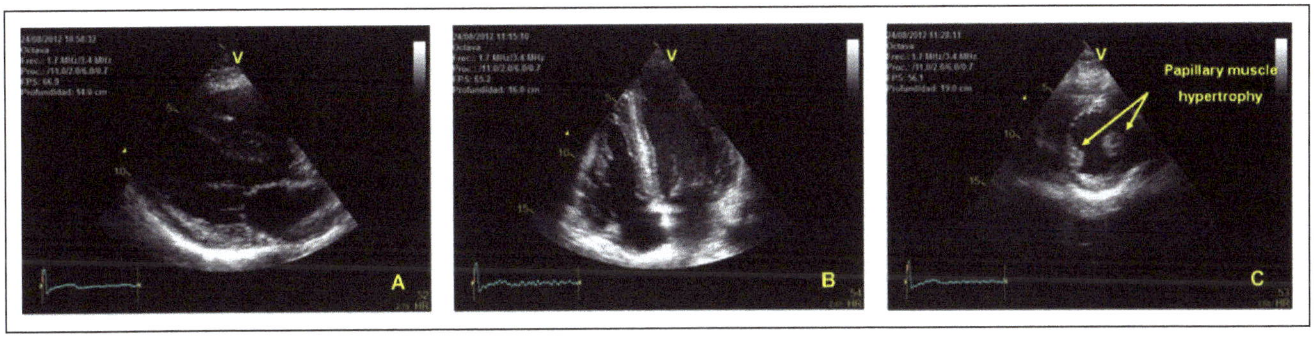

Figure 1. Doppler echocardiography in a patient with Fabry disease. A, Parasternal long axis (left). B, Apical 4-chamber view showing advanced cardiomyopathy with asymmetrical septal hypertrophy. C, Short-axis echo view (right) showing a prominent papillary muscle hypertrophy.

glycosphingolipids having galactose α-glycosidic terminal, especially globotriaosylceramide (GL-3; also abbreviated as Gb3) and the deacylated GL-3 (lyso-globotriaosylceramide [lyso-GL3]), which therefore accumulates mainly in the heart, skin, kidneys, blood vessels, peripheral nerves, and central nervous system. In the heart, the GL-3 deposits occur in cardiomyocytes, conduction system cells, valve fibroblasts, and endothelial cells of the different types of blood vessels. It has been shown that GL-3 deposits occur in only 3% of the myocardium, and the increased wall thickness is also due to hypertrophy of cardiomyocytes by mechanisms that are not fully determined.[18-26] For this reason, histologically FD cardiomyopathy is expressed by myocyte hypertrophy and vacuolization.[18-26]

Cardiac Involvement

The main manifestation of cardiac involvement in FD is the progressive thickening of the heart walls and therefore may be expressed as an HCM. The patients with FD may also present atrioventricular (AV) conduction disturbances, arrhythmias, valvular involvement, and coronary disease. Left ventricular hypertrophy is usually concentric but may also exhibit asymmetrical shapes (Figure 1). Patients with FD have also been recently described with other forms of phenotypic expression similar to HCM caused by mutations in genes encoding sarcomeric proteins. For example, there are reports of patients with FD expressed as apical HCM, HCM forms associated with midventricular obstruction, and even FD manifested as noncompaction cardiomyopathies.[27-29] Other relatively common finding in FD is the presence of prominent papillary muscles.[30] In the so-called cardiac FD variant, the heart may be the organ involved predominantly, and this presentation is usually more common in females.[31] The intracellular accumulation of GL-3 also occurs within the valves and vascular endothelium of the heart.[5,32,33] However, it is important to note that the earliest cardiovascular manifestations are pathophysiological changes involving the microvasculature, with arterial remodeling and intima–media thickening of the small and medium arterioles.[34-36]

Clinical Presentation and Confirmation of the Disease

Although imaging methods may lead to the suspicion of FD, it is very important to note that the diagnosis is predominantly clinical and is based on the search for extracardiac signs and symptoms, for this is an entity featuring systemic involvement.[3,5] Cardiologists must suspect the disease in patients with family history of heart disease, unexplained early death, premature stroke, chronic kidney disease, and absence of male-to-male transmission.[5] Many of the male patients develop a classic severe phenotype with early onset of the characteristic symptoms and signs of FD as the presence of angiokeratomas, acroparesthesias, hypohidrosis, tinnitus, and gastrointestinal symptoms. On physical examination, we must also look for the presence of cornea verticillata, proteinuria, and hearing loss.[5] As FD progresses patients also report symptoms related to the degree of cardiovascular impairment and renal failure, such as angina pectoris, dyspnea, and palpitations due to cardiac arrhythmias.[7-9] Heterozygous females may be affected and can express phenotype of FD ranging from asymptomatic to major involvement of different organs, and the worsening of the disease usually occurs later in life than in men.[7-10] However, the clinical diagnosis of FD can sometimes be difficult, as most of the signs and symptoms resemble those of other common diseases.[3] The most common detection method is the measurement of the αGAL activity in dried blood on filter paper (DBS).[37,38] However, any positive result on a DBS, must be confirmed by direct methods, such as the dosage of αGAL activity in leukocytes, serum, cultured fibroblasts, or by genotyping.[5,38] Although a decrease in activity of αGAL in DBS can confirm the diagnosis of FD in hemizygous males, this is not the most reliable diagnostic method in heterozygous females, since in this group of patients the enzyme activity levels may be within the normal range in a percentage close to 40.[38,39] For this reason, women with high clinical suspicion should undergo genotyping to confirm the diagnosis.[3,38,39] It should be underscored that currently, most laboratories worldwide performing genetic studies to investigate the cause of HCM include the gene encoding the enzyme αGAL in their panels.[3,4,40] When the mutation has been identified in the index case, targeted mutation analysis may be used to identify other affected family members.[3,4] Patients with a positive genotype but without

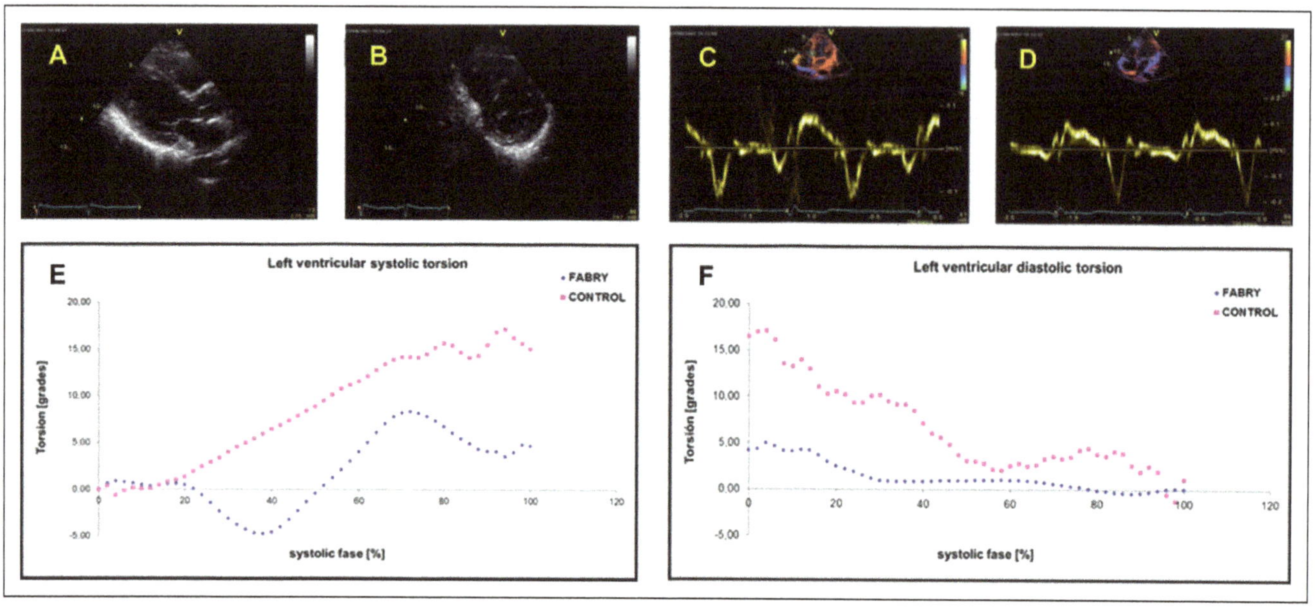

Figure 2. Doppler echocardiography in a 21-year-old asymptomatic patient with Fabry disease (FD). A and B, Parasternal long axis (left) and left parasternal short axis, respectively, with normal characteristics. C and D, Pulsed tissue Doppler of septal and lateral mitral annulus, respectively, with normal characteristics. E and F, Twisting and untwisting analysis comparing this patient with FD (blue dots), with average of 6 age-matched healthy individuals (red dots), showing twist and untwist alterations as early manifestations of FD.

phenotypic manifestations must be followed with annual clinical evaluation.[3-5] To date, hundreds of different FD mutations have been identified that explain the large variation in the residual enzyme activity and clinical presentation of FD.[5,41,42] Endomyocardial biopsies (EMBs) are not routinely included in the diagnosis of HCM; however, they are used in certain clinical scenarios where there is a suspicion of a deposit or infiltrative disease such as FD.[3] In these cases, identification of GL-3 deposits in the myocardium of patients undergoing EMB may be indicative of a diagnosis of FD.[5,43]

Early Diagnosis

It is essential to identify the early signs of cardiac involvement, as younger patients and patients with less renal involvement will benefit the most from enzyme replacement therapy (ERT).[44-47] Therefore, it is important that cardiologists think of FD even in the absence of LVH and also look for early signs of cardiac involvement in patients detected by family screening. In this sense, patients with FD should be evaluated with an electrocardiogram (ECG) because ventricular repolarization disorders and conduction abnormalities may occur several years before the patient develops LVH or other cardiovascular manifestations.[48-51] Moreover, changes in the tissue Doppler velocities also precede the development of LVH, and strain rate imaging and 2-dimensional speckle tracking echocardiography may evidence left ventricle, right ventricle, and left atrium dysfunction, even when conventional cardiac parameters are normal (Figure 2).[52-56] Endomyocardial biopsy and perfusion studies with dipyridamole infusion with ^{13}N-labeled ammonia by positron-emission tomography can reveal the presence of microvascular dysfunction, which is also an early sign of cardiac involvement and precedes the development of LVH.[34-36] Endomyocardial biopsy is the confirmatory tool for the diagnosis of cardiac involvement in cases in which doubts are raised, but the evaluation must be very cautious because certain drugs such as amiodarone, chloroquine, and tamoxifen have a storage pattern similar to FD.[57,58] Cardiologists now have a new method for detecting early cardiac involvement in FD, which is the magnetic resonance noncontrast myocardial T1 mapping that may show glycosphingolipid deposits before the onset of LVH, and it is also a useful method for differentiating FD from other causes of LVH.[59] The significant reduction in the values of noncontrast myocardial T1 is the most sensitive and specific parameter by resonance in patients with FD, regardless of gender, morphology, and left ventricular function.[59-62] The reduction in resonance noncontrast myocardial T1 values before the onset of LVH is associated with parameters of early diastolic and systolic dysfunction measured by echocardiography.[59-62] Regarding biomarkers, the N-terminal fragment of the pro-brain natriuretic peptide (NT-proBNP) is elevated in patients with diastolic dysfunction in the absence of LVH and increased in relation to the stage of the cardiac involvement.[26,63,64] Even when this is correct, the specificity of this finding should be taken carefully for different reasons; for example, NT-proBNP could be elevated due to chronic kidney disease in patients with FD. The lyso-GL3 is also found in increased concentrations in the plasma of patients with FD. It has been proposed that the lyso-GL3 favors GL-3 accumulation, the proliferation of smooth muscle cells in vitro, and may have deleterious effects on the intima and media of small arterioles.[18] The lyso-GL3 predicts clinically relevant FD in patients with mutations in *GLA* gene; this is especially useful for new mutations in women with normal αGAL activity.[41]

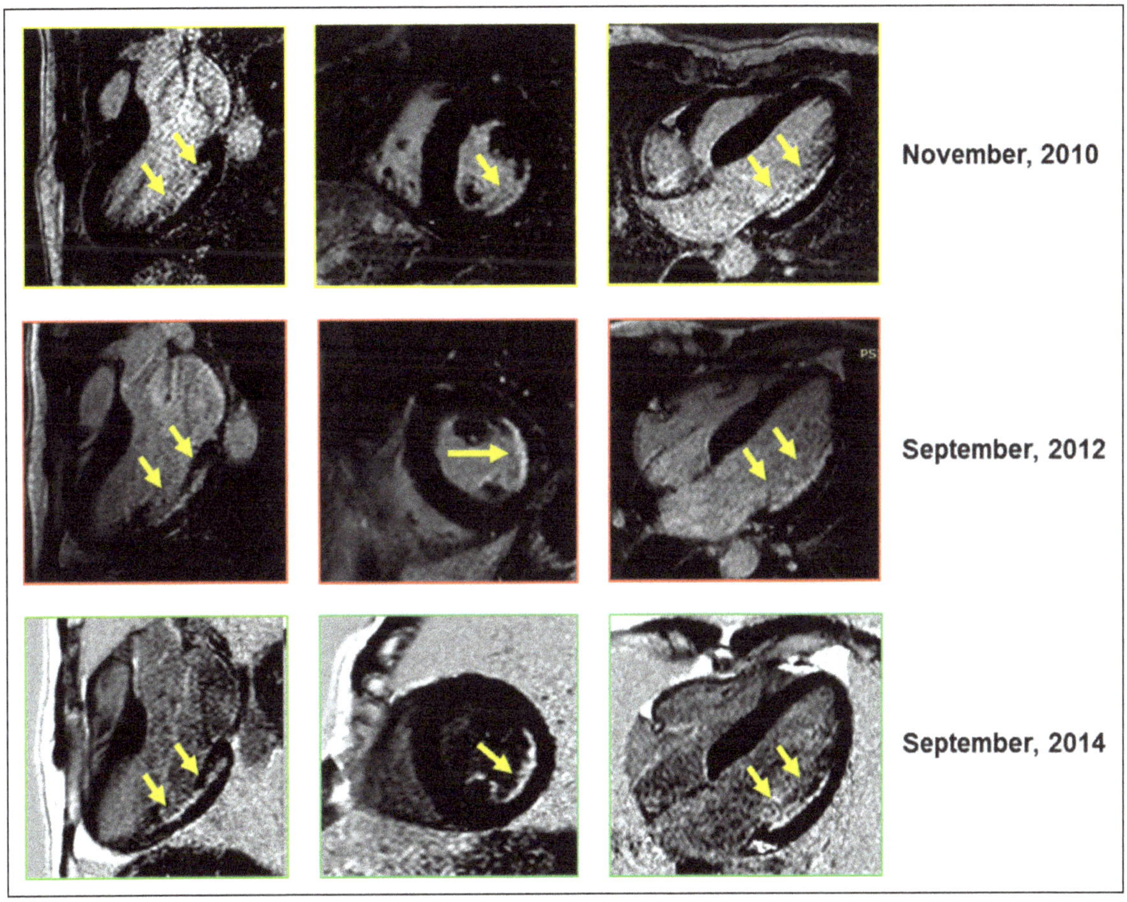

Figure 3. Cardiac magnetic resonance imaging (MRI) in patient with Fabry disease (FD) and history of inferolateral infarction—cardiac MRI is an excellent method to reveal the presence of fibrosis in FD, which is commonly located in the posterolateral basal and midlevel or subepicardial layers, but in this case, the late enhancement MRI shows subendocardial, anterolateral, and inferoposterior wall (basal and middle) enhancement in the area of circumflex coronary artery distribution (necrosis). Magnetic resonance imaging is an excellent method to guide the diagnosis, and on the other hand, it is one of the useful tools available to predict treatment response.

Prognosis and Treatment

Enzyme Replacement Therapy

Since 2001, ERT with recombinant human αGAL (rhαGAL) has been available to treat FD.[44-47,65,66] Two ERTs are currently available for FD; agalsidase-α and agalsidase-β, both administered intravenously every other week. Several studies have shown that the intravenous infusion of rhαGAL effectively reduces both plasma and urine GL-3 levels.[44-47,65,66] At cardiac level, ERT improves ventricular morphology and function and has effects on the conduction system but to optimize the benefits of ERT should be started early before irreversible organ damage occurs.[46,47,65,66] For this reason, it is fundamental to rule out FD in patients with HCM and to make an early diagnosis in affected family members.[47,65-67] Cardiac magnetic resonance imaging (MRI) is an excellent method to guide the diagnosis, and on the other hand, it is one of the useful tools available to predict treatment response (Figure 3). For example, cardiac MRI is an excellent method to reveal the presence of fibrosis in FD, which is commonly located in the posterolateral basal and midlevel or subepicardial layers.[68] Such fibrotic process begins at intramural level to then become transmural.[68,69] In patients without fibrosis or with involvement of only one segment, a reduction in LVH with ERT is observed with stabilized function and improved exercise capacity. In patients with FD having extensive fibrosis treated with ERT, LVH reduction is achieved; however, no improvement in left ventricular function is observed.[66] This cardiac replacement fibrosis is expressed by relevant electrical changes in the ECG, such as repolarization abnormalities at rest and during exercise testing, greater density of premature ventricular beat with Holter ECG. It is also one of the factors that influences exercise intolerance in these patients.[70] Women may develop fibrosis without LVH, and recently, this behavior in young male patients with FD has also been observed.[8,71] Typically, cardiologists tend to diagnose FD late, and unfortunately, cardiac involvement is the leading cause for the substantially increased morbidity and death in these patients.[32,72,73] In advanced stages of the disease, patients may develop conduction disorders, arrhythmias, progressive deterioration of ventricular function, and so on, which determine increased risk of stroke due to atrial

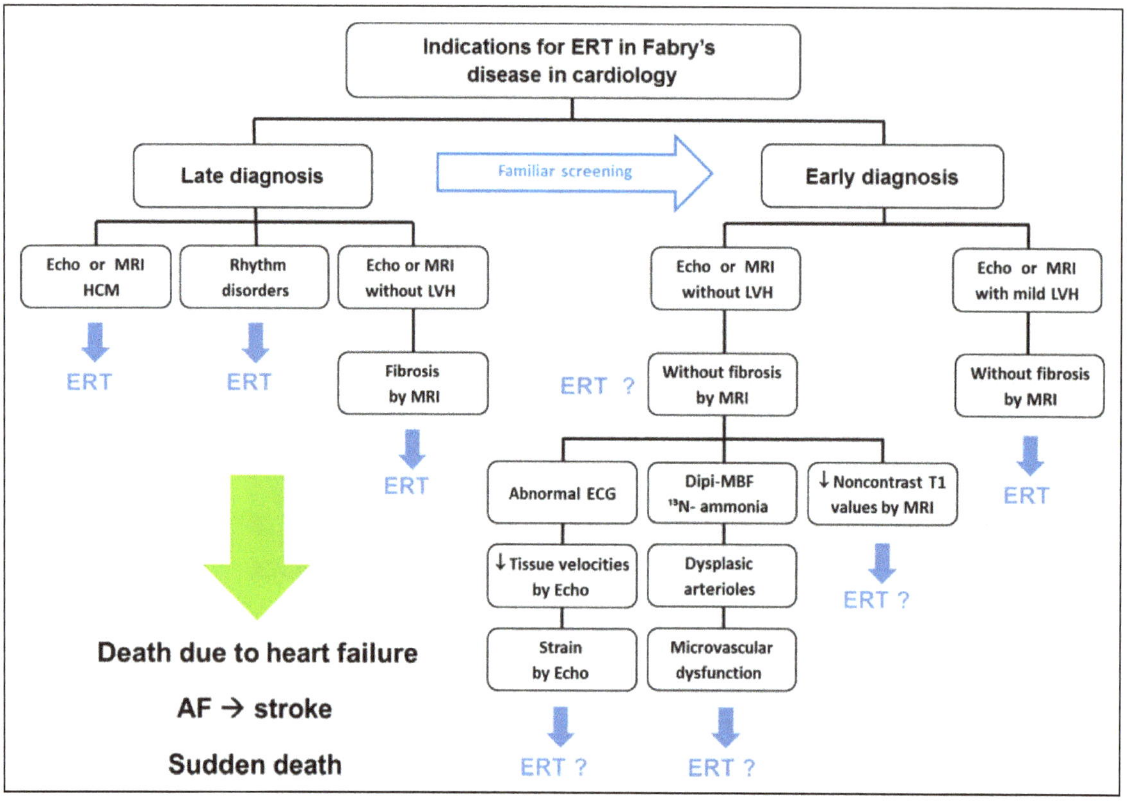

Figure 4. Indications for ERT in Fabry disease in cardiology. AF indicates atrial fibrillation; Dip-MBF, myocardial blood flow following dipyridamole infusion with ^{13}N-labeled ammonia by positron-emission tomography; ECG, electrocardiogram; Echo, echocardiogram; ERT, enzyme replacement therapy; HCM, hypertrophic cardiomyopathy; LVH, left ventricular hypertrophy; MRI, magnetic resonance imaging.

fibrillation (AF), death from heart failure, and SCD.[42,74] Patients who develop systolic dysfunction have an extensive replacement by fibrosis caused by severe microvascular dysfunction and metabolites identified as profibrotic whose levels may decrease with ERT.[34,75] Left ventricular geometry is altered in relation to the stage of the cardiomyopathy and predicts disease progression.[76-80]

Concomitant Treatment

In patients with heart failure and coronary or valve disease, it is important to add adjuvant drug therapy to ERT to improve the quality of life and survival. The first hemodynamic manifestation of cardiac involvement is usually diastolic dysfunction, which may take months or even years to cause symptoms. The conditions predisposing diastolic dysfunction, such as high blood pressure, should be treated appropriately. Blood pressure should be adequately controlled with angiotensin-converting enzyme (ACE) inhibitors or angiotensin receptor blockers (ARB) if ACE inhibitors are not tolerated, since a minimal increase in systolic blood pressure levels is associated with acceleration of fibrosis and adverse course of the disease.[63,81] In addition, we must take into account the nephroprotective effects of such treatment. Beta-blockers should be considered in asymptomatic patients with FD even in the absence of LVH but should be used with caution in patients who do not have pacemakers, since they can trigger conduction abnormalities. Patients with FD that evolved with systolic dysfunction should also be treated with ACE inhibitors (or ARB if ACE inhibitors are not tolerated) and diuretics since they contribute to improve symptoms, ventricular function, and therefore the prognosis of these patients.[76-80] Patients with coronary artery disease must receive aspirin and statins (see the next chapter in this issue of the *Journal* in relation to coronary disease in patients with FD). Patients with symptomatic sinus bradycardia and those with asymptomatic intermittent AV block, progressive conduction system abnormalities, or significant bradycardia should be treated with a pacemaker.[82] Septal reduction therapy with septal myectomy or septal alcohol ablation to improve symptoms may be considered in patients with a resting or provoked maximum left ventricular tract obstruction gradient of $\geq$50 mm Hg, who are severely symptomatic, despite maximum tolerated medical therapy.[1-3,12] Sequential AV pacing, with optimal AV interval to reduce the left ventricular outflow tract gradient may be considered in patients with contraindications for septal myectomy or septal alcohol ablation.[1-3] Patients who had an SCD episode should receive an implantable cardiac defibrillator (ICD) for secondary prevention.[2,3] Moreover, one of the biggest challenges cardiologists face is to identify the small percentage of patients with FD that may benefit from the implantation of an ICD for primary prevention of SCD.[82] This indication is currently based on expert opinion related to isolated case reports or small series, since the recommendations of major international HCM guidelines have not been validated in patients with FD.[2,3] Thus, for example, there have been reported cases of sustained ventricular tachycardia in patients with FD having apical aneurysms secondary to mid-ventricular obstruction; also it has been reported that fibrosis progression increased the risk of fatal ventricular arrhythmias.[83,84] In these patients, we must consider an ICD for primary prevention, and also we must evaluate this indication in patients with FD having left ventricular dysfunction or significant LVH who have an unexplained syncope, in those who have nonsustained ventricular tachycardia on Holter monitoring, and in those patients with a family history of SCD.[74,83,84] Regarding patients with FD having AF, the use of Score for Determining Stroke Risk for Those with Atrial Fibrillation (CHA2DS2-VASc) is not recommended in this population.[3] Given the high incidence of stroke, patients with FD and AF should receive oral anticoagulation for life, even when they recover sinus rhythm.[3] Implantable loop recorder or 48-hour ambulatory ECG monitoring every 6 to 12 months to detect AF should be considered in patients who are in sinus rhythm and have a left atrial diameter higher than or equal to 45 mm.[3] Orthotopic cardiac transplantation may be considered in selected patients who have systolic dysfunction and New York Heart Association functional Class III to IV symptoms despite optimal medical therapy.[1-3,76-80,85]

When to Start ERT in Cardiology?

Fabry disease is a multisystemic disease, and for that reason, it should be managed by a multidisciplinary team, and the decision to initiate ERT is based on the evaluation of symptoms, signs, and organ involvement. The decision to start ERT should be made jointly by a cardiologist and physician specialized in the other areas involved. Current information on genotype–phenotype correlations in FD is very limited, and it is not enough by itself to decide the initiation of ERT in the absence of other manifestations of the disease.[5] There is general agreement on the indication to start therapy in patients with FD having evidence of HCM, heart rhythm disorders (arrhythmias and/or conduction abnormalities), and in patients with evidence of fibrosis as shown by MRI even in the absence of LVH. It is also indicated in patients with mild to moderate LVH without evidence of fibrosis in the MRI, which was previously discussed, that is, they are those who will benefit more from the ERT. We should define more precisely which patients will benefit from ERT in the presence of cardiac involvement, with no development of LVH or have not expressed fibrosis by MRI[34,36,49] (Figure 4).

Conclusion

The heart is one of the organs that may be affected by FD, and FD is one of the causes of HCM. However, we should bear in mind that when a patient with FD develops HCM, it is because we have made a late diagnosis of the disease. Therefore, at this stage, patients have a higher rate of fatal and nonfatal events (stroke, death by heart failure, SCD) that may be avoided with an early diagnosis and the early initiation of ERT. However, in patients with irreversible organ damage, ERT contributes to the stabilization of the disease, delayed progression to severe heart complications, and improved survival. One of the most important contributions that cardiologists can make is to think about a diagnosis of FD in patients with cardiac manifestations preceding the development of LVH and conduct family screening to identify patients with early cardiac involvement which will benefit more from ERT. Patients with FD without cardiac manifestations of the disease should be evaluated annually by a cardiologist specialized in FD disease, regardless of the indication for ERT.

Acknowledgments

The authors would like to thank Ms Claudia Tarazona (medical translator and interpreter) for the revision of this document and also Eduardo Guevara and Horacio Di Nunzio, Favaloro Foundation University Hospital, for providing us with echocardiography and resonance images, respectively.

Declaration of Conflicting Interests

The author(s) declared the following potential conflicts of interest with respect to the research, authorship, and/or publication of this article: A.F. has received speaker's fees from Genzyme and J.P. from Genzyme, Shire, and Amicus.

Funding

The author(s) received no financial support for the research, authorship, and/or publication of this article.

References

1. Maron BJ, McKenna WJ, Danielson GK, et al. ACC/ESC clinical expert consensus document on hypertrophic cardiomyopathy: a report of the American College of Cardiology Task Force on Clinical Expert Consensus Documents and the European Society of Cardiology Committee for Practice Guidelines (Committee to Develop an Expert Consensus Document on Hypertrophic Cardiomyopathy). *Eur Heart J.* 2003;24(21):1965-1991.
2. Gersh BJ, Maron BJ, Bonow RO, et al. 2011 ACCF/AHA Guideline for the diagnosis and treatment of hypertrophic cardiomyopathy: executive summary: a report of the American College of Cardiology Foundation/American Heart Association Task Force on Practice Guidelines. *Circulation* 2011;124(24):2761-2796.
3. Elliott PM, Anastasakis A, Borger M, et al. 2014 ESC Guidelines on diagnosis and management of hypertrophic cardiomyopathy: the Task Force for the Diagnosis and Management of Hypertrophic Cardiomyopathy of the European Society of Cardiology. *Eur Heart J.* 2014;35(39):2733-2779.
4. Charron P, Arad M, Arbustini E, et al; European Society of Cardiology Working Group on Myocardial and Pericardial Diseases. Genetic counseling and testing in cardiomyopathies: a position statement of the European Society of Cardiology Working Group

on Myocardial and Pericardial Diseases. *Eur Heart J.* 2010; 31(22):2715-2726.
5. Yousef Z, Elliott PM, Cecchi F, et al. Left ventricular hypertrophy in Fabry disease: a practical approach to diagnosis. *Eur Heart J.* 2013;34(11):802-808.
6. Arad M, Maron BJ, Gorham JM, et al. Glycogen storage diseases presenting as hypertrophic cardiomyopathy. *N Engl J Med.* 2005; 352(4):362-372.
7. Wilcox WR, Oliveira JP, Hopkin RJ, et al; Fabry Registry. Females with Fabry disease frequently have major organ involvement: lessons from the Fabry Registry. *Mol Genet Metab.* 2008; 93(2):112-128.
8. Niemann M, Herrmann S, Hu K, et al. Differences in Fabry cardiomyopathy between female and male patients: consequences for diagnostic assessment. *JACC Cardiovasc Imaging.* 2011; 4(6):592-601.
9. Patel MR, Cecchi F, Cizmarik M, et al. Cardiovascular events in patients with Fabry disease natural history data from the Fabry registry. *J Am Coll Cardiol.* 2011;57(9):1093-1099.
10. Politei JM, Cabrera G, Amartino H, et al. Fabry disease in Argentina: an evaluation of patients enrolled in the Fabry Registry. *Int J Clin Pract.* 2013;67(1):66-72.
11. Sachdev B, Takenaka T, Teraguchi H, et al. Prevalence of Anderson-Fabry disease in male patients with late onset hypertrophic cardiomyopathy. *Circulation.* 2002;105(12):1407-1411.
12. Ommen SR, Nishimura RA, Edwards WD. Fabry disease: a mimic for obstructive hypertrophic cardiomyopathy? *Heart.* 2003;89(8):929-930.
13. Chimenti C, Pieroni M, Morgante E, et al. Prevalence of Fabry disease in female patients with late-onset hypertrophic cardiomyopathy. *Circulation.* 2004;110(9):1047-1053.
14. Monserrat L, Gimeno-Blanes JR, Marín F, et al. Prevalence of Fabry disease in a cohort of 508 unrelated patients with hypertrophic cardiomyopathy. *J Am Coll Cardiol.* 2007;50(25): 2399-2403.
15. Havndrup O, Christiansen M, Stoevring B, et al. Fabry disease mimicking hypertrophic cardiomyopathy: genetic screening needed for establishing the diagnosis in women. *Eur J Heart Fail.* 2010;12(6):535-540.
16. Hagège AA, Caudron E, Damy T, et al; FOCUS Study Investigators. Screening patients with hypertrophic cardiomyopathy for Fabry disease using a filter-paper test: the FOCUS study. *Heart.* 2011;97(2):131-136.
17. Elliott P, Baker R, Pasquale F, et al; ACES Study Group. Prevalence of Anderson-Fabry disease in patients with hypertrophic cardiomyopathy: the European Anderson-Fabry Disease survey. *Heart.* 2011;97(23):1957-1960.
18. Aerts JM, Groener JE, Kuiper S, et al. Elevated globotriaosylsphingosine is a hallmark of Fabry disease. *Proc Natl Acad Sci U S A.* 2008;105(8):2812-2817.
19. von Scheidt W, Eng CM, Fitzmaurice TF, et al. An atypical variant of Fabry's disease with manifestations confined to the myocardium. *N Engl J Med.* 1991;324(6):395-399.
20. Brakch N, Dormond O, Bekri S, et al. Evidence for a role of sphingosine-1 phosphate in cardiovascular remodeling in Fabry disease. *Eur Heart J.* 2010;31(1):67-76.
21. Elleder M, Bradová V, Smíd F, et al. Cardiocyte storage and hypertrophy as a sole manifestation of Fabry's disease. Report on a case simulating hypertrophic non obstructive cardiomyopathy. *Virchows Arch A Pathol Anat Histopathol.* 1990;417(5):449-455.
22. Barbey F, Brakch N, Linhart A, et al. Cardiac and vascular hypertrophy in Fabry disease: evidence for a new mechanism independent of blood pressure and glycosphingolipid deposition. *Arterioscler Thromb Vasc Biol.* 2006;26(4):839-844.
23. Rombach SM, Dekker N, Bouwman MG, et al. Plasma globotriaosylsphingosine: diagnostic value and relation to clinical manifestations of Fabry disease. *Biochim Biophys Acta.* 2010; 1802(9):741-748.
24. Shen JS, Meng XL, Moore DF, et al. Globotriaosylceramide induces oxidative stress and up-regulates cell adhesion molecule expression in Fabry disease endothelial cells. *Mol Genet Metab.* 2008;95(3):163-168.
25. Ashrafian H, Redwood C, Blair E, Watkins H. Hypertrophic cardiomyopathy: a paradigm for myocardial energy depletion. *Trends Genet.* 2003;19(5):263-268.
26. Coats CJ, Parisi V, Ramos M, et al. Role of serum N-terminal pro-brain natriuretic peptide measurement in diagnosis of cardiac involvement in patients with Anderson-Fabry disease. *Am J Cardiol.* 2013;111(1):111-117.
27. Caetano F, Botelho A, Mota P, Silva J, Leitão Marques A. Fabry disease presenting as apical left ventricular hypertrophy in a patient carrying the missense mutation R118C. *Rev Port Cardiol.* 2014;33(3):183.
28. Cianciulli TF, Saccheri MC, Fernández SP, Fernández CC, Rozenfeld PA, Kisinovsky I. Apical left ventricular hypertrophy and mid-ventricular obstruction in Fabry disease. *Echocardiography.* 2015;32(5):860-863.
29. Martins E, Pinho T, Carpenter S, et al. Histopathological evidence of Fabry disease in a female patient with left ventricular noncompaction. *Rev Port Cardiol.* 2014;33(9):565.
30. Niemann M, Liu D, Hu K, et al. Prominent papillary muscles in Fabry disease: a diagnostic marker? *Ultrasound Med Biol.* 2011; 37(1):37-43.
31. Nakao S, Takenaka T, Maeda M, et al. An atypical variant of Fabry's disease in men with left ventricular hypertrophy. *N Engl J Med.* 1995;333(5):288-293.
32. Putko BN, Wen K, Thompson RB, et al. Anderson-Fabry cardiomyopathy: prevalence, pathophysiology, diagnosis and treatment. *Heart Fail Rev.* 2015;20(2):179-191.
33. Weidemann F, Strotmann JM, Niemann M, et al. Heart valve involvement in Fabry cardiomyopathy. *Ultrasound Med Biol.* 2009;35(5):730-735.
34. Tomberli B, Cecchi F, Sciagrà R, et al. Coronary microvascular dysfunction is an early feature of cardiac involvement in patients with Anderson-Fabry disease. *Eur Heart Fail.* 2013;15(2): 1363-1373.
35. Frustaci A, Russo MA, Francone M, Chimenti C. Microvascular angina as prehypertrophic presentation of Fabry disease cardiomyopathy. *Circulation.* 2014;130(17):1530-1531.
36. Tschöpe C, Dominguez F, Canaan-Kühl S, et al. Endomyocardial biopsy in Anderson-Fabry disease: the key in uncertain cases. *Int J Cardiol.* 2015;190:284-286.

37. Chamoles NA, Blanco M, Gagilo D. Fabry disease: enzymatic diagnosis in dried blood spots on filter paper. *Clin Chim Acta*. 2001;308(1-2):195-196.
38. Gal A, Hughes DA, Winchester B. Toward a consensus in the laboratory diagnostics of Fabry disease—recommendations of a European expert group. *J Inherit Metab Dis*. 2011;34(2): 509-514.
39. Linthorst GE, Poorthuis BJ, Hollak CE. Enzyme activity for determination of presence of Fabry disease in women results in 40% false-negative results. *J Am Coll Cardiol*. 2008;51(21):2082.
40. Wheeler M, Pavlovic A, DeGoma E, Salisbury H, Brown C, Ashley EA. A new era in clinical genetic testing for hypertrophic cardiomyopathy. *J Cardiovasc Transl Res*. 2009;2(4):381-391.
41. Niemann M, Rolfs A, Störk S, et al. Gene mutations versus clinically relevant phenotypes: lyso-Gb3 defines Fabry disease. *Circ Cardiovasc Genet*. 2014;7(1):8-16.
42. Patel V, O'Mahony C, Hughes D, et al. Clinical and genetic predictors of major cardiac events in patients with Anderson-Fabry Disease. *Heart*. 2015;101(12):961-966.
43. Cooper LT, Baughman KL, Feldman AM, et al. The role of endomyocardial biopsy in the management of cardiovascular disease: a scientific statement from the American Heart Association, the American College of Cardiology, and the European Society of Cardiology Endorsed by the Heart Failure Society of America and the Heart Failure Association of the European Society of Cardiology. *Eur Heart J*. 2007;28(24):3076-3093.
44. Schiffmann R, Kopp JB, Austin HA III, et al. Enzyme replacement therapy in Fabry disease: a randomized controlled trial. *JAMA*. 2001;285(21):2743-2749.
45. Eng CM, Guffon N, Wilcox WR, et al; International Collaborative Fabry Disease Study Group. Safety and efficacy of recombinant human alpha-galactosidase A—replacement therapy in Fabry's disease. *N Engl J Med*. 2001;345(1):9-16.
46. Watt T, Burlina AP, Cazzorla C, et al. Agalsidase beta treatment is associated with improved quality of life in patients with Fabry disease: findings from the Fabry registry. *Genet Med*. 2010; 12(11):703-712.
47. Germain DP, Charrow J, Desnick RJ, et al. Ten-year outcome of enzyme replacement therapy with agalsidase beta in patients with Fabry disease. *J Med Genet*. 2015;52(5):353-358.
48. Havranek S, Linhart A, Urbanova Z, Ramaswami U. Early cardiac changes in children with Anderson-Fabry disease. *JIMD Rep*. 2013;11:53-64.
49. Namdar M, Steffel J, Vidovic M, , et al. Electrocardiographic changes in early recognition of Fabry disease. *Heart*. 2011; 97(6):485-490.
50. Kouris NT, Kontogianni DD, Pavlou MT, Babalis DK. Atrioventricular conduction disturbances in a young patient with Fabry's disease without other signs of cardiac involvement. *Int J Cardiol*. 2005;99(2):327-328.
51. Ikari Y, Kuwako K, Yamaguchi T. Fabry's disease with complete atrioventricular block: histological evidence of involvement of the conduction system. *Br Heart J*. 1992;68(3):323-325.
52. Pieroni M. Echocardiographic assessment of Fabry cardiomyopathy: early diagnosis and follow-up. *J Am Soc Echocardiogr*. 2011; 24(9):1033-1036.
53. Zamorano J, Serra V, Pérez de Isla L, et al. Usefulness of tissue Doppler on early detection of cardiac disease in Fabry patients and potential role of enzyme replacement therapy (ERT) for avoiding progression of disease. *Eur J Echocardiogr*. 2011; 12(9):671-677.
54. Saccheri MC, Cianciulli TF, Lax JA, et al. Two-dimensional speckle tracking echocardiography for early detection of myocardial damage in young patients with Fabry disease. *Echocardiography*. 2013;30(9):1069-1077.
55. Morris DA, Blaschke D, Canaan-Kühl S, et al. Global cardiac alterations detected by speckle-tracking echocardiography in Fabry disease: left ventricular, right ventricular and left atrial dysfunction are common and linked to worse symptomatic status. *Int J Cardiovasc Imaging*. 2015;31(2):301-313.
56. Shanks M, Thompson RB, Paterson ID, et al. Systolic and diastolic function assessment in Fabry disease patients using speckle-tracking imaging and comparison with conventional echocardiographic measurements. *J Am Soc Echocardiogr*. 2013;26(12): 1407-1414.
57. Smid BE, van der Tol L, Cecchi F, et al. Uncertain diagnosis of Fabry disease: consensus recommendation on diagnosis in adults with left ventricular hypertrophy and genetic variants of unknown significance. *Int J Cardiol*. 2014;177(2):400-408.
58. Roos JM, Aubry MC, Edwards WD. Chloroquine cardiotoxicity: clinicopathologic features in three patients and comparison with three patients with Fabry disease. *Cardiovasc Pathol*. 2002;11(5): 277-283.
59. Sado DM, White SK, Piechnik SK, et al. Identification and assessment of Anderson-Fabry disease by cardiovascular magnetic resonance noncontrast myocardial T1 mapping. *Circ Cardiovasc Imaging*. 2013;6(3):392-398.
60. Thompson RB, Chow K, Khan A, et al. T1 mapping with cardiovascular MRI is highly sensitive for Fabry disease independent of hypertrophy and sex. *Circ Cardiovasc Imaging*. 2013;6(5): 637-645.
61. Edwards NC, Teoh JK, Steeds RP. Hypertrophic cardiomyopathy and Anderson-Fabry disease: unraveling septal hypertrophy with T1-mapping CMR. *Eur Heart J*. 2014;35(28):1896.
62. Pica S, Sado DM, Maestrini V, et al. Reproducibility of native myocardial T1 mapping in the assessment of Fabry disease and its role in early detection of cardiac involvement by cardiovascular magnetic resonance. *J Cardiovasc Magn Reson*. 2014;16:99.
63. Krämer J, Bijnens B, Störk S, et al. Left ventricular geometry and blood pressure as predictors of adverse progression of Fabry Cardiomyopathy. *PLoS One*. 2015;10(11):e0140627.
64. Torralba-Cabeza MÁ, Olivera S, Hughes DA, Pastores GM, Mateo RN, Pérez-Calvo JI. Cystatin C and NT-proBNP as prognostic biomarkers in Fabry disease. *Mol Genet Metab*. 2011; 104(3):301-307.
65. Motwani M, Banypersad S, Woolfson P, Waldek S. Enzyme replacement therapy improves cardiac features and severity of Fabry disease. *Mol Genet Metab*. 2012;107(1-2):197-202.
66. Weidemann F, Niemann M, Breunig F, et al. Long-term effects of enzyme replacement therapy on Fabry cardiomyopathy: evidence for a better outcome with early treatment. *Circulation*. 2009; 119(4):524-529.

67. Weidemann F, Linhart A, Monserrat L, Strotmann J. Cardiac challenges in patients with Fabry disease. *Int J Cardiol.* 2010; 141(1):3-10.
68. Moon JC, Sachdev B, Elkington AG, et al. Gadolinium enhanced cardiovascular magnetic resonance in Anderson-Fabry disease. Evidence for a disease specific abnormality of the myocardial interstitium. *Eur Heart J.* 2003;24(23):2151-2155.
69. Sheppard MN. The heart in Fabry's disease. *Cardiovasc Pathol.* 2011;20(1):8-14.
70. Krämer J, Nordbeck P, Störk S, et al. Electrical changes in resting, exercise, and Holter electrocardiography in Fabry cardiomyopathy [Published online October 27, 2015]. *JIMD Rep.* 2015.
71. Sechi A, Nucifora G, Piccoli G, Dardis A, Bembi B. Myocardial fibrosis as the first sign of cardiac involvement in a male patient with Fabry disease: report of a clinical case and discussion on the utility of the magnetic resonance in Fabry pathology. *BMC Cardiovasc Disord.* 2014;14:86.
72. Kunkala MR, Aubry MC, Ommen SR, Gersh BJ, Schaff HV. Outcome of septal myectomy in patients with Fabry's disease. *Ann Thorac Surg.* 2013;95(1):335-337.
73. Geske JB, Jouni H, Aubry MC, Gersh BJ. Fabry disease with resting outflow obstruction masquerading as hypertrophic cardiomyopathy. *J Am Coll Cardiol.* 2014;63(17):e43.
74. Acharya D, Doppalapudi H, Tallaj JA. Arrhythmias in Fabry cardiomyopathy. *Card Electrophysiol Clin.* 2015;7(2):283-291.
75. Weidemann F, Sanchez-Niño MD, Politei J, et al. Fibrosis: a key feature of Fabry disease with potential therapeutic implications. *Orphanet J Rare Dis.* 2013;8:116.
76. Cecchi F, Olivotto I, Gistri R, Lorenzoni R, Chiriatti G, Camici PG. Coronary microvascular dysfunction and prognosis in hypertrophic cardiomyopathy. *N Engl J Med.* 2003;349:1027-1035.
77. Harris KM, Spirito P, Maron MS, et al. Prevalence, clinical profile, and significance of left ventricular remodeling in the end-stage phase of hypertrophic cardiomyopathy. *Circulation* 2006; 114(3):216-225.
78. Olivotto I, Cecchi F, Gistri R, et al. Relevance of coronary microvascular flow impairment to long-term remodeling and systolic dysfunction in hypertrophic cardiomyopathy. *J Am Coll Cardiol.* 2006;47(5):1043-1048.
79. Fernández A, Vigliano C, Casabé J H, et al; Favaloro Foundation. Comparison of prevalence, clinical course, and pathological findings of left ventricular systolic impairment versus normal systolic function in patients with hypertrophic cardiomyopathy. *Am J Cardiol.* 2011;108(4):548-555.
80. Olivotto I, Cecchi F, Poggesi C, Yacoub MH. Patterns of disease progression in hypertrophic cardiomyopathy: an individualized approach to clinical staging. *Circ Heart Fail.* 2012;5(4):535-546.
81. Warnock DG, Jain G. Blood pressure, proteinuria and nephropathy in Fabry disease. *Nephron Clin Pract.* 2011;118(1):c43-c48.
82. Frustaci A, Chimenti C. Images in cardiovascular medicine. Cryptogenic ventricular arrhythmias and sudden death by Fabry disease: prominent infiltration of cardiac conduction tissue. *Circulation.* 2007;116(12):e350-e351.
83. Poulin MF, Shah A, Trohman RG, Madias C. Advanced Anderson-Fabry disease presenting with left ventricular apical aneurysm and ventricular tachycardia. *World J Clin Cases.* 2015;3(6):519-524.
84. Krämer J, Niemann M, Störk S, et al. Relation of burden of myocardial fibrosis to malignant ventricular arrhythmias and outcomes in Fabry disease. *Am J Cardiol.* 2014;114(6):895-900.
85. Cantor WJ, Daly P, Iwanochko M, Clarke JT, Cusimano RJ, Butany J. Cardiac transplantation for Fabry's disease. *Can J Cardiol.* 1998;14(1):81-84.

12

Impact of Enzyme Replacement Therapy in a Patient Younger Than 2 Years Diagnosed With Maroteaux-Lamy Syndrome (MPS VI)

Johanna Acosta Guio, MD[1,2] and Gustavo AdolfoGiraldo-Ospina, MD[3]

Abstract

Introduction: Mucopolysaccharidosis type VI, also known as Maroteaux-Lamy syndrome (#OMIM 253200), is a rare autosomal recessive genetic disorder due to deficient activity of the enzyme N-acetylgalactosamine 4-sulfatase (arylsulfatase B) required for the breakdown of dermatan sulfate and chondroitin sulfate. **Patient:** Report of a female patient started on enzyme replacement therapy at 17 months of age. At the time of diagnosis (14 months), the patient presented mild corneal opacity and significant thoracolumbar kyphosis, but no visceral involvement or growth arrest. At 73 months of treatment, weight was normal, although the patient was in a low height percentile. The patient showed adequate neural development, with improvement in lumbar spine and joint involvement. Corneal compromise or valvular disease progression was not evident. **Conclusion:** Early and timely diagnosis and treatment with enzyme replacement therapy are essential, as the means to change the natural history of the disease, avoiding comorbidities and improving final prognosis.

Keywords

mucopolysaccharidosis type VI (MPS VI), Maroteaux-Lamy syndrome, enzyme replacement therapy, glycosaminoglycans

Introduction

Mucopolysaccharidoses (MPS) are a group of innate errors of metabolism of the complex molecule catabolism type. They are caused by a deficiency of a specific lysosomal enzyme that affects the normal catabolism of glycosaminoglycans (GAGs), leading to their accumulation in different organs and tissues and resulting in a number of complex signs and symptoms of multisystem disease.[1-3] Mucopolysaccharidosis type VI (MPS VI) or Maroteaux-Lamy syndrome (OMIM #253200) is a rare genetic disease of autosomal recessive inheritance caused by a deficiency of the N-acetylgalactosamine-4-sulfatase enzyme, also known as arylsulfatase B (ARSB), which hydrolyzes the sulfate fraction of the dermatan GAG.[1,2,4]

It is estimated that the incidence of MPS VI in the world ranges between 1 in 248 000 and 1 in 300 000 live births.[5] Nevertheless, Orphanet (http://www.orpha.net) reports a prevalence of 1 to 9 per 1 000 000. In Brazil, population data reveal that the incidence may be higher. A screening of a high-risk population with a diagnosis of MPS showed that 19% of this high-risk population was with MPS VI, although no ethnic group or founding effect was observed in the population.[6-8] In Colombia, there are no updated epidemiological data regarding the incidence of the disease in the population.

Patients with MPS VI exhibit a wide range of multisystem symptoms as part of a characteristically progressive and chronic course, affecting mainly their cardiorespiratory and skeletal systems, cornea, skin, liver, spleen, meninges, and brain.[3] The systemic involvement is very similar to the one observed in MPS I but, unlike that form of the disease, intelligence is not affected.

At present, galsulfase (recombinant form of human N-acetylgalactosamine [rhASB]; Naglazyme), an enzymatic replacement therapy (ERT), is the sole treatment approved for patients with MPS VI. Galsulfase has been approved by the regulatory agencies of the United States, the European Union,

[1] Instituto de Ortopedia Infantil Roosevelt, Bogotá, Colombia
[2] Instituto de Genética, Universidad Nacional, Bogotá, Colombia
[3] Facultad de Medicina, Universidad Pontificia Bolivariana, Clínica Universitaria Bolivariana, Medellín, Colombia

Corresponding Author:
Johanna Acosta Guio, Instituto de Ortopedia Infantil Roosevelt, Av. Circunvalar N. 17-50, PBX (571) 3534000 Bogotá, Colombia.
Email: joacaguio@hotmail.com

Australia, Brazil, Colombia, and other countries. The international management guidelines for MPS VI recommend galsulfase ERT as first-line treatment for patients with MPS VI.[7] In 2014, Giugliani et al, in a study about the natural history and treatment with galsulfase in patients with MPS VI, concluded that long-term galsulfase ERT improves survival, continued growth, endurance, and lung function. The treatment was also shown to help stabilize cardiac function and improve quality of life in patients with this disease. Even in patients with the most severe form of the disease, galsulfase ERT stabilizes endurance and lung function and improves survival. Early initiation of ERT may improve the clinical benefits in patients with MPS VI.[9]

This article reports the case of a 13-month-old Colombian patient with a clinical and biochemical diagnosis of MPS VI, started on ERT at 17 months of age. The article highlights the importance of early diagnosis for timely initiation of treatment, which results in a significant change in the progression of the disease and the quality of life for patients and families alike.

Case Report

This is a 13-month-old female patient born in Bogota, Colombia, to nonconsanguineous parents. The patient was the fourth pregnancy and received antenatal care. Ultrasound scans were within normal limits. The mother was delivered by cesarean section (37 weeks' gestation) due to preeclampsia. Weight and length at birth were 3200 g and 49 cm, respectively. Due to early jaundice, the neonate required admission to the neonatal care unit for management with phototherapy. From the time of birth, lumbar spine deformity prompted the mother to visit several pediatricians. Nevertheless, no workup or treatment was indicated. A pediatric orthopedic surgeon diagnosed hyperlordosis and scoliosis. The patient was referred to the medical genetics service. Parents reported normal neural development. The patient was asymptomatic at the time of the initial visit.

Family History

The patient has a half maternal sister, healthy; had a brother diagnosed with intrauterine growth restriction died at 18 days of birth of no clear cause; had a second sister died in uterus, at 7 months, with no cause of death identified. The mother reports no fetal hydrops or phenotypical abnormalities in either case.

Initial Physical Examination Findings

Weight (10 kg) and size (76 cm) were normal for age (Table 1). The patient had macrocephaly, broad forehead, mid-face hypoplasia, mildly coarse facies, thick eyebrows, anteverted nostrils, broad nasal bridge, epicanthal fold, mild corneal opacity, gingival hypertrophy, tonsillar hypertrophy, short mobile symmetrical neck, short chest, mild pectus excavatum, soft abdomen with no visceral enlargement, small reducible umbilical hernia, and bilateral reducible inguinal hernias. Joint mobility mildly impaired for elbow extension, and the patient had brachydactyly, no evidence of claw hand, no lower limb range of motion limitation, and evidence of lumbar kyphoscoliosis (Figure 1A). Several mongoloid spots located in the back and lumbar region.

Neurological Examination

Patient was alert with normal tone, normal gait, preserved strength, and sensation in the 4 limbs. Electrophoresis for MPS was performed with reported dermatan sulfate excretion, enzymatic activity for ARSB on filter paper was reported as 0.0, and leukocyte arylsulfatase at 0.71 (reference value of 115-226 nmol/mg/protein/h), confirming the diagnosis of Maroteaux-Lamy syndrome (MPS VI). Molecular sequencing of the ARSB gene identified the mutations giving rise to the disease on allele 1: c.1143-1G>C (IVS5-1g>c), as reported by Garrido et al,[10] and on allele 2: c.332 A>C (p.H111P), as reported by Giraldo et al[11] in patients with the severe phenotype.

Baseline Tests (Prior To Treatment Initiation)

Lumbar spine X-rays showed oval-shaped vertebral bodies and lumbar hyperlordosis. Echocardiography revealed mitral valve dysplasia with grade I prolapse and mild regurgitation, with mild aortic and tricuspid regurgitation. Total abdominal computed tomography scan showed no findings of enlarged organs. Brain magnetic resonance imaging (MRI) revealed enlarged perivascular spaces; brainstem auditory evoked potentials were within normal limits. Long-bone X-rays showed widening of the proximal and distal metaphyses. Cervical spine MRI and ribcage X-rays were normal (Table 2).

The ERT was initiated 3 months after diagnosis (17 months of age) using N-acetylgalactosamine 4-sulfatase, rhASB (galsulfase, Naglazyme) 1 mg/kg/wk intravenously (IV; total dose of 10 mg/wk). To date, there have been no reports of adverse reactions associated with the ERT. After 50 ERT infusions, the patient was within the normal percentiles for weight and height (87 cm, 12 kg) and head circumference was 48 cm. After 62 weeks of treatment, height, weight, and head circumference were 88 cm, 12.5 kg, and 48 cm, respectively, all within the low normal range. Later, there was a dip in height (Figure 2), but on the last follow-up (6 years of age), there is a trend toward recovery in the growth curve, with height, weight, and head circumference of 98.5 cm, 16.5 kg, and 48 cm, respectively (Figure 3). The patient has achieved therapeutic targets of improved joint mobility, corrected kyphoscoliosis with the use of a brace, and significantly improved corneal opacity, apnea/hypopnea syndrome, and adenoid infiltration. There is no evidence of valvular disease progression.

In summary, ERT has modified the natural history of the disease. Growth curves are within normal ranges and there is no organ enlargement (Figures 1 and 4). X-rays at 6 years of age show mild bony changes, but there is no evidence of severe bone disease such as dysostosis multiplex (Figure 5).

Table 1. Clinical Variants During the Course of the Treatment.

Parameter	Onset	49 Weeks ERT	62 Weeks ERT	98 Weeks ERT	110 Weeks ERT	122 Weeks ERT	133 Weeks ERT	136 Weeks ERT	149 Weeks ERT	160 Weeks ERT	172 Weeks ERT	196 Weeks ERT	206 Weeks ERT	219 Weeks ERT	231 Weeks ERT	270 Weeks ERT
Age	14 months	26 months	29 months	38 months	41 months	44 months	47 months	47.8 months	50 months	53 months	56 months	62 months	65 months	67 months	70 months	73 months
Weight	10 kg	12 kg	12.5 kg	13.2 kg	13.1 kg	12.2 kg	13.8 kg	14.2 kg	14 kg	14.4 kg	14 kg	14 kg	14.7 kg	14.7 kg	15.4 kg	16.5 kg
Size	76 cm	87 cm	88 cm	90 cm	91.5 cm	92 cm	94 cm	94.5 cm	94.5 cm	94.5 cm	94.5 cm	96.5 cm	96.5 cm	96.5 cm	96.5 cm	98.5 cm
Head circumference	46 cm	48.5 cm	48 cm	49.4 cm	47.5 cm	47.6 cm	47.5 cm	48 cm	49 cm	49 cm	49 cm	49 cm	48.5 cm	48.5 cm	48.5 cm	48 cm
Facial appearance	Mild coarse facies	Mild coarse facies	Mild coarse facies	Mild coarse facies	Mild coarse facies	Mild coarse facies	Mild coarse facies	Mild coarse facies	Mild coarse facies	Mild coarse facies	Mild coarse facies	Mild coarse facies	Mild coarse facies	Mild coarse facies	Mild coarse facies	Mild coarse facies
Chest	Mild pectus excavatum	Mild pectus excavatum		Mild pectus excavatum			Mild pectus excavatum			Mild pectus excavatum		Mild pectus excavatum				Bell-shaped chest, prominent inferior costal arches
Major joints	Mild limitation of elbow extension	No changes	No changes	No changes	No changes	Mild range of motion limitation at the elbows	No changes	No changes	No changes	Mild range of motion limitation at the elbows	No changes	No changes	No changes	No changes	Extension limitation at the elbows, mild gene valgum	No changes
Hands	Normal	Normal	Normal	Normal	Normal	Normal	Normal	Normal	Normal	Normal	Normal	Mild interphalangeal contractures in fourth digit of the right hand	No changes	Mild bilateral contractures in third, fourth, and fifth fingers	No changes	Mild bilateral contractures in third, fourth, and fifth fingers

Abbreviation: ERT, enzymatic replacement therapy.

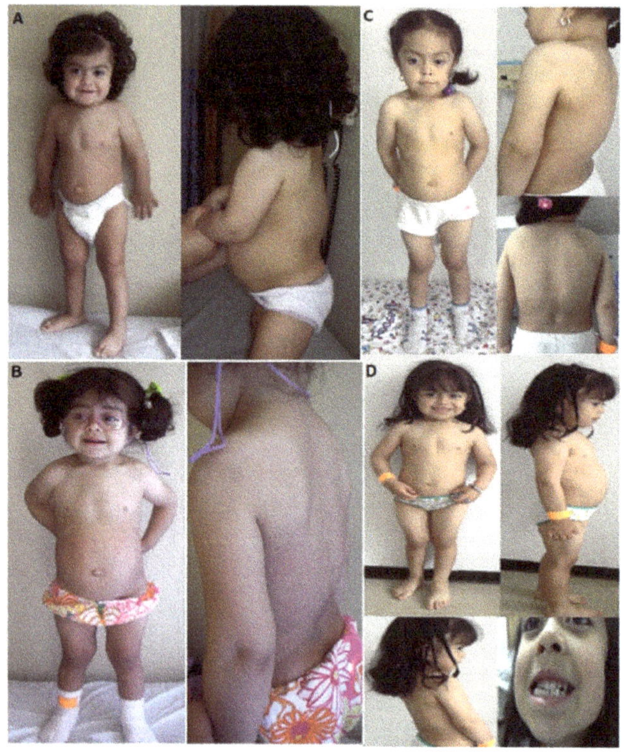

Figure 1. A, Patient at the time of diagnosis (16 months old), before initiating enzymatic replacement therapy (ERT). B, Patient at 28 months with no evidence of disease progression. C, Four-year-old patient: slow progression of the disease. D, Five-year-old patient: mild progression of the disease (without gingival hypertrophy or skeletal abnormality).

These changes include mild acetabular dysplasia, mild camptodactyly, and mild metaphyseal widening. Follow-up imaging tests have shown no evidence of hepatomegaly or splenomegaly, with oval-shaped vertebral bodies, and absence of scoliosis. Audiometry is normal. Brain MRI is normal and full spine MRI shows hyperlordosis and scoliosis. Echocardiography shows dysplastic aortic valve, mild aortic root dilatation, mitral dysplasia with regurgitation, and mild prolapse, with no improvement, but no worsening of cardiac involvement either. Follow-up parameters remained stable, but there was a small progression of clinical and paraclinical findings (Tables 1 and 2).

The patient has been followed up regularly by a multidisciplinary group. She goes to school and has a normal neurological development according to her age. The natural history of the disease was modified, and the patient showed improvement in airway and visual involvement, no progression of the valvular or skeletal disease, no visceral enlargement, and no changes in her facial phenotype.

Discussion

Doctors Maroteaux and Lamy first described MPS VI or Maroteaux-Lamy syndrome in 1963.[12] It is caused by mutations in the N-acetylgalactosamine-4-sulfatase or ARSB gene. This enzyme is responsible for removing the C4 ester sulfate group from the N-acetylgalactosamine sugar of dermatan sulfate and chondroitin 4-sulfateglycosaminoglycans (GAGs). Mutations in this gene cause ARSB enzyme deficiency and inadequate lysosomal GAG breakdown, eventually leading to GAG intralysosomal storage and urinary excretion.[8]

Patients with MPS VI exhibit a wide range of multisystem symptoms, including tracheobronchomalacia that contributes to respiratory problems, with frequent findings of obstructive sleep apnea. Cardiac compromise is responsible for morbidity and mortality in the vast majority of patients with MPS VI.[13]

Genotype identification may be important for predicting phenotype and therapeutic decision-making in some cases of MPS. Additionally, it can be used to provide genetic counseling on reproductive risks, thus contributing to lowering the recurrence of the disease.[3]

Before the advent of stem cell treatment and, in particular, ERT, treatment of patients diagnosed with MPS VI was palliative and symptomatic, aimed at managing and preventing complications.[3] The ERT with human recombinant N-acetylgalactosamine-sulfatase (rhASB) has shown to be effective in human phase II and phase III clinical trials, with significant improvement in endurance tests (12-minute walk, 3-minute stair climbing), increased joint range of motion, improved respiratory function tests, and reduced urine GAG excretion.[14,15] Enzyme replacement treatment was administered as a single dose of 1 mg/kg/wk infusion over a 4-hour period with antihistamine premedication in order to diminish the risk of secondary adverse events.[16] All clinical trials were done in patients older than 5 years to assess efficacy and safety. Since 2009, some papers have been published describing treatment in patients younger than 5 years,[16] with significant improvement in paraclinical parameters and in bone and joint parameters (scoliosis and joint mobility).

McGill et al described the case of 2 siblings with a diagnosis of MPS VI in utero. The first started treatment at 3.6 years, and the second at 8 weeks of life. At present, the first sibling has coarse facies, visceral enlargement, and bone and joint compromise, whereas the second patient shows mild signs and symptoms of the disease after 182 weeks of treatment (moderate pectus excavatum, mild restriction of shoulder flexion, normal hands and facial appearance).[16] Safety of the medication was demonstrated in patients younger than 5 years. Ribeiro et al have demonstrated the safety of ERT in patients younger than 1 year, with improvement in urine GAG excretion and functional status and a reduction of disease burden.[17]

In 2013, a study by Horovitz et al described 34 patients (21 males and 13 females) with MPS VI who started galsulfase ERT before 5 years, with a mean age at diagnosis of 28.5 months and a mean age at the start of therapy of 38.5 months. The study concluded that ERT with galsulfase at the prescribed dose of 1 mg/kg/wk IV was shown to be safe

Table 2. Laboratories and Imaging Studies During the Course of the Treatment.

Parameter	Onset	49 Weeks ERT	98 Weeks ERT	110 Weeks ERT	122 Weeks ERT	136 Weeks ERT	149 Weeks ERT	196 Weeks ERT	219 Weeks ERT	231 Weeks ERT	270 Weeks ERT
Age	14 months	25 months	38 months	41 months	44 months	47.8 months	50 months	62 months	67 months	70 months	73 months
Spine X-ray	Hyperlordosis, oval-shaped vertebral bodies	Oval-shaped vertebral bodies, improved hyperlordosis	Not done	No scoliotic curve, significant improvement of kyphotic curve, oval-shaped vertebral bodies	Not done	Not done	Not done	Significant improvement of scoliosis and lordosis oval-shaped vertebral bodies	Not done	Not done	No evidence of scoliosis, oval-shaped vertebral bodies
Echocardiogram	Mitral dysplasia, grade I prolapse, mild mitral, tricuspid, and aortic regurgitation	Mild aortic root dilatation, mitral valve dysplasia with regurgitation and mild prolapse, mild left ventricular dilatation	Not done	Moderate left ventricular hypertrophy and dilatation, grade II aortic insufficiency, mitral valve with grade II-III insufficiency	Left ventricular hypertrophy and dilatation, mitral valve prolapse, mild grade II insufficiency, grade II aortic insufficiency, left atrial dilatation	Not done	Moderate concentric left ventricular hypertrophy, mild aortic insufficiency, mild mitral prolapse and moderate insufficiency	Mild-to-moderate concentric left ventricular hypertrophy, thickened tricuspid, mild insufficiency, mild compromise of thickened, myxomatous anterior mitral leaflet, mitral prolapse, mild tricuspid regurgitation, FEV1 65%	Mild compromise of thickened, myxomatous anterior mitral leaflet, severe regurgitation, thickened tricuspid aortic valve severe, mild insufficiency, severe left atrial and ventricular dilatation, left ventricular diastolic diameter 4, 3 cm, mild-to-moderate left ventricular concentric hypertrophy	Not done	Moderate mitral insufficiency; ring diameter 2.4 cm, tricuspid 2.32, mild left heart dilatation, tricuspid aortic valve, mild insufficiency, no stenosis, mild tricuspid regurgitation FEV1 79%
Audiometry	Normal	Not done	Not done	Not done	Not done	Not done	Not done	Not done	Not done	Not done	Normal
Liver on abdominal ultrasound	Normal liver size	Not done	Liver slightly increased in size	Not done	Not done	Not done	Not done	Not done	Not done	Not done	Normal
Brain MRI	Enlarged perivascular spaces	Not done	Not done	Not done	Not done	Not done	Normal	Not done	Not done	Not done	Within normal limits
Spine MRI	Radiology report within normal limits	Not done	Not done	Not done	Not done	Not done	Mild cervical spine stenosis of the foramen magnum odontoid peg hypoplasia, dural thickening, hypoplasia of the posterior arch of C1. Lumbar hypoplasia of L1 and L2. Mil thoracic spine scoliosis	Not done	Not done	Not done	Not done
Auditory evoked potentials	Normal	Not done	Not done	Not done	Not done	Not done	Normal	Not done	Normal right ear. Prolonged absolute latencies of the left ear conductive hearing loss	Not done	Normal
Hip X-ray	Not done	Mild bilateral acetabular dysplasia	Not done	Not done	Not done	Not done	Not done	Not done	Not done	Mild bilateral acetabular dysplasia	Not done
Others						Gait analysis: Gait pattern with minor abnormalities of joint kinematics with no significant functional impact	Polysomnography: IAH 2 still mild		Normal liver and kidneys on abdominal CT scan		Normal bone density according to age

Abbreviations: MRI, magnetic resonance imaging; LVE, Left ventricular ejection fraction; AHI, Apnea hypoapnea index.

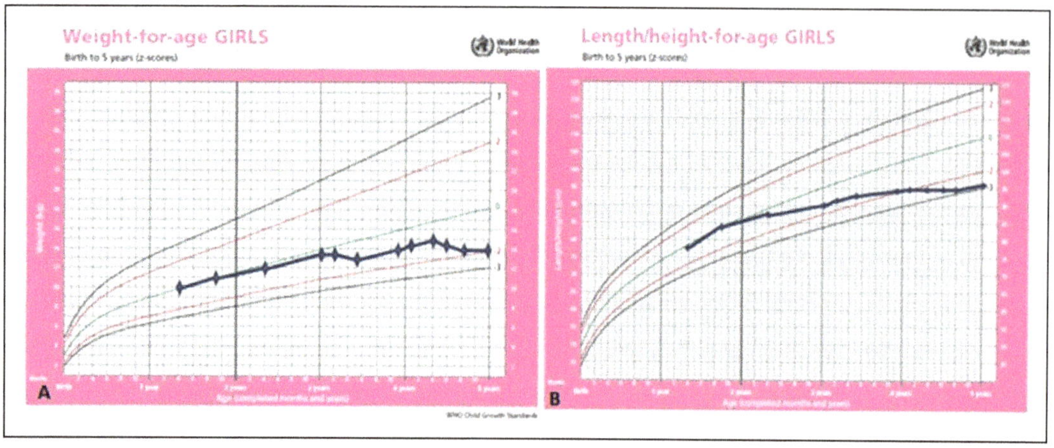

Figure 2. World Health Organization growth tables for girls 5 years of age. A, Weight curve for the patient from 5 years. B, Height curve for the patient from 5 years.

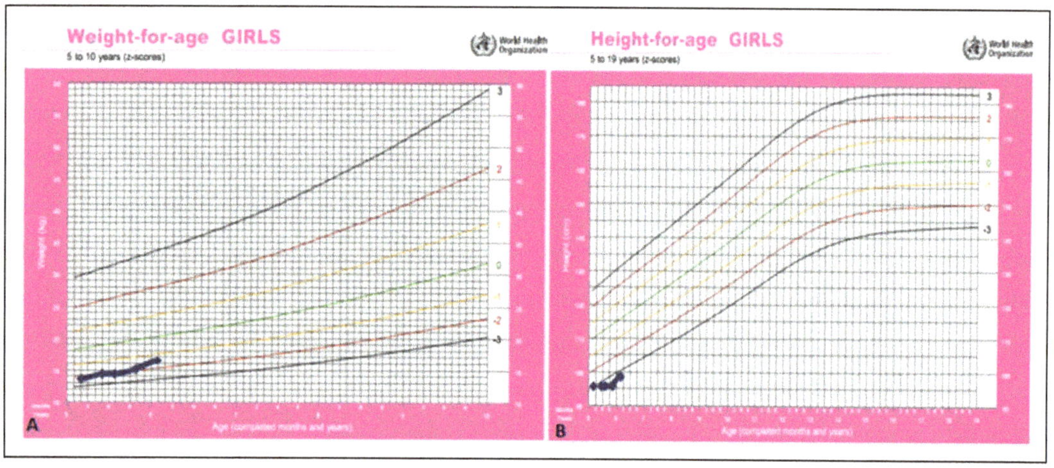

Figure 3. World Health Organization growth tables for girls up to 5 years of age. A, Weight curve for the patient from 16 months to 5 years. B, Height curve for the patient from 16 months to 5 years.

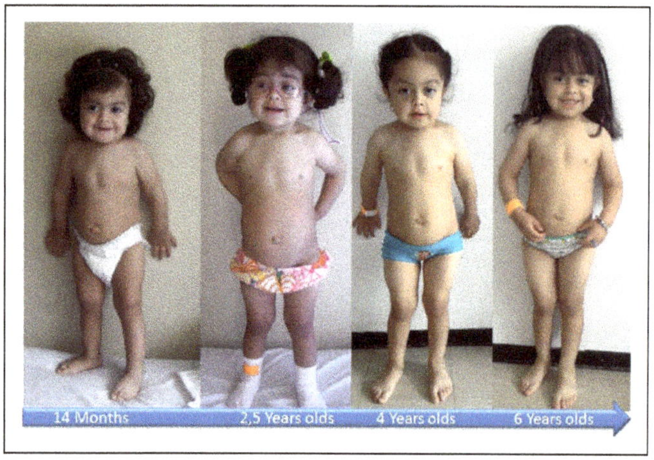

Figure 4. At different time points, the patient did not show significant progression of the disease.

and effective in slowing the progression and/or improving the burden of the disease in small children with MPS VI. The results of the study in this young cohort of patients include early recognition of the subtler symptoms associated with the slowly progressing form of the disease, which must be a priority to ensure early diagnosis and treatment. Patients must be followed closely, particularly in relation to cardiorespiratory compromise and spinal cord compression.[18]

In this case report, early diagnosis (biochemical) was made at 13 months and treatment was started at 17 months. Later, the molecular diagnosis identified c.1143-1G>C (IVS5-1g>c) and c.332 A>C (p.H111P) mutations, which have been reported in patients with the severe phenotype.[10,11] However, timely and adequate management has led to a clear arrest in the progression of the disease. Although the patient does not have a normal height, she is still within her growth percentile, but there is evidence of visceral, ocular, respiratory, and skeletal impact.

Lysosomal storage diseases are progressive, multisystem, and degenerative genetic disorders characterized by chronic deposit of macromolecules. The importance of an early initiation of ERT in patients diagnosed with lysosomal storage diseases is increasing, as ERT clearly avoids the progressive accumulation of metabolites, which could lead to cellular

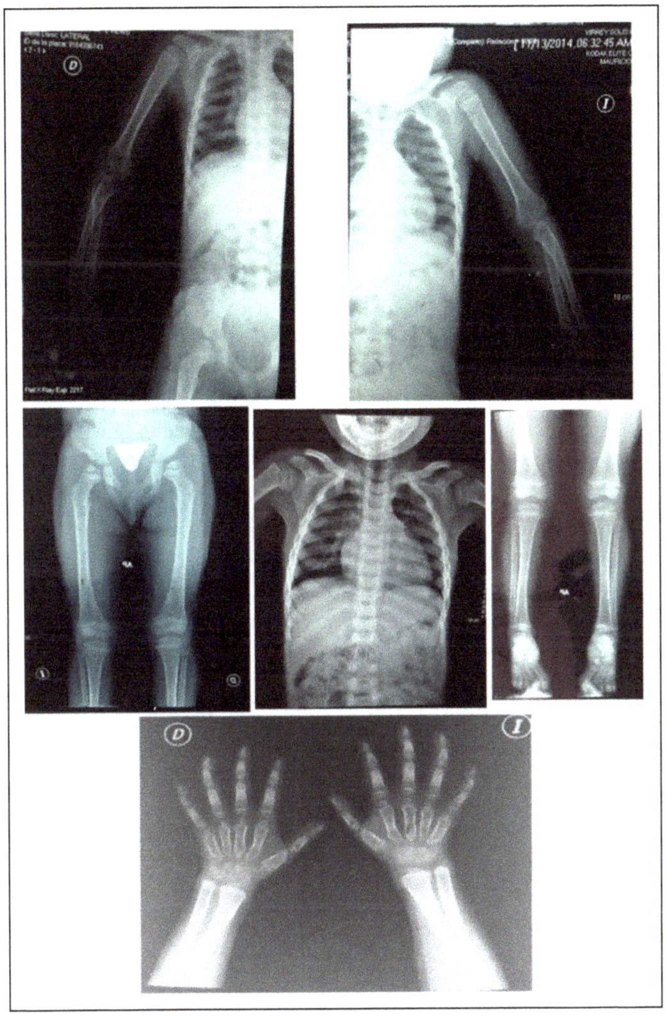

Figure 5. X-rays of the long bones and chest showing evidence of thickening of the clavicles, ribs, with slight paddle deformity due to proximal thinning and distal widening, acetabular hip dysplasia, and hand camptodactyly with mild widening of the proximal metacarpal metaphysis.

death. Thus, early initiation of ERT prevents disease progression and clinical and functional deterioration of the patient.

There are only a few reports in the indexed medical literature about MPS VI treatment. Among these reports, the one published by Lin et al stands out. It reports a case series of Taiwanese patients treated long term with galsulfase. One of the patients started the treatment at a similar age (16 months) as the one mentioned in this report.[19]

It is important to emphasize that this is the first case of MPS VI, treated before 2 years of age, reported in Colombia. This case demonstrates the importance of an early diagnosis and brings up the discussion about the convenience of performing newborn screening for lysosomal storage diseases.[20]

Conclusion

As has been shown in prior studies, and in this case report, ERT with galsulfase in patients younger than 5 years diagnosed with MPS VI is safe and effective and has a favorable impact on the natural course of the disease. This therapy has shown to improve bone and joint involvement, maintain an adequate growth curve, and frequently prevent visceral, respiratory, and cardiac compromise. The article emphasizes the importance of initiating ERT as early as possible in order to achieve the therapeutic objectives described above.

This is the first article on the Colombian population, and one of the very few published regarding the Latin American population, that reports early management of a lysosomal storage disease.

Ethical Considerations

The patient's guardian signed the informed consent for making pictures and visual recording of medical genetics with the support of Roosevelt Institute. He authorizes their use in medical publications (including articles, books, and online publications) and accepts that images may be seen by the public, besides medical and scientific researchers, who use these publications as part of their professional training.

Declaration of Conflicting Interests

The author(s) declared the following potential conflicts of interest with respect to the research, authorship, and/or publication of this article: Biomarin Colombia LTDA sponsored the translation and publication of this article.

Funding

The author(s) received no financial support for the research, authorship, and/or publication of this article.

References

1. Matalon R, Arbogast B, Dorfman A. Deficiency of chondroitin sulfate N-acetylgalactosamine 4-sulfate sulfatase in Maroteaux-Lamy syndrome. *Biochem Biophys Res Commun*. 1974;61(4): 1450-1457.
2. Valayannopoulos V, Nicely H, Harmatz P, Turbeville S. Mucopolysaccharidosis VI. *Orphanet J Rare Dis*. 2010;5:5.
3. Giugliani R, Federhen A, Rojas MV, et al. Mucopolysaccharidosis I, II, and VI: brief review and guidelines for treatment. *Genet Mol Biol*. 2010;33(4):589-604.
4. Neufeld E, Muenzer J. The mucopolysaccharidoses. In: Scriver C, Beaudet A, Valle D, Sly W, eds. *The Metabolic and Molecular Bases of Inherited Disease*. 8th ed. New York, NY: McGraw-Hill; 2001:3421-3452.
5. El Dib RP, Pastores GM. A systematic review of new advances in the management of mucopolysaccharidosis VI (Maroteaux-Lamy syndrome): focus on galsulfase. *Biologics*. 2009;3:459-468.
6. Coelho JC, Wajner M, Burin MG, Vargas CR, Giugliani R. Selective screening of 10,000 high-risk Brazilian patients for the detection of inborn errors of metabolism. *Eur J Pediatr*. 1997;156(8): 650-654.
7. Giugliani R, Harmatz P, Wraith JE. Management guidelines for mucopolysaccharidosis VI. *Pediatrics*. 2007;120(2):405-418.

8. Karageorgos L, Brooks DA, Pollard A, et al. Mutational analysis of 105 mucopolysaccharidosis type VI patients. *Hum Mutat.* 2007;28(9):897-903.
9. Giugliani R, Lampe C, Guffon N, et al. Natural history and galsulfase treatment in mucopolysaccharidosis VI (MPS VI, Maroteaux-Lamy syndrome)—10-year follow-up of patients who previously participated in an MPS VI Survey Study. *Am J Med Genet A.* 2014;164A(8):1953-1964.
10. Garrido E, Chabás A, Coll MJ, et al. Identification of the molecular defects in Spanish and Argentinian mucopolysaccharidosis VI (Maroteaux-Lamy syndrome) patients, including 9 novel mutations. *Mol Genet Metab.* 2007;92(1-2):122-130.
11. Giraldo GA, Ayala-Ramírez P, Prieto JC, García-Robles R, Acosta JC. Molecular findings of Colombian patients with type VI mucopolysaccharidosis (Maroteaux-Lamy syndrome). *Meta Gene.* 2015;7:83-89.
12. Maroteaux P, Leveque B, Marie J, Lamy M. A new dysostosis with urinary elimination of chondroitin sulfate B [in French]. *Presse Med.* 1963;71:1849-1852.
13. Braunlin EA, Harmatz PR, Scarpa M, et al. Cardiac disease in patients with mucopolysaccharidosis: presentation, diagnosis and management. *J Inherit Metab Dis.* 2011;34(6):1183-1197.
14. Harmatz P, Ketteridge D, Giugliani R, et al. Direct comparison of measures of endurance, mobility, and joint function during enzyme-replacement therapy of mucopolysaccharidosis VI (Maroteaux-Lamy syndrome): results after 48 weeks in a phase 2 open-label clinical study of recombinant human N-acetylgalactosamine 4-sulfatase. *Pediatrics.* 2005;115(6): e681-e689.
15. Harmatz P, Giugliani R, Schwartz I, et al. Enzyme replacement therapy for mucopolysaccharidosis VI: a phase 3, randomized, double-blind, placebo-controlled, multinational study of recombinant human N-acetylgalactosamine 4-sulfatase (recombinant human arylsulfatase B or rhASB) and follow-on, open-label extension study. *J Pediatr.* 2006;148(4):533-539.
16. McGill JJ, Inwood AC, Coman DJ, et al. Enzyme replacement therapy for mucopolysaccharidosis VI from 8 weeks of age—a sibling control study. *Clin Genet.* 2010;77(5):492-498.
17. Ribeiro E AA, Giuliani L, Horovitz D, et al. Experience in treating very young mucopolysaccharidosis VI patients with ERT. *J Inherit Metab Dis.* 2010;33 suppl:1.
18. Horovitz DD, Magalhães TS, Acosta A, et al. Enzyme replacement therapy with galsulfase in 34 children younger than five years of age with MPS VI. *Mol Genet Metab.* 2013;109(1):62-69.
19. Lin HY, Chuang CK, Wang CH, et al. Long-term galsulfase enzyme replacement therapy in Taiwanese mucopolysaccharidosis VI patients: a case series. *Mol Genet Metab Rep.* 2016;7: 63-69.
20. Giugliani R. Newborn screening for lysosomal diseases: current status and potential interface with population medical genetics in Latin America. *J Inherit Metab Dis.* 2012;35(5):871-877. doi:10.1007/s10545-011-9436-z. PubMed PMID:22231381.

13

An Adaptation of the Profile of Mood States for Use in Adults With Phenylketonuria

Elizabeth D. Bacci, PhD[1], Kathleen W. Wyrwich, PhD[2], Katharine S. Gries, PhD[1], Yinpu Chen, PhD[3], Rishabh Jain, MS[3], Laurel Konkol, MS[3], Markus J. Merilainen, MD[3], and Haoling H. Weng, MD[3]

Abstract

Adults with phenylketonuria (PKU) experience disturbances in mood. This study used qualitative and quantitative techniques to adapt the 65-item Profile of Mood States (POMS) for the assessment of key mood domains in adults with PKU. First, cognitive interviews on 58 POMS items (excluding 7 Friendliness domain items) among 15 adults and adolescents (age ≥ 16 years) with PKU were conducted to eliminate items poorly understood or considered irrelevant to PKU; 17 items were removed. Next, the remaining POMS items were quantitatively examined (Mokken scaling and Rasch analysis) in 115 adult patients with PKU. An additional 21 items were removed iteratively, resulting in the 20-item draft PKU-POMS. Finally, the psychometric properties of the draft PKU-POMS were examined. The instrument displayed strong psychometric properties (reliability, validity, and responsiveness) over 6 domains (Anxiety, Depression, Anger, Activity, Tiredness, and Confusion) and all items were well understood in the final cognitive interviews with 10 adults with PKU.

Keywords

phenylketonuria, profile of mood states, patient-reported outcome, psychometric, item reduction, cognitive interview

Introduction

Phenylketonuria (PKU; Online Mendelian Inheritance in Man 261600 and 261630]) is a rare autosomal recessive inborn error of metabolism in which the body is deficient in the phenylalanine (Phe) hydroxylase enzyme and as a result is unable to process the amino acid Phe. If untreated, Phe will accumulate in the body and cause mental retardation (in children), microcephaly, delayed speech, delayed social skills, psychiatric symptoms, and behavioral abnormalities.[1] Uncontrolled blood Phe levels in adulthood are also associated with executive dysfunction; lack of concentration; anxiety; depression; and a variety of behavioral, psychiatric, and mood problems.[2-5] ten Hoedt and colleagues[6] conducted a randomized double-blind, placebo-controlled cross-over study of Dutch patients with PKU to determine the effect of high Phe levels on mood using a revised version of the Profile of Mood States (POMSr) instrument designed to provide data on 5 categories of mood states: tension, depression, anger, vigor, and fatigue.[7] Results indicated that when patients were in the high Phe intake period, their overall mood was worse ($p = .017$), and they were more fatigued ($p = .021$) and less vigorous ($p = .006$) than when in the placebo period, providing evidence of the potential importance of the POMS and mood symptoms in understanding the effects of Phe intake in adults with PKU. However, no patient-reported outcome (PRO) measure of mood symptoms has been developed specifically for patients with PKU.

The original 65-item POMSr PRO, developed in 1971, has been used across various therapeutic areas for the assessment of a respondent's transient and variable moods; however, it has never been used with patients with PKU.[8] The 65-item POMS is a self-administered evaluation that uses a 5-point Likert scale ranging from 0 (*Not at all*), 1 (*A little*) 2 (*Moderately*), 3 (*Quite*

[1] Evidera, Inc, Seattle, WA, USA
[2] Evidera Inc, Bethesda, MD, USA
[3] BioMarin Pharmaceuticals Inc, Novato, CA, USA

Corresponding Author:
Elizabeth D. Bacci, Evidera, Inc, 1417 4th Avenue, Suite 510, Seattle, WA 98101, USA.
Email: elizabeth.bacci@evidera.com

a bit), to 4 (*Extremely*). Mood states are interpreted though 6 mood domains: tension-anxiety (9 items), depression-dejection (15 items), anger-hostility (12 items), vigor-activity (8 items), fatigue-inertia (7 items), and confusion-bewilderment (7 items). The POMS user manual contains the full list of these items.[8] The remaining 7 items relate to the friendliness domain; however, subsequent analyses by the POMS developers showed evidence that the friendliness domain is considered too weak to be scored.[9] Although widely used, the POMS instrument has been subjected to various revisions in order to reduce the number of items or to better adapt the instrument for the assessment of mood symptoms in a specific target patient population[10-14] or specific culture.[7,15-18] These studies used either qualitative or quantitative research techniques to modify the instrument, resulting in a reduced number of items, the addition of items, or the reconfiguration of the domain structure. Limited validation research has been conducted to assess the psychometric properties of some of the reduced or adapted POMS instruments; no extensive validation research has been conducted on any one version.[19-21]

Aims

The aim of the current study was to use qualitative and quantitative analytic techniques to adapt the 65-item POMS for the assessment of key mood states in adults with PKU and to assess the psychometric properties of this revised instrument, as this instrument was not developed or validated specifically for use in patients with PKU.

Methods

A multistep process that incorporated both qualitative and quantitative analyses was used to develop the PKU-POMS. This process consisted of 3 phases: (1) qualitative assessment of item comprehensibility, acceptability, and relevance to adults with PKU; (2) quantitative assessment of item and domain performance and item reduction; and (3) quantitative and qualitative assessment of the draft items.

Phase 1: Qualitative Assessment of Item Comprehensibility, Acceptability, and Relevance to Adults With PKU

In phase 1, one-on-one qualitative (mixture of in person and telephone) interviews were conducted in the United States among individuals with PKU in order to determine if any of the 58 POMS items (after removal of the seven friendliness items) should be removed due to the lack of comprehension, acceptability, and relevance to patients with PKU.

Patient population. Participants were eligible to participate if they were English speaking, 16 years of age or older, diagnosed with PKU, and were not currently taking or had not taken any medication intended to treat PKU (eg, levodopa, pegvaliase, Kuvan, BH4, and neutral amino acid) in the past 4 weeks. Participants were recruited through the distribution of study fliers; in person or via e-mail to patients attending the 2014 National PKU Alliance Conference and posted to a study Web site. This study was approved by the Ethical and Independent Review Services Institutional Review Board (http://www.eandireview.com/).

Procedures and analysis. Study staff trained on the conduct of patient interviews conducted one-on-one cognitive debriefing interviews with participating patients using a semi-structured interview guide, which involved asking the participants questions about the 58 POMS items to address the comprehensiveness, acceptability, and relevance to patients with PKU. Following completion of the interviews, 2 study staff members independently reviewed the cognitive debriefing portion of the interview transcripts to determine if any of the POMS items should be removed based on established thresholds. Items were considered for removal if >25% of respondents did not understand the item, did not think the item was acceptable because it was not a "good word to use," or did not find the item relevant to PKU. Only the items retained through this analysis were included in the analyses in phase 2 (quantitative assessment).

Phase 2: Quantitative Assessment of Item and Domain Performance and Item Reduction

In phase 2, a series of iterative quantitative analyses were conducted in order to assess item and domain performance of the retained POMS items from phase 1, and to remove poorly performing items, as needed, to achieve acceptable measurement properties in patients with PKU. This phase consisted of 3 steps including (1) examination of item-level descriptive and domain structure, (2) item reduction using Mokken scale assessment (MSA), and (3) finally item evaluation using Rasch analysis.

Data source. The pegvaliase (BMN 165) clinical development program was designed to demonstrate the safety and efficacy of pegvaliase in the treatment of adult patients with PKU. Data were used from PRISM-1 study (formerly referred to as BMN 165-301)—a phase 3, open-label, randomized study designed to further characterize the safety of pegvaliase of individuals being treated in induction, titration, and maintenance dose regimens in adults with PKU who have not had previous exposure to pegvaliase (ClinicalTrials.gov: NCT01819727). Study participants were 18 to 70 years old and recruited from 32 study sites in the United States. Individuals were required to have a diagnosis of PKU with blood Phe concentration >600 μmol/L at screening and average blood Phe concentration of >600 μmol/L over the past 6 months per medical history. The analytic population for the current analysis included all enrolled patients who completed a POMS assessment at day 1.

Step 1: Examination of item-level descriptive and domain structure. The frequency and percentage of each response category was assessed, as well as the mean, percentages of minimum and maximum responses for floor and ceiling effects[22] (ie, >50% of participants selecting a response of 0 or 4), and percentage missing. An item was flagged for further investigation and possible removal if it exhibited floor/ceiling effects or excessive missingness (>5% missing), as this is indicative that the range of available response options are not appropriate for the patient population.

To understand the domain structure of the reduced POMS prior to further quantitative analyses to assess the instrument, confirmatory factor analysis (CFA) was conducted. The CFA was conducted to model the fit of the items to each of the 6 POMS domains separately. The following statistics and threshold values were used to evaluate model fit: comparative fit index (CFI) $\geq$0.90, root mean square error of approximation (RMSEA) $\leq$0.10, and weighted root mean square residual (WRMR) $\leq$0.05. Acceptable item fit was demonstrated if items had a factor loading $\geq$0.40.[23,24]

Step 2: Item reduction using MSA. The MSA is a nonparametric method of data reduction that uses a probabilistic, hierarchical search procedure to identify the best subset of similar items within a measurement scale or domain of items.[25] The model assumes that the data are defined by unidimensionality (ie, 1 latent trait is being measured), local monotonicity (ie, as a person's mood decreases, the chance of giving a response indicating improved mood should never increase), and local independence (ie, responses to any 2 items should be independent and not depend on any other aspects of the respondent or items). Loevinger's coefficient H[26] was used to assess the scalability of the POMS items within each domain, and the 6 domains within the overall instrument. Mokken[27] proposed an interpretation of this scalability coefficient: H > 0.5 indicates a strong scale, 0.4 < H < 0.5 indicates a medium scale, and 0.3 < H < 0.4 indicates a weak scale. Items with loadings <0.4 were considered candidates for item removal. An iterative process of item removal was used by removing items within a domain one by one and checking the scalability coefficients for each iterative revision. This process continued until no items had loadings below 0.4 and the scalability coefficient for each domain was considered medium or strong.

Step 3: Final item evaluation using Rasch analysis. Following the Mokken scaling analysis, separate Rasch analyses were conducted using the reduced sets of items within each of the 6 POMS domains. Rasch analysis was selected to determine if each item and domain fit the Rasch measurement model,[28] which has scaling properties of linear and interval measurement.[29] With the Rasch model, the probability of a positive response is modeled as a logistic function of the simultaneous difference between a patient's PKU severity and the severity that is measured by that item response. The following parameters were examined to determine acceptable Rasch model fit: (1) threshold ordering (ie, determine if each item's response category probability distributions indicate the proper ordering of response category shifts across all categories); (2) residual fit statistics to assess item redundancy and multidimensionality (ie, evidence that an item is being affected by some other dimension other than the latent trait the scale is measuring); and (3) χ^2 item fit of the observed data to the model. Individual item test of fit showed the χ^2 probability for each item, where items with P < .05 were considered ill fitting. Items with high negative residuals (<−3.0) indicated an overfitting item, wherein the information provided by this item did not add additional value to the measure. High positive residuals (>3.0) indicated that the item was underfitting, indicating that the item had a poor model fit and the response categories were underdiscriminating or not discriminating differences in severity.[30] Failure to meet these standard thresholds can be indicative of a flawed item in need of revision or removal.

An iterative series of Rasch models were fit and examined in relation to the thresholds above, such that within each iteration, the previous iteration's most problematic item(s) was removed, continuing as long as there was poor fit of the Rasch model. However, to increase domain reliability, all efforts were made to retain at least 3 items per domain.[31] The remaining items were deemed the final items to compose the draft POMS for use in patients with PKU (ie, PKU-POMS) subjected to a final quantitative and qualitative confirmatory assessment in phase 3.

Phase 3: Quantitative and Qualitative Assessment of the Draft Items

In phase 3, the psychometric properties of the draft PKU-POMS were assessed using data from PRISM-1 study. These assessments included internal consistency reliability using Cronbach's α (day 1); convergent validity using Pearson's correlations between scores on each PKU-POMS domain and scores on the Attention-Deficit Hyperactivity Disorder Rating Scale-IV (ADHD RS-IV) and plasma Phe values (day 1); and responsiveness using Pearson's correlations between change from day 1 to end of study (EOS) on each PKU-POMS domain and change in the ADHD RS-IV and plasma Phe. Plasma Phe was selected for use in the validation analyses as exploratory, because although it is an objective measure of patients' health in this patient population, it was unknown if changes in mood states would correspond to changes in Phe.

Finally, one-on-one cognitive interviews were conducted via telephone to investigate the acceptability of the draft PKU-POMS in adults with PKU, including the relevance of all retained items as well as the understandability of the instructions, recall period, response options, item content, and domains. The patient population was a separate, but highly similar, patient population of the initial qualitative interviews conducted in phase 1 (with the same inclusion/exclusion criteria required for participation), in order to ensure that the final draft instrument is understood in the same population in which it was created and validated.

Results

Phase 1: Qualitative Assessment of Item Comprehensibility, Acceptability, and Relevance to Patients With PKU

Interviews were conducted with 9 women (60%) and 6 men (40%) with PKU (mean age: 30.4 ± 12.9 years). All participants were diagnosed with PKU during the first year of life, and the majority were currently following a Phe-restricted diet (93.3%). Only 2 participants (13.3%) reported a formal diagnosis of anxiety, and 2 (13.3%) reported a formal diagnosis of depression.

Seventeen POMS items were identified that were not well understood (eg, Muddled, Shaky), not acceptable as a good word to use (eg, Bushed, Bewildered), or not relevant to patients with PKU (eg, Unworthy, Guilty). These 17 items were removed from the proposed PKU-POMS, as detailed in Table 1, resulting in 41 remaining items.

Table 1. POMS Items Removed From Revised POMS Following PKU Patient Interviews.[a]

POMS Domain (Number of Items)	Items Removed
Vigor-activity (8)	Q56. Full of pep
	Q60. Carefree
	Q63. Vigorous
Confusion-bewilderment (7)	Q37. Muddled
	Q50. Bewildered
Tension-anxiety (9)	Q2. Tense
	Q10. Shaky
	Q16. On edge
	Q27. Restless
Fatigue-inertia (7)	Q11. Listless
	Q65. Bushed
Anger-hostility (12)	Q12. Peeved
	Q24. Spiteful
Depression-dejection (15)	Q9. Sorry for things done
	Q18. Blue
	Q23. Unworthy
	Q62. Guilty

Abbreviations: PKU, phenylketonuria; POMS, profile of mood states.
[a]N = 15

Phase 2: Quantitative Assessment of Item and Domain Performance and Item Reduction

Data from a total of 115 patients with PKU were available for the analysis from PRISM-1 study. Patient demographic characteristics are presented in Table 2.

Table 2. Sociodemographic and Clinical Characteristics at Day 1.[a]

	Day 1
Age, years	
n	115
Mean (SD)	29.1 (8.8)
Median (range)	28.0 (16–51)
Sex, n (%)	
Male	59 (51.3%)
Female	56 (48.7%)
Race, n (%)	
American Indian or Alaska Native	1 (0.9%)
Black or African American	3 (2.6%)
White or Caucasian	109 (94.8%)
Other	2 (1.7%)
Plasma Phe level at day 1 (μmol/L)	
n	114
Mean (SD)	1217 (389.0)
Median (range)	1211 (510–2330)
ADHD RS-IV at day 1	
n	114
Mean (SD)	9.9 (5.7)
Median (range)	9.5 (0–26)

Abbreviations: ADHD RS-IV, Attention Deficit Hyperactivity Disorder Rating Scale IV; Phe, phenylalanine; SD, standard deviation.
[a]N = 115.

Step 1. Examination of item-level descriptive and domain structure. Descriptive statistics for the 41 remaining POMS items are shown in Table 3. At day 1, 14 of the 41 items displayed floor effects (ie, item where ≥50% of sample responded "not at all"), while no items displayed ceiling effects (ie, item where ≥50% of sample responded "extremely"). No items exhibited missingness >2%.

The CFA was conducted using the retained 41 items, yielding estimates of global model fit for each individual POMS domain. Using thresholds for acceptable fit, global model fit was found to be unacceptable for all 6 POMS domains (Table 4). In addition, the items weary, alert, and efficient were found to have low item loadings (ie, <0.40). The findings of lack of domain and item-level fit indicated that these 41 remaining POMS items did not conform to the 6-domain structure of the original POMS in this patient population, and informed the item analyses that followed.

Step 2: Item reduction using MSA. The MSA was conducted to assess item fit to each domain as well as the scalability of each of the 6 domains to the overall model. Using the H coefficient as an indicator of scalability, the depression-dejection and fatigue-inertia domains were found to be strong, tension-anxiety and anger-hostility were found to be medium, and vigor-activity and confusion-bewilderment were found to be weak (column 1 of Table 5).

In addition, each domain included at least 1 item that had a low item loading (ie, H < 0.40). Items with low item scalability coefficients were removed from each domain, one at a time, and the fit of the domain reassessed. This iterative process continued within each domain separately until all items demonstrated a loading above 0.4 and each domain had an H value indicative of a strong scale (column 2 of Table 5). Specifically, in the first iteration of the MSA analysis, the following items were removed by domain: alert (vigor-activity), relaxed (tension-anxiety), efficient and uncertain about things (confusion-bewilderment), weary (fatigue-inertia), rebellious (anger-hostility), and terrified

Table 3. Descriptive Statistics of POMS at Day 1.[a,b]

Item	n	Mean (SD)	Frequency, n (%)					
			Not At All (Floor)	A Little	Moderately	Quite a Bit	Extremely (Ceiling)	Missing
Angry	115	1.1 (1.1)	40 (34.8%)	38 (33.0%)	27 (23.5%)	6 (5.2%)	4 (3.5%)	
Worn out	115	2.1 (1.2)	11 (9.6%)	28 (24.3%)	29 (25.2%)	31 (27.0%)	16 (13.9%)	
Unhappy	114	1.0 (1.0)	42 (36.5%)	47 (40.9%)	15 (13.0%)	7 (6.1%)	3 (2.6%)	1 (0.9%)
Lively	115	2.2 (1.0)	6 (5.2%)	21 (18.3%)	42 (36.5%)	33 (28.7%)	13 (11.3%)	
Confused	115	1.0 (1.0)	47 (40.9%)	36 (31.3%)	22 (19.1%)	7 (6.1%)	3 (2.6%)	
Sad	115	1.0 (1.1)	46 (40.0%)	39 (33.9%)	17 (14.8%)	8 (7.0%)	5 (4.3%)	
Active	115	2.4 (1.1)	4 (3.5%)	22 (19.1%)	33 (28.7%)	40 (34.8%)	16 (13.9%)	
Grouchy	115	1.3 (1.2)	33 (28.7%)	40 (34.8%)	26 (22.6%)	8 (7.0%)	8 (7.0%)	
Energetic	115	2.1 (1.1)	10 (8.7%)	23 (20.0%)	41 (35.7%)	28 (24.3%)	13 (11.3%)	
Panicky	115	1.0 (1.2)	50 (43.5%)	33 (28.7%)	18 (15.7%)	8 (7.0%)	6 (5.2%)	
Hopeless	115	0.5 (0.9)	**80 (69.6%)**	18 (15.7%)	13 (11.3%)	2 (1.7%)	2 (1.7%)	
Relaxed	115	2.1 (1.1)	7 (6.1%)	28 (24.3%)	36 (31.3%)	34 (29.6%)	10 (8.7%)	
Uneasy	115	1.2 (1.1)	37 (32.2%)	34 (29.6%)	29 (25.2%)	10 (8.7%)	5 (4.3%)	
Unable to concentrate	115	1.5 (1.2)	28 (24.3%)	33 (28.7%)	26 (22.6%)	19 (16.5%)	9 (7.8%)	
Fatigued	115	1.9 (1.2)	15 (13.0%)	37 (32.2%)	21 (18.3%)	31 (27.0%)	11 (9.6%)	
Annoyed	115	1.8 (1.2)	17 (14.8%)	29 (25.2%)	36 (31.3%)	23 (20.0%)	10 (8.7%)	
Discouraged	115	1.2 (1.2)	45 (39.1%)	33 (28.7%)	20 (17.4%)	8 (7.0%)	9 (7.8%)	
Resentful	115	0.5 (0.9)	**75 (65.2%)**	24 (20.9%)	12 (10.4%)	3 (2.6%)	1 (0.9%)	
Nervous	115	1.6 (1.2)	26 (22.6%)	36 (31.3%)	23 (20.0%)	22 (19.1%)	8 (7.0%)	
Lonely	114	0.9 (1.2)	**62 (53.9%)**	26 (22.6%)	12 (10.4%)	8 (7.0%)	6 (5.2%)	1 (0.9%)
Miserable	115	0.6 (1.1)	**79 (68.7%)**	18 (15.7%)	7 (6.1%)	8 (7.0%)	3 (2.6%)	
Cheerful	115	2.3 (1.0)	3 (2.6%)	20 (17.4%)	40 (34.8%)	39 (33.9%)	13 (11.3%)	
Bitter	115	0.5 (0.8)	**69 (60.0%)**	31 (27.0%)	13 (11.3%)	2 (1.7%)		
Exhausted	115	1.8 (1.3)	19 (16.5%)	33 (28.7%)	27 (23.5%)	22 (19.1%)	14 (12.2%)	
Anxious	115	1.8 (1.2)	18 (15.7%)	33 (28.7%)	28 (24.3%)	23 (20.0%)	13 (11.3%)	
Ready to fight	115	0.6 (1.0)	**77 (67.0%)**	20 (17.4%)	10 (8.7%)	6 (5.2%)	2 (1.7%)	
Gloomy	115	0.8 (1.1)	**63 (54.8%)**	30 (26.1%)	10 (8.7%)	8 (7.0%)	4 (3.5%)	
Desperate	115	0.3 (0.8)	**91 (79.1%)**	13 (11.3%)	8 (7.0%)	2 (1.7%)	1 (0.9%)	
Sluggish	115	1.5 (1.3)	33 (28.7%)	30 (26.1%)	24 (20.9%)	20 (17.4%)	8 (7.0%)	
Rebellious	115	0.6 (0.9)	**69 (60.0%)**	31 (27.0%)	8 (7.0%)	6 (5.2%)	1 (0.9%)	
Helpless	115	0.4 (0.8)	**86 (74.8%)**	17 (14.8%)	7 (6.1%)	4 (3.5%)	1 (0.9%)	
Weary	115	0.8 (0.8)	50 (43.5%)	43 (37.4%)	20 (17.4%)	1 (0.9%)	1 (0.9%)	
Alert	114	2.4 (1.0)	3 (2.6%)	19 (16.5%)	37 (32.2%)	42 (36.5%)	13 (11.3%)	1 (0.9%)
Deceived	114	0.5 (0.9)	**83 (72.2%)**	15 (13.0%)	9 (7.8%)	5 (4.3%)	2 (1.7%)	1 (0.9%)
Furious	114	0.7 (1.2)	77 (67.0%)	16 (13.9%)	11 (9.6%)	2 (1.7%)	8 (7.0%)	1 (0.9%)
Efficient	113	2.1 (1.1)	9 (7.8%)	23 (20.0%)	35 (30.4%)	38 (33.0%)	8 (7.0%)	2 (1.7%)
Bad-tempered	114	0.9 (1.1)	**58 (50.4%)**	27 (23.5%)	15 (13.0%)	10 (8.7%)	4 (3.5%)	1 (0.9%)
Worthless	113	0.5 (0.9)	**84 (73.0%)**	12 (10.4%)	11 (9.6%)	6 (5.2%)		2 (1.7%)
Forgetful	114	1.6 (1.3)	24 (20.9%)	35 (30.4%)	30 (26.1%)	12 (10.4%)	13 (11.3%)	1 (0.9%)
Terrified	114	0.4 (0.7)	**80 (69.6%)**	24 (20.9%)	7 (6.1%)	3 (2.6%)		1 (0.9%)
Uncertain about things	114	1.7 (1.3)	25 (21.7%)	25 (21.7%)	30 (26.1%)	22 (19.1%)	12 (10.4%)	1 (0.9%)

Abbreviations: POMS, profile of mood states; SD, standard deviation.
[a]Boldface values indicate items with floor effects (>50%).
[b]N = 115.

(depression-dejection). In the second iteration of the MSA analysis, cheerful (vigor-activity) and resentful (anger-hostility) were removed. Finally, in the third iteration of the MSA analysis, only bitter (anger-hostility) was removed. A total of 10 items were removed in step 2, resulting in 31 remaining items.

Step 3: Final item evaluation using Rasch analysis. The fit of the remaining 31 items to the Rasch measurement model was then assessed, separately within each POMS domain (Table 6). This analysis demonstrated that the fit of each item within the vigor-activity and tension-anxiety domains met the established thresholds for the Rasch measurement model. For the confusion-bewilderment domain, the fit of each item was acceptable according to the fit residuals and χ^2 values; however, the response thresholds for forgetful were found to be disordered. Specifically, moving from a response of 0 (Not at all) to a 1 (A little) and from 1 (A little) to 2 (Moderately) corresponded to a linear increase in the latent trait of experiencing a confused mood state, but moving from a 3 (Quite a bit) to 4 (Extremely) was actually associated with a lesser experience of a confused mood state. By collapsing response options of Extremely with Quite a bit, the thresholds for this item were ordered, and the fit

Table 4. Confirmatory Factor Analysis of POMS at Day 1.

PKU-POMS Domain, Item	Standardized Coefficient or Model Fits (RMSEA, CFI, WRMR)[a]
Vigor-activity	0.14, 0.97, 0.53
Lively	0.72
Active	0.72
Energetic	0.82
Cheerful	0.57
Alert	0.35
Tension-anxiety	0.17, 0.96, 0.66
Panicky	0.79
Relaxed	−0.35
Uneasy	0.69
Nervous	0.82
Anxious	0.77
Confusion-bewilderment	0.00, 1.00, 0.26
Confused	0.62
Unable to concentrate	0.80
Efficient	−0.28
Forgetful	0.87
Uncertain about things	0.59
Fatigue-inertia	0.09, 1.00, 0.39
Worn out	0.84
Fatigued	0.81
Exhausted	0.90
Sluggish	0.73
Weary	0.30
Anger-hostility	0.12, 0.95, 0.86
Angry	0.70
Grouchy	0.71
Annoyed	0.79
Resentful	0.70
Bitter	0.70
Ready to fight	0.76
Rebellious	0.62
Deceived	0.78
Furious	0.84
Bad-tempered	0.80
Depression-dejection	0.08, 0.99, 0.68
Unhappy	0.78
Sad	0.86
Hopeless	0.85
Discouraged	0.86
Lonely	0.84
Miserable	0.85
Gloomy	0.85
Desperate	0.77
Helpless	0.75
Worthless	0.93
Terrified	0.56

Abbreviations: CFI, comparative fit index; EOS, end of study; PKU, phenylketonuria; POMS, profile of mood states; RMSEA, root mean square error of approximation; WRMR, weighted root mean square residual.
[a]Model fit thresholds for acceptable fit included CFI ≥0.90, RMSEA ≤0.10, and WRMR ≤0.05.

of all items in this domain found acceptable. For the fatigue-inertia domain, fatigued was also found to have disordered thresholds, but the removal of this item rather than collapsing item response thresholds increased the performance of this domain overall.

For the remaining 2 domains (anger-hostility and depression-dejection), a more iterative series of Rasch analyses were conducted to arrive at best fit due to the large number of problematic items within these domains in fitting the Rasch measurement model (Table 6). The selection of items to remove was based on the performance of each item in relation to established thresholds, the possibility of collapsing response options, and considering the distribution of each item (eg, presence of high floor effects [>50%]; Table 3). In the anger-hostility domain, 4 items demonstrated disordered thresholds in the initial Rasch analysis. To improve fit, all items were removed but the 3 without floor effects (angry, grouchy, and annoyed), but in the resulting model, grouchy remained disordered. After collapsing the response options of quite a bit and extremely in grouchy, an acceptable fit was found for this domain. For depression-dejection, 6 items displayed threshold disordering in the initial Rasch analysis, and 7 displayed high floor effects. The set of 3 items without floor effects (unhappy, sad, and discouraged) fit the Rasch model well with no threshold disordering. In order to retain at least 4 items, all removed items were reintroduced one by one with the 3 remaining items, and the fit of the items and domain reassessed. Only the reincorporation of lonely performed adequately and was included in the final depression-dejection domain.

Overall, 11 items were removed using Rasch analysis; the Rasch model parameters and item fit statistics of the remaining 20 items are provided in Table 6. A final MSA within each domain of the remaining 20 items was also conducted (column 3 of Table 5); all item loadings were acceptable and the scalability coefficient indicated that all items and scales were medium to strong. Given acceptable scalability and fit to the Rasch model, these remaining 20 items were used to compose the draft PKU-POMS. The 6 domains were renamed to reflect the remaining items after removal of items from phases 1 and 2 as follows: anxiety, depression, anger, activity, tiredness, and confusion (formerly tension-anxiety, depression-dejection, anger-hostility, vigor-activity, fatigue-inertia, and confusion-bewilderment, respectively).

Phase 3: Quantitative and Qualitative Assessment of Draft Items

Psychometric assessment of the draft 20-item PKU-POMS indicated that each domain demonstrated high internal consistency (Cronbach's $\alpha = 0.75\text{-}0.87$). Pearson's correlations between each domain and the ADHD RS-IV (except activity and depression) were statistically significant. Correlations with plasma Phe levels were not statistically significant (Table 7). Finally, when using correlations with the ADHD RS-IV inattentiveness scores as the primary analysis of responsiveness, all PKU-POMS domains (except depression) exhibited responsiveness to change from day 1 to EOS (Table 7). Correlations with plasma Phe were treated as exploratory and demonstrated support for the responsiveness of anxiety, depression, and confusion domains.

Finally, cognitive interviews were conducted with 5 women and 5 men with PKU (mean age: 27.2 ± 4.6 years).

Table 5. Mokken Scaling Assessment Results.[a]

PKU-POMS Domain, Item	Initial MSA H Scaling Coefficient[b]	Final MSA (Pre-Rasch Analysis) H Scaling Coefficient[b]	Final MSA (Post-Rasch Analysis) H Scaling Coefficient[b]
Tension-anxiety	Fit of item to domain	Fit of item to domain	Fit of item to domain
Full-scale H	0.46 (0.06)	0.57 (0.06)	0.57 (0.06)
Panicky	0.53 (0.06)	0.56 (0.07)	0.56 (0.07)
Relaxed	0.28[c] (0.08)	—[c]	—[c]
Uneasy	0.47 (0.07)	0.51 (0.07)	0.51 (0.07)
Nervous	0.52 (0.06)	0.60 (0.06)	0.60 (0.06)
Anxious	0.49 (0.06)	0.60 (0.06)	0.59 (0.06)
Vigor-activity			
Full-scale H	0.39 (0.06)	0.55 (0.07)	0.54 (0.07)
Lively	0.43 (0.07)	0.49 (0.09)	0.48 (0.09)
Active	0.41 (0.06)	0.55 (0.07)	0.54 (0.07)
Energetic	0.47 (0.06)	0.61 (0.06)	0.60 (0.06)
Cheerful	0.38 (0.07)	—[d]	—[d]
Alert	0.24[c] (0.08)	—[c]	—[c]
Confusion-bewilderment			
Full-scale H	0.39 (0.06)	0.55 (0.07)	0.55 (0.07)
Confused	0.40 (0.07)	0.49 (0.1)	0.49 (0.10)
Unable to concentrate	0.47 (0.06)	0.58 (0.07)	0.58 (0.07)
Efficient	0.21[c] (0.08)	—[c]	—[c]
Forgetful	0.50 (0.05)	0.59 (0.07)	0.59 (0.06)
Uncertain about things	0.37[c] (0.07)	—[c]	—[c]
Fatigue-inertia			
Full-scale H	0.53 (0.05)	0.65 (0.05)	0.67 (0.05)
Worn out	0.59 (0.05)	0.69 (0.05)	0.71 (0.05)
Fatigued	0.57 (0.05)	0.63 (0.06)	—[e]
Exhausted	0.62 (0.04)	0.69 (0.05)	0.68 (0.06)
Sluggish	0.53 (0.06)	0.58 (0.06)	0.63 (0.06)
Weary	0.23[c] (0.09)	—[c]	—[c]
Anger-hostility			
Full-scale H	0.47 (0.05)	0.53 (0.05)	0.612(0.06)
Angry	0.46 (0.07)	0.51 (0.07)	0.63 (0.06)
Grouchy	0.47 (0.06)	0.49 (0.07)	0.58 (0.08)
Annoyed	0.55 (0.06)	0.57 (0.06)	0.63 (0.06)
Resentful	0.41 (0.07)	—[d]	—[d]
Bitter	0.43 (0.08)	—[d]	—[d]
Ready to fight	0.47 (0.06)	0.49 (0.07)	—[e]
Rebellious	0.39[c] (0.08)	—[c]	—[c]
Deceived	0.47 (0.07)	0.47 (0.07)	—[e]
Furious	0.51 (0.06)	0.56 (0.07)	—[e]
Bad-tempered	0.53 (0.05)	0.58 (0.05)	—[e]
Depression-dejection			
Full-scale H	0.59 (0.05)	0.63 (0.05)	0.68 (0.06)
Unhappy	0.58 (0.07)	0.61 (0.07)	0.66 (0.07)
Sad	0.65 (0.05)	0.67 (0.05)	0.72 (0.06)
Hopeless	0.62 (0.06)	0.65 (0.06)	—[e]
Discouraged	0.65 (0.06)	0.68 (0.06)	0.66 (0.06)
Lonely	0.61 (0.06)	0.65 (0.06)	0.68 (0.06)
Miserable	0.60 (0.07)	0.63 (0.07)	—[e]
Gloomy	0.63 (0.06)	0.64 (0.06)	—[e]
Desperate	0.50 (0.09)	0.51 (0.09)	—[e]
Helpless	0.52 (0.08)	0.51 (0.09)	—[e]
Worthless	0.65 (0.06)	0.67 (0.06)	—[e]
Terrified	0.32[c] (0.07)	—[c]	—[c]

Abbreviations: MSA, Mokken scaling assessment; PKU, phenylketonuria; POMS, profile of mood states.
[a]N = 110.
[b]Low scalability defined as H coefficient <0.40.
[c]Items removed after iteration 1 of MSA.
[d]Items removed after iterations 2 and 3 of MSA.
[e]Items removed through Rasch analysis.

Table 6. Initial and Final Rasch Model Parameters.

PKU-POMS Domain, Item	Category Threshold Parameters				Fit Residual	Item Fit χ^2	χ^2, *P* Value
	a1	a2	a3	a4			
A. Initial Rasch Model Parameters Item Fit of 31 Items Retained After Mokken Scaling Analysis[a,b]							
Vigor-activity							
Lively	−2.45	−0.82	0.91	2.37	1.09	0.51	.77
Active	−2.34	−0.30	0.79	2.95	0.63	1.92	.38
Energetic	−2.62	1.05	0.74	1.82	−0.54	1.84	.40
Tension-anxiety							
Panicky	−0.73	0.24	1.03	1.46	−0.03	0.73	.70
Uneasy	−1.27	−0.34	1.18	1.56	1.20	0.94	.62
Nervous	−1.99	−0.36	−0.11	1.80	−0.12	2.41	.30
Anxious	−2.51	−0.80	−0.20	1.01	−0.34	0.56	.76
Confusion-bewilderment							
Confused	−0.88	0.11	1.33	2.12	1.42	0.88	.64
Unable to concentrate	−1.85	−0.51	0.20	1.26	−0.30	1.97	.37
Forgetful[c]	−2.23	−0.61	0.73	0.33	−0.42	1.70	.43
Fatigue-inertia							
Worn out	−3.25	−0.85	−0.013	1.88	−0.28	2.38	.31
Fatigued[c]	−2.70	0.02	−0.069	2.39	0.55	0.51	.78
Exhausted	−2.08	−0.40	0.57	1.96	−0.44	2.69	.26
Sluggish	−0.89	−0.042	0.71	2.76	1.27	1.45	.48
Anger-hostility							
Angry[c]	−1.78	−0.47	1.32	0.92	0.257	1.77	.41
Grouchy[c]	−2.13	−0.56	0.83	0.06	1.3	1.24	.54
Annoyed	−3.70	−1.56	−0.23	0.70	0.095	1.13	.57
Ready to fight	0.12	0.32	0.34	1.89	−0.676	1.53	.47
Deceived[c]	0.53	0.18	0.54	1.31	−0.161	0.90	.64
Furious[c]	0.24	−0.04	1.62	−1.19	−0.628	2.34	.31
Bad-tempered	−0.85	−0.12	0.17	1.56	−1.232	4.42	.11
Depression-dejection							
Unhappy	−3.28	−0.31	0.09	1.32	0.87	0.73	.69
Sad	−2.84	−0.80	0.03	0.70	−0.37	2.55	.28
Hopeless[c]	−0.73	−0.68	2.16	1.03	−0.46	0.83	.66
Discouraged[c]	−2.88	1.24	−0.11	−0.31	−0.08	0.34	.84
Lonely	−1.80	−0.53	−0.51	0.46	0.24	0.41	.81
Miserable[c]	−0.79	−0.06	−0.53	1.29	−0.02	1.49	.48
Gloomy[c]	−1.84	−0.20	−0.32	0.98	−0.13	1.75	.42
Desperate[c]	0.04	−0.22	1.57	1.24	0.83	0.82	.66
Helpless	−0.41	0.14	0.55	1.47	0.80	0.88	.65
Worthless[c]	−0.22	−0.72	0.66	7.59	−1.33	3.80	.15
B. Final Rasch Model Parameters and Item Fit of 20 Items in Draft PKU-POMS[b,d]							
Activity							
Lively	−2.45	−0.82	0.91	2.37	1.09	0.51	.77
Active	−2.34	−0.30	0.79	2.95	0.63	1.92	.38
Energetic	−2.62	1.05	0.74	1.82	−0.54	1.84	.40
Anxiety							
Panicky	−0.73	0.24	1.03	1.46	−0.03	0.73	.69
Uneasy	−1.27	−0.34	1.18	1.56	1.20	0.94	.62
Nervous	−1.99	−0.36	−0.11	1.80	−0.128	2.42	.30
Anxious	−2.51	−0.80	−0.17	1.01	−0.34	0.56	.76
Confusion							
Confused	−0.76	0.24	1.548774	2.19	1.36	1.17	.56
Unable to concentrate	−1.71	−0.38	0.365705	1.45	−0.41	1.98	.37
Forgetful	−2.10	−0.45	0.336567	—[e]	−0.08	2.70	.26
Tiredness							
Worn out	−3.41	−0.92	−0.14	2.00	−0.11	3.13	.21
Exhausted	−2.09	−0.47	0.42	2.08	0.32	0.89	.64
Sluggish	−1.04	−0.19	0.75	3.00	1.07	0.55	.76

(continued)

Table 6. (continued)

PKU-POMS Domain, Item	Category Threshold Parameters a1	a2	a3	a4	Fit Residual	Item Fit χ^2	χ^2, *P* Value
Anger							
Angry	−1.40	−0.05	2.00	3.19	0.05	1.52	.47
Grouchy	−1.85	−0.04	0.86	—[e]	1.40	0.24	.89
Annoyed	−2.9	1.25	0.12	1.68	−0.08	0.30	.86
Depression							
Unhappy	−2.53	0.14	0.86	2.76	0.74	1.10	.58
Sad	−2.15	−0.22	0.54	2.04	−0.36	2.56	.28
Discouraged	−2.05	−0.66	0.32	0.45	0.18	0.46	.79
Lonely	−1.02	−0.14	0.02	1.65	0.19	1.00	.61

Abbreviations: PKU, phenylketonuria; POMS, profile of mood states.
[a]Items examined in Rasch analyses were those retained as acceptable items from Mokken scaling.
[b]Separate Rasch analyses were conducted within each of the 6 domains.
[c]Indicates disordered thresholds.
[d]Items examined in Rasch analyses were a reduced set from those retained from both Mokken scaling and the first Rasch analysis.
[e]The response option for "extremely" was collapsed with "quite a bit" in final model.

All 10 participants were diagnosed with PKU during the first year of life, and all were currently following a Phe-restricted diet. Of the 10 participants, 4 (40%) reported a formal diagnosis of anxiety and 2 (20%) reported a formal diagnosis of depression. The interviews demonstrated that the final 20 items in the draft PKU-POMS were relevant and well understood by patients with PKU. The instructions, recall period, response options, item content, and domains were found to be comprehensive, clear, and relevant, with no revisions needed.

Discussion

The original 65-item POMS is a widely used instrument for the assessment of mood states, and multiple revised versions of the measure have been created in order to adapt the measure to a specific patient population[10-14] or specific culture.[7,15-18] However, no known PRO for the assessment of mood states, or revised version of the POMS, has been created for patients with PKU. Additionally, the content validity and psychometric properties of the POMS in patients with PKU has not been investigated previously. Thus, in the current study, a 3-phase, mixed qualitative and quantitative approach was used to assess the content validity, revise the original POMS for use specifically in patients with PKU, and assess the psychometric properties of the new PKU-POMS.

In phase 1, cognitive interviews with adults with PKU were conducted on the POMS to identify and remove items that were poorly understood, thought to be unacceptable as appropriate words to describe the patient's mood state, or considered irrelevant to patients with PKU. In total, 17 items were removed across all 6 domains from the 58 original POMS items (excluding the 7 friendliness domain items). As noted above, previous investigations conducted on multiple patient populations have reduced the original POMS by removing poorly performing items. All 17 items removed in the present study correspond to other independent item reduction studies where the same POMS items have been removed, such as sorry for things done,[7,12,16,32] shaky,[7,12,14,17] unworthy,[12-15,17,18] muddled,[7,13,18,33] and carefree.[7,12-14,18] These findings provide further support for the removal of the selected items in the current investigation using input from adults and adolescents (≥16 years) with PKU.

In phase 2, the remaining items were assessed quantitatively first using MSA and then Rasch analysis. Using MSA, an iterative process was used to remove the worst items within weak domains until all domains and all items achieved at least a moderate scalability level, and an additional 10 POMS items were removed. Following the MSA analysis, Rasch analyses were conducted on the reduced 31-item POMS, again using an iterative process within each of the 6 domains, to remove all misfitting items. Much like in phase 1, all items removed through the quantitative analysis had previously been identified as poorly performing items and removed through other revisions of the POMS, such as ready to fight,[7,12,13,33] miserable,[12,13,18] and helpless.[13,14,16] The MSA technique is a useful nonparametric approach for the development of questionnaires to measure health constructs,[34] which relies on less stringent statistical assumptions compared to Rasch analysis.[35] By coupling these 2 approaches in the development of the PKU-POMS, the current study was able to first identify the most problematic items within each domain and then more specifically assess the fit of the remaining items and domains to the stricter Rasch measurement model. The fit of the draft 20-item PKU-POMS to the Rasch measurement model and scalability was found acceptable.

In phase 3, the psychometric properties of the draft 20-item PKU-POMS were examined, and cognitive interviews among adults with PKU were conducted to investigate the acceptability of the draft instrument in the target population. These analyses demonstrated that the revised domains were internally consistent and provided preliminary support for the

Table 7. PKU-POMS Convergent Validity and Responsiveness Assessed Using Pearson's Correlations Between PKU-POMS and ADHD RS-IV and Plasma Phe Levels.

	Convergent Validity[a]				Responsiveness[b]			
	ADHD RS-IV		Plasma Phe		ADHD RS-IV		Plasma Phe	
PKU-POMS Domain	N	Pearson's *r*	N	Pearson's *r*	N	Pearson's *r*	N	Pearson's *r*
Activity	114	−0.04	114	−0.06	65	−0.40[c]	52	−0.25
Anxiety	114	0.33[d]	114	0.09	65	0.43[d]	52	0.34[c]
Confusion	114	0.60[e]	114	0.09	65	0.52[e]	52	0.47[d]
Tiredness	114	0.28[c]	114	0.17	65	0.34[c]	52	0.15
Anger	114	0.31[d]	114	0.08	65	0.32[c]	52	0.26
Depression	114	0.15	114	0.00	65	0.21	52	0.32[c]

Abbreviations: ADHD RS-IV, Attention-Deficit Hyperactivity Disorder Rating Scale IV; EOS, end of study; Phe, phenylalanine; PKU, phenylketonuria; POMS, profile of mood states.
[a]Convergent validity assessed using values at day 1.
[b]Responsiveness assessed using change scores from day 1 to EOS.
[c]$P < .05$.
[d]$P < .001$.
[e]$P < .0001$.

convergent validity and responsiveness of the measure. Finally, cognitive interviews on the draft PKU-POMS indicated that the measure is clear and easy to understand, with all items being relevant to patients with PKU. Additionally, patients believed that the revised domain labels accurately reflected the items contained within each domain. Thus, through this adaptation process, the PKU-POMS is shorter and less burdensome for patients to complete compared to the original 65-item POMS, and is clear, relevant, and easy for patients with PKU to understand.

Various research studies in the patients with PKU have demonstrated that even with early initiation of treatment, there is still an increased prevalence for various psychiatric, neurocognitive, and behavioral problems, including problems with mood,[2-5] and that these psychiatric problems are associated with increases in Phe. Using the Brief Symptom Inventory (BSI), Bilder and colleagues[36] assessed the psychiatric symptom patterns in 64 patients with PKU, finding that 6 of the 7 subscales of the BSI were elevated in patients with PKU. Further, in a systematic review of 10 published intervention and case reports, there was a clear association between reductions in Phe with marked reductions in psychiatric symptoms in all studies.[37] However, no instruments of psychiatric symptoms used in any of the clinical studies identified were developed specifically for use in adults with PKU. The revised PKU-POMS developed through 3 phases of qualitative and quantitative research with adults having PKU can help more clearly elucidate the relationships between Phe and mood symptoms and serve as a valid, reliable, and responsive measure of changes in mood symptoms in clinical studies of PKU.

The strengths of this study included the use of both qualitative and quantitative methods to adapt the POMS for use in patients with PKU. However, certain limitations of the study should be noted. Specifically, the participants recruited for phase 1 included only patients taking part in the National PKU Alliance Conference or saw the recruitment flier online via a study Web site. Thus, it is unknown if these findings generalize to a broader sample of adults with PKU. Additionally, the sample size in the PRISM-1 study at the EOS was limited (n = 65), and the psychometric validation analyses utilized the same data with which the quantitative data reduction analyses were conducted. Thus, a follow-up psychometric validation study on the PKU-POMS in a separate sample of patients with PKU will be used to further inform the usefulness and psychometric properties of this instrument.

Conclusion

A detailed, 3-phase item reduction process incorporating qualitative and quantitative techniques yielded the 20-item PKU-POMS instrument. This new instrument is designed for the assessment of treatment efficacy on change in mood states in clinical trials of adult patients with PKU.

Acknowledgments

The authors thank the National PKU Alliance for their support, and the participants who contributed to this research.

Declaration of Conflicting Interests

The author(s) declared potential conflict of interest with respect to the following research, authorship, and/or publication of this article: Yinpu Chen, Rishabh Jain, Laurel Konkol, Markus Merilainen, and Holly Weng are employees of BioMarin Pharmaceuticals and receive financial support in terms of salary and stock.

Funding

The author(s) disclosed receipt of the following financial support for the research, authorship, and/or publication of this article: Elizabeth Bacci, Kathleen Wyrwich, and Katharine Gries are employees of Evidera, which received financial support from BioMarin Pharmaceuticals in connection with the study development and execution as well as the manuscript development.

References

1. Kaufman S. An evaluation of the possible neurotoxicity of metabolites of phenylalanine. *J Pediatr*. 1989;114(5):895-900.
2. Moyle JJ, Fox AM, Arthur M, Bynevelt M, Burnett JR. Meta-analysis of neuropsychological symptoms of adolescents and adults with PKU. *Neuropsychol Rev*. 2007;17(2):91-101.
3. Pietz J, Fatkenheuer B, Burgard P, Armbruster M, Esser G, Schmidt H. Psychiatric disorders in adult patients with early-treated phenylketonuria. *Pediatrics*. 1997;99(3):345-350.
4. Smith I, Knowles J. Behaviour in early treated phenylketonuria: a systematic review. *Eur J Pediatr*. 2000;159(suppl 2):S89-S93.
5. Waisbren S. Phenylketonuria. In: Goldstein S, Reynolds CR, eds. *Handbook of Neurodevelopmental and Genetic Disorders in Children*. New York, NY: Guilford Press; 1999:433-458.
6. ten Hoedt AE, de Sonneville LM, Francois B, et al. High phenylalanine levels directly affect mood and sustained attention in adults with phenylketonuria: a randomised, double-blind, placebo-controlled, crossover trial. *J Inherit Metab Dis*. 2011; 34(1):165-171.
7. Wald FD, Mellenbergh GJ. [The shortened version of the Dutch translation of the Profile of Mood States (POMS)]. *Ned Tijdschr voor Psychol*. 1990;45(2):86-90.
8. McNair DM, Lorr M, Droppleman LF. *Manual for the Profile of Mood States*. San Diego, CA: Educational and Industrial Testing Services; 1971.
9. McNair DM, Heuchert J, Shilony E. *Profile of Mood States (POMS): Technical Update*. Tonawanda, NY: Multi-Health Systems, Inc; 2003.
10. Heuchert JP, McNair DM. *POMS 2 ®: Profile of Mood States Second Edition*. Tonawanda, NY: Multi-Health Systems, Inc; 2012.
11. Cranford JA, Shrout PE, Iida M, Rafaeli E, Yip T, Bolger N. A procedure for evaluating sensitivity to within-person change: can mood measures in diary studies detect change reliably? *Pers Soc Psychol Bull*. 2006;32(7):917-929.
12. Shacham S. A shortened version of the Profile of Mood States. *J Pers Assess*. 1983;47(3):305-306.
13. Sutherland HJ, Lockwood GA, Cunningham AJ. A simple, rapid method for assessing psychological distress in cancer patients. *J Pyschosoc Oncol*. 1989;7(1-2):31-43.
14. Terry PC, Lane AM, Lane HJ, Keohane L. Development and validation of a mood measure for adolescents. *J Sports Sci*. 1999;17(11):861-872.
15. Fernandez EMA, Fernandez CA, Pesqueria GS. Adaptation of the profile of mood states into Spanish with a sample athletes. *Psicothema*. 2002;14(4):708-713.
16. Netz Y, Zeav A, Arnon M, Daniel S. Translating a single-word items scale with multiple subcomponents—a Hebrew translation of the Profile of Mood States. *Isr J Psychiatry Relat Sci*. 2005; 42(4):263-270.
17. Perczek R, Carver CS, Price AA, Pozo-Kaderman C. Coping, mood, and aspects of personality in Spanish translation and evidence of convergence with English versions. *J Pers Assess*. 2000; 74(1):63-87.
18. Shin YH. A study on verification of the profile of mood states (POMS) for Korean elders. *J Korean Acad Nurs*. 1996;26(4):743-758.
19. Albani C, Blaser G, Geyer M, et al. [The German short version of "Profile of Mood States" (POMS): psychometric evaluation in a representative sample]. *Psychother Psychosom Med Psychol*. 2005;55(7):324-330.
20. Curran SL, Andrykowski MA, Studts JL. Short Form of the Profile of Mood States (POMS-SF): Psychometric Information. *Psychol Assess*. 1995;7(1):80-83.
21. Fillion L, Gagnon P. French adaptation of the shortened version of the Profile of Mood States. *Psychol Rep*. 1999;84(1):188-190.
22. Moret L, Nguyen JM, Pillet N, Falissard B, Lombrail P, Gasquet I. Improvement of psychometric properties of a scale measuring inpatient satisfaction with care: a better response rate and a reduction of the ceiling effect. *BMC Health Serv Res*. 2007;7:197.
23. Steiger JH. Understanding the limitations of global fit assessment in structural equation modeling. *Pers Indiv Differ*. 2007;42(5): 893-898.
24. Yu CY. *Evaluating Cutoff Criteria of Model Fit Indices for Latent Variable Models with Binary and Continuous Outcomes* [doctoral dissertation]. Los Angeles, CA: University of California; 2002.
25. van Shurr WH.Mokken scale analysis: between the Guttman scale and parametric item response theory. *Polit Anal*. 2003;11(2): 139-143.
26. Loevinger J. The technic of homogeneous tests compared with some aspects of scale analysis and factor analysis. *Psychol Bull*. 1948;45(6):507-529.
27. Mokken RJ. *A Theory and Procedure of Scale Analysis*. The Hague/Berlin: Mouton/De Gruyter; 1971.
28. Rasch G. *Probabilistic Models for Some Intelligence and Attainment Tests*. (Republished). Chicago, IL: The University of Chicago Press; 1980.
29. Embretson SE, Reise SP. *Item Response Theory for Psychologists*. Mahwah, NJ: Lawrence Erlbaum Associates; 2000.
30. Linacre JM. What do infit and outfit mean-square and standardized mean? *Rasch Meas Trans*. 2002;16(2):878.
31. Bollen KA. *Structural Equations with Latent Variables*. Hoboken, NJ: John Wiley and Sons; 1989.
32. Andrade E, Arce C, Torrado J, Garrido J, De Francisco C, Arce I. Factor structure and invariance of the POMS Mood State Questionnaire in Spanish. *Span J Psychol*. 2010;13(1):444-452.
33. Grove JR, Prapavessis H. Preliminary evidence for the reliability and validity of an abbreviated Profile of Mood States. *Int J Sport Psychol*. 1992;23(2):93-109.
34. Stochl J, Jones PB, Croudace TJ. Mokken scale analysis of mental health and well-being questionnaire item responses: a non-parametric IRT method in empirical research for applied health researchers. *BMC Med Res Methodol*. 2012;12:74.
35. Sijtsma K, Molenaar IW. *Introduction to Nonparametric Item Response Theory*. London, UK: Sage Publications; 2002.
36. Bilder DA, Burton BK, Coon H, et al. Psychiatric symptoms in adults with phenylketonuria. *Mol Genet Metab*. 2013;108(3):155-160.
37. Bilder DA, Noel JK, Baker ER, et al. A systematic review (SR) of the effectiveness of reducing blood phenylalanine (Phe) levels in adults with phenylketonuria (PKU) on neuropsychiatric symptoms. *J Inherit Metab Dis*. 2014;37(suppl 1):S27-S185; Abstract P-069.

14

SUMA Technology and Newborn Screening Tests for Inherited Metabolic Diseases in Cuba: An Overview of the First 30 Years

Ernesto Carlos González Reyes, PhD[1], Elisa M. Castells, MSc[1], Amarilys Frómeta, MSc[1], Ana Luisa Arteaga, MD[2], Lesley Del Río, MSc[1], Yileidis Tejeda, MSc[1], Pedro L. Pérez, LT[1], Mary Triny Segura, BSc[1], Pedro Almenares, MSc[1], Yenitse Perea, MSc[1], Niurka M. Carlos, MSc[3], René Robaina, MD, PhD[1], and José L. Fernández-Yero, MD, PhD[4]

Abstract

The ultramicroanalytic system (SUMA), created in the 1980s, is a complete system of reagents and instrumentation to perform ultramicroassays combining the sensitivity of the micro-enzyme-linked immunosorbent assay (ELISA) tests with the use of ultramicrovolumes. This technology permitted establishing large-scale newborn screening programs (NSPs) for metabolic and endocrine disorders in Cuba. This article summarizes the main results of the implementation during the 30 years of SUMA technology in NSP for 5 inherited metabolic diseases, using ultramicroassays developed at the Department of Newborn Screening at the Immunoassay Center. Since 1986, SUMA technology has been used in the Cuban NSP for congenital hypothyroidism, initially studying thyroid hormone in cord serum samples. In 2000, a decentralized program for the detection of hyperphenylalaninemias using heel dried blood samples was initiated. These successful experiences permitted including protocols for screening congenital adrenal hyperplasia, galactosemia, and biotinidase deficiency in 2005. A program for the newborn screening of CH using the thyroid-stimulating hormone Neonatal ultramicro-ELISA was fully implemented in 2010. Nowadays, the NSP is supported by a network of 175 SUMA laboratories. After 30 years, more than 3.8 million Cuban newborns have been screened, and 1002 affected children have been detected. Moreover, SUMA technology has been presented in Latin America for over 2 decades and has contributed to screen around 17 million newborns. These results prove that developing countries can develop appropriate diagnostic technologies for making health care accessible to all.

Keywords

SUMA, technology, newborn screening, UMTEST, UMELISA

Introduction

From January 1959, health and human life became a constant concern of the Cuban reality. Sociopolitical changes in the island brought a different conception of health services, being conceived by the state as an integrated system, with emphasis on disease prevention and universal access to services. This conception has significantly impacted on the progresses of medicine in Cuba.[1-2]

Among the efforts to advance this concept, the creation and opening of the Immunoassay Center (CIE) in 1987 are included, an organization in charge of developing and producing kits for diagnostic purposes where its leading products are the ultramicroanalytic system (SUMA) or SUMA technology,[3] part of BioCubaFarma business group, which gathers major

[1] Department of Newborn Screening, Immunoassay Center, Cubanacan, Havana, Cuba
[2] National Programs Department, TecnoSuma Internacional SA Cubanacan, Havana, Cuba
[3] Immunoassay Center, Cubanacan, Havana, Cuba
[4] Center of Molecular Immunology, Atabey, Havana, Cuba

Corresponding Author:
Ernesto Carlos González Reyes, PhD, Department of Newborn Screening, Immunoassay Center, 134 Street and 25 Avenue, Cubanacan, Playa, Havana, Cuba.
Email: ernesto.gonzalez@cie.cu

centers for scientific research and production in the area of biotechnology and the pharmaceutical industry in our country.

In the late 1970s, a small group of young researchers from the National Center for Scientific Research (CNIC), with the aim of contributing to the reduction in infant mortality in Cuba and by the existing need in the country of counting on economical and reliable methods for diagnosis, began to develop a sustainable test for the quantification of serum α-fetoprotein in pregnant women.[4]

This small group, led from the beginning by Dr Jose Luis Fernandez Yero, who became later CIE's Founding-Director for 25 years, laid out a strategy to achieve a type of test that would be compatible with the conditions of a country with limited financial resources and underdeveloped infrastructure; it should also have had low operating costs and could be easily adapted to the Cuban health system. That is how the SUMA technology was born, an own health technology and especially "appropriate" to the conditions and realities of the country.[3-4] In the 1980s, the development of the SUMA technology created the basis for establishing large-scale newborn screening programs (NSPs) for metabolic and endocrine disorders in Cuba.

Newborn screening programs are essential, preventive public health programs for early identification of disorders in newborns that can affect the quality of their life and expectancy. Early detection, diagnosis, and treatment of certain genetic, metabolic, or infectious congenital disorders can lead to significant reductions in death, disease, and associated disabilities.[5,6]

This article reviews the main results on the implementation of this technology in NSP for 5 inherited metabolic disorders: congenital hypothyroidism (CH), congenital adrenal hyperplasia (CAH), biotinidase deficiency (BIOT), phenylketonuria (PKU), and galactosemia (GAL), using ultramicroassays, developed for almost 3 decades in the Department of Newborn Screening at the CIE. Besides, the article approaches the main challenges that SUMA technology, applied to the newborn screening, will be facing in the next years.

Methodology

Ultramicroassays for Neonatal Screening Supported by SUMA Technology

The SUMA technology is a complete system of reagents and instrumentation to perform ultramicro-enzyme-linked immunosorbent assay (UMELISA) or ultramicrotest (UMTEST), which comprises fully computerized spectrofluorometers for automatic reading, validation, interpretation, and quantification of results, plate washers, manual and automatic punchers, and reagent kits designed to perform UMTESTs (10-30 μL volumes of samples and reagents). The technology is manufactured by the CIE, Havana, Cuba, and it combines the sensitivity of the micro-ELISA tests with the use of ultramicrovolumes.[7] Since the birth of the methodology, the development and use of dedicated software for each of the tests have been a complementary tool that gave independence and added value to the technology.[8]

Currently, neonatal SUMA's assays include a set of 8 kits for newborn diagnosis of inherited metabolic diseases that CIE provides for the Cuban National Health Care System. Six of them use dried blood spots (DBS) on filter paper and the other 2 use serum samples. At present, the latter kits (TSH UMELISA and T4 UMELISA) are used for the confirmation of CH.

This article focuses on the characteristics of assays using DBS samples collected between the 5th and 7th days of age, with analytical quality evaluated and certified, and comparable with other existing commercial methods.[9]

Thyroid-stimulating hormone (TSH) NEONATAL UMELISA, an ultramicroassay developed by CIE to determine neonatal TSH levels in DBS, is a sandwich-type, heterogeneous enzyme immunoassay using as solid-phase UMELISA strips (10 μL of solution per well) coated with monoclonal antibodies anti-TSH beta chain. Dried blood spots are eluted with a solution that contains sheep polyclonal anti-TSH/alkaline phosphatase conjugate, and the eluate is placed in the coated reaction opaque polystyrene UMELISA plates, where an antibody/TSH/antibody–enzyme complex is formed. A posterior washing of the plates eliminates the unbound conjugate and other components of the samples. When the fluorogenic substrate (4-metilumbeliferil phosphate) is added to the wells, the enzyme of the conjugate hydrolyzes it, and subsequent fluorescence intensity will be in proportion to TSH concentrations in the samples.[10]

The thyroxine (T4) Neonatal UMELISA is an additional competitive ultramicromethod for CH screening, designed for the determination of total T4 in DBS, where the natural antigen and the enzyme-labeled antigen compete for a limited number of binding sites on the antibody. This assay uses as a solid-phase UMELISA strips coated with specific rabbit polyclonal anti-T4 antibodies. The DBS are eluted with a solution that contains the T4/alkaline phosphatase conjugate, and the eluate is placed in the coated reaction opaque polystyrene UMELISA plates. When samples are incubated in the reaction wells, antibody–antigen or antibody–antigen–enzyme complex are formed. A posterior washing of the plates eliminates the unbound conjugate and other components of the samples. When the fluorogenic substrate is added to the wells, the conjugated enzyme hydrolyzes it so that the intensity of fluorescence will be inversely proportional to the total T4 concentrations present in the samples.[11]

The UMTEST PKU is a modification of the traditional McCaman and Robin method to determine the concentration of phenylalanine (Phe) in DBS. This ultramicrofluorometric test, supported in the SUMA technology, requires less time and volume than the traditional method by McCaman et al. The test is based on the reaction of Phe present in the sample with ninhydrin, in optimal conditions of pH and temperature, forming a low-level fluorescent complex. With the addition of copper ions, this complex becomes fluorescent, increasing its intensity due to the previous addition of L-leucyl-L-alanine to the reaction. The intensity of the emitted fluorescence is proportional to Phe concentration in the mixture.[7]

Table 1. Ultramicroanalytic System (SUMA) Assays and Disorders Included in the Cuban Newborn Screening Program.[a]

Disorder	Analyte	Kits	Year Introduced	Cutoff
CH	TSH[b]	TSH Neonatal UMELISA	1986	15 mUI/L
PKU	Phe	UMTEST PKU	2000	240 μmol/L
Congenital adrenal hyperplasia	17α-hydroxyprogesterone (17OHP)	17OH progesterone UMELISA	2005	55 nmol/L
Galactosemia	Galactose	UMTEST GAL	2005	10 mg/dL
Biotinidase deficiency	Biotinidase activity	UMTEST biotinidase	2005	Qualitative decision (total and partial deficiency)

Abbreviations: GAL, galactosemia; Phe, phenylalanine; PKU, phenylketonuria; TSH, thyroid-stimulating hormone; UMELISA, ultramicro-enzyme-linked immunosorbent assay; UMTEST, ultramicrotest.
[a]Source: Newborn screening programs (NSP) database network of SUMA laboratories, Immunoassay Center.
[b]Since 1986 to 2010 NSP for congenital hypothyroidism (CH) used the TSH UMELISA in cord serum samples.

Initially, these 3 assays used 5-mm DBS samples, standards, and controls.[12] With the increase in tests done in NSP, it was necessary to use smaller blood punches in order to make a more rational use of the samples, so these kits were modified into 3-mm DBS discs at the beginning of this century.

The 17-hydroxyprogesterone (17OHP) Neonatal UMELISA is a simple and rapid competitive UMELISA assay designed to determine 17OHP levels in DBS. The assay is based on competition between 17OHP in blood specimens and 17OHP-alkaline phosphatase conjugate for a limited number of binding sites on specific rabbit polyclonal anti-17OHP antibodies. Standards, control, and samples blood spots are eluted with 17OHP-alkaline phosphatase conjugate in a danazol solution, and the eluates are placed in the coated reaction opaque polystyrene UMELISA plates. When samples are incubated in the strip wells, an antibody/17OHP or antibody/17OHP-alkaline phosphatase conjugate complex is formed. A posterior washing of the plates eliminates the unbound components. When the fluorogenic substrate (4-metilumbeliferil phosphate) is added to the wells, the enzyme of the conjugate hydrolyzes it, and subsequent fluorescence intensity will be inversely proportional to the amount of 17OHP in the sample. The 17OHP Neonatal UMELISA described initially used 40 μL of eluting solution,[13] which it was subsequently modified to 70 μL in the year 2010.

The UMTEST GAL is a simple, rapid, quantitative UMTEST based on the fluorometric method introduced by Fujimura et al adapted to SUMA technology for the detection of total galactose (GAL) in DBS. A methanol/acetone/water solution is used for deproteination. Galactosemia and galactose-1-phosphate are determined by measuring the change in fluorescence of nicotinamide adenine dinucleotide (reduced form $NADH^{+}H$) at 450 nm, treated with β-galactose dehydrogenase and alkaline phosphatase. Both reactions occur in optimal conditions of pH and temperature. The resulting fluorescence is directly proportional to the amount of GAL in DBS.[14] The ultramicroassay described initially used 70 μL of deproteination solution, which was subsequently modified to 30 μL in the year 2014.

In all quantitative assays described, automatic validation and interpretation of the results are done using a dedicated SUMA assay software.[8] The UMTEST BIOTINIDASE is a simple qualitative visual ultramicroassay based on the colorimetric method introduced by Heard et al for the detection of BIOT in dried blood samples spotted on filter paper using N-biotinyl-p-aminobenzoate (B-PAB) as a substrate. According to the controls and samples evaluation, the ultramicroassay could clearly discriminate between normal newborns and those ones with low or absent biotinidase enzymatic activity. Results are obtained by a simple visual inspection of the colorimetric reaction. Those samples that developed a purple color are considered to have a normal biotinidase activity, and therefore, they are normal. The samples that developed a clear purple color are considered to have low biotinidase activity, and it was suspected that they are partial deficient. Those that present light yellow color are considered to have little or none activity, and they are classified as profound deficient. The ultramicroassay described initially used 40 μL of B-PAB,[15] which was subsequently modified to 70 μL in the year 2007. Table 1 shows the SUMA assays and the cutoff values used for the newborn screening of the 5 disorders included in the Cuban NSP.

Cuban NSP Strategy

Cuban NSP is managed by the Ministry of Public Health through its Program for Comprehensive Care for Women and Children, which coordinate the actions of the health institutions in charged for the diagnosis, confirmation, control of the cases, treatment, follow-up of patients, and attention to families. The algorithm of the Cuban NSP is shown in Figure 1.

Newborn screening tests were initially conducted by a national laboratory network made up by 32 laboratories. In the year 2010, all municipalities had at least a SUMA laboratory, which operated as a comprehensive active screening center for studying people according to their age, physical condition, and risk of contracting transmissible and nontransmissible diseases, in coordination with the primary health-care system, through polyclinics and family doctors. Thus, the number of laboratories covering the entire national territory performing neonatal screening tests has increased up to 175.

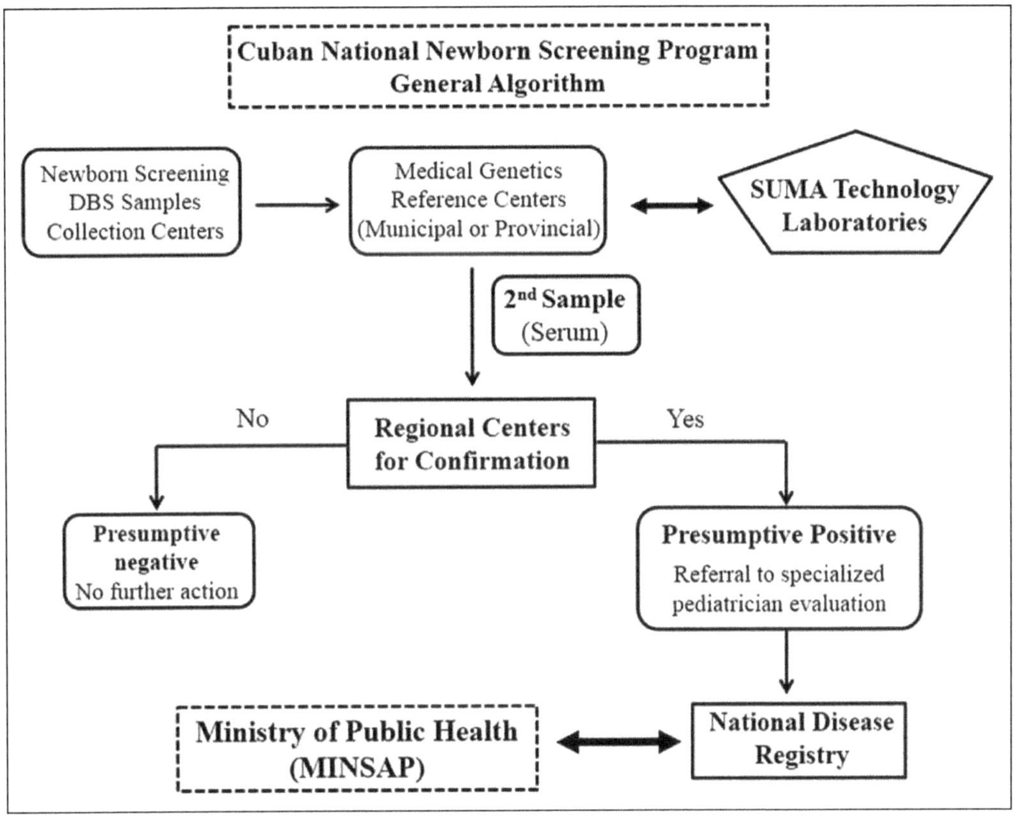

Figure 1. Cuban National Newborn Screening Program Algorithm.

Technical and analytical assistance, replacement, and upgrading of equipment and reagents are supplied by Tecnosuma Internacional SA (TISA), which manages 5 regional technical assistance centers spread throughout the country.

The DBS samples are collected in the municipal collection centers preferably between the 5th and 7th days of life and sent to medical genetics reference centers, which are responsible for recording the data, and sent DBS samples to laboratories within 72 hours. Specimens are analyzed quickly after arrival in order to have the results ready in <24 hours. Thyroid-stimulating hormone, Phe, Gal, 17OHP, and BIOT activity are measured by the SUMA technology test for newborn screening previously described.

All newborns with a positive screening test are referred immediately for biochemical and clinical confirmation and follow-up at the regional pediatric centers. These institutions of the health system are nationally controlled by the National Institute of Endocrinology (CH and CAH) and the National Medical Genetics Center (GAL, PKU, and BIOT).

Confirmation is performed on serum samples that are sent to referral centers. Infants with negative serum results with respect to the cutoff value used for a given analyte are considered as simple false positives, and no other further investigations are made. Generally, patients with a positive confirmation serum result are referred to Provincial Pediatric Specialized Services for starting treatment. The DNA testing is only performed on PKU and CAH patients to study phenotype–genotype correlation.[16,17]

In the specific case of the CAH program, due to the high false-positive rate (FPR), neonates with serum 17OHP levels ≥ cutoff value without clinical signs are considered as hyper-17OHP infants and are submitted to clinical and biochemical follow-up monitoring until the normalization of hormone values. Treatment with hydrocortisone is begun in all newborns with 17OHP levels ≥ cutoff value and clinical or biochemical signs of CAH. Patients with suggestive salt-wasting crises are given fludrocortisone doses.

Some quality indicators of the Cuban NSP were analyzed. The NSP database network of SUMA laboratories was reviewed from 1986 to December 2015 to determine the number of live births, screened infants, and confirmed cases. In addition, the number of positives (true and false positives) was recorded to calculate the positive predictive value (PPV) of the screening test and the incidence of the disorders. Further indicators such as coverage of the program, time of collection, percentage of unsatisfactory or invalid specimens, sample transit, and processing time in the laboratory and delivery time of results were evaluated in the period 2010 to 2015.

Results

Cuban NSP Results

In Cuba, the Cuban NSP using SUMA technology was initiated with an original development strategy, organizational model, and technological resources by a research and

Table 2. Some Main Results of the Cuban Newborn Screening Program (1986-2015).[a]

Disorder	Newborns Screened	Cases Detected	Positive Predictive Value (%)	Incidence
Congenital hypothyroidism	3 873 709	884	2.30	1:4382
Phenylketonuria	1 545 295	33	0.90	1:46 827
Congenital adrenal hyperplasia	1 264 964	61	0.31	1:20 737
Galactosemia	1 212 782	12	0.14	1:101 065
Biotinidase deficiency	1 249 534	12	0.84	1:104 127

[a]Source: Newborn screening program (NSP) database network of ultramicroanalytic system (SUMA) laboratories, Immunoassay Center.

development-closed cycle through which scientific findings and technological developments are part of a combined effort to solve a specific health problem with feedback to improve it. The program was organized to be incorporated into the existing health-care system and make the most efficient use of limited resources. The evolution and the main results of the Cuban NSP are shown in Table 2.

The program for CH began in May 1986 and since 1988 has spread throughout the country. After Canada, Cuba was a leading pioneer nation of the Americas that provided a program with full coverage of the CH detection for newborn babies.

Until 2007, the study of TSH was exclusively done in cord serum using the TSH UMELISA,[18] when a pilot program for the implementation of the TSH Neonatal UMELISA was started.

In this case, SUMA technology has made possible to provide early detection of CH to all the Cuban children born since that date. Through December 31, 2015, a total of 3 847 656 children had been studied, of which 868 had that pathology at birth. Quality control in NSP requires precise assessment of target variables of development of the children, which should be identified and defined operationally throughout the entire program. The NSP for CH has made efforts to complement all the specialities. Nowadays, when the TSH value in DBS samples is over 15 mUI/L, the result is considered positive, and this leads to collection of a second sample for the determination of TSH and T4 in serum. Until this result is known, therapy with L-T4 is begun. If the confirmation tests are positives, the infant is continued on this treatment and evaluated by a team that includes an endocrinologist, a psychologist, and a technician specialized in psychological testing. All patients are followed by a pediatric multidisciplinary team until the adult age.

Coordinators of the NSP have emphasized the value of studying the neurodevelopment in infants with CH, providing complementary data for the clinical management of the patients and continuous feedback to determine screening program efficacy and performance. The follow-up of the patients provides information that could lead to new means for optimal intervention in these and other affected children.[19,20]

If they had not been detected by the screening provided with the SUMA test and provided with the medical treatment required by these cases, those children would had developed severe mental retardation due to the low levels of thyroid hormone production.

During 2000, the Ministry of Health has been reformulating the NSP for the gradual introduction of UMTEST PKU allowing the decentralization of the Cuban program for the detection of hyperphenylalaninemias using heel dried blood samples. Guthrie's BIA was used in Cuba, since 1983 until 2000,[21] with an incidence of 1:50 000.[22] A pilot program for the newborn screening of hyperphenylalaninemias started in that year using the UMTEST PKU.[7]

This ultramicrofluorometric test, supported in the SUMA technology, is a simple, specific, precise, accurate, and rapid assay that permits the processing of many samples at low cost and guarantees efficiency and reliable results. The UMTEST PKU requires less time and volume than the traditional method by McCaman et al.[23] With regard to the Guthrie's BIA, previously used in the Cuban neonatal PKU screening program, it needs over 16 hours to perform the assay, while the total time required by the UMTEST PKU is about 2 hours. The diagnosis and treatment time are reduced, and the newborn screening quality is increased using the ultramicrofluorometric method. In addition, the UMTEST PKU gives the possibility of automatic validation and interpretation from data processing and permits the development of decentralized programs for the neonatal screening of hyperphenylalaninemias. The analytical performance characteristics of this method and its practical application in the Cuban PKU NSP have demonstrated its suitability for the neonatal screening of PKU.[7]

These successful experiences permitted developing screening programs for CAH, Gal, and BIOT in 2005. Additionally, a decentralized NSP for CH in DBS using the TSH Neonatal UMELISA was fully implemented in 2010.

As shown in Table 2, after 30 years, more than 3.8 million Cuban newborns have been screened with this technology, and 1002 affected children have been detected. The current global incidence of inherited metabolic diseases identified by the Cuban NSP screening program was 2.02 per 10 000 live births (1:4890), with an annual rate of 25 cases/year. In the program, the age at serum sampling for the confirmatory testing was conducted between 9.0 to 20.0 days with a mean of 13.7 $\pm$ 9.9 days. The mean age for the start of the treatment was estimated at 21.8 $\pm$ 9.6 days.

The PPV and FPR are 2 aspects of the program that should be analyzed. The percentage of false positives among screened infants is maintained below 0.70% for the majority of the disorders, except for CAH screening. Table 2 shows that in general the PPVs in the programs are low, being higher only for CH screening. In some cases (Gal, PKU, and BIOT), this is related to the low incidence of these disorders, but in CH and

Table 3. Cuban Quality Newborn Screening Program Indicators (2010-2015).[a]

Program Indicator	2010	2011	2012	2013	2014	2015
% NSP coverage	98.2	98.5	98.9	99.3	99.1	99.2
Unsatisfactory specimens	0.61	0.97	0.41	0.35	0.37	0.35
% Sample collection (5-6 days)	88.8	93.4	93.8	93.5	94.4	95.8
% Sample transit <72 hours	61.5	63.9	80.3	82.5	83.4	91.1
% Processing time <48 hours	98.7	97.7	98.1	98.0	97.7	99.3
% Report laboratory results <24-72 hours	99.8	99.5	98.6	99.2	97.8	98.6

Abbreviation: NSP, newborn screening program.
[a]Source: Newborn screening program (NSP) database network of ultramicroanalytic system (SUMA) laboratories, Immunoassay Center.

CAH programs, there exists other factors that influence the PPV values.

In 2010, with the implementation of TSH UMELISA Neonatal in the Cuban NSP for CH, there was a marked decrease in the FPR. In the period 1986 to 2010, detecting TSH in cord serum samples, the FPR was 1.14%, whereas the use of DBS samples and the introduction of TSH UMELISA Neonatal diminished this rate to 0.21%. Thus, the PPV increased from 2.2 % to 5.8% in the last 6 years.

However, the magnitude of false-positive results generated in the CAH screening program has represented a great challenge for the public health system. In December 2015, the FPR for the CAH program was 1.54%. That's why, in spite of the incidence of the disease, the PPV has been very low. A previous work had analyzed that a unique cutoff value of 55 nmol/L (calculated by 98th percentile) is used in the program, and more than 50% of false-positive results occurred in infants with a birth weight (BW) <2500 g or gestational age (GA) <37 weeks and was concluded that using an optimized cutoff level for BW or GA could lead to a reduction in the percentage of recalled babies and improve the PPV.[24] Taking into consideration these studies, 3 different cutoff values using BW and GA were applied in the Cuban NSP for CAH since November 2015.

Some Cuban NSP efficiency indicators in the period 2010 to 2015 are summarized in Table 3. In this study period, the program was able to achieve over 98% coverage. By the end of 2013, the coverage reached values higher than 99%, which have been maintained for the last 3 years. The analysis done to the rest of the indicators gathered in Table 3 shows that in spite of counting on a decentralized program, the percentage of unsatisfactory specimens has appropriately progressed in the last years, whereas an adequate and sustained work is observed collecting samples between the fifth and sixth day of life, processing time in the laboratory before 48 hours and informing the results in less than 72 hours.

Nevertheless, diminishing of sample transit to the laboratory is an important issue to work in because this is an essential element that would improve significantly the efficiency of the program, favoring the quality of the samples due to temperature excursions to which they may be subjected and increase the diagnostic opportunity of the program.

Finally, it should be mentioned that SUMA neonatal kits are regularly monitored for accuracy of results. Monthly, all laboratories in Cuba and most in Latin America participate in the Integral Scheme for Assurance and External Quality Assessment (EIAEEC) implemented since 1988 and provided by TISA.[25,26] Additionally, some SUMA laboratories are integrated in International monitoring External Quality Assurance Schemes, such as the US Center for Disease Control Newborn Screening Quality Assurance Program[27] and External Quality Assurance Program for NBS (PEEC-PN) from Argentina.[28] It is important to emphasize that the EIAEEC, as part of the SUMA technology, was the first EQAS for NBS, implemented in Latin America in 1988, and plays an important role because it includes the entire region.[28]

Presence of SUMA Technology in Latin America and Other World Regions

From the consolidation of SUMA technology, and always with the main objective to guarantee national health programs, CIE has also dedicated to propose, design, and expand health programs in other countries, mainly in the Latin American region.

In Latin America, a sustained and significant growth in newborn screening activities has been palpable through the last 20 years, highlighted by the implementation of new national or regional NSP, the increases in the percentage of population covered, the expansion of the diseases included in the screening panels, and the increased involvement of the government and public health authorities.[6,29]

In 1990, within this context, TISA is created who is in charge of marketing, extending health programs across the country, and makes them function stably, safely, and with the required quality.

The SUMA technology was installed in Brazil for the first time,[30] and then other countries such as Colombia, Mexico, Venezuela, Peru, Ecuador, Nicaragua, Bolivia, China, and Angola have followed. At present, more than 750 SUMA technology laboratories are installed worldwide.

Moreover, SUMA technology, which has been present in Latin America for 2 decades, has contributed to screening more than 17 million newborns, and more than 5000 affected patients have been detected during that period.

Challenges of the SUMA Technology

In Cuba, the implementation of SUMA technology has provided a model of a successful public health NSP for the past

30 years. However, this way has not been without its difficulties and challenges.

The SUMA technology and its application in the NSP have important challenges. Projects for the development of new tests and to improve existing ones together with assimilation and development of new technologies give continuity to the efforts for continuous improvement in neonatal screening in the country.

First, it is necessary to develop new affordable methods to complete the diseases included in the basic newborn screening panel and begin working on the development of methodologies to quickly count on with an expanded sustainable newborn screening panel in Cuba.

In this sense, in 2016, regional pilot screening projects are planning to test new assays for cystic fibrosis and maple urine disease supported in the SUMA technology. Successful results will permit proposing to the Ministry of Health to expand NSP of these disorders to the national territory.

Along with this, it should be considered to decrease the time of collection of the sample at 3 to 5 days of life, which would increase the diagnostic opportunity of the program and favor the future introduction of other diseases to the NSP, where time collection is crucial to ensure reliable results.

Second, although SUMA technology emerged as a semiautomatic technology mainly intended for laboratories of low and medium sample processing capacity, the global trend toward centralization of the newborn screening laboratories, increasing the amount of samples to be processed, it has made necessary the automation of this technology.

That is why a new automated analyzer for Neonatal Screening of SUMA technology SUMAutoLab has been developed.[31] The instrument presents a robotic arm for liquid handling with ceramic-coated stainless steel tips, a robotic arm to transport the plates to the various devices, programmable temperature incubators, shakers, plate washer, and fluorescence reader. The equipment is controlled by specific software that optimally schedules the different tasks and provides the necessary information both in preparation and during the run. The SUMAutoLab will allow the customers to increase efficiently the volume of sample processing in the laboratory, and it also results in more reliable and accurate diagnoses, drastically reducing the number of handling errors by operators.[31]

Finally, the assimilation of new technologies when economically possible will favor the detection of new analytes, will increase the number of diseases, and will improve the protocols for newborn screening, confirmation, and follow-up. For example, it is known that PKU screening could be dramatically improved by adding a Phe/tyrosine (tyr) ratio, but unfortunately, the current technology does not allow us to apply this methodology. However, since 2010, an high-performance liquid chromatography method for simultaneously quantifying serum Phe and tyr is used to perform confirmatory and differential diagnosis of hyperphenylalaninemias, as well as biochemical monitoring of Cuban PKU patients.[32]

Current economic conditions (mainly related to communications and transport) do not allow us to centralize the neonatal screening. In the future, with the introduction of a greater number of diseases to this program and the use of more expensive technologies (eg, tandem mass spectrometry), it will require to reevaluate the algorithm of the current NSP.

Final Considerations

Since the second half of the 20th century, the world is witnessing an unprecedented scientific–technological progress in all spheres of society. Impact of technologies in clinical practice and in the organization and delivery of services has been exponential, and today, it is possible to have more and better diagnostic and therapeutic prevention methods.[33]

Contemporary world health situation demands the society to place in the foreground of analysis issues like equity, health promotion, and prevention, quality of care, ethical dilemmas, technological needs recognition, and the use of appropriate technologies as key factors for the development of adequate national health policies.[4,34-36]

Today, when referring to appropriate technologies, it should prevail the idea that their use must be determined by national technological capabilities and its correspondence with the social, economic, political, and cultural context of a particular country or region.[4,33] Thus, the solutions for massive and free application of preventive diagnostic systems and treatment of inherited metabolic disorders in the developing world could not come only from by simple technological assimilation because the economic implications would be unaffordable for those countries.

Therefore, in the case of Cuba, it was necessary to find own technological solutions adapted to its conditions of development and socioeconomic infrastructure, to thereby further progress in improving its public health system.[1-3]

The profound political, social, and economic changes that occurred in Cuba since 1959 have led to a significant improvement in the quality of life that shows health indicators of developed countries. In Cuba, health is seen as a strategic objective in the growth and development of society, where the state assumes full responsibility for the health care of the entire population.[1-3]

The SUMA technology is a genuine product of the Cuban technical–scientific revolution, developed in the early 80s of the last century as a response to a problem of our own health conditions of development: the need for making early diagnosis of diseases in large populations.[3,4]

For almost 3 decades, the CIE has developed and commercialized SUMA technology, an appropriate methodology for diagnosis, to solve major health problems, introducing and maintaining quality indicators comparable with similar technologies in the field of clinical diagnostic.

Health programs supported by SUMA technology products include prenatal and neonatal screening, epidemiological surveillance, blood certification, and nontransmissible chronic diseases, giving a solution to the variety of diagnosis made in the laboratory.[3,4]

Specifically, in the field of neonatal screening, through the development and implementation of SUMA technology, NSP for inherited metabolic diseases have been functioning in Cuba for more than 30 years and have expanded their coverage and now reach more than 99% of newborns.

In this manner, Cuban NSPs have been a triumph of public health system; through these programs, each year infants born with potentially devastating but treatable diseases are identified, treated, and preserved from an early death or mental retardation.

Conclusions

Genetics and immunology have experienced major scientific and technological progress in recent times, mainly in the industrialized world. The development of these sciences and the diagnosis of inherited metabolic diseases differ in Cuba in relation to other developing countries of the region and the world, given the advantages of our social and public health models.

This article has reviewed main elements related to the design and development of SUMA technology, an own and appropriate diagnostic procedure, which has largely allowed improving health indicators of the Cuban people over the last 30 years, being the main incentive for the continuous progress of this technology.

The creation of the CIE and the implementation of SUMA technology marked a significant moment in the scientific development of the Caribbean Island. In 2015, Cuba reached the lowest infant mortality rate in America, a figure that ratifies it as a leading country in this indicator, internationally regarded as a reflection of the health of the population and sociocultural development.

In these results, it has been important the expansion of NSP for 5 inherited metabolic disorders using SUMA technology, which places Cuba among the most developed in the region in the field of neonatal screening and demonstrate that developing countries can develop own and appropriate diagnostic technologies, that correctly applied can make health care accessible to all.

Acknowledgments

The authors would like to thank all employees who have served for 3 decades from Immunoassay Center. Also thank all the people and institutions from the Cuban public health system, who have been the most responsible for the results reported in this article.

Declaration of Conflicting Interests

The author(s) declared no potential conflicts of interest with respect to the research, authorship, and/or publication of this article.

Funding

The author(s) received no financial support for the research, authorship, and/or publication of this article.

References

1. Cooper RS, Kennelly JF, Orduñez P. Health in Cuba. *Int J of Epidemiol*. 2006;35(4):817-824.
2. Fernández JA, Díaz J. Some theoretical considerations on the active inquiry. *Revista Cubana de Medicina General Integral*. 2009;25(4):107-116.
3. Sánchez A, Gorry C. Immunodiagnostics: the convergence of biotech and public health. *MEDICC Review*. 2013;15(1):7-10.
4. Reed G. Generating appropriate technologies for health equity. *MEDICC Review*. 2009;11(1):14-17.
5. Wilcken B, Wiley V. Fifty years of newborn screening. *J Paediatr Child Health*. 2015;51(1):103-107.
6. Therrell BL, Padilla CD, Loeber G, et al. Current status of newborn screening worldwide: 2015. *Semin Perinatol*. 2015;39(3):171-187.
7. González EC, Frómeta A, del Río L, et al. Cuban neonatal screening of phenylketonuria using an ultramicro-fluorometric test. *Clin Chim Acta*. 2009;402(1-2):129-132.
8. Carlos N, Rego A, Fernández-Yero JL, Sistachs V. Perinatal screening and data processing with the SUMA® technology in Cuba. *Biotecnología Aplicada*. 2014;31(4):311-316.
9. Newborn Screening Quality Assurance Program: Current reports. Web site. http://www.cdc.gov/labstandards/nsqap_reports.html. Published July 2015. Updated July 31, 2015. Accessed February 15, 2016.
10. Herrera D, González EC, Pérez PL, Frómeta A. Normalización del UMELISA TSH NEONATAL® a discos de 3 mm. *CENIC Ciencias Biológicas*. 2006;37(2):119-124.
11. Castells E, González EC, Frómeta A, et al. Modified T4 Neonatal UMELISA® to 3 mm discs for a more rational use of dried blood newborn samples on filter paper. *Biotecnología Aplicada*. 2013; 30(2):137-141.
12. Marrero N, Portuondo M, Lardoeyt R, Tassé D, Lantigua A. Screening for congenital hypothyroidism, phenylketonuria, galactosemia and biotinidase deficiency in a sample of mentally retarded patients in the city of Havana. *Rev Neurol*. 2003; 36(10):913-916.
13. González EC, Marrero N, Pérez PL, et al. An enzyme immunoassay for determining 17α-hydroxyprogesterone in dried blood spots on filter paper using an ultramicroanalytical system. *Clin Chim Acta*. 2008;394(1-2):63-66.
14. Frómeta A, González EC, Castells E, et al. Quantitative ultramicrotest for newborn screening of galactosemia in Cuba. *J Perinat Med*. 2011;39(1):77-81.
15. González EC, Marrero N, Frómeta A, et al. Qualitative colorimetric ultramicroassay for the detection of biotinidase deficiency in newborns. *Clin Chim Acta*. 2006;369(1):35-39.
16. Gutierrez E, Barrios B, Gutierrez R, Damiani A. Molecular characterization of Cuban patients with phenylketonurias. *Rev Cubana Pediatr*. 2002;75(2):101-105.
17. Santana EE, Collazo T, Tamayo VJ, Motes M, Betancourt Y. Genotype phenotype correlation in patients with congenital adrenal hyperplasia diagnosed by neonatal screening. *Rev Ciencias Médicas*. 2015;19(5):830-839.
18. Frómeta A, Barrios M, Hernández O, Lugo E, Baloy A. Influencia de algunos factores asociados con el embarazo y el parto en la

concentración de hormona estimulante de la tiroides (TSH) en suero del cordón umbilical. *Biomédica*. 2001;21(3):242-247.

19. Álvarez MA, Guell R, Gonzalez J, et al. Neuropsychological development during the first two years in children with congenital hypothyroidism screened at birth: the Cuban experience. *Screening*. 1992;1(3):167-173.
20. Álvarez M, Carvajal F, Renón A, et al. Differential effect of fetal, neonatal and treatment variables on neurodevelopment in infants with congenital hypothyroidism. *Horm Res*. 2004;61(1):17-20.
21. Heredero L, Atencio G, Vega JL, Gutiérrez E, Damiani A. Early diagnosis of phenylketonuria in Cuba: preliminary report. *Rev Cuba Pediatr*. 1986;58(1):27-33.
22. Martínez L, Robaina Z, García S, Gutiérrez E. The Cuban program for neonatal screening of phenylketonuria. Twenty years of experience: the clinical and social attention. *Rev Cuba Genet Comunit*. 2008;2(1):45-51.
23. McCaman MW, Robins E. Fluorimetric method for determination of phenylalanine in serum. *J Lab Clin Med*. 1962;59(5):885-890.
24. González EC, Carvajal F, Frómeta A, et al. Newborn screening for congenital adrenal hyperplasia in Cuba: six years of experience. *Clin Chim Acta*. 2013;421:73-78.
25. Rizo D, González A, González E, et al. Standardisation of external multicontrols in dried blood spots (TSH-T4-PHE-GAL-17-OHP-BIOT) for neonatal screening. EQAnews. *Int J Qual Assur*. 2003;14(3):43-50.
26. Rego A, Pérez H, López L, Carlos N. Integral evaluation of quality in diagnostic laboratory networks. *Biotecnol Apl*. 2009;26(2):151-155.
27. De Jesús VR, Mei JV, Cordovado SK, Cuthbert CD. The Newborn Screening Quality Assurance Program at the Centers for Disease Control and Prevention: thirty-five year experience assuring newborn screening laboratory quality. *Int J Neonatal Screen*. 2015;1(1):13-26.
28. Borrajo GJC, Mazziota D. Control de calidad en programas de pesquisa neonatal. In: Colombo M, Cornejo V, Raimann E, eds. *Errores Innatos en el Metabolismo del Niño*. 2nd ed. Santiago, Chile: Editorial Universitaria; 2003:385-402.
29. Borrajo GJC. Newborn screening in Latin America at the beginning of the 21st century. *J Inherit Metab Dis*. 2007;30(4):466-481.
30. Frómeta A, Lechuga MF, Pérez PL, et al. Desenvolvimento do UMELISA TSH neonatal para dosagem de TSH em sangue coletado em papel filtro. *Rev Bras Anál Clín*. 1996;28(4):202-204.
31. Frías GR, Toledano A, Iglesias A, et al. SUMAutoLab: automatic Analyzer of SUMA1 Technology for Neonatal Screening (P047). Book of Abstracts X Latin American Congress of Inborn Errors of Metabolism and Neonatal. *JIEMS*. January–December 2015; 3: 28. doi:10.1177/2326409815613261.
32. Contreras J, Alonso E, Fuentes LE. HPLC for confirmatory diagnosis and biochemical monitoring of Cuban patients with hyperphenylalaninemias. *MEDICC Review*. 2015;17(1):23-28.
33. Howitt P, Darzi A, Yang GZ, et al. Technologies for global health. *Lancet*. 2012:380(9840):507-535.
34. Kerruish NJ, Robertson SP. Newborn screening: new developments, new dilemmas. *J Med Ethics*. 2005;31(7):393-398.
35. McCabe LL, Therrell BL, McCabe ERB. Newborn screening: rationale for a comprehensive, fully integrated public health system. *Molecular Genetics and Metabolism*. 2002;77(4):267-273.
36. Sinha SR, Barry M. Health technologies and innovation in the global health arena. *N Engl J Med*. 2011;365(9):779-782.

15

Mechanistic Bases of Neurotoxicity Provoked by Fatty Acids Accumulating in MCAD and LCHAD Deficiencies

Alexandre U. Amaral, PhD[1,2], Cristiane Cecatto, MSc[1], Janaína C. da Silva, PhD[1], Alessandro Wajner, PhD[1], and Moacir Wajner, MD, PhD[1,3,4]

Abstract

Fatty acid oxidation defects (FAODs) are inherited metabolic disorders caused by deficiency of specific enzyme activities or transport proteins involved in the mitochondrial catabolism of fatty acids. Medium-chain fatty acyl-CoA dehydrogenase (MCAD) and long-chain 3-hydroxyacyl-CoA dehydrogenase (LCHAD) deficiencies are relatively common FAOD biochemically characterized by tissue accumulation of medium-chain fatty acids and long-chain 3-hydroxy fatty acids and their carnitine derivatives, respectively. Patients with MCAD deficiency usually have episodic encephalopathic crises and liver biochemical alterations especially during crises of metabolic decompensation, whereas patients with LCHAD deficiency present severe hepatopathy, cardiomyopathy, and acute and/or progressive encephalopathy. Although neurological symptoms are common features, the underlying mechanisms responsible for the brain damage in these disorders are still under debate. In this context, energy deficiency due to defective fatty acid catabolism and hypoglycemia/hypoketonemia has been postulated to contribute to the pathophysiology of MCAD and LCHAD deficiencies. However, since energetic substrate supplementation is not able to reverse or prevent symptomatology in some patients, it is presumed that other pathogenetic mechanisms are implicated. Since worsening of clinical symptoms during crises is accompanied by significant increases in the concentrations of the accumulating fatty acids, it is conceivable that these compounds may be potentially neurotoxic. We will briefly summarize the current knowledge obtained from patients with these disorders, as well as from animal studies demonstrating deleterious effects of the major fatty acids accumulating in MCAD and LCHAD deficiencies, indicating that disruption of mitochondrial energy, redox, and calcium homeostasis is involved in the pathophysiology of the cerebral damage in these diseases. It is presumed that these findings based on the mechanistic toxic effects of fatty acids may offer new therapeutic perspectives for patients affected by these disorders.

Keywords

fatty acid oxidation defects, MCAD deficiency, LCHAD deficiency, medium-chain fatty acids, long-chain 3-hydroxy fatty acids, mitochondrial dysfunction, oxidative stress

Introduction

Medium-chain fatty acyl-CoA dehydrogenase (MCAD) and long-chain 3-hydroxyacyl-CoA dehydrogenase (LCHAD) deficiencies are among the most common fatty acid oxidation defects (FAODs) that are caused by deficient activities of MCAD and LCHAD, respectively. The biochemical hallmark of these disorders is tissue accumulation of medium-chain fatty acids (MCFAs) and long-chain 3-hydroxy fatty acids (LCHFAs) and their carnitine derivatives.

Medium-Chain Acyl-CoA Dehydrogenase Deficiency

Medium-chain acyl-CoA dehydrogenase (E.C. 1.3.99.3) deficiency (OMIM # 201450) is the most common FAOD with a

[1] Programa de Pós-Graduação em Ciências Biológicas: Bioquímica, Instituto de Ciências Básicas da Saúde, Universidade Federal do Rio Grande do Sul, Porto Alegre, Rio Grande do Sul, Brazil
[2] Departamento de Ciências Biológicas, Universidade Regional Integrada do Alto Uruguai e das Missões, Erechim, Rio Grande do Sul, Brazil
[3] Departamento de Bioquímica, Instituto de Ciências Básicas da Saúde, Universidade Federal do Rio Grande do Sul, Porto Alegre, Rio Grande do Sul, Brazil
[4] Serviço de Genética Médica, Hospital de Clínicas de Porto Alegre, Porto Alegre, Rio Grande do Sul, Brazil

Corresponding Author:
Alexandre U. Amaral, PhD, Departamento de Ciências Biológicas, Universidade Regional Integrada do Alto Uruguai e das Missões, Avenida Sete de Setembro, 1621, CEP 99709-910, Erechim, Rio Grande do Sul, Brazil.
Email: alexandreamaral@uricer.edu.br

prevalence of around 1:10 000 newborns. It is caused by a defect in MCAD, leading to the accumulation of octanoate, decanoate, cis-4-decenoate, and their respective carnitine derivatives. Lactic acidosis has been also found in the affected patients, especially during episodes of metabolic decompensation.[1,2] Clinical presentation usually occurs during fasting or metabolic stress and is characterized by lethargy, seizures, and coma. Progressive encephalopathy with brain abnormalities is commonly found in many untreated patients.[3] Muscle weakness and rhabdomyolysis during acute episodes can also be observed.[4,5] Death may occur in 25% of patients with MCAD deficiency undiagnosed in the first presentation. In this context, diagnosis is usually performed by the detection of increased octanoylcarnitine concentrations in blood and medium-chain dicarboxylic acids and glycine derivatives in urine.[1]

An important measure for MCAD deficiency treatment is to reverse catabolism and sustain anabolism by administrating high amount of carbohydrates and to prescribe frequent meals and fasting avoidance to prevent episodes of decompensation. On the other hand, L-carnitine sometimes coupled to riboflavin supplementation may be helpful in MCAD deficiency, as well as for very long-chain acyl-CoA dehydrogenase (VLCAD) and multiple acyl-CoA dehydrogenase deficiencies, although this is still controversial.[6,7] L-Carnitine administration may increase urinary excretion of accumulating toxic metabolites by its property of binding to these compounds and correct L-carnitine deficiency,[8-10] whereas riboflavin was shown to activate octanoyl-CoA dehydrogenase in lymphocytes from patients with MCAD deficiency,[9,11] as well as the respiratory chain.[12] On the other hand, newborn screening of MCAD deficiency has dramatically improved the clinical course of the disease, significantly preventing mortality and morbidity.[13]

Long-Chain 3-Hydroxyacyl-CoA Dehydrogenase Deficiency

Long-chain 3-hydroxyacyl-CoA dehydrogenase (EC 1.1.1.211) deficiency (OMIM # 609016) is FAOD with an approximate prevalence of 1:50 000 newborns.[14] Laboratory and clinical features include hypoglycemia, metabolic acidosis, hyperlacticacidemia, hyperammonemia, skeletal myopathy, hypotonia, cardiomyopathy, and hepatopathy. Mortality is mainly caused by cardiac decompensation and liver failure and may be as high as 80%.[15] Milder cases surviving into adolescence and adulthood usually present hypotonia, seizures, mental retardation, hypoglycemia, cardiomyopathy, peripheral neuropathy, and retinopathy.[15,16] Metabolic crises are characterized by encephalopathy with seizures, hypoketotic hypoglycemia, vomiting, and dehydration precipitated by infections. Diagnosis of LCHAD deficiency is performed by identification of high urinary excretion of dicarboxylic acids with a hydroxyl group and their carnitine derivatives in blood.[1]

Therapy is based on the prevention of fasting and acute infections, as well as a high carbohydrate consumption at frequent intervals associated with medium-chain triglyceride supplementation.[17] The use of L-carnitine as adjuvant therapy is also controversial and may even aggravate the clinical condition possibly by generating toxic long-chain carnitine derivatives.[18,19] It is emphasized that patients affected by LCHAD deficiency are difficult to treat since many of them present severe clinical manifestations despite the use of an appropriate diet and medications.[20]

Table 1. Potential Pathogenetic Mechanisms Underlying Brain Damage in Fatty Acid Oxidation Disorders (FAOD).

Pathogenetic Mechanisms	Possible Causes	References
Energy deficiency	Mitochondrial dysfunction Hypoketotic hypoglycemia Loss or deficiency of carnitine and CoA β-Oxidation blockage	21,24
Oxidative stress	Respiratory chain inhibition Misfolded protein	22,23
Hyperammonemia	Reduction of hepatic ATP availability from fatty acid oxidation	21,25
Lipotoxicity	Toxicity of fatty acids and carnitine derivatives altering cellular functions	21

Potential Mechanisms of Neurotoxicity in FAOD

Although the pathophysiology of FAOD is still poorly known, brain dysfunction has been attributed to inadequate energy supply due to hypoketotic hypoglycemia, as well as by the toxic effects of high ammonia levels that occur in some patients with these disorders. However, other pathomechanisms seem to be implicated in their pathogenesis. In this context, observations of disturbed redox homeostasis in tissues from patients with MCAD deficiency[9] and more recently neurotoxic properties of the accumulating fatty acids and/or carnitine derivatives may represent contributory factors to FAOD pathophysiology.[21,22] In the present review, we focus on the role of disrupted mitochondrial homeostasis and oxidative stress observed in humans with MCAD and LCHAD deficiencies. We also provide animal experimental data demonstrating that disruption of mitochondrial functions is caused by the fatty acids found at high concentrations in tissues of the affected patients. This is consistent with the observations showing that symptomatology worsening is associated with substantial increase in the concentrations of the potentially toxic fatty acids, particularly during catabolic crises. Table 1 displays the proposed major pathomechanisms of brain damage in FAOD.[21-25]

It should be stressed that neural cells express β-oxidation enzyme activities at low levels, especially the thiolase activity that is nearly absent in this tissue, explaining the inability of brain to oxidize fatty acid to sustain ATP generation.[26,27] However, the presence of β-oxidation pathway enables neural cells to potentially produce and accumulate fatty acids in patients affected by MCAD and LCHAD deficiencies. On the other hand, although brain lipid composition is high, central nervous system is capable of synthesizing only a few nonessential fatty acids, so that both essential and some nonessential fatty acids must enter into the brain from the blood to be incorporated into complex lipids. Short-chain and medium-chain fatty acids with less than 12 carbons can be efficiently transported from the systemic circulation to the brain by passive diffusion through the blood–brain barrier (BBB), whereas long-chain fatty acids are less soluble and must be transported in the nonionized form linked to fatty acid transport proteins to cross the BBB. The protein-mediated transport is carried out by specific protein transporters expressed on the cell membrane, including the fatty acid transport proteins 1 to 6, the fatty acid translocase/CD36, and the plasma membrane fatty acid–binding protein.[28-30]

Disruption of Mitochondrial Homeostasis in MCAD and LCHAD Deficiencies

Mitochondria are essential for cellular homeostasis and survival, since they play critical roles in energy (ATP) production and intracellular transfer, as well as in the regulation of redox and calcium homeostasis, fatty acid oxidation, and apoptosis.[31,32] Oxidative phosphorylation (OXPHOS) is the major source of cellular ATP and reactive oxygen species (ROS) formation.[33] Reactive oxygen species have essential functions in cellular signaling mainly by regulating the expression/activity of many genes and enzymes. However, when at high concentrations, ROS become toxic to the cell causing oxidative damage to mitochondrial proteins, lipids, and DNA that may lead to a cascade of apoptosis or necrosis.[34] Oxidative damage and elevated intracellular calcium concentrations cause mitochondrial stress and collapse of internal membrane potential in a process called mitochondrial permeability transition that also leads to cell death.[35]

Brain is highly dependent on OXPHOS for energy production and therefore is highly susceptible to alterations in mitochondrial function. When OXPHOS is compromised, ATP synthesis is decreased and free radical production increased, potentially leading to cell damage. Thus, it is expected that disordered mitochondrial functions is associated with encephalopathy.

Available human studies point to mitochondrial dysfunction as an important mechanism in the pathogenesis of brain damage in patients affected by MCAD and LCHAD deficiencies. This is consistent with the observations of hyperlacticacidemia, decreased activity of respiratory chain complexes, oxidative stress biomarkers, mitochondrial morphological abnormalities, and rhabdomyolysis that have been demonstrated in patients affected by these diseases.[5,9,23,36-43] However, the exact underlying mechanisms of mitochondrial deregulation are still unclear in these disorders.

Fatty Acid Toxicity

Table 2 shows potential mechanisms of mitochondrial disruption. Long-chain fatty acids that are routinely present in plasma of normal individuals were shown to have cytotoxic effects at high concentrations, impair ATP generation, uncouple OXPHOS, inhibit the respiratory chain, depolarize mitochondria by their protonophoric properties, induce oxidative stress, and have permeability transition.[44-49] Medium-chain fatty acid effects on mitochondrial functions are less studied, but may similarly affect mitochondrial respiration and disturb the translocation of ADP in mitochondria.[50] Therefore, it is feasible that the fatty acids that accumulate in tissues of patients with MCAD and LCHAD deficiencies (Table 3) may similarly induce cellular toxicity. This presumption is supported by mounting evidence of deleterious effects on mitochondrial functions attributed to these compounds. We present below evidence that lipotoxicity caused especially by the principal fatty acids accumulating in MCAD and LCHAD deficiencies may contribute decisively to disrupt mitochondrial homeostasis in brain tissue.

Table 2. Toxicity of Fatty Acids Commonly Found in High-Concentration Human Plasma.

Fatty Acid	Mitochondrial Homeostasis Disruption	References
Palmitic acid, stearic acid	Inhibition of oxidative phosphorylation in fibroblasts	47
	Uncoupler of oxidative phosphorylation in liver	44
	Induction of permeability transition in liver	48,49
Oleic acid, palmitoleic acid	Reduction of Na^+, K^+—ATPase activity in purified enzyme	46
	Decrease of Ca^{2+}—ATPase activity in human red cell membranes	45

Table 3. Major Fatty Acids Accumulating in Medium-Chain Acyl-CoA Dehydrogenase (MCAD) and Long-Chain 3-Hydroxyacyl-CoA Dehydrogenase (LCHAD) Deficiencies.

FAOD	Fatty Acids
MCAD deficiency	Octanoic acid, decanoic acid, cis-4-decenoic acid
LCHAD deficiency	3-Hydroxydodecanoic acid, 3-hydroxytetradecanoic acid, 3-hydroxypalmitic acid

Abbreviations: FAOD, fatty acid oxidation defect.

Evidence That Mitochondrial Dysfunction Is Caused by the Major Fatty Acids Accumulating in MCAD and LCHAD Deficiencies

It can be seen in Table 4 that the MCFAs accumulating in MCAD deficiency deregulate various crucial mitochondrial functions in the brain. It has been demonstrated that MCFA, particularly decanoic and cis-4-decenoic acids, behave as uncouplers of OXPHOS and metabolic inhibitors, as well as inductors of mitochondrial permeability transition and oxidative stress.[51-56] These effects may be associated at least partly

Table 4. Disruption of Brain Mitochondrial Homeostasis Provoked by the Major Medium-Chain Fatty Acids Accumulating in Medium-Chain Acyl-CoA Dehydrogenase (MCAD) Deficiency.

Accumulating Fatty Acids	Mitochondrial Homeostasis Disruption	References
Octanoic acid; decanoic acid; cis-4-decenoic acid	Uncoupling of oxidative phosphorylation	51,54,55
	Metabolic inhibition	54,55
	Decrease of NAD(P)H content	54,55
	Respiratory chain and creatine kinase activities inhibition	54,56-58
	Induction of oxidative stress	52,53
	Decrease of Ca^{2+} retention capacity	56
	Induction of permeability transition	56

Table 5. Disruption of Brain Mitochondrial Homeostasis Provoked by the Major Long-Chain 3-Hydroxy Fatty Acids Accumulating in Long-Chain 3-Hydroxyacyl-CoA Dehydrogenase (LCHAD) Deficiency.

Accumulating Fatty Acids	Mitochondrial Homeostasis Disruption	References
3-Hydroxydodecanoic acid	Uncoupling of oxidative phosphorylation	61
	Induction of oxidative stress	63
3-Hydroxytetradecanoic acid; 3-hydroxypalmitic acid	Uncoupling of oxidative phosphorylation	61
	Induction of oxidative stress	63
	Decrease of NAD(P)H content	61
	Decrease of Ca^{2+} retention capacity	62
	ATP production impairment	62
	Induction of permeability transition	62

with the blockage of the respiratory chain provoked by MCFA that may stimulate superoxide and other ROS production[54,56-58] and with the protonophoric action of these fatty acids due to the transbilayer movement of undissociated (linked to protons) fatty acids through the mitochondrial inner membrane toward the mitochondrial matrix.[59,60]

Mitochondrial dysfunction has also been suggested as an important pathomechanism involved in the neurological symptoms that affect individuals with LCHAD deficiency since there are clear human evidences of mitochondrial damage in these patients. Furthermore, the major hydroxylated fatty acids accumulating in LCHAD deficiency deregulate crucial mitochondrial functions such as maintenance of membrane potential, NAD(P)H redox status, and calcium retention capacity (Table 5). They also uncouple the OXPHOS, induce mitochondrial permeability transition pore opening, and provoke metabolic inhibition in forebrain of adolescent rats,[61,62] besides inducing oxidative stress.[63] These data allied to previous observations demonstrating that long-chain 3-hydroxyacyl-CoA derivatives inhibiting ATP production in human fibroblasts support the hypothesis that LCHFAs disrupt energy and redox mitochondrial homeostasis, probably representing a relevant underlying mechanism in the pathophysiology of the cerebral alterations observed in LCHAD deficiency.

Taken together, the available data strongly indicate that the major fatty acids accumulating in MCAD and LCHAD deficiencies probably contribute to the pathogenesis and perhaps symptomatology of affected patients, by disrupting mitochondrial homeostasis, especially during catabolic situations in which their concentrations significantly increase in blood and other tissues due to accelerated lipolysis. Figure 1 depicts the potential mechanisms involved in FAOD pathophysiology, emphasizing the important role of lipotoxicity provoked by the accumulating metabolites inducing deregulation of mitochondrial homeostasis.

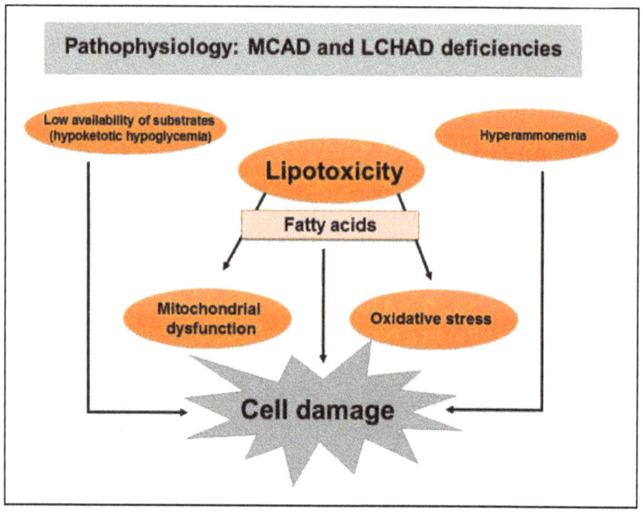

Figure 1. Lipotoxicity as an important pathomechanism involved in the brain damage of medium-chain acyl-CoA dehydrogenase (MCAD) and long-chain 3-hydroxyacyl-CoA dehydrogenase (LCHAD) deficiencies.

Concluding Remarks

Growing evidence obtained from human and animal studies revealed that disturbance of mitochondrial functions associated with oxidative stress at least partly caused by accumulating fatty acids is involved in the pathophysiology of MCAD and LCHAD deficiencies. It is presumed that this pathomechanism possibly contribute to the chronic and neurologic symptoms seen in these defects. Moreover, although it is difficult to evaluate the relative contribution of the toxic fatty acids in the neuropathology of these diseases, it is conceivable that there may be a synergistic action between the toxicity of these metabolites, hyperammonemia, and hypoketotic hypoglycemia (energy deficit) leading to brain damage. It is expected that the development of new drugs targeting the mitochondrion, initially in animal models and thereafter as adjuvant therapeutic approaches for the patients, may become an important focus in the future. In this context, bezafibrate, which activates the peroxisome proliferator-activated receptor that induces transcription of various enzymes involved in mitochondrial fatty acid oxidation,[64] was shown to normalize impaired β-oxidation in skin fibroblast from patients with various FAOD,[65-68] as well as improve the clinical symptoms of late-onset type glutaric acidemia type II.[69] Similar effects were attributed to the antioxidant and anti-inflammatory natural compound resveratrol with positive effects on mitochondrial energy metabolism[70,71] improving mitochondrial fatty acid oxidation capacities in fibroblasts from patients with VLCAD and carnitine palmitoyltransferase II deficiency.[72,73] Thus, these compounds may represent potential novel candidates for the treatment of these diseases by a dual mechanism, improving fatty acid oxidation and counteracting oxidative stress.[73]

Declaration of Conflicting Interests

The author(s) declared no potential conflicts of interest with respect to the research, authorship, and/or publication of this article.

Funding

The author(s) disclosed receipt of the following financial support for the research and/or authorship of this article: The research activity in the authors' laboratories was supported in parts by research grants from Conselho Nacional de Desenvolvimento Científico e Tecnológico (CNPq) 404883/2013-3, Fundação de Amparo à Pesquisa do Estado do Rio Grande do Sul (FAPERGS) 2266-2551/14-2.

References

1. Roe CR, Ding J. Mitochondrial fatty acid oxidation disorders. In: Scriver CR, Beaudet AL, Sly WS, Valle D, eds. *The Metabolic and Molecular Bases of Inherited Disease*. Columbus, OH: McGraw-Hill; 2005.
2. Derks TG, Reijngoud DJ, Waterham HR, et al. The natural history of medium-chain acyl CoA dehydrogenase deficiency in the Netherlands: clinical presentation and outcome. *J Pediatr*. 2006; 148(5):665-670.
3. Touma EH, Charpentier C. Medium chain acyl-CoA dehydrogenase deficiency. *Arch Dis Child*. 1992;67(1):142-145.
4. Iafolla AK, Thompson RJ, Jr, Roe CR. Medium-chain acylcoenzyme A dehydrogenase deficiency: clinical course in 120 affected children. *J Pediatr*. 1994;124(3):409-415.
5. Ruitenbeek W, Poels PJ, Turnbull DM, et al. Rhabdomyolysis and acute encephalopathy in late onset medium chain acyl-CoA dehydrogenase deficiency. *J Neurol Neurosurg Psychiatry*. 1995; 58(2):209-214.
6. Spiekerkoetter U, Bastin J, Gillingham M, Morris A, Wijburg F, Wilcken B. Current issues regarding treatment of mitochondrial fatty acid oxidation disorders. *J Inherit Metab Dis*. 2010;33(5):555-561.
7. Behin A, Acquaviva-Bourdain C, Souvannanorath S, et al. Multiple acyl-CoA dehydrogenase deficiency (MADD) as a cause of late-onset treatable metabolic disease. *Rev Neurol (Paris)*. 2016;172(3):231-241.
8. Lee PJ, Harrison EL, Jones MG, et al. L-Carnitine and exercise tolerance in medium-chain acyl-coenzyme A dehydrogenase (MCAD) deficiency: a pilot study. *J Inherit Metab Dis*. 2005; 28(2):141-152.
9. Derks TG, Touw CM, Ribas GS, et al. Experimental evidence for protein oxidative damage and altered antioxidant defense in patients with medium-chain acyl-CoA dehydrogenase deficiency. *J Inherit Metab Dis*. 2014;37(5):783-789.
10. Antozzi C, Garavaglia B, Mora M, et al. Late-onset riboflavin-responsive myopathy with combined multiple acyl coenzyme A dehydrogenase and respiratory chain deficiency. *Neurology*. 1994;44(11):2153-2158.
11. Duran M, Cleutjens CB, Ketting D, et al. Diagnosis of medium-chain acyl-CoA dehydrogenase deficiency in lymphocytes and liver by a gas chromatographic method: the effect of oral riboflavin supplementation. *Pediatr Res*. 1992;31(1):39-42.
12. Olsen RK, Konarikova E, Giancaspero TA, et al. Riboflavin-responsive and non-responsive mutations in FAD synthase cause multiple acyl-CoA dehydrogenase and combined respiratory-chain deficiency. *Am J Hum Genet*. 2016;98(6):1130-1145.
13. Lindner M, Gramer G, Haege G, et al. Efficacy and outcome of expanded newborn screening for metabolic diseases—report of 10 years from South-West Germany. *Orphanet J Rare Dis*. 2011;6:44.
14. Hagenfeldt L, Venizelos N, von Dobeln U. Clinical and biochemical presentation of long-chain 3-hydroxyacyl-CoA dehydrogenase deficiency. *J Inherit Metab Dis*. 1995;18(2):245-248.
15. Spiekerkoetter U. Mitochondrial fatty acid oxidation disorders: clinical presentation of long-chain fatty acid oxidation defects before and after newborn screening. *J Inherit Metab Dis*. 2010; 33(5):527-532.
16. Tyni T, Rapola J, Paetau A, et al. Pathology of long-chain 3-hydroxyacyl-CoA dehydrogenase deficiency caused by the G1528C mutation. *Pediatr Pathol Lab Med*. 1997;17(3):427-447.
17. Spiekerkoetter U, Lindner M, Santer R, et al. Treatment recommendations in long-chain fatty acid oxidation defects: consensus from a workshop. *J Inherit Metab Dis*. 2009;32(4):498-505.
18. Rocchiccioli F, Wanders RJ, Aubourg P, et al. Deficiency of long-chain 3-hydroxyacyl-CoA dehydrogenase: a cause of lethal myopathy and cardiomyopathy in early childhood. *Pediatr Res*. 1990; 28(6):657-662.
19. Treem WR, Shoup ME, Hale DE, et al. Acute fatty liver of pregnancy, hemolysis, elevated liver enzymes, and low platelets syndrome, and long chain 3-hydroxyacyl-coenzyme A dehydrogenase deficiency. *Am J Gastroenterol*. 1996;91(11):2293-2300.
20. Spiekerkoetter U, Lindner M, Santer R, et al. Management and outcome in 75 individuals with long-chain fatty acid oxidation defects: results from a workshop. *J Inherit Metab Dis*. 2009;32(4): 488-497.
21. Olpin SE. Pathophysiology of fatty acid oxidation disorders and resultant phenotypic variability. *J Inherit Metab Dis*. 2013;36(4): 645-658.
22. Olsen RK, Cornelius N, Gregersen N. Genetic and cellular modifiers of oxidative stress: what can we learn from fatty acid oxidation defects? *Mol Genet Metab*. 2013;110(suppl):S31-S39.

23. Enns GM, Bennett MJ, Hoppel CL, et al. Mitochondrial respiratory chain complex I deficiency with clinical and biochemical features of long-chain 3-hydroxyacyl-coenzyme A dehydrogenase deficiency. *J Pediatr*. 2000;136(2):251-254.
24. Spiekerkoetter U, Wood PA. Mitochondrial fatty acid oxidation disorders: pathophysiological studies in mouse models. *J Inherit Metab Dis*. 2010;33(5):539-546.
25. Baruteau J, Sachs P, Broue P, et al. Clinical and biological features at diagnosis in mitochondrial fatty acid beta-oxidation defects: a French pediatric study of 187 patients. *J Inherit Metab Dis*. 2013;36(5):795-803.
26. Yang SY, He XY, Schulz H. Fatty acid oxidation in rat brain is limited by the low activity of 3-ketoacyl-coenzyme A thiolase. *J Biol Chem*. 1987;262(27):13027-13032.
27. Reichmann H, Maltese WA, DeVivo DC. Enzymes of fatty acid beta-oxidation in developing brain. *J Neurochem*. 1988;51(2): 339-344.
28. Miller JC, Gnaedinger JM, Rapoport SI. Utilization of plasma fatty acid in rat brain: distribution of [14C]palmitate between oxidative and synthetic pathways. *J Neurochem*. 1987;49(5): 1507-1514.
29. Hamilton JA. New insights into the roles of proteins and lipids in membrane transport of fatty acids. *Prostaglandins Leukot Essent Fatty Acids*. 2007;77(5-6):355-361.
30. Mitchell RW, Hatch GM. Fatty acid transport into the brain: of fatty acid fables and lipid tails. *Prostaglandins Leukot Essent Fatty Acids*. 2011;85(5):293-302.
31. McBride HM, Neuspiel M, Wasiak S. Mitochondria: more than just a powerhouse. *Curr Biol*. 2006;16(14):R551-R560.
32. Bueler H. Mitochondrial dynamics, cell death and the pathogenesis of Parkinson's disease. *Apoptosis*. 2010;15(11):1336-1353.
33. Lemasters JJ, Qian T, Bradham CA, et al. Mitochondrial dysfunction in the pathogenesis of necrotic and apoptotic cell death. *J Bioenerg Biomembr*. 1999;31(4):305-319.
34. Kroemer G, Reed JC. Mitochondrial control of cell death. *Nat Med*. 2000;6(5):513-519.
35. Kowaltowski AJ, de Souza-Pinto NC, Castilho RF, Vercesi AE. Mitochondria and reactive oxygen species. *Free Radic Biol Med*. 2009;47(4):333-343.
36. Tyni T, Majander A, Kalimo H, Rapola J, Pihko H. Pathology of skeletal muscle and impaired respiratory chain function in long-chain 3-hydroxyacyl-CoA dehydrogenase deficiency with the G1528C mutation. *Neuromuscul Disord*. 1996;6(5):327-337.
37. Ventura FV, Ruiter JP, IJlst L, de Almeida IT, Wanders RJ. Lactic acidosis in long-chain fatty acid beta-oxidation disorders. *J Inherit Metab Dis*. 1998;21(6):645-654.
38. Das AM, Fingerhut R, Wanders RJ, Ullrich K. Secondary respiratory chain defect in a boy with long-chain 3-hydroxyacyl-CoA dehydrogenase deficiency: possible diagnostic pitfalls. *Eur J Pediatr*. 2000;159(4):243-246.
39. Feillet F, Steinmann G, Vianey-Saban C, et al. Adult presentation of MCAD deficiency revealed by coma and severe arrhythmias. *Intensive Care Med*. 2003;29(9):1594-1597.
40. Wakabayashi M, Kamijo Y, Nakajima T, et al. Fatty acid accumulation and resulting PPARalpha activation in fibroblasts due to trifunctional protein deficiency. *PPAR Res*. 2012;2012:371691.
41. Diekman EF, van der Pol WL, Nievelstein RA, et al. Muscle MRI in patients with long-chain fatty acid oxidation disorders. *J Inherit Metab Dis*. 2014;37(3):405-413.
42. Najdekr L, Gardlo A, Madrova L, et al. Oxidized phosphatidylcholines suggest oxidative stress in patients with medium-chain acyl-CoA dehydrogenase deficiency. *Talanta*. 2015;139:62-66.
43. Wajner M, Amaral AU. Mitochondrial dysfunction in fatty acid oxidation disorders: insights from human and animal studies. *Biosci Rep*. 2015;36(1):e00281.
44. Berry MN, Clark DG, Grivell AR, Wallace PG. The calorigenic nature of hepatic ketogenesis: an explanation for the stimulation of respiration induced by fatty acid substrates. *Eur J Biochem*. 1983;131(1):205-214.
45. Davis FB, Davis PJ, Blas SD, Schoenl M. Action of long-chain fatty acids in vitro on Ca2+-stimulatable, Mg2+-dependent ATPase activity in human red cell membranes. *Biochem J*. 1987;248(2):511-516.
46. Swarts HG, Schuurmans Stekhoven FM, De Pont JJ. Binding of unsaturated fatty acids to Na+, K(+)-ATPase leading to inhibition and inactivation. *Biochim Biophys Acta*. 1990;1024(1):32-40.
47. Ventura FV, Ruiter JP, Ijlst L, Almeida IT, Wanders RJ. Inhibition of oxidative phosphorylation by palmitoyl-CoA in digitonin permeabilized fibroblasts: implications for long-chain fatty acid beta-oxidation disorders. *Biochim Biophys Acta*. 1995;1272(1):14-20.
48. Sultan A, Sokolove PM. Palmitic acid opens a novel cyclosporin A-insensitive pore in the inner mitochondrial membrane. *Arch Biochem Biophys*. 2001;386(1):37-51.
49. Mironova GD, Gritsenko E, Gateau-Roesch O, et al. Formation of palmitic acid/Ca2+ complexes in the mitochondrial membrane: a possible role in the cyclosporin-insensitive permeability transition. *J Bioenerg Biomembr*. 2004;36(2):171-178.
50. Schonfeld P, Wojtczak AB, Geelen MJ, Kunz W, Wojtczak L. On the mechanism of the so-called uncoupling effect of medium- and short-chain fatty acids. *Biochim Biophys Acta*. 1988;936(3): 280-288.
51. Parker WD, Jr, Haas R, Stumpf DA, Eguren LA. Effects of octanoate on rat brain and liver mitochondria. *Neurology*. 1983; 33(10):1374-1377.
52. Schuck PF, Ceolato PC, Ferreira GC, et al. Oxidative stress induction by cis-4-decenoic acid: relevance for MCAD deficiency. *Free Radic Res*. 2007;41(11):1261-1272.
53. Schuck PF, Ferreira GC, Moura AP, et al. Medium-chain fatty acids accumulating in MCAD deficiency elicit lipid and protein oxidative damage and decrease non-enzymatic antioxidant defenses in rat brain. *Neurochem Int*. 2009;54(8):519-525.
54. Schuck PF, Ferreira Gda C, Tonin AM, et al. Evidence that the major metabolites accumulating in medium-chain acyl-CoA dehydrogenase deficiency disturb mitochondrial energy homeostasis in rat brain. *Brain Res*. 2009;1296:117-126.
55. Schuck PF, Ferreira Gda C, Tahara EB, et al. Cis-4-decenoic acid provokes mitochondrial bioenergetic dysfunction in rat brain. *Life Sci*. 2010;87(5-6):139-146.
56. Amaral AU, Cecatto C, da Silva JC, et al. Cis-4-decenoic and decanoic acids impair mitochondrial energy, redox and Ca(2+) homeostasis and induce mitochondrial permeability transition

pore opening in rat brain and liver: possible implications for the pathogenesis of MCAD deficiency. *Biochim Biophys Acta*. 2016; 1857(9):1363-1372.

57. Kim CS, Roe CR, Ambrose WW. L-Carnitine prevents mitochondrial damage induced by octanoic acid in the rat choroid plexus. *Brain Res*. 1990;536(1-2):335-338.
58. Reis de Assis D, Maria Rde C, Borba Rosa R, et al. Inhibition of energy metabolism in cerebral cortex of young rats by the medium-chain fatty acids accumulating in MCAD deficiency. *Brain Res*. 2004;1030(1):141-151.
59. Wojtczak L, Schonfeld P. Effect of fatty acids on energy coupling processes in mitochondria. *Biochim Biophys Acta*. 1993;1183(1): 41-57.
60. Schonfeld P, Wojtczak L. Fatty acids as modulators of the cellular production of reactive oxygen species. *Free Radic Biol Med*. 2008;45(3):231-241.
61. Tonin AM, Ferreira GC, Grings M, et al. Disturbance of mitochondrial energy homeostasis caused by the metabolites accumulating in LCHAD and MTP deficiencies in rat brain. *Life Sci*. 2010;86(21-22):825-831.
62. Tonin AM, Amaral AU, Busanello EN, et al. Mitochondrial bioenergetics deregulation caused by long-chain 3-hydroxy fatty acids accumulating in LCHAD and MTP deficiencies in rat brain: a possible role of mPTP opening as a pathomechanism in these disorders? *Biochim Biophys Acta*. 2014;1842(9):1658-1667.
63. Tonin AM, Grings M, Busanello EN, et al. Long-chain 3-hydroxy fatty acids accumulating in LCHAD and MTP deficiencies induce oxidative stress in rat brain. *Neurochem Int*. 2010;56(8):930-936.
64. Barish GD, Narkar VA, Evans RM. PPAR delta: a dagger in the heart of the metabolic syndrome. *J Clin Invest*. 2006;116(3): 590-597.
65. Djouadi F, Bonnefont JP, Thuillier L, et al. Correction of fatty acid oxidation in carnitine palmitoyl transferase 2-deficient cultured skin fibroblasts by bezafibrate. *Pediatr Res*. 2003; 54(4):446-451.
66. Djouadi F, Aubey F, Schlemmer D, et al. Bezafibrate increases very-long-chain acyl-CoA dehydrogenase protein and mRNA expression in deficient fibroblasts and is a potential therapy for fatty acid oxidation disorders. *Hum Mol Genet*. 2005;14(18): 2695-2703.
67. Yamaguchi S, Li H, Purevsuren J, et al. Bezafibrate can be a new treatment option for mitochondrial fatty acid oxidation disorders: evaluation by in vitro probe acylcarnitine assay. *Mol Genet Metab*. 2012;107(1-2):87-91.
68. Djouadi F, Habarou F, Le Bachelier C, et al. Mitochondrial trifunctional protein deficiency in human cultured fibroblasts: effects of bezafibrate. *J Inherit Metab Dis*. 2016;39(1):47-58.
69. Yamada K, Kobayashi H, Bo R, et al. Efficacy of bezafibrate on fibroblasts of glutaric acidemia type II patients evaluated using an in vitro probe acylcarnitine assay. *Brain Dev*. 2017; 39(1):48-57.
70. Lagouge M, Argmann C, Gerhart-Hines Z, et al. Resveratrol improves mitochondrial function and protects against metabolic disease by activating SIRT1 and PGC-1alpha. *Cell*. 2006;127(6): 1109-1122.
71. Mercader J, Palou A, Bonet ML. Resveratrol enhances fatty acid oxidation capacity and reduces resistin and retinol-binding protein 4 expression in white adipocytes. *J Nutr Biochem*. 2011; 22(9):828-834.
72. Bastin J, Lopes-Costa A, Djouadi F. Exposure to resveratrol triggers pharmacological correction of fatty acid utilization in human fatty acid oxidation-deficient fibroblasts. *Hum Mol Genet*. 2011; 20(10):2048-2057.
73. Aires V, Delmas D, Le Bachelier C, et al. Stilbenes and resveratrol metabolites improve mitochondrial fatty acid oxidation defects in human fibroblasts. *Orphanet J Rare Dis*. 2014;9:79.

16

Newborn Screening Quality Assurance Program for CFTR Mutation Detection and Gene Sequencing to Identify Cystic Fibrosis

Miyono M. Hendrix, MS[1], Stephanie L. Foster, BS[1], and Suzanne K. Cordovado, PhD[1]

Abstract

All newborn screening laboratories in the United States and many worldwide screen for cystic fibrosis. Most laboratories use a second-tier genotyping assay to identify a panel of mutations in the CF transmembrane regulator (*CFTR*) gene. Centers for Disease Control and Prevention's Newborn Screening Quality Assurance Program houses a dried blood spot repository of samples containing *CFTR* mutations to assist newborn screening laboratories and ensure high-quality mutation detection in a high-throughput environment. Recently, *CFTR* mutation detection has increased in complexity with expanded genotyping panels and gene sequencing. To accommodate the growing quality assurance needs, the repository samples were characterized with several multiplex genotyping methods, Sanger sequencing, and 3 next-generation sequencing assays using a high-throughput, low-concentration DNA extraction method. The samples performed well in all of the assays, providing newborn screening laboratories with a resource for complex *CFTR* mutation detection and next-generation sequencing as they transition to new methods.

Keywords

cystic fibrosis, *CFTR*, mutation, newborn screening, next-generation sequencing

Introduction

Cystic fibrosis (CF) is one of the most common autosomal recessive disorders that affects approximately 1:4000 people of Western European, North American, and Australasian descent. When CF is identified and treated early, patients avoid many of the devastating clinical consequences, allowing for improved growth, reduced hospitalizations, and longer life span, which resulted in the US Centers for Disease Control and Prevention (CDC) recommending that CF be included in newborn screening panels in the United States.[1,2] Newborn screening for CF begins with an immunoassay that measures the pancreatic enzyme immunoreactive trypsinogen (IRT), which is elevated in newborns affected with CF.[3,4] Since IRT can be elevated for reasons other than CF, this test alone does not have the specificity required for newborn screening. In 1989, scientists discovered the CF transmembrane regulator (*CFTR*) gene on chromosome 7.[5] Defects in the *CFTR* gene that alter structure, function, or expression of this protein can lead to malfunctions or disease processes in the lungs, upper respiratory tract, gastrointestinal tract, pancreas, liver, sweat glands, and genitourinary tract.[6]

All US states and many international programs have implemented routine newborn screening for CF. Most US programs use an algorithm that involves at least 1 initial measurement of IRT from a dried blood specimen (DBS) taken from all newborns and then testing for a panel of *CFTR* mutations on a subset of babies with elevated IRT.[7,8] The panel of *CFTR* mutations can be variable between programs but typically includes the American College of Medical Genetics (ACMG) recommended 23 mutations and often additional mutations.[7-10] Newborns with either 1 or 2 *CFTR* mutations are considered screen positive by most programs and are sent to CF care centers for diagnostic

[1] Centers for Disease Control and Prevention, Atlanta, GA, USA

Corresponding Author:
Suzanne K. Cordovado, PhD, Centers for Disease Control and Prevention, 4770 Buford Highway, MS F24, Atlanta, GA, USA.
Email: scordovado@cdc.gov

workup. Although this algorithm has a relatively low false-negative rate, it has quite a high false-positive rate with most babies being carriers of 1 *CFTR* mutation and do not display any symptoms associated with CF. As an example, the state of Wisconsin reported a false-positive rate as high as a 90%[11] and the New York state found as high as a 94% false-positive rate (excludes screen positives with no mutations identified).[12] The false-positive rates vary between programs most often because of the differences in the IRT cutoff but sometimes because of the mutation panels used. Currently, the only US program that identifies a screen positive as 2 identified *CFTR* mutations is the state of California, which initially tests for a panel of *CFTR* mutations in babies with elevated IRT. If a newborn has only 1 mutation from the California panel, the *CFTR* gene is sequenced and only those babies with 2 mutations are sent for clinical evaluation. Using this algorithm, California reported that 34% of their screen-positive newborns were CF, 53% had a milder form of *CFTR*-related metabolic syndrome (CRMS), and 13% were carriers with complex mutations.[13]

False CF-positive results, while unavoidable in newborn screening, cause parental anxiety, unnecessary clinical testing, and downstream genetic counseling.[14-17] Thus, there are ongoing efforts to redefine a positive newborn screening test such that it requires the identification of 2 CF-causing *CFTR* mutations[18] similar to what is being done in California.[13] Since there are >2000 mutations or variants in the *CFTR* gene with more still being discovered,[19,20] the requirement of identifying 2 CF-causing mutations would likely necessitate either gene sequencing or a greatly expanded genotyping panel of *CFTR* mutations. As the complexity of *CFTR* mutation detection in newborn screening expands, there is a need for more extensively characterized dried blood spot quality assurance materials to ensure that high levels of accuracy are maintained in these analytical measurements.

The CDC's Newborn Screening Quality Assurance Program (NSQAP) provides DBS proficiency testing to United States and international laboratories for both IRT (N = 215 laboratories, quarter 1 of 2016) and *CFTR* mutation detection (N = 68 laboratories, quarter 1 of 2016).[21,22] The NSQAP's CF DNA DBS repository, made from CF patient and family blood samples, contains a wide variety of *CFTR* mutations including the 23 recommended by ACMG as well as 47 additional mutations. Each repository sample is characterized extensively by CDC's Molecular Quality Improvement Program Laboratories using Sanger sequencing and commonly used genotyping methods to ensure robust performance in newborn screening laboratories. As the complexity of CF molecular methods continues to evolve, CDC has performed a comprehensive evaluation and characterization of the CF DNA DBS repository samples using a diverse array of genotyping and next-generation sequencing methods that would be amenable in the newborn screening laboratory environment.

Materials and Methods

Samples

Samples from 198 patients and family members affected by CF were collected from CF care centers located in Maryland, Ohio, and Wisconsin[22] and more recently in California in collaboration with the Sequoia Foundation and the California Department of Public Health. All blood was collected in EDTA blood collection tubes from adult donors with at least 1 *CFTR* mutation (Becton Dickinson, Franklin Lakes, New Jersey) and shipped to CDC, where blood was spotted on to Whatman 903 filter paper (Piscataway, New Jersey) to create dried blood spots (75 μL) for quality assurance. This project was approved by the institutional review boards of all participating CF care centers, and the CDC's Office of Science at the National Center for Environmental Health determined that CDC was not involved with human subjects under 45 CFR 66.012(d).b because all specimens are deidentified and cannot be traced back to the donor.

Newborn Screening Quality Assurance Program CF DNA Proficiency Testing (PT) Program

Each participating laboratory received 5 blind-coded proficiency testing specimens 4 times a year, and laboratories reported both the genotyping results and clinical assessments to CDC. These results were evaluated based on the program's stated mutation panel and molecular algorithm. Programs were informed to assume all samples have an elevated IRT that would trigger their algorithm to test for *CFTR* mutations. To ensure accurate grading, each programs provided descriptive information including *CFTR* genotyping/sequencing method, mutation detected or exons sequenced if not using a commercial method, secondary/confirmatory method, description of when and how a secondary/confirmatory method is used, and DNA extraction method.[23]

DNA Extraction and Quantitation

Genomic DNA was extracted from 250-μL whole blood (EDTA anticoagulant) using the Qiagen QIACube Micro spin columns and resuspended in 100 μL of Tris-buffered EDTA (Valencia, California). The DNA was quantified using the NanoDrop spectrophotometer (Wilmington, Delaware) and diluted to 10 ng/μL for direct use only in Sanger sequencing. Genomic DNA was also extracted from one 3.2-mm DBS punch using the Qiagen Generation DNA Purification and Elution Solutions. The punch was washed 2 times for 15 minutes in 150 μL of DNA Purification Solution followed by one 15-minute wash with 150 μL of DNA Elution Solution. All washes were performed at room temperature with slight agitation. Genomic DNA was eluted from the punch in 50 μL of DNA Elution Solution after incubating at 99°C for 15 minutes. All assays other than Sanger sequencing used DNA extracted from DBS. When quantification of DNA extracted from DBS punches was required, a real-time polymerase chain reaction (PCR) of the *RNase P* gene using the TaqMan RNaseP Control Reagents was used (Thermo Fisher Scientific, Waltham, Massachusetts). The standard curve was made from human genomic DNA (Roche Applied Science, Penzberg, Germany).

CFTR Genotyping

Following the manufacturer' instructions, the NSQAP samples were genotyped and analyzed using 3 commercially available products: InPlex CF Molecular Test 40+4 (Hologic, Marlborough, Massachusetts), xTAG CF39v2 and CF60v2 kits (Luminex, Austin, Texas), and the MiSeqDx CF 139-variant assay (Illumina, San Diego, California). The InPlex CF Molecular test 40+4 followed the manufacturer's instruction for the in vitro diagnostic (IVD) InPlex CF Molecular Test IVD with 1 modification—the second cycling step during the amplification process was increased from 12 to 14 cycles. The DNA volume used for the Hologic InPlex CF Molecular Test 40+4, both the Luminex xTAG 39 and 60 kits, and the MiSeqDx CF 139-variant assay kit was 5 μL of the Generation extraction's 50 μL total volume (5-10 ng DNA). Samples were also analyzed using 45 unique TaqMan *CFTR* single-nucleotide polymorphism (SNP) assays that include all but the I148T (c.443T>C) and D1270N (c.3808G>A) mutations in the InPlex CF Molecular Test 40+4 assay and the addition of the I506V (c.1516A>G) and I507V (c.1519A>G) variants. Each 10 μL reaction consisted of 1× DurAmp v2 Master Mix (Thermo Fisher Scientific), 1× of SNP genotyping probe mix, and 1 μL of the Generation extraction's 50 μL total volume (1-2 ng DNA). All run data were loaded into Thermo Fisher Scientific's Genotyper software and analyzed with Hardy-Weinberg analysis with noted exceptions. Hardy-Weinberg analysis was disabled for the F508del (c.1521_1523delCTT), I507del (c.1519_1521delATC), I506V (c.1516A>G), I507V (c.1519A>G), F508C (c.1523T>G), 5T (c.1210-12[5]), and 9T (c.1210-12[9]) assays. (Note: since the writing of this manuscript, the Hologic Inplex CF assays have been recalled and discontinued.)

Next-Generation Sequencing of *CFTR*

Ion AmpliSeq CFTR Panel on the Ion Torrent PGM. Target regions of the *CFTR* gene were amplified in 2 amplicon pools that covered all exons, untranslated regions (UTRs), and regions of interest in introns 12 and 22 and bar-coded using a custom Ion AmpliSeq *CFTR* Panel and IonXpress bar codes (Thermo Fisher Scientific). Each pool required 6 μL of Generation extracted genomic DNA (5-50 ng/pool; average: 18 ng/pool) and was quantitated, pooled, amplified, enriched, and sequenced on a 318 chip according to manufacturer's instructions. Data from the Ion PGM (Thermo Fisher Scientific) were processed and aligned to the human genome reference sequence (hg19, build GRCh37). In order to determine the level of sequence coverage for the targeted genomic region, the manufacturer provided Coverage Analysis plug-in (v4.0-r73765) was utilized. Variants were called and annotated using the Variant Caller plug-in (v4.0-r73742) with a customized hotspot file consisting of 240 unique variants also provided by the manufacturer. The custom hotspot file is available upon request. The data were visually inspected using Integrative Genomics Viewer (IGV) from the Broad Institute (Cambridge, Massachusetts).[24,25] All analyzed data from the Ion PGM were then compared for concordance against the Sanger sequence data.

Swift Biosciences Accel-Amplicon CFTR Panel for Illumina Platforms. Target regions of the *CFTR* gene were amplified in a single amplicon pool that covered all exons, UTRs, and regions of interest in introns 12 and 22 known to contain mutations 1811+1.6kbA>G (c.1679+1.6kbA>G) and 3849+10kbC>T (c.3717+12191C>T) using the Accel-Amplicon *CFTR* Panel for the Illumina MiSeq Platform (Swift Biosciences, Ann Arbor, Michigan). The genomic DNA input was between 10 and 30 ng, and the libraries were prepared according to the manufacturer's instructions. The libraries were diluted by 1:100 000 and quantified using KAPA Biosciences Library Quantification kit KK4835 (Wilmington, Massachusetts) according to the manufacturer's recommendation on the QuantStudio 12K Flex (Thermo Fisher Scientific). Libraries were diluted to either 2 or 4 nmol/L and pooled together for denaturing and subsequent loading on to the MiSeq flow cell at a final concentration of 12 to 16 pmol/L . The samples were run on the MiSeqDx instrument research mode using either the MiSeq Reagent Kit v2 Standard (300 cycles) or MiSeq Reagent kit v2 Micro (300 cycles; Illumina).

As an open system, data from the Accel-Amplicon *CFTR* Panel were processed using several freeware bioinformatic tools to create a custom analytical pipeline. The first step was to trim the 5′- and 3′-anchored primers using Cutadapt.[26] The data were then aligned to the human genome reference sequence (hg19, build GRCh37) using Burrows-Wheeler Aligner BWA-MEM version 0.7.5a-r405,[27] and variants were extracted using FreeBayes version v1.0.2[28] and GATK version 3.5 (3.5.0-g36282e4)[29] using a Browser Extensible Data (BED) file supplied by the manufacturer to limit the sequence area of interest. The data were also visually inspected using IGV. All analyzed data were then compared for concordance against the Sanger sequence data.

Sanger Sequencing of *CFTR*

Sanger sequencing was performed for all exons, intron/exon borders, and a region of interest in intron 22 known to contain mutation 3849+10kbC>T (c.3717+12191C>T). The *CFTR* gene was amplified using primer sets (RSS000010013) described in the National Center for Biotechnology Information's Probe database. Each region was amplified from 5 to 10 ng of genomic DNA in a 10 μL reaction, using 10 pmol each of forward and reverse primers in the RSS000010013 primer sets, and 1× HotStarTaq Master Mix (Qiagen, Valencia, California). Cycling conditions were as follows: 10-minute denaturing step at 95°C; 40 cycles at 95°C for 30 seconds, 62°C for

Table 1. DNA Extration Methods Used by the 2016 Quarter 1 CF DNA PT Participants.

DNA Extraction Methods Used by CF DNA PT Participants	No. of Laboratories
Qiagen QIAamp spin columns (manual or robotic)	5
Qiagen magnetic bead kit (EZ1 or BioSprint 96)	2
Qiagen Generation DNA purification and DNA elution solutions	22
Sigma Aldrich Extract-N-Amp	3
In-house alkaline lysis prep	7
In-house boiling prep	6
In-house lysis boiling prep	1
Other	11
No response	6

Abbreviation: CF, cystic fibrosis.

30 seconds, and 72°C for 1 minute; 10-minute extension at 72°C, followed by a 4°C hold. Unused primers and nucleotides were removed using ExoSAP-IT (Affymetrix, Santa Clara, CA), and sequencing was performed using BigDye Terminator Ready Reaction kit, version 1.1. The cycle sequencing reaction consisted of 1 μL of BigDye Terminator, 1.5 μL of 5× sequencing buffer, 3.2 pmol primer, and 1 μL of PCR product. Additional primers sets not covered by the RSS000010013 were also amplified and cycle sequenced as previously described.[30] Excess BigDye terminators were removed using BigDye XTerminator, and samples were electrophoresed on the 3730 DNA Analyzer (Thermo Fisher Scientific) using the run module BDx_Rapid-Seq36_POP7 (Thermo Fisher Scientific). Sequence data were analyzed using the SeqScape software (Thermo Fisher Scientific) with GenBank *CFTR* genomic reference sequence NG_016465.

Results

The CDC's NSQAP sends DBS samples to participating laboratories engaged in CF newborn screening 4 times a year. Based on the information collected from the 63 laboratories that reported data for quarter 1 of 2016, the most commonly used method of DNA extractions was the Qiagen Generation DNA Purification and Elution Solution method (Table 1). This method is a relatively crude extraction that often results in a lower concentration of DNA. Thus, the Generation DNA extraction method was used in this study to validate the various genotyping and sequencing methods. The primary and secondary genotyping/sequencing methods reported by the laboratories for this quarter included 27 different methods that were either commercially available or laboratory developed. The number of mutations that each method detects is reported in Table 2 and ranged from 1 to 139 detected mutations for genotyping assays and 2 to an unlimited number of detected mutations for Sanger and next-generation sequencing methods.

DNA was extracted from a 3.2-mm punch taken from a DBS that contains approximately 3 μL of blood. Since newborn screening laboratories do not typically quantify DNA, a prescribed volume of extracted DNA was used in most of the assays rather than a set concentration or quantity. In order to better define the working range of DNA concentrations for the assays not commonly used in newborn screening laboratories, DNA extracts were quantified using real-time PCR, and the average quantity and range of concentrations are presented in Table 3.

All genotyping method results were compared with Sanger sequence data and found to have 100% concordance with the mutations included in their panels (Table 4 includes ACMG recommended mutations and variants, and Table 5 includes expanded panel mutations beyond the ACMG recommended). The CFTRdele2,3 (c.54-5940_273+10250del21kb) mutation detected by the xTAG CF60v2 kit was confirmed using the CF 139-variant assay kit because this mutation is not detectable using Sanger sequencing. The xTAG CF kits conditionally report the intron 9 poly T status (c.1210-12[5], c.1210-12[7], and c.1210-12[9]) when an R117H (c.350G>A) mutation is present, whereas these data can be seen for all samples using the InPlex 40+4 assay. Similarly, the F508C (c.1523T>G), I506V (c.1516A>G), and I507V (c.1519A>G) variants are assayed, but results are only displayed when the software designates a "Mut D" call (indicating no normal sequence detected) for F508del (c.1521_1523delCTT) and/or I507del (c.1519_1521delATC) for the xTAG kits, but the F508C (c.1523T>G) is shown for all InPlex 40+4 samples. These variants when analyzed by the genotyping assays were 100% concordant with Sanger sequence data (Tables 4 and 5). For this study, only TaqMan Genotyping assays corresponding to the InPlex CF Molecular test 40+4 kit were assayed, however, additional *CFTR* mutation probe sets are available and can be used to create a more customized panel.

Three next-generation sequencing methods and 2 instrument platforms (MiSeqDx and Ion Torrent PGM) were used to characterize the CF DNA DBS repository. Both the MiSeqDx *CFTR* 139-variant genotyping assay and the AmpliSeq *CFTR* gene sequencing panel have a developed bioinformatics pipeline for analysis on their respective instruments, whereas the Accel-Amplicon *CFTR* panel, which is still in development, was analyzed using freeware bioinformatics tools.[26-29] The results from all 3 next-generation sequencing methods were 100% concordant with Sanger sequence. Since Sanger sequencing cannot detect the CFTR dele2,3 mutation in the MiSeqDx *CFTR* 139-variant assay, this sample was compared with the xTAG CF60v2 and also found to be 100% concordant (Tables 4 and 5).

The MiSeqDx *CFTR* 139-variant next-generation sequencing assay which can accommodate up to 48 samples per flow cell had a density range between 473 ± 11 and 983 ± 9 K/mm^2, with an average quality score ≥Q30 of 88.6% for read 1 and 79.9% for read 2. The Ion AmpliSeq *CFTR* libraries were pooled and run on six 318 chips; five 318 chips were loaded with 20 samples, and one 318 chip was loaded with 32 samples. The average mapped reads for the 5 chips with 20 samples was 276 939, and 97.2% of reads were on target with a read depth of 2 476 and a uniformity of 88.1%. The 318 chip with 32 samples had 102 862 mapped reads and 94.8% reads on target with a read depth of 705 and uniformity of 88.3%. The Ion AmpliSeq *CFTR* Panel was designed to distinguish the intron 9 PolyT 5

Table 2. Primary and Secondary Genotyping Methods and Number of Mutations/Variants Detected by each Method for the 2016 Quarter 1 CF DNA PT Participants.

	Labs using Genotyping/ Sequencing Method				Mutations/Variants Detected by Genotyping/ Sequencing Methods				
Genotyping/Sequencing Methods	# labs using as primary method	# labs using as secondary method	U.S. labs	non-U.S. labs	# mutations detected	# ACMG mutations	# expanded mutations	variants (F508C, I506V, I507V)	Intron 9 (5/7/9T)
Hologic CF InPlex® Molecular Test—ACMG	3	1	4	0	23	23	1[a]	F508C	5/7/9T
Hologic CF InPlex® Molecular Test 40+4	20	6	19	1	40[b]	23	19	F508C	5/7/9T
Luminex Molecular Diagnostics xTAG® CF—ACMG only	0	0	0	0	23	23	0	Yes	5/7/9T
Luminex Molecular Diagnostics IVD xTAG® CF39 v2	7	4	5	2	39	23	16	Yes	5/7/9T
Luminex Molecular Diagnostics xTAG® CF60 v2	1	0	1	0	60	23	37	Yes	5/7/9T
Luminex Molecular Diagnostics xTAG® CF71 v2	0	0	0	0	71	23	48	Yes	5/7/9T
Luminex Platform and Laboratory Developed Test	1	0	1	0	40	15	25	No	No
Elucigene Diagnostics Elucigene® CF4v2	1	0	0	1	4	4	0	No	No
Elucigene Diagnostics Elucigene® CF30v2	3	0	0	3	29	19	10	No	No
Elucigene Diagnostics Elucigene® CFEU2v1	1	1	0	1	51	23	27	No	5/7/9T
Abbott Molecular CF Genotyping Assay v3	2	1	0	4	32	23	9	Yes	5/7/9T
Fujirebio INNO–LiPA® Strip 19	0	1	0	1	19	12	7	No	No
Fujirebio INNO–LiPA® Strips 17+19	3	2	0	3	36	23	13	No	5/7/9T
Sequenom® assays other than HerediT™ CF (MALDI-TOF Mass Spectrometry)	1	1	0	3	12-42	11-21	1-21	No	No
ViennaLab Diagnostics GmbH CF StripAssay®	1	0	0	1	34	23	11	No	5/7/9T
Allele-specific Oligonucleotide PCR	2	0	1	1	1-9	1-9	0	No	No
High Resolution Melt Technology	2	0	0	2	3-11	3-8	0-3	Unknown	No
Real-time PCR Allelic Discrimination Assay (ie TaqMan®)	2	0	2	0	1	1	0	No	No
In-house Amplification Refractory Mutation System	1	1	0	1	1	1	0	No	No
In-house single nucleotide primer extension assay	1	0	0	1	12	10	1	No	5/7/9T
PCR/Heteroduplex Analysis/Gel Electrophoresis	0	2	0	2	1	0	1	No	No
Capillary Electrophoresis	0	1	0	1	3	3	0	No	No
Amplification and Restriction Fragment Length Polymorphism Analysis (PCR-RFLP)	2	1	0	2	5-9	4-8	1-1	No	No
Amplification and Polyacrylamide Gel Electrophoresis (PCR-PAGE)	0	0	0	1	1	1	0	excludes variants	No
Next-generation sequencing—Illumina MiSeqDx™ Cystic Fibrosis 139 Variant Assay	1	0	0	1	139	23	113	Yes	5/7/9T
Next-generation sequencing—Multiplicom Molecular Diagnostics CFTR MASTR™ v2	2	0	0	1	varies[c]	20-23[c]	varies[c]	varies[c]	varies[c]
Next-generation sequencing—Ion AmpliSeq™ CFTR Community Panel	0	1	0	1	varies[c]	23	varies[c]	Yes	5T
All other gene sequencing protocols including Sanger and Next Gen	5	5	1	8	varies[c]	2-23	varies[c]	Yes[c]	5/7/9T[d]
Other—Hydrolysis probe	1	0	0	1	4	4	0	No	No
Other—LiGHT SNiP	0	1	0	1	7	7	0	No	No

[a] The 2183AA>G mutation is used for the interpretation of the 2184delA mutation and is not reported.
[b] Note that the InPlex 40+4 contains two non CF causing variants, I148T (c.443T>C) and D1270N (c.3808G>A) are not counted in these numbers.
[c] Varies by the sequencing technology used and/or whether filters are applied to mask certain results.
[d] Intron 9 - 5/7/9T detetable by Sanger if included in assay.

(c.1210-12[5]) from the 7 and 9T (c.1210-12[7] and c.1210-12[9]), so Poly T7 and 9 were not called using the bioinformatics pipeline. The AmpliSeq results were 100% concordant with Sanger sequence for all mutations and variants (Tables 4 and 5). In 1 sample, the Variant Caller plug-in did not make an automated call for an F508del/F508C (c.1521_1523delCTT/c.1523T>G) compound heterozygous sample. The F508del (c.1521_1523delCTT) was classified by the automated analysis as a no call, likely because of the complexity in the region when these mutations are present in the same sample. Examination of the sequence data did detect the presence of this mutation, and the correct genotype was called manually. In addition, an I507del/F508del (c.1519_1521delATC /c.1521_1523delCTT) sample required visual inspection for the final call for similar reasons. Since the results presented here are based on chemistry and algorithms from 2013, it is predicted that newer chemistries and algorithms may improve these calls.

The Accel-Amplicon *CFTR* panel libraries were run on the MiSeqDx in Research Run mode using 2 flow cells. A library of 94 samples was loaded on a micro flow cell and produced a density of 1299 $\pm$ 10 K/mm^2 with a read quality of $\geq$Q30 of 88.8% for read 1 and 84.3% for read 2. A second library of 74 samples was loaded on a standard flow cell and produced a density of 698 $\pm$ 10 K/mm^2 with read quality of $\geq$Q30 for 90.2% of read 1 and 80.4% for read 2. There was an average of 115 611 mapped reads with 87.2% of reads on target with a read depth of 1142 and 74.9% uniformity. Both FreeBayes[28] and GATK[29] was used to make variant calls because they produced different call frequencies. The output from both programs was used along with visualization of the data for analysis. As with the AmpliSeq assay, a sample containing I507del/F508del (c.1519_1521delATC /c.1521_1523delCTT) required visually inspection for the final call again due to the complexity in the region when these mutations are presented in the same sample.

In addition to the mutations listed in Tables 4 and 5, 8 additional mutations in our CF DNA DBS repository that cannot be detected by any of the IVD genotyping assay were observed. These mutations can only be detected by Sanger and some of the next-generation sequencing methods. They include the following mutations: 124del23bp (c.-9_14del23), 185+4A>T (c.53+4A>T), F311del (c.933_935delCTT), 1288insTA (c.1153_1154dupTA), 2105-2117del13insAGAAA (c.1973_1985del13insAGAAA), L967S (c.2900T>C), M1101R (c.3302T>G), and S1235R (c.3705T>G). There was 100% concordance between all methods where the mutation was run, however, more complex mutations such as the 2105-2117del13insAGAAA (c.1973_1985del13insA-GAAA) had to be visually inspected and manually called for both the AmpiSeq and Accel-Amplicon assays, and the 124del23bp (c.-9_14del23) was analyzed with no primer trimming for Accel-Amplicon (Note: only the normal sequence of this mutation was sequenced using the AmpliSeq assay in this study).

A summary of DNA quantity inputs, single-run capacity and assay time requirements, data analysis software, and mutation reports for each method is presented in Table 3. DNA quantity inputs are not reported for the xTAG CF and InPlex CF kits because DNA is not typically quantified prior to use in newborn screening laboratories, rather each run uses 5 μL of a 50-μL Generation DNA extraction from a 3.2-mm DBS punch. Library prep time, which is only reported for next-generation sequencing assays, includes PCR setup and run time, whereas PCR setup and run time is only reported for genotyping assays. Analysis time for Sanger sequencing and next-generation sequencing is not included in this table because it may vary depending on the software and pipeline utilized. The OpenArray mentioned with TaqMan Genotyping was not used in this study, however, it is included in the table as it is an available option. All methods except Sanger sequencing were executed using DNA extracted from a 3.2-mm punch taken from a DBS using the Generation DNA extraction method.

Discussion

All US states and many international laboratories screen their newborn population for CF with the majority using second-tier CFTR mutation detection assay as part of their screening algorithm. Although these programs have been very effective,[7,8] CF newborn screening has a low-positive predictive value with >90% false-positives. The reason for the low-positive predictive value is that most programs use a panel of only 23 to 40 CF-causing mutations, and a screen-positive sample only has to contain 1 *CFTR* mutation.[12,18,31] As CF is a recessive disease, carriers of a single *CFTR* mutation are initially flagged as false-positives. In order to increase the positive predictive value of the CF screen to reduce the burden on the CF care centers, some newborn screening programs are exploring more comprehensive mutation detection assays with the goal of a screen positive being defined as babies with elevated IRT and 2 CF-causing mutations. A 2-mutation detection strategy could increase the false-negative rate if the panel of *CFTR* mutations was not sufficiently large enough to address the spectrum of mutations across diverse ethnic populations. Using variants identified by CFTR2 project,[32] a study by Baker et al found that a panel of 162 mutations was not sufficiently comprehensive to capture all babies identified by the current algorithm in Wisconsin.[18] Expanding the CFTR2 panel of mutations to 276 mutations and variants, 2 babies with known mutations in the Wisconsin study would still have been reported as false negatives.[33] With an increasingly diverse ethnic population occurring in the most US state populations, it is expected that a predefined expanded panel of mutations approach will likely be insufficient to define a screen positive as 2 *CFTR* mutations, resulting in the continued high false-positive rates.

To address the limitations of genotyping panels, gene sequencing methods enable every base within the *CFTR* gene to be screened. Currently, there are 2 distinct sequencing methodologies used. The older, more established method uses Sanger sequencing and is currently being used for newborn screening in the US state of California.[34] Next-generation sequencing is the second and more recent technology that enables more comprehensive and higher throughput screening of CF samples.

Table 3. Comparison of Method Input DNA Required, Mutations Detected, Number of Reactions, Run Time, and Run Capacity.[a]

Method	No. Mutations/ Variants Detected	No. Reactions	DNA Volume Used in Study[b]	Avgerage DNA Qty Used Per Reaction (Min-Max)[b]	Library Prep Time	PCR Setup and Run Time	Post-PCR Processing/ Run Time	Instrument Run Time	Total Run Time	Single-Run Capacity[c]	System Dedicated Software	Mutation Report
Sanger	Unlimited in regions amplified	42 PCR rxns86 cycle sequencing	42 μL (1 μL/ PCR rxn)	5-10 ng	NA	3 hours	4 hours	14.5 hours	21.5 hours	Nine 384-well plates (+2, 96-well plates with varying run conditions)	Y SeqScape	Does not distinguish variants from defined mutations—requires expert interpretation
Ion AmpliSeq CFTR Community Panel	Unlimited in regions amplified	2 Pools	12 μL (6 μL/ pool)	18.2 ng (0.76-8.98 ng/μL)	4-6 hours	NA	6-7 hours	2-7 hours (dependent on chip size)	12-20 hours	Eight 314 chip (500×) Forty-nine 316 chip (500×) Ninety-six 318 chip (500×)	Y Coverage Analysis Variant Caller	CFTR2 defined mutations and variants listed in Hotspot file are annotated (Legacy and HGVS)—novel mutations and variants require expert interpretation
Swift Biosciences Accel-Amplicon CFTR Panel	Unlimited in regions amplified	1 Pool	5-10 μL	19.3 ng (0.55-5.21 ng/μL)	2.5 hours	NA	1.5 hours	28 hours	32 hours	Forty-eight Nano flow cell (400×) Forty-eight Micro flow cell (1600×)	N[d] Freeware: Cutadapt, BWA-MEM, FreeBayes, GATK	Does not distinguish variants from defined mutations—requires expert interpretation
MiSeqDx Cystic Fibrosis 139-Variant Assay	139	1 Pool	5 μL	8.95 ng (0.55-3.88 ng/μL)	5 hours	NA	3 hours	28 hours	36 hours	Forty-eight flow cells	Y MiSeq Reporter	Defined mutations identified
Hologic InPlex CF Molecular Test 40+4	42 + 2 variants	1 rxn	5 μL	Not quantified	NA	2.5 hours	1 hour	5 minutes	3.5 hours	8 Cards	Y Call Reporting Software	Defined mutations identified
Luminex xTAG CF39v2 kit	39 + 4 variants	1 rxn	5 μL	Not quantified	NA	2 hours	3.5 hours	1 hour	6.5 hours	Ninety-six 96-well plates	Y TDAS CFTR	Defined mutations identified
Luminex xTAG CF60v2 kit	60 + 4 variants	1 PCR rxns 2 ASPE rxns	5 μL	Not quantified	NA	2 hours	4 hours	1 hour	7 hours	Forty-eight 96-well plates	Y TDAS CFTR	Defined mutations identified
Thermo Fisher Scientific TaqMan SNP Genotyping	44	45 rxns	45 μL[e] (1 μL/mutation)	1.59 ng (0.62-4.82 ng/μL)	NA	15 minutes - 96-well plate 30 minutes - 384-well plate 30 minutes - OpenArray plate	NA	1.5 hours	~2 hours - 96-well plate ~2 hours - 384-well plate ~4 hours - OpenArray plate	Two 96-well plates Eight 384-well plate Forty-eight OpenArray plates (64 assay format)	Y Genotyper	Defined mutations identified—some mutations require interpretation using multiple probes (intron 9-5/7/9T and I507del and F508del region)

Abbreviations: ASPE, allele specific primer extension; CF, cystic fibrosis; CFTR, CF transmembrane regulator; DBS, dried blood specimen; HGVS, human genome variation society; NA, not available; NBS, newborn screening; PCR, polymerase chain reaction; rxn, reaction; SNP, single-nucleotide polymorphism.

[a]The run times in this table are based on our laboratory's experience, however it does not include analysis of the data. The Bioinformatics are described in the materials and methods.

[b]Typically DNA is not quantitated prior to use in NBS labs, so some of the quantities are estimated based on average known concentration of DNA extracted from adult DBS.

[c]The single-run capacity indicates the number of samples that can be loaded onto an instrument at a time.

[d]The Accel-Amplicon CFTR panel is still in development, the company plans on offering a Bioinformatic pipeline (T. Harkins, personal communication, March 29, 2016).

[e]OpenArray was not performed in this study. The manufacturer recommended input is 2.5 μL of DNA exctracted from DBS.

Table 4. ACMG Recommended Mutations found in the CF DNA DBS Repository Samples as Characterized by Next-Generation Sequencing and Mutation Analysis.

Mutation (Legacy Name)	Mutation (HGVS)	Sanger	AmpliSeq CFTR Community Panel	Accel-Amplicon CFTR Panel	CF 139-Variant Assay	InPlex CF 40+4	xTAG CF39v2 kit	xTAG CF60v2 kit	TaqMan SNP Genotyping
F508del	**c.1521_1523delCTT**	+	+	+	+	+	+	+	+
I507del	**c.1519_1521delATC**	+	+	+	+	+	+	+	+
G542X	**c.1624G>T**	+	+	+	+	+	+	+	+
G85E	**c.254G>A**	+	+	+	+	+	+	+	+
R117H	**c.350G>A**	+	+	+	+	+	+	+	+
621+1G>T	**c.489+1G>T**	+	+	+	+	+	+	+	+
711+1G->T	**c.579+1G>T**	+	+	+	+	+	+	+	+
R334W	**c.1000C>T**	+	+	+	+	+	+	+	+
R347P	**c.1040G>C**	+	+	+	+	+	+	+	+
A455E	**c.1364C>A**	+	+	+	+	+	+	+	+
1717-1G>A	**c.1585+1G>A**	+	+	+	+	+	+	+	+
R560T	**c.1679G>C**	+	+	+	+	+	+	+	+
R553X	**c.1657C>T**	+	+	+	+	+	+	+	+
G551D	**c.1652G>A**	+	+	+	+	+	+	+	+
1898+1G>A	**c.1766+1G>A**	+	+	+	+	+	+	+	+
2184delA	**c.2052delA**	+	+*	+	+	+	+	+	+
2789+5G>A	**c.2657+5G>A**	+	+	+	+	+	+	+	+
3120+1G>A	**c.2988+1G>A**	+	+	+	+	+	+	+	+
R1162X	**c.3484C>T**	+	+	+	+	+	+	+	+
3659delC	**c.3528delC**	+	+	+	+	+	+	+	+
3849+10kbC>T	**c.3717+12191C>T**	+	+	+	+	+	+	+	+
W1282X	**c.3846G>A**	+	+	+	+	+	+	+	+
N1303K	**c.3909C>G**	+	+	+	+	+	+	+	+
F508C	c.1523T>G	+	+	+	nr	+	nr	nr	+
T5	c.1210-12[5]	+	+	+	CR	+	CR	CR	+
T7	c.1210-12[7]	+	ND	+	CR	+	CR	CR	+
T9	c.1210-12[9]	+	ND	+	CR	+	CR	CR	+

Abbreviations: ACMG, American College of Medical Genetics; CF, cystic fibrosis; CFTR, CF transmembrane regulator; CR, conditionally reported with an R117H present; ND, not distinguishable; nr, not reported but used for correct mutation interpretation; SNP, single-nucleotide polymorphism; +, mutations detected; +*, not assayed in this study but detectable by method.

[a]Boldface entries indicates ACMG mutations.

Although these approaches solve the issue of being able to identify uncommon mutations particularly in minority populations,[34] it creates a new issue, which is the identification of babies who do not have CF but rather CRMS.[35] The Cystic Fibrosis Foundation describes CRMS as infants with hypertrypsinogenemia on newborn screening who have sweat chloride values <60 mmol/L and up to 2 CFTR mutations, at least 1 of which is not clearly categorized as CF causing.[36]

This study demonstrates that NSQAP's CF DNA DBS repository is appropriate for use with CF screening assays as they are performed today both in the United States and internationally. These repository samples would also support next-generation sequencing assays for *CFTR* if programs choose to modify their screening algorithms to require 2 *CFTR* mutations. The input DNA is a critical component to all molecular tests and the DNA extraction methods reported from NSQAP participants range from a very crude methanol boil preparation to a more purified extraction involving column purification. The majority of US programs use a commercially available simple purification that involves wash steps followed by a boil step (Table 1). In addition, the CF DNA DBS repository samples used in this study have a lower DNA yield than newborn DBS because they were made from adult blood that has a lower average white blood cell count than newborns (7.4×10^6 per mL of blood vs 1.9×10^7 per mL of blood, respectively).[37]

All of the genotyping and sequencing methods tested on the repository samples provided robust and accurate results using the crude DNA extraction and is consistent with previous studies involving next-generation *CFTR* analysis using newborn DBS.[11,38-40] Currently, the most commonly used genotyping assays in the United States, xTAG CF39v2 and InPlex CF 40+4, have defined mutation panels of 39 and 40 mutations, respectively. Since the InPlex CF 40+4 will be discontinued in early 2016 (note that the InPlex CF 23 will continue to be available), we also tested a custom TaqMan panel of mutations that mirrors the *CFTR* mutations in the InPlex CF 40+4. The TaqMan approach is different from the other genotyping approaches in that each mutation is a separate assay allowing for the easy addition or deletion of mutations. This approach requires more input DNA if it is performed in a 384-well format as presented here. There is a higher throughput version available for the OpenArray platform, however, it was not tested in

Table 5. Mutations Excluding ACMG Recommended Mutations Found in the CF DNA DBS Repository Samples as Characterized by Next-Generation Sequencing and Mutation Analysis.

Mutation (Legacy Name)	Mutation (HGVS)	Sanger	AmpliSeq CFTR Community Panel	Accel-Amplicon CFTR Panel	CF 139-Variant Assay	InPlex CF 40+4	xTAG CF39v2 kit	xTAG CF60v2 kit	TaqMan SNP Genotyping
394delTT	c.262_263delTT	+	+*	+	+	+	+	+	+
A559T	c.1675G>A	+	+	+	+	NA	+	+	AV
S549N	c.1646G>A	+	+	+	+	+	+	+	+
2183AA>G	c.2051_2052delAAinsG	+	+	+	+	+	+	+	+
2307insA	c.2175_2176insA	+	+*	+	+	+	+	+	AV
Y1092X	c.3276C>A or c.3276C>G	+	+	+	+	+	+	+	+
3876delA	c.3744delA	+	+	+	+	+	+	+	+
3905insT	c.3773dupT	+	+	+	+	+	+	+	+
CFTR dele2,3	c.54-5940_273+10250del21kb	NA	NA	NA	+	NA	NA	+	AV
E60X	c.178G>T	+	+	+	+	+	NA	+	+
R75X	c.223C>T	+	+	+	+	NA	NA	+	AV
406-1G>A	c.274-1G>A	+	+*	+	+	NA	NA	+	AV
L206W	c.617T>G	+	+	+	+	NA	NA	+	AV
935delA	c.803delA	+	+*	+	NA	NA	NA	+	AV
Q493X	c.1477C>T	+	+	+	+	+	NA	+	+
Q890X	c.2668C>T	+	+	+	+	NA	NA	+	AV
1677delTA	c.1545_1546delTA	+	+	+	+	NA	NA	+	AV
2055del9>A	c.1923_1931del9insA	+	+	+	NA	NA	NA	+	AV
R1158X	c.3472C>T	+	+	+	+	NA	NA	+	AV
R1066C	c.3196C>T	+	+	+	+	NA	+	+	AV
W1089X	c.3266G>A	+	+	+	+	NA	NA	+	AV
D1152H	c.3454G>C	+	+	+	NA	+	NA	+	+
3791delC	c.3659delC	+	+*	+	+	NA	NA	+	AV
D1270N	c.3808G>A	+	+	+	NA	+	NA	NA	NA
Q39X	c.115C>T	+	+*	+	+	NA	NA	NA	AV
663delT	c.531delT	+	+	+	+	NA	NA	NA	AV
P205S	c.613C>T	+	+	+	+	NA	NA	NA	AV
1154 insTC	c.1022_1023insTC	+	+*	+	+	NA	NA	NA	AV
1248+1G>A	c.1116+1G>A	+	+	+	+	NA	NA	NA	AV
L467P	c.1400T>C	+	+*	+	+	NA	NA	NA	AV
S492F	c.1475C>T	+	+	+	+	NA	NA	NA	AV
1812-1G>A	c.1680-1G>A	+	+	+	+	NA	NA	NA	AV
2184insA	c.2052dupA	+	+	+	+	NA	NA	NA	NA
3121-1G>A	c.2989-1G>A	+	+	+	+	NA	NA	NA	AV
3272-26A>G	c.3140-26A>G	+	+	+	+	NA	NA	NA	AV
R1066H	c.3197G>A	+	+	+	+	NA	NA	NA	AV
W1204X	c.2611G>A or c.3612G>A	+	+	+	+	NA	NA	NA	AV
G1244E	c.3731G>A	+	+*	+	+	NA	NA	NA	AV

Abbreviations: AV, assay available but not evaluated in this study; CF, cystic fibrosis; CFTR, CF transmembrane regulator; NA, not available in assay; SNP, single-nucleotide polymorphism; +, mutations detected; +*, specimen containing mutation not assayed but normal region sequenced in this study.

this study. The next-generation sequencing approaches used in this study were selected to test the utility and robustness of crude low-concentration DNA with different next-generation sequencing platforms and library preparation assays. Although the US Food and Drug Administration (FDA)-approved CF 139-Variant Assay uses next-generation sequencing technology, it reports a genotype for a defined panel of mutations and variants. The mutation panel is not diverse enough to define a positive newborn screen positive as having 2 *CFTR* mutations; Illumina does offer an FDA-approved *CFTR* gene sequencing assay that was not tested in this study. Given the similar technology and work flow, it is anticipated that this method would also work well with DNA extracted from DBS. The *CFTR* gene next-generation sequencing assays tested in this study were the AmpliSeq *CFTR* Community Panel on the Ion Torrent PGM and the Accel-Amplicon *CFTR* Panel on the MiSeq. The Accel-Amplicon *CFTR* Panel can also be made for use with the Ion Torrent PGM.

The general trend of increasing population diversity, new technology introductions allowing for expanded mutation screening or gene sequencing, and the varying sizes of newborn screening programs are just 3 of many factors contributing to the complexities of newborn screening for CF. In addition, the current newborn screening algorithms have a high false-positive rate, prompting some programs to consider whether the definition of a CF screen positive should be redefined. The NSQAP offers quality assurance tools and services to newborn screening laboratories as they explore transitioning from one technology to another to meet their changing needs. The CF DNA DBS repository provides laboratories with representative samples with rare *CFTR* mutations for robust testing and evaluation purposes. The study presented here is a comprehensive characterization of these DBS samples and highlights their utility for a diverse range of methods being used in CF newborn screening today as well as next-generation sequencing assays that can be used in the future.

Acknowledgments

The findings and conclusions in this report are those of the authors and do not necessarily represent the views of the Centers for Disease Control and Prevention. Use of trade names and commercial sources is for identification only and does not constitute endorsement by the US Department of Health and Human Services or US Centers for Disease Control and Prevention. Special thanks to manufacturer collaborators Clarence Lee, PhD and Warren Tom from Life Technologies (now Thermo Fisher Scientific); Tim Harkins, PhD and Julie Laliberte, PhD, from Swift Biosciences; and Junko Stevens, PhD, Jordan Lang, and Lauren Tracey from Thermo Fisher Scientific. We also thank our partners who have helped collect patient samples for the CF DNA DBS repository which includes Dr Phillip M. Farrell from the University of Wisconsin School of Medicine and Public Health, Dr Peter Mogayzel from the CF Center at Johns Hopkins Medical Institutions, Dr Michael Konstan from Rainbow Babies and Children's Hospital and Case Western Reserve University School of Medicine, Martin Kharrazi, PhD from the California Department of Public Health, and Charlene Sacramento from Sequoia Foundation. In addition, we thank the patients and families who generously donated blood. Without them, this program would not be possible.

Declaration of Conflicting Interests

The author(s) declared no potential conflicts of interest with respect to the research, authorship, and/or publication of this article.

Funding

The author(s) disclosed receipt of the following financial support for the research, authorship, and/or publication of this article: Stephanie Foster was funded by the Research Participation Program at the Centers for Disease Control and Prevention (CDC), National Center for Environmental Health's Division of Laboratory Sciences, administered by the Oak Ridge Institute for Science and Education through an interagency agreement between the U.S. Department of Energy and CDC.

References

1. Grosse SD, Boyle CA, Botkin JR, et al. Newborn screening for cystic fibrosis: evaluation of benefits and risks and recommendations for state newborn screening programs. *MMWR Recomm Rep.* 2004;53(RR-13):1-36.
2. Dijk FN, Fitzgerald DA. The impact of newborn screening and earlier intervention on the clinical course of cystic fibrosis. *Paediatr Respir Rev.* 2012;13(4):220-225.
3. Crossley JR, Elliott RB, Smith PA. Dried-blood spot screening for cystic fibrosis in the newborn. *Lancet.* 1979;1(8114):472-474.
4. Hammond KB, Abman SH, Sokol RJ, Accurso FJ. Efficacy of statewide neonatal screening for cystic fibrosis by assay of trypsinogen concentrations. *N Engl J Med.* 1991;325(11): 769-774.
5. Riordan JR, Rommens JM, Kerem B, et al. Identification of the cystic fibrosis gene: cloning and characterization of complementary DNA. *Science.* 1989;245(4922):1066-1073.
6. Welsh MJ, Ramsey BW, Accurso FJ, Cutting GR. Cystic Fibrosis. In: Scriver CR, Beaudet AL, Sly WS, Valle D, eds. *The Metabolic and Molecular Bases of Inherited Disease.* Vol 3. 8th ed. New York, NY: McGraw-Hill; 2001:5121-5188.
7. Comeau AM, Parad RB, Dorkin HL, et al. Population-based newborn screening for genetic disorders when multiple mutation DNA testing is incorporated: a cystic fibrosis newborn screening model demonstrating increased sensitivity but more carrier detections. *Pediatrics.* 2004;113(6):1573-1581.
8. Gregg RG, Wilfond BS, Farrell PM, Laxova A, Hassemer D, Mischler EH. Application of DNA analysis in a population-screening program for neonatal diagnosis of cystic fibrosis (CF): comparison of screening protocols. *Am J Hum Genet.* 1993;52(3):616-626.
9. Ranieri E, Lewis BD, Gerace RL, et al. Neonatal screening for cystic fibrosis using immunoreactive trypsinogen and direct gene analysis: four years' experience. *BMJ.* 1994;308(6942): 1469-1472.
10. Grody WW, Cutting GR, Klinger KW, Richards CS, Watson MS, Desnick RJ. Laboratory standards and guidelines for population-based cystic fibrosis carrier screening. *Genet Med.* 2001;3(2): 149-154.
11. Baker MW, Groose M, Hoffman G, Rock M, Levy H, Farrell PM. Optimal DNA tier for the IRT/DNA algorithm determined by CFTR mutation results over 14 years of newborn screening. *J Cyst Fibros.* 2011;10(4):278-281.
12. Kay DM, Maloney B, Hamel R, et al. Screening for cystic fibrosis in New York State: considerations for algorithm improvements. *Eur J Pediatr.* 2016;175(2):181-193.
13. Kharrazi M, Yang J, Bishop T, et al. Newborn screening for cystic fibrosis in California. *Pediatrics.* 2015;136(6):1062-1072.
14. Tluczek A, Koscik RL, Farrell PM, Rock MJ. Psychosocial risk associated with newborn screening for cystic fibrosis: parents' experience while awaiting the sweat-test appointment. *Pediatrics.* 2005;115(6):1692-1703.
15. La Pean A, Farrell MH, Eskra KL, Farrell PM. Effects of immediate telephone follow-up with providers on sweat chloride test timing after cystic fibrosis newborn screening identifies a single mutation. *J Pediatr.* 2013;162(3):522-529.
16. Castellani C, Picci L, Scarpa M, et al. Cystic fibrosis carriers have higher neonatal immunoreactive trypsinogen values than non-carriers. *Am J Med Genet A.* 2005;135(2):142-144.

17. Wells J, Rosenberg M, Hoffman G, Anstead M, Farrell PM. A decision-tree approach to cost comparison of newborn screening strategies for cystic fibrosis. *Pediatrics*. 2012;129(2):e339-e347.
18. Baker MW, Atkins AE, Cordovado SK, Hendrix M, Earley MC, Farrell PM. Improving newborn screening for cystic fibrosis using next-generation sequencing technology: a technical feasibility study. *Genet Med*. 2016;18(3):231-238.
19. Pratt VM, Caggana M, Bridges C, et al. Development of genomic reference materials for cystic fibrosis genetic testing. *J Mol Diagn*. 2009;11(3):186-193.
20. Tsui L. Cystic Fibrosis Mutation Database. 2010; Web site. http://genet.sickkids.on.ca/. Updated April 25, 2011. Accessed January 26, 2016.
21. Li L, Zhou Y, Bell CJ, Earley MC, Hannon WH, Mei JV. Development and characterization of dried blood spot materials for the measurement of immunoreactive trypsinogen. *J Med Screen*. 2006;13(2):79-84.
22. Earley MC, Laxova A, Farrell PM, et al. Implementation of the first worldwide quality assurance program for cystic fibrosis multiple mutation detection in population-based screening. *Clin Chim Acta*. 2011;412(15-16):1376-1381.
23. Newborn Screening Quality Assurance Program (NSQAP) Cystic Fibrosis Mutation Detection. Web site. https://www.cdc.gov/lab standards/pdf/nsqap/nsqap_CysticFibrosisMDFeb2016.pdf. Published February 1, 2016.
24. Robinson JT, Thorvaldsdottir H, Winckler W, et al. Integrative genomics viewer. *Nat Biotechnol*. 2011;29(1):24-26.
25. Thorvaldsdottir H, Robinson JT, Mesirov JP. Integrative Genomics Viewer (IGV): high-performance genomics data visualization and exploration. *Brief Bioinform*. 2013;14(2): 178-192.
26. Martin M. Cutadapt removes adapter sequences from high-throughput sequencing reads. *EMBnet. journal*. 2011;17(1): 10-12.
27. Li H, Durbin R. Fast and accurate short read alignment with Burrows-Wheeler transform. *Bioinformatics*. 2009;25(14): 1754-1760.
28. Garrison E, Marth G. Haplotype-based variant detection from short-read sequencing[published online July 24, 2012]. *Genomics*. 2012.
29. McKenna A, Hanna M, Banks E, et al. The Genome Analysis Toolkit: a MapReduce framework for analyzing next-generation DNA sequencing data. *Genome Res*. 2010;20(9): 1297-1303.
30. Cordovado SK, Hendrix M, Greene CN, et al. CFTR mutation analysis and haplotype associations in CF patients. *Mol Genet Metab*. 2012;105(2):249-254.
31. (CLSI) CaLSI. *Newborn Screening for Cystic Fibrosis: Approved Guideline*. Wayne, PA: Clinical and Laboratory Standards Institute; 2011.
32. Sosnay PR, Siklosi KR, Van Goor F, et al. Defining the disease liability of variants in the cystic fibrosis transmembrane conductance regulator gene. *Nat Genet*. 2013;45(10):1160-1167.
33. Clinical and Functional Translation of CFTR (CFTR2). Web site. http://www.cftr2.org/. Accessed February 9, 2016.
34. Kammesheidt A, Kharrazi M, Graham S, et al. Comprehensive genetic analysis of the cystic fibrosis transmembrane conductance regulator from dried blood specimens—implications for newborn screening. *Genet Med*. 2006;8(9):557-562.
35. Prach L, Koepke R, Kharrazi M, et al. Novel CFTR variants identified during the first 3 years of cystic fibrosis newborn screening in California. *J Mol Diagn*. 2013;15(5):710-722.
36. Cystic Fibrosis F, Borowitz D, Parad RB, et al. Cystic Fibrosis Foundation practice guidelines for the management of infants with cystic fibrosis transmembrane conductance regulator-related metabolic syndrome during the first two years of life and beyond. *J Pediatr*. 2009;155(6 suppl): S106-S116.
37. Engorn B, Flerlage J, eds. *The Harriet Lane Handbook: A Manual For Pediatric House Officers*. 20th ed. Philadelphia: Elsevier Saunders; 2015.
38. Hughes EE, Stevens CF, Saavedra-Matiz CA, et al. Clinical sensitivity of cystic fibrosis mutation panels in a diverse population. *Hum Mutat*. 2016;37(2):201-208.
39. Loukas YL, Thodi G, Molou E, Georgiou V, Dotsikas Y, Schulpis KH. Clinical diagnostic Next-Generation sequencing: the case of CFTR carrier screening. *Scand J Clin Lab Invest*. 2015;75(5): 374-381.
40. Lefterova MI, Shen P, Odegaard JI, et al. Next-generation molecular testing of newborn dried blood spots for cystic fibrosis. *J Mol Diagn*. 2016;18(2):267-282.

17

Potential Therapeutic Targets of the Endocannabinoid System in Common Neurodegenerative Disorders and Organic Acidemias

Gabriela Aguilera, MSc[1,2] and Abel Santamaria, PhD[1]

Abstract

The cannabinoid chemistry is currently being addressed in preclinical approaches as a viable therapeutic alternative for the management of a wide range of signs, symptoms, and some biochemical hallmarks of many neurological pathologies (such as neuroinflammation and neurodegeneration). This clinical orientation is grounded on the consistent promissory profile that cannabinoid compounds have shown, and the great necessity of feasible options to undergo such disorders. Even though at early research stages, metabolic disorders are starting to rise as potential targets of cannabinoid alternatives; approaches in this term could, in turn, aim to modulate the endocannabinoid response for therapeutic purposes. This review recalls the pathologic scenarios endured in the course of neurological diseases of high occurrence and the most typical metabolic disorders, while discussing the neuroprotective mechanisms of cannabinoid agonists in the central nervous system, and the potential targets of the endocannabinoid system and metabolic disorders.

Keywords

endocannabinoid system, organic acidemias, neurodegenerative disorders, therapeutic mechanisms, cannabinoids

Introduction

Neurodegenerative diseases, such as Alzheimer disease (AD), Parkinson disease (PD), and multiple sclerosis (MS), are few examples of an enriched acquisition of disorders that have been studied for several decades. From its very first description, our comprehension of the intrinsic mechanisms behind such conditions has experienced substantial growth. Such a progress involves many overlapping mechanisms, including deposition and aggregation of misfolded proteins, resulting in progressive degeneration of nerve cells. Undoubtedly, such a setup has presented a unique opportunity for the alternative proposals of pathophysiological mechanisms and drug targets as well as novel pharmacological strategies in the generation of new drugs.

Frequently Expressed Neurodegenerative Disorders

As revised elsewhere, consistent pathological hallmarks of AD comprise the extracellular deposits of β-amyloid peptide, which is associated with cell death, and the consequent behavioral, memory, and cognitive alterations. Additionally, the formation of intracellular neurofibrillary tangles of tau protein constitutes a second distinctive characteristic of AD, and such a process is associated with detriment in neuronal communication. Furthermore, the role of activated microglia at the senile plaque's fringe has been related with the antioxidant defense in AD brains.[1–5] On the other hand, PD constitutes a second major example of the most notorious

[1] Laboratorio de Aminoácidos Excitadores, Instituto Nacional de Neurología y Neurocirugía, Mexico City, Mexico
[2] Departamento de Ciencias Biológicas y de la Salud, Universidad Autónoma Metropolitana-Iztapalapa, Mexico City, Mexico

Corresponding Authors:
Gabriela Aguilera, MSc, Laboratorio de Aminoácidos Excitadores, Instituto Nacional de Neurología y Neurocirugía, Insurgentes Sur 3877, Ciudad de México 14269, Mexico City, Mexico.
Abel Santamaria, PhD, Departamento de Ciencias Biológicas y de la Salud, Universidad Autónoma Metropolitana-Iztapalapa, Mexico City 09340, Mexico.
Emails: absada@yahoo.com; aguilerag@icloud.com

neurodegenerative diseases, and its characteristic motor and nonmotor signs are the result of a progressive loss of dopaminergic neurons residing principally in the *substantia nigra pars compacta* and their endings at the striatum.[6,7] Moreover, the pathological processes associated with the disease encompass the alteration of non-dopaminergic neurotransmitters and associated events,[8] and more importantly, dopaminergic metabolism as an intracellular source of reactive oxygen species (ROS). To complete the brief count, MS is a demyelinating disorder of the central nervous system (CNS) apparently caused by particular genotypes and environmental stimuli; it often stands out for its motor exacerbation manifestations, or "relapses," which are followed by "remissions." As known, MS leads to immune attack to the CNS and severe damage to oligodendrocytes—the glial cells that form myelin—as well as progressive inflammation throughout the brain and meninges. Therefore, the progression of the disease results in neuronal dysfunction and irreversible disability.[9–12] Hence, countless efforts are being concentrated into the research and comprehension of these and many more neurodegenerative diseases, as therapeutics still face important challenges ranging from timely and accurate diagnoses to the generation of novel and effective therapies. For this reason, several pathogenic mechanisms are continuously being suggested and include mostly oxidative stress, local/generalized neuroinflammation, mitochondrial energy depletion, and so on, and the current ideology contemplates these examples, either running simultaneously or converging through time, as a feasible mechanism that leads to the progression observed typically in neurodegenerative diseases.[6,13]

Organic Acidurias

Generically, organic acidurias (OAs) have been described as a family of inheritable disorders due to defects in metabolic pathways of amino acid degradation. These disorders are characterized by the tissue accumulation and high urinary excretion of organic acids, including glutaric acid (GA), 3-hydroxyglutaric acid (3-OHGA), methylglutaric acid (MGA), methylmalonic acid (MMA), propionic acid (PA), and so on, with special deleterious consequences to the brain.[14] Indeed, OAs are among the major causes of brain damage and other alterations in children.[15–18] In high-risk groups, the frequency of OAs is much higher than in the general population.[19] Features such as age of onset and the severity of illness seem to depend on the accumulated levels of specific toxic metabolites. Some environmental factors, including metabolic distress and infections, are known to accelerate the severity of the clinical manifestations of these diseases, probably because of the dramatic increase in the accumulating metabolites.

Diagnosis of OA

Clinical characteristics in patients with OAs include mental retardation, seizures, coma, lethargy, vomiting, hypotonia, hepatomegaly, and cardiac malfunction. An early and accurate diagnosis (1-3 days) helps to prevent chronic events, such as mental retardation and physical dysfunction.[20] Two common laboratory features of OAs are hyperammonemia and metabolic acidosis. Other common biochemical events include hypoglycemia and ketonuria.

The OAs exclusively or predominantly affecting the brain are also known as "cerebral" OAs and are characterized by severe neurological manifestations.[18] Increased amounts of organic acids in the urine of patients with OAs are crucial for an accurate diagnosis. Current analytical methods to achieve diagnosis or OAs are gas chromatography/mass spectrometry that in some cases can be improved by tandem mass spectrometry, enzyme assays, and DNA analysis. Proton nuclear magnetic resonance and dinitrophenyl hydrazine tests can be also employed, although they are not conclusive of diagnosis.[20]

Treatment

With a timely and accurate diagnosis, some OAs can be effectively treated, whereas many others do not reach a real treatment. Nutritional therapy provides essential nutrients to preserve and recover physical and mental conditions,[21] restricting the amino acids that generate the accumulating organic acids. Therefore, while alternative amino acid–based therapies constitute a constant source of energy and nutrients that can promote anabolism and growth,[20] dietary precursors of GA (mainly lysine) have to be avoided in glutaric aciduria type I (GA-I).[22] Since carnitine deficiency is also common in these disorders and helps to increase the excretion of organic acids, L-carnitine is usually supplemented.[23] Acute crises in OAs are generally treated with dialysis, correction of electrolyte imbalances and acidosis, brain perfusion, and control of oxygen and glucose levels.[20] Glycine and carnitine are also given as detoxifying treatments. Classical OAs inherited as autosomal recessive pattern include GA-I, PAcidemia, MMAcidemia, among others.

Glutaric Aciduria Type I

The GA-I is a cerebral OA caused by a deficiency of glutaryl-CoA dehydrogenase (McKusick 23167; OMIM # 231670). Untreated patients show increased concentrations of GA (500-5000 μmol/L) and 3-OHGA (40-200 μmol/L) in body fluids and tissues, especially in the CNS.[24,25] Frontotemporal cortical atrophy at birth, progressive spongy formation, leukoencephalopathy, and acute damage of the caudate/putamen, are characteristically seen in this disorder during encephalopathy, that occur between 6 months and 4 years of age.[26,27] Although the pathogenic mechanisms responsible for neurological sequelae in GA-I are not fully established, several in vitro and in vivo studies suggest that the accumulating organic acids induce excitotoxicity, oxidative stress, and energy metabolism impairment.[28–32]

Methylmalonic Acidemia and Propionic Acidemia

Methylmalonic acidemia (MMAcidemia) and propionic acidemia (PAcidemia) are caused by a severe deficiency of methylmalonyl-CoA mutase (EC 5.4.99.2) and propionyl-CoA carboxylase activities (EC 6.4.1.3) and are biochemically characterized by predominant blood accumulation of MM (1-2.5 mmol/L) and PA (5 mmol/L), respectively. Clinical presentation of both OAs is similar and includes lethargy, psychomotor delay/mental retardation, focal and generalized convulsions, vomiting, dehydration, hepatomegaly, hypotonia, and encephalopathy, all leading to coma and death.[33] Cerebral magnetic resonance imaging shows delayed myelination (progressive cortical atrophy) and hypodensity of the basal ganglia.[34,35] It has been suggested that brain injury due to MMAcidemia and PAcidemia is mainly related with the toxic effects exerted by the accumulating metabolites. In this context, it has been demonstrated that MMA causes impairment of brain mitochondrial energy metabolism, as well as alterations in the redox status and glutamatergic neurotransmission.[36–38] Neurotoxic effects of PA have also been reported in rat brain and human preparations.[39–47]

The Endocannabinoid System: Overview

The endocannabinoid system (ECS) has been known and increasingly recognized for about 2 decades. Given the emerging knowledge achieved throughout the history of *Cannabis* use, together with the evolving hypotheses of the overall role of cannabinoid (CB) circuitry in the human body, the ECS is now addressed as a rich matrix of receptors, ligands, and associated molecules involved in many physiological and pathological conditions.[48–52] The ECS recruits a mechanism of intercellular communications that would execute modulatory actions in brain and peripheral systems; examples of physiological actions in which CB signaling might be associated include mood regulation (depression and anxiety),[53] control of intestinal motility,[52] urinary tract physiology,[54] vasorelaxation of healthy vasculature,[55] interference of the production of proinflammatory cytokines, and probably other immune functional activities as well as the maintenance of the immune homeostatic balance.[56] In addition, the role of CB signaling has been associated with crucial functions throughout the CNS development (both prenatal and postnatal),[50] which might play a relevant role under pathological contexts.

The ECS begins with the CB receptors 1 and 2 (CB1 and CB2, respectively), which are highly distributed within the CNS as well as in peripheral tissues. Both receptors belong to the superfamily of transmembrane-domain Guanosine triphosphate (GTP)-binding protein-coupled receptors, and it is known that they are associated with numerous cellular processes, such as the inhibition of synaptic transmission and the inhibition of the adenylate cyclase activity, resulting in the regulation of neurotransmitter release through its activation.[50] Opposite to the recurring hydrophilic cations associated with the Class A-G protein-coupled receptors' group, its ligands have a lipophilic nature derived from the arachidonic acid,[48,53] such as fatty acid ethanolamides or glycerols found in countless CBs of endogenous nature.[49] As such, CB1 receptors are vastly expressed in the CNS, comparing in density with that of γ-aminobutyric acid or even glutamate-gated ion channels[50]; in this form, areas such as basal ganglia (caudate, putamen, globus pallidus, substantia nigra, etc), cerebellum, and hippocampus display great number of receptors and consequently a higher endocannabinoid activity.[49] On the other hand, CB2 subtype is highly expressed in the overall immune system, with great density in B lymphocytes, but quantitatively decreasing in natural killer cells, microglia, and T lymphocytes.[56] Given such diverse distribution, the role of CB1 receptors is mainly associated with pain, inflammation, and many other responses, while CB2 receptors might have the potential as immunomodulators in various immune processes. As expected, these receptors possess an overall fixed structure of an extracellular N-terminus domain, 7 transmembrane α-helixes, and an intracellular C-terminus domain. Under the circumstances of ongoing immune processes, receptor activation stimulates the interaction with G proteins and ultimately upholds the Guanosine diphosphate/GTP exchange and further dissociation of the corresponding subunits.[49]

Following the definition of the receptors, several molecules bind to CB1 and CB2 receptors and constitute ligands of endogenous or synthetic nature. Research efforts have led to the recognition and characterization of many molecules, and such progress has yielded a vast number of studies aiming to explore its potential under pathological defies. To date, 2 endogenous ligands of the CB system have been a matter of great interest: anandamide (AEA) and 2-arachidonylglycerol (2-AG). Both constitute elements of biological and physiological relevance under many circumstances, especially when considering that both are associated with the neurotransmitter-release inhibition through the adenylate cyclase inhibition.[57] Besides these molecules, other examples of endogenous ligands—and some data supporting its participation in significant biochemical events—include 2-arachidonylglycerol ether (noladin ether),[58–61] N-arachidonyl-dopamine,[62] virodhamine,[63] and so on. On the other hand, the synthetic CB counterparts are frequently classified for its study. Such classification led in 2002 to a group of 4 components that remains valid nowadays: classic CBs (HU-210,[64] nabilone,[65,66] cannabidiol,[67,68] and other); nonclassic CBs (CP-47,497,[69,70] CP-55,244,[71] and CP-55,940[69]), aminoalkylindoles (R-(+)-WIN 55,212-2,[72] and JWH-015[73]), and eicosanoids (AEA[74] as the most notable as well as methanandamide[75] and arachidonoyl-2-chloroethylamide[76]) to name a few, that account as synthetic eicosanoids.[77]

Besides these main components, the ECS is enriched by a number of synthesis and degrading enzymes, transporter molecules, and minor intermediates that complete the arrangement. In this form, many molecular mechanisms take place in order to execute CB receptor signaling in anterograde and retrograde directions, as well as the corresponding cycles of synthesis, transport, and inactivation/degradation of CB agonists, which ultimately represent processes that are not entirely understood but yet remain enthralling and promissory.

Possible Neuroprotective Mechanisms of CBs in the Brain

The ECS was first recognized around the 80s, and emerging data have confirmed its relevance and intricate association with brain physiology and pathology ever since. As discussed previously, circuitry hierarchy of CB is settled with the CB1 (widely expressed in the CNS) and CB2 (both CNS and periphery) receptors, and the differential distribution points out the therapeutic potential of the ECS in neurological diseases. Although the constitutive expression of the receptors in the CNS plays a vital and consistent role in physiology, the inducible expression can also be provoked with prior inflammatory insult. Currently, the connection between the ECS and neurological diseases is not entirely understood; nevertheless, copious information proposes ECS' hypofunction and overall dysregulation as the cause of some notorious symptoms of neurological diseases, especially when considering its neuroprotective and prohomeostatic functions, which drives the system as a whole to a potential link to mood and anxiety alterations,[78,79] major motor disorders such as PD or HD,[80,81] and other pathologies (Figure 1). Hence, most therapeutic approaches bet on pharmacological methodologies that alter the CB pathway or explore the endogenous increase in specific CB compounds that trigger desired responses.

As mentioned previously, CBs exert its biological functions through the activation of CB1 and CB2 receptors. The 2 most noticeable CBs of endogenous nature include the AEA and 2-AG but also include diacylglycerol, diacylglycerol lipase, fatty acid amidehydrolase (FAAH), monoacylglycerol lipase, N-acylphosphatidylethanolamine, and so on. Moreover, AEA and 2-AG represent endogenous ligands released "on demand," that subsequently suffer a hydrolysis process by the FAAH; consequently, the reduction in the normal levels of FAAH is associated with AEA concentration, which ultimately impacts the inhibitory effect of nociceptors.[82] Likewise, the neuroprotective assets of some endocannabinoids were first drawn from findings confirming that synthesis of AEA or 2-AG is Ca^{2+} influx dependent, implying therefore that endogenous CB tone would be determined as a response to intracellular calcium levels.[2] In this form, there is a precise distribution of CBs within the CNS and peripheral tissues, and together with the density of receptors and correlated molecules, the postactivation responses of ECS suggest the neuroprotective role of the CB matrix.

The state of knowledge of CB circuitry, along with its connection with pathological processes, discloses a great number of events that occur as part of the onset and progression of disease under many scenarios. As expected, the description of the involvement of CB signaling in pathological scenarios is currently engaged with the assessment of experimental data. Neurological diseases face challenging scenarios consisting essentially of lack of effectiveness of present pharmacological alternatives and limited emerging therapeutic proposals. Thus, the close relationship of these disorders and the ECS has directed attention to the exploration of CB chemistry to assess its antihyperkinetic, anti-inflammatory, and neuroprotective qualities through alternatives such as the effective expression of CBs, enhancement of CB synthesis, and so on, further leading to the control of motor activity and some other processes.[83,84] As a result, there is a special interest in the study of the risks and benefits implied in the use of CB-derived compounds in neurological pathology; in fact, motor-related disorders, neurodegenerative diseases, and some low-incidence pathologies show improvement under CB-administration schemes evidenced by the reduction of detrimental processes, such as excitotoxicity, oxidative stress, and inflammation.[57,81] This setup qualifies diseases from degenerative contexts such as AD, PD, and HD as ideal targets for experimental approaches but also reflects in disorders of low incidence—and rising awareness—such as OAs (GA-I, PAcidemia, MMAcidemia, etc).[85]

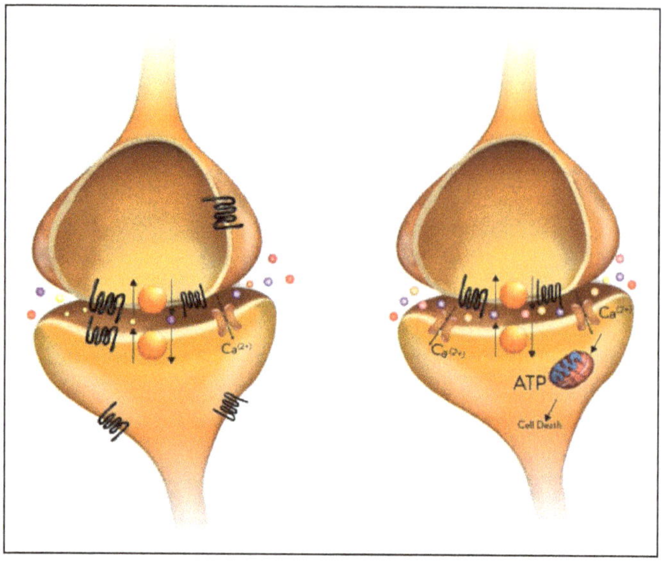

Figure 1. Alterations of the endocannabinoid system under pathological conditions. The image on the left is a conceptual representation of physiological conditions of pre- and postsynaptic neurons, with proportioned and functional CB1 (black) and CB2 (textured) receptors, transporters, and endogenous molecules such as anandamide (red dots), 2-arachidonoylglycerol (light yellow dots) and glutamate (purple dots). Conversely, the right image shows typical alterations of the endocannabinoid arrangement in pathological conditions, with fewer CB1 and CB2 receptors, decrease in the cannabinoid tone of anandamide and 2-arachidonoylglycerol, increase in glutamate levels, as well as the presence of glutaric (pink dots) and quinolinic (orange small dots) acids, 2 intermediates of metabolic pathways that may accumulate under pathological conditions and exert toxic effects. CB1 indicates cannabinoid receptor 1; CB2, cannabinoid receptor 2.

Particular effects evoked after CB activation have attracted interest due to its advantageous applications. One of the most prominent is the antinociceptive response produced by CBs, which are mainly exerted through CB1 receptors.[86,87] Furthermore, such effects are taken to a new high when proposing the neuroprotective strategies of the CB elements in the brain. As known, the elucidation of the mechanisms that underlie the pathogenesis of neurological diseases constitutes exceptional dilemmas that therapeutics need to address. For example, a promissory finding applicable in neurodegenerative contexts involves the hypotheses in which cell survival, specifically neuronal type, is closely connected to the ECS, given that neuronal insult triggers repair mechanisms and endogenous production of CBs, such as AEA.[88] In fact, specific detrimental proteins present in neurodegenerative diseases (ie, Aβ) evoke localized and eventually general neuronal degeneration, which is also manifested in function impairment; then again, this deleterious conditions are reported to induce the production of endocannabinoids such as 2-AG, so that its neuroprotective qualities can be exerted.[89]

Moreover, the ECS experiences downregulation of CBs as part of the hallmarks of some neurological diseases on early stages (usually previous to diagnosis), whereas advanced phases exhibit important receptor loss in the basal ganglia; in this form, both traits are consistent with initial hypokinetic manifestations versus advanced hyperkinetic symptoms experienced by patients in diseases such as PD or HD.[90,91] In addition, neurological pathologies of different nature show changes in the CB chemistry, as the alteration of receptors in purinergic signaling is known to be related to the decay of endocannabinoid level, thus reducing its protective qualities.[4]

Potential Therapeutic Targets of the ECS in Neurodegenerative Disorders and OAs: Experimental Evidence

The aforementioned findings are currently under study with a therapeutic orientation, as the status of many neurological diseases highlights the relevance of the ECS in these pathologies. Research has led so far to great amount of information in regard to the ECS involvement in common neurological diseases such as AD, PD, MS, to name a few. Aside of the pathophysiological hallmark of AD, which has been addressed extensively, our knowledge of the participation of endocannabinoid elements has settled in several notions: Hippocampus expresses several subpopulations of CB1r, all of which contribute actively to the memory processes that suffer the deleterious effects during the neurodegenerative course of the disease. In fact, published works have stated the connection of neuronal cell survival and the CB chemistry. Such statements are possible given that such circuitry enables repair mechanisms to avoid or diminish oxidative injury or apoptotic events and could, in any given time, reduce the negative effects of molecules such as Aβ in AD. Moreover, the characteristic cognitive alterations due to hippocampal dent might be modulated by the ECS through anti-inflammatory and antioxidant means—and overall neuroprotective mechanisms—in this form, several experimental strategies explored the scopes and limitations of the ECS under the pathological hallmarks of AD and continue to provide valuable information in these regards.[88,89,92] Aside of the classical signs of AD, the overactivation of the *N*-methyl-D-aspartate receptor (NMDAr) and the consequent dysregulation of Ca^{2+} influx converge in the degenerative course of the disease. Accordingly, available information strongly suggests that the activation of CB1r could trigger protective actions along with the inhibition of excessive Ca^{2+} entry; such approaches propose hitherto the upregulation of the most prominent endogenous CBs as well as the reduction in the excitotoxic events resulting from the excessive Ca^{2+} influx. Moreover, the synthesis of AEA and 2-AG is known to be Ca^{2+} dependent, therefore rendering its constitutive concentration, as well as the CB response, as a factor directly related to the Ca^{2+} load.[2,93]

Progress has also been achieved in regard to some other neurodegenerative disorders. Notorious motor symptoms (dyskinesias, bradykinesia, tremor, rigidity, etc) accompany the development of PD; its disabling potential reduces dramatically the quality of life of the people facing the condition, reason why such symptoms constitute a major target of new therapies. As seen with some typical brain disorders, the ECS endures central alterations that occur along with the numerous degenerative processes of the disease; more precisely, early stages of PD—often presymptomatic—are associated with downregulation or desensitization of CB1r, which ultimately led to oxidative stress and excitotoxic/inflammatory events, while an upregulation of endocannabinoid agonists and receptors (CB1r specifically) is attained on advanced stages due to the influence of dopamine depletion on substantia nigra and, consequently, the striatum.[90] Under these circumstances, frequent proposals imply timely administration of molecules to inhibit the endogenous degradation of CBs in order to reduce the classic motor symptoms of PD.[94] Moreover, NMDAr antagonists are emerging as feasible options to mediate overactivation of such receptors, the consequent toxic events, and the cellular damage associated with it.

Contrasting hypotheses have risen in regard to MS, a disease that deals with severe immune attack and reportedly face a reduction in the CBs of endogenous nature as a result of the alteration of purinergic receptors[4] and, altogether, would contribute to the pathologic components of MS. The increasing awareness of CB potential has led to numerous preclinical evaluations exploring its properties, and even some advanced clinical studies following the same goal. As such, the improvement in disabling symptoms, such as spasticity and overall quality of life, might be achieved through synthetic CBs, given that such motor symptoms seem to be CB1r dependent[95]; in fact, most of the explored applications suggest the administration of *Cannabis* derivatives to enhance endocannabinoid signaling.[96]

As evident, these are examples of highly prevalent diseases of great interest in biomedical research, and their pathophysiological hallmarks are rather understood and studied acutely. However relevant, the awareness of and overall progress made in metabolic disorders have not shown such growth, and CB chemistry began to represent eventful alternatives only recently in this matter. The exploration of the potential modulation of some elements of the ECS and specific metabolic disorders just started to emerge and has been addressed only once with experimental purposes. In 2015, Colín-González and colleagues[85] published a synthetic approach used to evaluate the effect of a synthetic CB on early markers of some OAs, based on the understanding that its genesis comes with the convergence of events such as excitotoxicity and oxidative stress. In this form, the protective effects of WIN 55,212-2 (a synthetic CBr agonist) were evaluated in regard to its capacity to prevent oxidative damage, lipid peroxidation, decrease in antioxidant defense, and mitochondrial dysfunction, all of them being known early markers of metabolic diseases (GA, 3-OHGA, MMA, and PA as distinctive metabolites of the most typical metabolic disorders). The referred study led to interesting findings, as WIN 55,212-2 exhibited protective effects on markers related with GA-I and MMAcidemia, evaluated in terms of the prevention of mitochondrial dysfunction, formation of ROS, and lipid peroxidation in rat brain synaptosomes; the aforementioned findings support unequivocally the protective role of CBs in the toxic events present at early stages of OAs as a novel approach to assess the modulatory potential of CB compounds.[85] By the same authors, a second effort in publishing process confirmed the effective prevention of the toxicity induced by 3-MGA in brain synaptosomes elicited by low concentrations of WIN 55,212-2 when used as pretreatment (for as long as 30 minutes and prior to toxic insult).[97] Given the lack of experimental designs involving OAs and its toxic early metabolites, the future is headed toward the integration of the viable CB alternatives existing at this point into proficient experimental approaches to assess and exploit the effects of the modulation of the CB chemistry.

Concluding Remarks

As seen, the promissory character of CBs has shown remarkable properties that might enable the reduction in oxidative stress and a number of neuroinflammatory markers, while reestablishing brain homeostasis and restorative mechanisms contribute actively. In conclusion, therapeutic approaches adopting endocannabinoid strategies for common neurodegenerative diseases and even for a group of inherited metabolic disorders known as organic acidemias, that are characterized by severe impairment of the CNS. This approach may undoubtedly possess incalculable potential, and yet the necessity of additional research and conclusive data are imperative in order to clarify its participation in the pathological picture of such conditions.

Acknowledgments

The authors wish to express gratitude to Prof Moacir Wajner for his valuable comments and suggestions.

Declaration of Conflicting Interests

The author(s) declared no potential conflicts of interest with respect to the research, authorship, and/or publication of this article.

Funding

The author(s) received no financial support for the research, authorship, and/or publication of this article.

References

1. Grotenhermen F, Müller-Vahl K. The therapeutic potential of cannabis and cannabinoids. *Dtsch Arztebl Int*. 2012;109(29-30): 495-501.
2. Cabranes A, Venderova K, de Lago E, et al. Decreased endocannabinoid levels in he brain and beneficial effects of agents activating cannabinoid and/ or canilloid receptors in a rat model of multiple sclerosis. *Neurobiol Dis*. 2005;20(2):207-217.
3. Pazos MR, Sagredo O, Fernández-Ruiz J. The endocannabinod system in Huntington's disease. *Curr Pharm Des*. 2008;14(23): 2317-2325.
4. Riedel G, Davies SN. Cannabinoid function in learning, memory and plasticity. *Handb Exp Pharmacol*. 2005;(168):445-477.
5. Shoemaker J, Seely K, Reed R, Crow J, Prather P. The CB2 cannabinoid agonist AM-1241 prolongs survival in a transgenic mouse model of amyotrophic lateral sclerosis when initiated at symptom onset. *J Neurochem*. 2007;101(1):87-98.
6. Lastres-Becker I, Molina-Holgado F, Ramos J, Mechoulam R, Fernández-Ruiz J. Cannabinoids provide neuroprotection against 6-hydroxydopamine toxicity in vivo and in vitro: relevance to Parkinson's disease. *Neurobiol Dis*. 2005;19(1): 96-107.
7. Salama M, Arias-Carrión O. Natural toxins implicated in the development of Parkinson's disease. *Ther Adv Neurol Disord*. 2011;4(6):361-373.
8. Dray A. Neuropathic pain: emerging treatments. *Br J Anaesth*. 2008;101(1):48-58. doi:10.1093/bja/aen107.
9. Aso E, Ferrer I. Cannabinoids for treatment of Alzheimer's disease: moving toward the clinic. *Front Pharmacol*. 2014;5:1-11. doi:10.3389/fphar.2014.00037.
10. Leung L. Cannabis and its derivatives: review of medical use. *J Am Board Fam Med*. 2011;24(4):452-462. doi:10.3122/jabfm.2011.04.100280.
11. Fernández-Ruiz J. The endocannabinoid system as a target for the treatment of motor dysfunction. *Br J Pharmacol*. 2009;156(7): 1029-1040. doi:10.1111/j.1476-5381.2008.00088.x.
12. García C, Palomo-Garo C, García-Arencibia M, Ramos J, Pertwee R, Fernández-Ruiz J. Symptom-relieving and neuroprotective effects of the phytocannabinoid Δ9-THCV in animal models of Parkinson's disease. *Brain J Pharmacol*. 2011; 163(7):1495-1506.
13. Bates G, Dorsey R, Gusella J, et al. Huntington's disease. *Nat Rev Dis Prim*. 2015;1:15005.
14. Orzand P, Gascon G. Organic acidurias: a review. Part I. *J Chil Neurol*. 1991;6(3):196-219.
15. Chalmers R, Lawson A. *Organic Acids in Man. Analytical Chemistry, Biochemistry and Diagnosis of the Organic Acidurias*. London: Chapman Hall. 1982.
16. Wajner M, Wannmacher C, Gaidzinski D, Dutra Filho C. Detection of inborn errors of metabolism in patients of pediatric intensive care units of Porto Alegre, Brazil. Comparison between the

prevalence of such disturbances in a selected and an unselected sample. *Braz J Genet*. 1986;9:331-340.
17. Wajner M, Barschak A, Luft A, Pires R, Grillo E, Lohr A. Organic aciduria: diagnosis in high risk Brazilian patients. *J Petiatr*. 2001; 77(5):401-406.
18. Hoffman G, Gibson K, Trefz F, Nyhan W, Bremer H, Rating D. Neurological manifestations of organic acid disorders. *Eur J Pediatr*. 1994;153(suppl 1):94-100.
19. Wanmacheer C, Wajner M, Giugliani R, Giugliani E, Costa M, Giugliani M. Detection of metabolic disorders among high-risk patients. *Rev Bras Genet*. 1982;5:187-194.
20. Vaidyanathan K, Narayanan M, Vasudevan D. Organic acidurias: an updated review. *Ind J Clin Biochem*. 2011;26(4):319-325.
21. Yannicelli S. Nutrition therapy of organic acidaemias with amino acid-based formulas: emphasis on methylmalonic and propionic acidaemia. *J Inherit Metab Dis*. 2006;29(2-3):281-287.
22. Thompson G, Chalmers R. Increased urinary metabolite excretion during fasting in dosorders of propionate metabolism. *Pediatr Res*. 1990;27(4 pt 1):413-416.
23. Chalmers R, Stacey T, Tracey B. L-Carnitine: insufficiency in disorders of organic acid metabolism: response to L-carnitine by patients with methylmalonic aciduria and 3-hydroxy-3-methylglutaric aciduria. *J Inherit Metab Dis*. 1984;7(suppl 2): 109-110.
24. Kölker S, Greenberg C, Linder M, Muller E, Naughten E, Hoffmann G. Emergency treatment in glutaryl-CoA dehydrogenase deficiency. *J Inherit Metab Dis*. 2004;27(6):893-902.
25. Sauer U. Metabolic networks in motion: ^{13}C-based flux analysis. *Mol Syst Biol*. 2006;2:62.
26. Amir N, El-Peleg O, Shalev R, Christensen E. Glutaric aciduria type I: clinical heterogeneity and neuroradiologic features. *Neurology*. 1987;37(10):1654-1657.
27. Hoffmann G, Zschocke J. Glutaric aciduria type I: from clinical, biochemical and molecular diversity to successful therapy. *J Inherit Metab Dis*. 1999;22(4):381-391.
28. Flott-Rahmel B, Falter C, Schluff P, et al. Nerve cell lesions caused by 3-hydroxyglutaric acid: a possible mechanism for neurodegeneration in glutaric acidemia I. *J Inherit Metab Dis*. 1997;20(3):387-390.
29. Latini A, Borba Rosa R, Scussiato K, Llesuy S, Belló-Klein A, Wajner M. 3-Hydroxyglutaric acid induces oxidative stress and decreases the antipxidant defenses in cerebral cortex of young rats. *Brain Res*. 2002;956(2):367-373.
30. de Oliveira Marques F, Hagen M, Pederzolli C, et al. Glutaric acid induces oxidative stress in brain of young rats. *Brain Res*. 2003; 964(1):153-158.
31. Wajner M, Kölker S, Souza D, Hoffmann G, de Mello C. Modulation of glutamatergic and GABAerigic neurotransmission in glutaryl-CoA dehydrogenase deficiency. *J Inherit Metab Dis*. 2004;27(6):825-828.
32. Sauer S, Okun J, Schwab M, et al. Bioenergetics in glutaryl-coenzyme A dehydrogenase deficiency: a role for glutaryl-coenzyme A. *J Biol Chem*. 2005;280(23):21830-21836.
33. Deodato F, Boenzi S, Santorello F, Dionisi-Vici C. Methylmalonic and propionic aciduria. *Am J Med Genet*. 2006;142C(2): 104-112.
34. Brismar J, Ozand P. CT and MR of the brain in the diagnosis of organic acidemias. Experiences from 107 patients. *Brain Dev*. 1994;16(suppl):104-124.
35. Chemelli A, Hugl B, Klocker J, et al. Endovascular repair of isolated iliac artery aneurysms. *J Endovasc Ther*. 2010;17(4): 492-503.
36. Kölker S, Hoffmann G, Okun J. Congenital glutamine deficiency with glutamine synthetase mutations. *N Engl J Med*. 2006; 354(10):1093-1094.
37. Stellmer F, Keyser B, Burckhardt B, et al. 3-Hydroxyglutaric acid is transported via the sodium-dependent dicarboxylate transporter NaDC3. *J Mol Med*. 2007;85(7):763-770.
38. Sauer S, Opp S, Hoffmann G, Koeller D, Okun J, Kölker S. Therapeutic modulation of cerebral L-lysine metabolism in a mouse model of glutaric aciduria type I. *Brain*. 2011;134(pt 1): 157-170.
39. Wyse A, Brusque A, Silva C, Streck E, Wajner M, Wannamacher C. Inhibition of Na^+, K^+-ATPase from rat brain cortex by propionic acid. *Neuroreport*. 1998;9(8):1719-1721.
40. Brusque A, Mello C, Buchanan D, et al. Effect of chemically induced propionic acidemia on neurobehavioral development of rats. *Pharmacol Biochem Behav*. 1999;64(3):529-534.
41. de Mattos-Dutra A, Meirelles R, Bevilaqua de Rocha B, et al. Methylmalonic and propionic acids increase the in vitro incorporation of 32P into cytoskeletal proteins from cerebral cortex of young rats through NMDA glutamate receptors. *Brain Res*. 2000; 856(1-2):111-118.
42. Fontella F, Pulrolnik V, Gassen E, et al. Propionic and L-methylmalonic acids induce oxidative stress in brain of young rats. *Neuroreport*. 2000;11(3):541-544.
43. Pettenuzzo L, Schuck P, Fontella F, et al. Ascorbic acid prevents cognitive deficits caused by cronic administration of propionic acid to rats in the water maze. *Pharmacol Biochem Behav*. 2002;73(3):623-629.
44. Trindade V, Brusque A, Raasch J, et al. Ganglioside alterations in the central nervous system of rats chronically injected with methylmalonic and propionic acids. *Metab Brain Dis*. 2002; 17(2):93-102.
45. Rigo F, Pasquetti L, Malfatti C, et al. Propionic acid induces convulsions and protein carbonylation in rats. *Neurosci Lett*. 2006;408(2):151-154.
46. RIbas G, Manfredini V, de Marco M, et al. Prevention by L-carnitine of DNA damage induced by propionic acid and L-methylmalonic acids in human peripheral leukocytes in vitro. *Mutat Res*. 2010;702(1):123-128.
47. Ribas G, Manfredini V, de Mari J, et al. Reduction of lipid and protein damage in patients with disorders of propionate metabolism under treatment: a possible protective role of L-carnitine supplementation. *Int J Dev Neurosci*. 2010;28(2):127-132.
48. Gómez-Ruiz M, Hernández M, De Miguel R, Ramos JA. An overview on the biochemistry of the cannabinoid system. *Mol Neurobiol*. 2007;36(1):3-14. doi:10.1007/s12035-007-0015-0.
49. Reggio PH. NIH public access: author manuscript. endocannabinoid binding to the cannabinoid receptors: what is known and what remains unknown. *Curr Med CHem*. 2010;17(14): 1468-1486.

50. Basavarajappa B, Nixon RA, Arancio O. HHS public access. 2016;9(4):448-462.
51. Alger BBE. Getting high on the endocannabinoid system. *Cerebrum* 2013;2013:1-14.
52. Di Marzo V, Piscitelli F. Gut feelings about the endocannabinoid system. *Neurogastroenterol Motil.* 2011;23(5):391-398. doi:10.1111/j.1365-2982.2011.01689.x.
53. Wyrofsky R, Mcgonigle P, Van Bockstaele EJ. HHS public access. *Expert Opin Drug Discov.* 2015;10(1):17-36. doi:10.1517/17460441.2014.966680.Drug.
54. Izzo AA, Muccioli GG, Ruggieri MR, Schicho R. Endocannabinoids and the digestive tract and bladder in health and disease. 2015:423-447. doi:10.1007/978-3-319-20825-1.
55. Sullivan SEO. Endocannabinoids and the cardiovascular system in health and disease. 2015:393-422. doi:10.1007/978-3-319-20825-1.
56. Cabral GA, Ferreira GA, Jamerson MJ. Endocannabinoids and the immune system in health and disease. 2015. doi:10.1007/978-3-319-20825-1.
57. Sanchez-mut JV, Gräff J. Epigenetic alterations in Alzheimer's disease. 2015;9:1-17. doi:10.3389/fnbeh.2015.00347.
58. Jones E, Kirkham T. Noladin ether, a putative endocannabinoid, enhances motivation to eat after acute systemic. *Br J Pharmacol.* 2012;166(6):1815-1821. doi:10.1111/j.1476-5381.2012.01888.x.
59. Shoemaker JL, Joseph BK, Ruckle MB, Mayeux PR, Prather PL, Rock L. The endocannabinoid noladin ether acts as a full agonist at human CB2 cannabinoid receptors. 2005;314(2):868-875. doi:10.1124/jpet.105.085282.al.
60. Duncan M, Millns P, Smart D, Wright JE, Kendall DA, Ralevic V. Noladin ether, a putative endocannabinoid, attenuates sensory neurotransmission in the rat isolated mesenteric arterial bed via a non-CB 1/CB 2 Gi/o linked receptor. *Br J Pharmacol.* 2004;(142):509-518. doi:10.1038/sj.bjp.0705789.
61. Oka S, Tsuchie A, Tokumura A, et al. Ether-linked analogue of 2-arachidonoylglycerol (noladin ether) was not detected in the brains of various mammalian species. *J Neurochem.* 2003;85(6):1374-1381. doi:10.1046/j.1471-4159.2003.01804.x.
62. Bisogno T, Melck D, Bobrov MY, et al. N-acyl-dopamines: novel synthetic CB1 cannabinoid-receptor ligands and inhibitors of anandamide inactivation with cannabimimetic activity in vitro and in vivo. *Biochem J.* 2000;351(pt 3):817-824.
63. Porter AC, Sauer JM, Knierman MD, et al. Characterization of a novel endocannabinoid, virodhamine, with antagonist activity at the CB1 receptor. *J Pharmacol Exp Ther.* 2002;301(3):1020-1024.
64. Hruba L, Mcmahon LR. NIH public access. *NIH Public Access Author Manuscr.* 2014;727(210):35-42. doi:10.1016/j.ejphar.2014.01.041. The.
65. Zajac DM, Sikkema SR, Chandrasena R. Nabilone for the treatment of dementia-associated sexual disinhibition. *Prim Care Companion CNS Disord.* 2015;17(1):8-10. doi:10.4088/PCC.14l01695.
66. Turcotte D, Doupe M, Torabi M, et al. NEUROPATHIC PAIN SECTION original research articles nabilone as an adjunctive to gabapentin for multiple sclerosis-induced neuropathic pain: a randomized controlled trial. *Pain Med.* 2015;16(1):149-159.
67. Giacoppo S, Rajan TS, Galuppo M, Pollastro F, Grassi G, Bramanti P. Purified Cannabidiol, the main non-psychotropic component of *Cannabis sativa*, alone, counteracts neuronal apoptosis in experimental multiple sclerosis. *Eur Rev Med Pharmacol Sci.* 2015;19(24):4906-4919.
68. Walsh SK, Hepburn CY, Keown O, Astrand A, Lindblom A, Ryberg E, Hjorth S, Leslie SJ, Greasley PJ, Wainwright CL. Pharmacological profiling of the hemodynamic effects of cannabinoid ligands: a combined in vitro and in vivo approach. *Pharmacol Res Perspect.* 2015;3(3):e00143.
69. Huffman JW, Thompson ALS, Wiley JL, Martin BR. Synthesis and pharmacology of 1-deoxy analogs of CP-47,497 and CP-55,940. *NIH Public Access Author Manuscr.* 2008;16(1):322-335.
70. Samano KL, Poklis JL, Lichtman AH, Poklis A. Development of a high-performance liquid chromatography–tandem mass spectrometry method for the identification and quantification of CP-47, 497, CP-47, 497-C8 and JWH-250 in mouse brain. *J Anal Toxicol.* 2014;38(6):307-314.
71. Griffin G, Wray E, Martin B, Abood M. Cannabinoid agonists and antagonists discriminated by receptor binding in rat cerebellum. *Br J Pharmacol.* 1999;128(3):684-688.
72. Rodríguez-Arias M, Roger-Sánchez C, Vilanova I, et al. Effects of cannabinoid exposure furing adolescence on the conditioned rewarding effects of WIN 55212-2 and cocaine in mice: influence of the novelty-seeking trait. *Neural Plast.* 2016:6481862.
73. Hanlon K, Lozano-Ondoua A, Imaretiya P, et al. Modulation of breast cancer cell viability by a cannabinoid receptor 2 agonist, JWH-015, is calcium dependent. *Breast Cancer (Dove Med Press.* 2016;8:59-71.
74. Jacome-Sosa M, Vacca C, Mangat R, et al. Vaccenic acid supresses intestinal inflammation by increasing anandamide and related N-acylethanolamines in the JCR: LA-cp rat. *J Lipid Res.* 2016;57(4):638-649.
75. Wiley J, Mathew Walentiny D, Vann R, Baskfield C. Dissimilar cannabinoid substitution patterns in mice trained to discriminate Δ(9)-tetrahydrocannabinol or methanandamide from vehicle. *Behav Pharmacol.* 2011;22(5-6):480-488.
76. Price T, Patwardhan A, Akopian A, Hargreaves K, Flores C. Moduation of trigeminal sensory neuron activity by the dual cannabinoid-vanilloid agonists andandamide, N-arachidonoyl-dopamine and arachidonoyl-2-chloroethylamide. *Br J Pharmacol.* 2004;141(7):1118-1130.
77. Howlett AC, Barth F, Bonner TI, et al.; International Union of Pharmacology. XXVII. classification of cannabinoid receptors. *Pharmacol Rev.* 2002;54(2):161-202.
78. Badgy G, Juhasz G, Gonda X. A new clinical evidence-based gene–environment interaction model of depression. *Neuropsychopharmacol Hung.* 2012;14(4):213-220.
79. Hermanson DJ, Hartley ND, Gamble-George J, et al. Substrate-selective COZ-2 inhibition decreases anxiety via endocannabinoid activation. *Nat Neurosci.* 2013;16(9):1291-1298.
80. Esposito E, Impellizzeri D, Mazzon E, Paterniti I, Cuzzocrea S. Neuroprotective activities of palmitoylethanolamide in an animal model of Parkinson's disease. *PLoS One.* 2012;7(8):e41880.
81. Fernández-Ruiz J. The endocannabinoid system as a target of the treatment of motor dysfunction. *Br J Pharmacol.* 2009;156(7):1029-1040.

82. Malek N, Kucharczyk M, Starowicz K. Alterations in the anandamide metabolism in the development of neuropathic pain. *Biomed Res Int*. 2014:686908.
83. Di Iorio G, Lupi M, Sarchione F, et al. The endocannabinoid system: a putative role in neurodegenerative diseases. *Int J High Risk Behav Addict*. 2013;2(3):100-106. doi:10.5812/ijhrba.9222.
84. Schrot RJ, Hubbard JR, Schrot RJ, Hubbard JR. Annals of medicine cannabinoids: medical implications. 2016;3890. doi:10.3109/07853890.2016.1145794.
85. Colín-González AL, Paz-Loyola AL, Serratos IN, et al. The effect of WIN 55,212-2 suggests a cannabinoid-sensitive component in the early toxicity induced by organic acids accumulating in glutaric acidemia type I and in related disorders of propionate metabolism in rat brain synaptosomes. *Neuroscience*. 2015;310:578-588.
86. Ulugöl A. The endocannabinoid system as a potential therapeutic target for pain modulation. *Balkan Med J*. 2014;31(2):115-120. doi:10.5152/balkanmedj.2014.13103.
87. Blazquez C, Chiarlone A, Sagredo O, et al. Loss of striatal type 1 cannabinoid receptors is a key pathogenic factor in Huntington's disease. *Brain*. 2011;134 (pt 1):119-136.
88. Juranek JK, Daffu GK, Wojtkiewicz J, Lacomis D, Kofler J, Schmidt AM. Receptor for advanced glycation end products and its inflammatory ligands are upregulated in amyotrophic lateral sclerosis. *Front Cell Neurosci*. 2015;9:485.
89. Scotter EL, Goodfellow CE, Graham ES, Dragunow M, Glass M. Neuroprotective potential of CB1 receptor agonists in an vivo model of Huntington's disease. *Brain J Pharmacol*. 2010; 160(3):747-761.
90. Takahashi KA, Castillo PE. The CB1 cannabinoid receptor mediates glutamatergic synamptic supression in the hippocampus. *Neuroscience*. 2006;139(3):795-802.
91. Domaradzki J. The impact of Huntington's disease on family carers: a literatyre overview. *Psychiatr Pol*. 2015;49(5):931-944.
92. Panlilio L V, Justinova Z, Goldberg SR. Animal models of cannabinoid reward. *Br J Pharmacol*. 2010;160(3):499-510. doi:10.1111/j.1476-5381.2010.00775.x.
93. Renton A, Chio A, Traynor B. State of play in amyotrophic lateral sclerosis genetics. *Nat Neurosci*. 2014;17(1):17-23.
94. Meissner W, Frasier M, Gasser T, et al. Priorities in Parkinson's disease research. *Nat Reviees Drug Discov*. 2011;10(5):377-393.
95. Morandi E, Tarlinton R, Gran B. Multiple sclerosis between genetics and infections: human endogenous retroviruses in monocytes and macrophages. *Front Immunol*. 2015;6:647.
96. Furukawa Y, Anzai I, Akiyama S, et al. Conformational disorder of the most immature Cu, Zn-superoxide dismutase leading to amyotrophic lateral sclerosis. *J Biol Chem*. 2016;291(8): 4144-4155.
97. Santamaría A, Colín-González AL, Paz-Loyola AL, et al. Experimental evidence that 3-methylglutaric acid disturbs mitochondrial function and induced oxidative stress in rat brain synaptosomes: new converging mechanisms. *Neurochem Res*. 2016;41(10): 2619-2626.

18

Diagnosis and Management of Classical Homocystinuria in Brazil: A Summary of 72 Late-Diagnosed Patients

Soraia Poloni, PhD[1,2], Giovana W. Hoss, MD[2,3], Fernanda Sperb-Ludwig, PhD[2,3], Taciane Borsatto, PhD[2,3], Maria Juliana R. Doriqui, MD[4], Emília K.E.A Leão, PhD[5,6], Ney Boa-Sorte, PhD[5,6], Charles M. Lourenço, PhD[7,8], Chong A. Kim, PhD[9], Carolina F. M. de Souza, PhD[10], Helio Rocha, MD[11], Marcia Ribeiro, PhD[11], Carlos E. Steiner, PhD[12], Carolina A. Moreno, PhD[12], Pricila Bernardi, MD[13], Eugenia Valadares, PhD[14], Osvaldo Artigalas, MD[15,16], Gerson Carvalho, MD[17], Hector Y. C. Wanderley, MD[18], Vânia D'Almeida, PhD[19], Luiz C. Santana-da-Silva, PhD[20], Henk J. Blom, PhD[21], and Ida V. D. Schwartz, PhD[1,2,3,10]

Abstract

This study described a broad clinical characterization of classical homocystinuria (HCU) in Brazil. This was a cross-sectional, observational study including clinical and biochemical data from 72 patients (60 families) from Brazil (South, n = 13; Southeast, n =

[1] Post-Graduation Program in Medical Sciences, Universidade Federal do Rio Grande do Sul, Porto Alegre, Brazil
[2] Laboratory of Basic Research and Advanced Investigations in Neurosciences (BRAIN), Hospital de Clínicas de Porto Alegre, Porto Alegre, Brazil
[3] Post-Graduation Program in Genetics and Molecular Biology, Universidade Federal do Rio Grande do Sul, Porto Alegre, Brazil
[4] Complexo Hospitalar Materno-Infantil do Maranhão, São Luis, Brazil
[5] Complexo Hospitalar Professor Edgard Santos, Salvador, Brazil
[6] Universidade do Estado da Bahia, Salvador, Brazil
[7] Hospital das Clínicas de Ribeirão Preto, Ribeirão Preto, Brazil
[8] Centro Universitário Estácio de Ribeirão Preto, Ribeirão Preto, Brazil
[9] Universidade de São Paulo, São Paulo, Brazil
[10] Medical Genetics Service, Hospital de Clínicas de Porto Alegre, Porto Alegre, Brazil
[11] Universidade Federal do Rio de Janeiro, Rio de Janeiro, Brazil
[12] Universidade Estadual de Campinas, Campinas, Brazil
[13] Universidade Federal de Santa Catarina, Florianópolis, Brazil
[14] Universidade Federal de Minas Gerais, Belo Horizonte, Brazil
[15] Hospital da Criança Conceição, GHC, Porto Alegre, Brazil
[16] Hospital Materno-Infantil Presidente Vargas, Porto Alegre, Brazil
[17] Hospital de Apoio de Brasília, Brasília, Brazil
[18] Escola Superior de Ciências da Santa Casa de Misericórdia de Vitória, Vitória, Brazil
[19] Department of Psychobiology, Universidade Federal de São Paulo, São Paulo, Brazil
[20] Universidade Federal do Pará, Belém, Brazil
[21] Laboratory for Clinical Biochemistry and Metabolism, University Medical Center, Freiburg, Germany

Corresponding Author:
Giovana W. Hoss, Ms, Universidade Federal do Rio Grande do Sul, R. Ramiro Barcelos, 2350, Porto Alegre, 90040, Brazil.
Email: giovana.weber@gmail.com

37; Northeast, n = 8; North, n = 1; and Midwest, n = 1). Parental consanguinity was reported in 42% of families. Ocular manifestations were the earliest detected symptom (53% of cases), the main reason for diagnostic suspicion (63% of cases), and the most prevalent manifestation at diagnosis (67% of cases). Pyridoxine responsiveness was observed in 14% of patients. Only 22% of nonresponsive patients on treatment had total homocysteine levels <100 μmol/L. Most commonly used treatment strategies were pyridoxine (93% of patients), folic acid (90%), betaine (74%), vitamin B12 (27%), and low-methionine diet + metabolic formula (17%). Most patients diagnosed with HCU in Brazil are late diagnosed, express a severe phenotype, and poor metabolic control. Milder forms of HCU are likely underrepresented due to underdiagnosis.

Keywords
classical homocystinuria, CBS deficiency, homocysteine, pyridoxine responsiveness, diagnosis

Introduction

Classical homocystinuria (HCU; OMIM 236200) is an inborn error of methionine metabolism caused by deficient activity of cystathionine β-synthase (CβS; EC 4.2.1.22). Cystathionine β-synthase deficiency leads to massive accumulation of homocysteine and methionine and low levels of cysteine.[1,2] Homocystinuria was first described in 1962[3]; since then, many advances in treatment and early diagnosis, including newborn screening, have improved prognosis dramatically.[4–6] However, diagnosis and management of HCU is still a major challenge in developing countries, where newborn screening is unavailable and access to health-care services is often poor and unequal.[7]

From a clinical standpoint, the classic signs of HCU are lens dislocation, thromboembolism, mental retardation, psychiatric disorders, osteoporosis, and marfanoid features.[8] Established treatment strategies include supplementation of pyridoxine (CβS cofactor), folic/folinic acid, betaine, and a methionine-restricted diet supplemented with an essential amino acids admixture free of methionine.[9] Novel therapies with chaperones and enzyme replacement are currently under development.[10–12] Usually, patients who respond to pyridoxine supplementation exhibit a milder phenotype and have a better prognosis.[8]

The worldwide prevalence of HCU is estimated to be 1:100 000.[13] However, several mild and late presentation phenotypes have been described,[14–16] raising the issue of whether HCU is largely underdiagnosed. Newborn screening for HCU is performed in some countries with high incidence of the disease, such as Ireland and Qatar.[5,17] Usually, newborn screening is performed by the determination of methionine on filter paper. However, this method has a large percentage of false negatives (up to 50%), since pyridoxine-responsive HCU may not present with hypermethioninemia in the first days of life.[18,19] In Brazil, the prevalence of HCU is unknown, and the disease is not included in the National Neonatal Screening Program.

Brazil is a very large country with over 200 million inhabitants, and the country is characterized by intense admixture.[20,21] The country also has one of the world's largest publicly funded health-care systems, the Unified Health System (*Sistema Único de Saúde*), which was established to provide equitable and comprehensive care to all users. However, betaine and the methionine-free amino acid formulation are not available through Unified Health System, and few centers across the country offer biochemical testing for diagnosis and management of this condition. Furthermore, several factors make diagnosis and management of HCU within the Brazilian health system a major challenge; hence, a substantial number of patients with this treatable condition are believed to remain undiagnosed and thus untreated. Within this context, the present study sought to establish a broad clinical characterization of HCU in Brazil through a survey on diagnosis and management of a representative patient population that is being followed at several centers nationwide.

Materials and Methods

The present study was approved by the local research ethics committee. Collection procedures for the study were conducted only after participants or their caregivers had agreed to take part in the investigation and provided written informed consent.

Patients

The study sample comprised 72 Brazilian patients with a diagnosis of HCU, from 60 different families. Diagnosis was in general made on clinical symptoms followed by clear elevations in homocysteine and methionine. Mutation analyses was performed in 35 of the 72 patients.[22] Families from all 5 regions of Brazil were represented: South (n = 13), Southeast (n = 37), Northeast (n = 8), North (n = 1), and Midwest (n = 1). Patients were recruited through contact with physicians involved in care and/or research activities at medical genetics centers across the country. A structured questionnaire containing queries regarding diagnosis, consanguinity, treatment strategies, metabolic control, and current health condition of patients with HCU was sent to 15 medical centers that had agreed to participate in the study. Clinical data regarding diagnosis were available only for 28 patients.

All 72 patients had delayed diagnoses: 62 patients had been diagnosed after clinical suspicion and biochemical findings consistent with HCU (hyperhomocysteinemia and hypermethioninemia), and the remaining 10 had been diagnosed on family screening. Each of the participating centers used a different protocol for determination of pyridoxine responsiveness. For the purposes of this study, patients were classified as

Table 1. Classical Homocystinuria in Brazil: A Summary of Clinical Findings at Diagnosis.[a]

	Total (N = 72)	Pyridoxine Responsive: Yes (n = 10)	Pyridoxine Responsive: No (n = 61)	P
Current age, years	19 (5-45)	23 (14-35)	18 (5-45)	.120
Age at first symptom onset, years	5 (0-20)	2 (0.2-15)	5 (0.7-20)	.316
Age at diagnosis, years	10 (1-39)	11 (4-34)	9 (1-39)	.545
Systems affected at diagnosis, %				
Ocular	72	50	75	.100
CNS	60	70	59	.497
Skeletal	60	40	54	.401
Vascular	15	20	14	.625

Abbreviation: CNS, central nervous system.
[a]N = 72, data expressed as the median (range) or percentage. In 1 patient, pyridoxine responsiveness could not be determined, data from this patient were used alone in the whole-group analysis.

responsive if they achieved homocysteine levels <50 µmol/L on pyridoxine alone or pyridoxine + folic acid (regardless of the number of weeks since testing). All other patients were classified as nonresponsive to pyridoxine.

Target total homocysteine levels on treatment were set according HCU guidelines,[9] which were <50 µmol/L for pyridoxine-responsive patients and <100 µmol/L for nonresponsive patients. Treatment adherence was determined by the subjective impressions of the care team at each medical center.

Statistical Analysis

Statistical analysis was performed using SPSS for Windows, version 18.0 (SPSS Inc, Chicago, Illinois). Asymmetrically distributed variables were expressed as the median (range). The Mann-Whitney *U* test (continuous variables) or χ^2 test (categorical variables) was used to assess between-group differences. Values of $P < .05$ were considered significant.

Results

Of the 72 patients included, 55% were male. Two patients were already deceased at the time of inclusion in the study (presumably due to thromboembolic events). The patients belonged to 60 families; parental consanguinity was reported in 25 (42%) families. Median age at assessment was 19 years. The youngest patient was aged 5, and the oldest was 45. Regarding pyridoxine responsiveness, 61 (85%) patients were classified as nonresponsive and 10 (13.8%) as responsive. In 1 patient, pyridoxine responsiveness was not reported/determined.

Journey to Diagnosis

The very first symptom noticed by families and/or physicians was visual impairment (mainly due to *ectopia lentis*) in 53% of the cases, followed by developmental delay (22% of cases), seizures (11% of cases), and isolated thromboembolic episodes (9.5% of cases). Table 1 reports clinical features at diagnosis for the sample as a whole and stratified by pyridoxine responsiveness.

The median time elapsed between symptom onset and diagnosis was 5 years (maximum, 34 years). One-third of the patients had 3 or more systems already affected at the time of diagnosis. The main clinical findings leading to investigation of HCU are represented in Figure 1. Eye disease, the most prevalent symptom at diagnosis (67% of cases), accounted for 63% of referrals for HCU investigation.

Management

Current clinical and biochemical data were available for 44 patients, of whom 7 were responsive and 37 were nonresponsive to pyridoxine. The median length of follow-up was 6 years (range, 0-27 years). Table 2 describes clinical manifestations and biochemical control in this group of patients. Ocular manifestations were more prevalent among pyridoxine-nonresponsive patients (71% vs 97%, $P = .01$). *Ectopia lentis* was the most common complication in our sample, affecting 91% of patients at the time of study inclusion.

Pyridoxine-responsive patients had significantly lower total homocysteine levels at study inclusion ($P < .001$). Only 22% of nonresponsive patients achieved target total homocysteine levels (<100 µmol/L) on treatment, while all responsive patients (n = 7) had total homocysteine <50 µmol/L. Treatment adherence was reported as appropriate in 44% of patients.

Regarding treatment strategies, 93% of patients were on pyridoxine supplementation, 90% on folic acid, 74% on betaine, 27% on vitamin B12, and only 17% on a low-methionine diet + metabolic formula.

Discussion

The present report provides the largest clinical profile of patients with HCU ever studied in Brazil to date. Clinical data of 72 patients (60 unrelated) from 15 medical genetics centers across Brazil were analyzed. Most families lived in the South and Southeast regions of the country. These regions are home to 57% of the country's population (http://www.ibge.gov.br/) and, compared to other regions of Brazil, have higher rates of access to health-care services and procedures. The fact that patients from other regions, particularly the North (n = 1) and Midwest (n = 1), were underrepresented suggests high rates of HCU underdiagnosis and/or limited access to care in these regions.[7]

A high proportion of pyridoxine-nonresponsive patients with HCU was found in our study (85%). Nonresponsive patients usually present a more severe phenotype, have more complications, and younger ages .[6,8,23] In our study, this proportion exceeded rates described worldwide of approximately 50%.[8] In countries where the proportion of nonresponsive patients is disproportionately high, such as Qatar and Ireland,

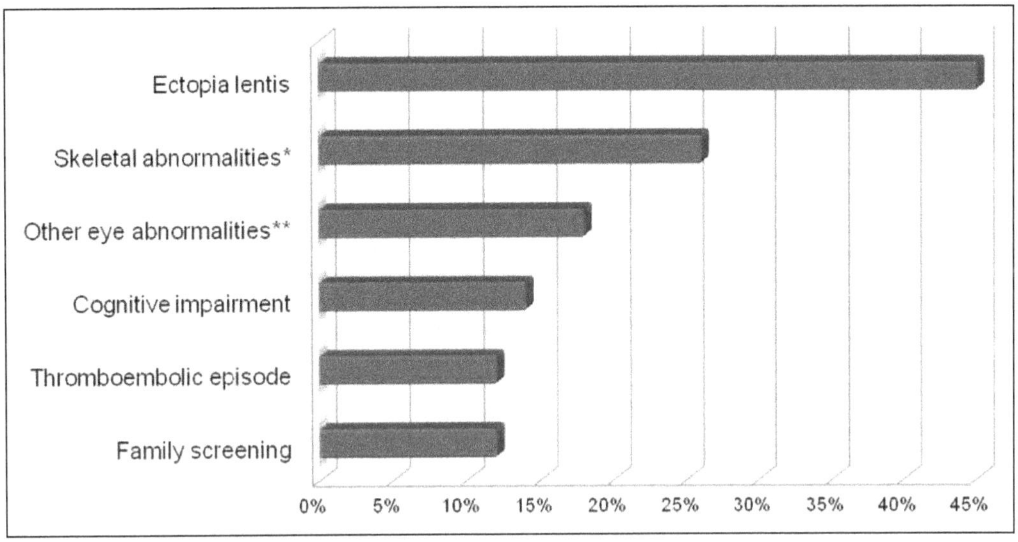

Figure 1. Main reasons for clinical suspicion of classical homocystinuria in our sample (N = 72). *Including marfanoid habitus, **Other than *ectopia lentis*.

Table 2. Classical Homocystinuria in Brazil: Clinical and Biochemical Profile of Patients on Treatment at the Time of Study Inclusion.[a]

		Pyridoxine Responsive		
	Total (n = 44)	Yes (n = 7)	No (n = 37)	*P*
Current age, years	16	19 (14-35)	16 (5-37)	.182
Homocysteine, μmol/L	168	19 (14-34)	212 (9-455)	<.001
Methionine, μmol/L	131	27 (23-650)	218 (6-881)	.065
Clinical manifestations, %				
Ocular	93	71	97	.013
CNS	70	86	68	.318
Skeletal	61	57	62	.803
Vascular	25	14	27	.475

Abbreviation: CNS, central nervous system.
[a]n = 44, data expressed as the median (range) or percentage; reference ranges: homocysteine, 5-15 μmol/L; methionine, 5-30 μmol/L.

specific genotypes are highly prevalent and account for these discrepancies .[24,25] In a previous study of our group, we explored in more depth the genotype of 35 patients with HCU who are also included in the current study.[22]

Our results show there is no single molecular basis for the high prevalence of HCU nonresponsive phenotypes in Brazil. In fact, the most prevalent mutation in that study (p.Ile278Thr) is a pyridoxine-responsive mutation. Another genetic study of 14 Brazilian patients with HCU showed similar results.[26] These findings rather suggest underdiagnosis of pyridoxine-responsive patients in Brazil who express milder phenotypes with fewer symptoms and later onset of clinical presentation.[6,8] In our study, no significant differences in age at symptom onset or age at diagnosis were found between pyridoxine-responsive and nonresponsive patients; however, we believe our analysis was underpowered because of the low number of pyridoxine-responsive patients (n = 10 vs n = 61, respectively).

The high prevalence of ocular manifestations at diagnosis and their predominant contribution to diagnostic suspicion reinforce the importance of eye disease in HCU. *Ectopia lentis* is usually the earliest manifestation of HCU, occurring in half of all untreated patients by age 10 years and in over 90% by age 24 years.[8] No significant difference in the prevalence of ocular manifestations at diagnosis was found between responsive and nonresponsive patients (75% vs 50%, P = .10), although the lack of significance could also be explained by the small sample size. However, this finding is consistent with previous reports in the literature.[8]

Skeletal and neurologic manifestations were also highly prevalent at diagnosis, affecting more than half of patients of our cohort. The lower prevalence of vascular events at diagnosis is consistent with the natural history of HCU, in which such manifestations usually occur in general at a later age.[8] However, vascular disease may have been underrepresented due to the high lethality of thromboembolic events. The relative large time gap between symptom onset to diagnosis (median, 5 years) and the presence of multiple clinical manifestations attest to the difficulty in establishing a definitive diagnosis in these patients.

The main strategies and goals of HCU treatment have been recently established in the first guidelines for the diagnosis and management of CβS deficiency.[9] Early diagnosis and early treatment are the key to prevent clinical manifestations and improve prognosis.[4,18]In the present study, current clinical and biochemical data were obtained from 44 patients in treatment. There was a clear difference in metabolic control between the groups: Responsive patients had low and even near-normal homocysteine and methionine levels, whereas most nonresponsive patients had persistently high homocysteine levels (>100 μmol/L) despite multiple treatment strategies. This difficulty in achieving metabolic control in pyridoxine-nonresponsive patients has been reported elsewhere.[18,27,28]

The high rate of betaine supplementation and comparatively low use of methionine-restricted diet in the nonresponsive patients may be attributed to several factors: (1) difficulties in obtaining the metabolic formula, which is expensive and not provided by the Unified Health System in Brazil;[29] (2) low adherence to dietary methionine restriction, particularly in patients with a late diagnosis; and (3) limited training of health-care professionals in dietary prescription. In a European survey of 181 patients with pyridoxine-nonresponsive HCU, 66% were on dietary treatment, that is, twice as many as in the present study.[30] Homocystinuria guidelines clearly state that betaine should not be considered a first-line treatment for HCU-nonresponsive patients but used as adjunct treatment in those who cannot achieve target levels of homocysteine by other means.[9] While dietary therapy dramatically reduces methionine and homocysteine and normalizes cysteine, betaine supplementation reduces homocysteine but increases methionine levels.[31,32] In animal models, betaine is less effective at preventing clinical manifestations,[33] and its efficacy declines over time.[34] In humans, there are no studies of the long-term efficacy of betaine supplementation alone in HCU.

In conclusion, this study provides the first broad clinical characterization of HCU in Brazil. All patients described here were late diagnosed, and most expressed a severe phenotype associated with nonresponsiveness to pyridoxine, early and multisystem clinical manifestations, and poor metabolic control. Limitations of this study include the underrepresented number of patients responsive to pyridoxine, and the number of patients coming from some regions of the country. We believe that our findings will contribute to the development of protocols and guidelines to improve diagnosis and management of HCU in Brazil.

Authors' Note

Soraia Poloni and Giovana Weber Hoss contributed equally to this article. Soraia Poloni, Giovana W. Hoss, Fernanda Sperb-Ludwig, Taciane Borsatto, and Ida V. D. Schwartz made substantial contributions to the conception and design, acquisition of data, analysis, and interpretation of data; Maria Juliana R. Doriqui, Emilia K.E.A Leão, Charles M. Lourenço, Chong A. Kim, Carolina F. M. Souza, Helio Rocha, Marcia Ribeiro, Carlos E. Steiner, Carolina A. Moreno, Pricila Bernardi, Eugenia Valadares, Osvaldo Artigalas, Gerson Carvalho, Hector Y. C. Wanderley, Ney Boa Sorte, and Luiz C. Santana-da-Silva made substantial contributions to the acquisition of data and were involved in revising the manuscript. Ida V. D. Schwartz and Henk J. Blom were involved in the analysis and interpretation of data and critically revising the manuscript for important intellectual content. All authors have given final approval of the version to be published and agreed to be accountable for all aspects of the work in ensuring that questions related to the accuracy or integrity of any part of the work are appropriately investigated and resolved.

Acknowledgments

The authors thank Prof. Roberto Giugliani, Rede EIM Brasil, Simone Allan Arede, and Associação Brasileira de Homocistinúria for their assistance with patient diagnosis and follow-up.

Declaration of Conflicting Interests

The author(s) declared the following potential conflicts of interest with respect to the research, authorship, and/or publication of this article. I. Schwartz and V. D'Almeida are National Council of Scientific and Technological Development (CNPq) research productivity fellows.

Funding

The author(s) disclosed receipt of the following financial support for the research, authorship, and/or publication of this article: Financial support for this study was provided by CNPq, CAPES, DAAD, and FIPE-HCPA.

References

1. Stipanuk MH, Ueki I. Dealing with methionine/homocysteine sulfur: cysteine metabolism to taurine and inorganic sulfur. *J Inherit Metab Dis*. 2011;34(1):17-32.
2. Blom HJ, Smulders Y. Overview of homocysteine and folate metabolism. With special references to cardiovascular disease and neural tube defects. *J Inherit Metab Dis*. 2011;34(1):75-81.
3. Carson NA, Neill DW. Metabolic abnormalities detected in a survey of mentally backward individuals in Northern Ireland. *Arch Dis Child*. 1962;37:505-513.
4. Yap S, Rushe H, Howard PM, Naughten ER. The intellectual abilities of early-treated individuals with pyridoxine-nonresponsive homocystinuria due to cystathionine beta-synthase deficiency. *J Inherit Metab Dis*. 2001;24(4):437-447.
5. Naughten ER, Yap S, Mayne PD. Newborn screening for homocystinuria: Irish and world experience. *Eur J Pediatr*. 1998; 157(suppl 2):S84-S87.
6. Skovby F, Gaustadnes M, Mudd SH. A revisit to the natural history of homocystinuria due to cystathionine beta-synthase deficiency. *Mol Genet Metab*. 2010;99(1):1-3.
7. Stopa SR, Malta DC, Monteiro CN, Szwarcwald CL, Goldbaum M, Cesar CLG. Use of and access to health services in Brazil, 2013 National Health Survey. *Rev Saude Publica*. 2017;51(suppl 1):3s.
8. Mudd SH, Skovby F, Levy HL, et al. The natural history of homocystinuria due to cystathionine beta-synthase deficiency. *Am J Hum Genet*. 1985;37(1):1-31.
9. Morris AA, Kožich V, Santra S, et al. Guidelines for the diagnosis and management of cystathionine beta-synthase deficiency. *J Inherit Metab Dis*. 2017;40(1):49-74.
10. Singh LR, Chen X, Kozich V, Kruger WD. Chemical chaperone rescue of mutant human cystathionine beta-synthase. *Mol Genet Metab*. 2007;91(4):335-342.
11. Kopecká J, Krijt J, Raková K, Kožich V. Restoring assembly and activity of cystathionine β-synthase mutants by ligands and chemical chaperones. *J Inherit Metab Dis*. 2011;34(1):39-48.
12. Majtan T, Hůlková H, Park I, et al. Enzyme replacement prevents neonatal death, liver damage, and osteoporosis in murine homocystinuria. *FASEB J*. 2017;31(12):5495-5506.
13. Moorthie S, Cameron L, Sagoo GS, Bonham JR, Burton H. Systematic review and meta-analysis to estimate the birth prevalence of five inherited metabolic diseases. *J Inherit Metab Dis*. 2014; 37(6):889-898.

14. Magner M, Krupková L, Honzík T, Zeman J, Hyánek J, Kožich V. Vascular presentation of cystathionine beta-synthase deficiency in adulthood. *J Inherit Metab Dis*. 2011;34(1):33-37.
15. Quintas S, Dotor-García Soto J, Alonso-Cerezo MC, Carreras MT. Late diagnosis of homocystinuria in an adult after extensive cerebral venous thrombosis. *Pract Neurol*. 2018;18(1):49-51.
16. Woods E, Dawson C, Senthil L, Geberhiwot T. Cerebral venous thrombosis as the first presentation of classical homocystinuria in an adult patient. *BMJ Case Rep*. 2017;2017.
17. Zschocke J, Kebbewar M, Gan-Schreier H, et al. Molecular neonatal screening for homocystinuria in the Qatari population. *Hum Mutat*. 2009;30(6):1021-1022.
18. Yap S, Naughten E. Homocystinuria due to cystathionine beta-synthase deficiency in Ireland: 25 years' experience of a newborn screened and treated population with reference to clinical outcome and biochemical control. *J Inherit Metab Dis*. 1998;21(7):738-747.
19. Huemer M, Kožich V, Rinaldo P, et al. Newborn screening for homocystinurias and methylation disorders: systematic review and proposed guidelines. *J Inherit Metab Dis*. 2015;38(6):1007-1019.
20. Moura RR, Coelho AV, Balbino VeQ, Crovella S, Brandão LA. Meta-analysis of Brazilian genetic admixture and comparison with other Latin America countries. *Am J Hum Biol*. 2015;27(5):674-680.
21. Kehdy FS, Gouveia MH, Machado M, et al. Origin and dynamics of admixture in Brazilians and its effect on the pattern of deleterious mutations. *Proc Natl Acad Sci U S A*. 2015;112(28):8696-8701.
22. Poloni S, Sperb-Ludwig F, Borsatto T, et al. CBS mutations are good predictors for B6-responsiveness: a study based on the analysis of 35 Brazilian Classical Homocystinuria patients. *Mol Genet Genomic Med*. 2018;6(2):160-170.
23. Mudd SH, Levy HL, Kraus JP. Disorders of transulfuration. In: Scriver CR, Beaudet AL, Sly WS, Valle D, eds. *The Metabolic and Molecular Bases of Inherited Disease*. 8th ed. New York: McGraw Hill; 2001.
24. El-Said MF, Badii R, Bessisso MS, et al. A common mutation in the CBS gene explains a high incidence of homocystinuria in the Qatari population. *Hum Mutat*. 2006;27(7):719.
25. Gallagher PM, Ward P, Tan S, et al. High frequency (71%) of cystathionine beta-synthase mutation G307 S in Irish homocystinuria patients. *Hum Mutat*. 1995;6(2):177-180.
26. Porto MP, Galdieri LC, Pereira VG, et al. Molecular analysis of homocystinuria in Brazilian patients. *Clin Chim Acta*. 2005;362(1-2):71-78.
27. Yap S, Boers GH, Wilcken B, et al. Vascular outcome in patients with homocystinuria due to cystathionine beta-synthase deficiency treated chronically: a multicenter observational study. *Arterioscler Thromb Vasc Biol*. 2001;21(12):2080-2085.
28. Yap S, Naughten ER, Wilcken B, et al. Vascular complications of severe hyperhomocysteinemia in patients with homocystinuria due to cystathionine beta-synthase deficiency: effects of homocysteine-lowering therapy. *Semin Thromb Hemost*. 2000;26(3):335-340.
29. Chieffi AL, Barradas RCB, Golbaum M. Legal access to medications: a threat to Brazil's public health system? *BMC Health Serv Res*. 2017;17(1):499.
30. Adam S, Almeida MF, Carbasius Weber E, et al. Dietary practices in pyridoxine non-responsive homocystinuria: a European survey. *Mol Genet Metab*. 2013;110(4):454-459.
31. Lawson-Yuen A, Levy HL. The use of betaine in the treatment of elevated homocysteine. *Mol Genet Metab*. 2006;88(3):201-207.
32. Komrower GM. Dietary treatment of homocystinuria. *Am J Dis Child*. 1967;113(1):98-100.
33. Gupta S, Wang L, Kruger WD. Betaine supplementation is less effective than methionine restriction in correcting phenotypes of CBS deficient mice. *J Inherit Metab Dis*. 2016;39(1):39-46.
34. Maclean KN, Jiang H, Greiner LS, Allen RH, Stabler SP. Long-term betaine therapy in a murine model of cystathionine beta-synthase deficient homocystinuria: decreased efficacy over time reveals a significant threshold effect between elevated homocysteine and thrombotic risk. *Mol Genet Metab*. 2012;105(3):395-403.

The Incidence of Transient Neonatal Tyrosinemia Within a Mexican Population

Alexandra V. Zea-Rey, MD[1,2], Héctor Cruz-Camino, BSc[2,3], Diana L. Vazquez-Cantu, BSc[1,2], Valeria M. Gutiérrez-García, BSc[1], Jesús Santos-Guzmán, PhD[1], and Consuelo Cantú-Reyna, MD[1,2,3]

Abstract

Transient neonatal tyrosinemia (TNT) is a form of hypertyrosinemia produced by the immaturity of 4-hydroxyphenylpyruvate dioxygenase (4-HPPD), a high intake of phenylalanine and tyrosine, and a relative ascorbic acid deficiency. Our objectives are to determine the incidence of TNT in Mexican newborns and to correlate it based on their sex, gestational age, and weight for gestational age to determine whether these are risk factors that predict the development of TNT. A cross-sectional descriptive study was conducted from January 2006 to August 2017. We analyzed 175 976 of newborn screening reports and found that the overall incidence of TNT was 1 (0.29%) in 342 newborns. It is more prevalent in preterm infants and in small for gestational age newborns (0.35%).The TNT incidence was determined in this Mexican population, and it was established as the most frequently occurring amino acid defect. We propose that pediatricians intentionally search for this pathology to offer patients access to adequate and timely treatment.

Keywords

4-hydroxyphenylpyruvate dioxygenase deficiency, transient neonatal tyrosinemia, newborn, incidence, Latin America

Introduction

Transient neonatal tyrosinemia (TNT) is a form of hypertyrosinemia, which is the most common pathology of amino acid metabolism. It is produced by a combination of several factors including the immaturity of 4-hydroxyphenylpyruvate dioxygenase (4-HPPD), which results from alterations in its synthesis; TNT is also caused by an elevated intake of phenylalanine and tyrosine, and an ascorbic acid deficiency.

Scant information has been published on the etiology of TNT in the last 20 years; therefore, recent epidemiological figures, both nationally and internationally, remain unknown. Also, it has not been possible to establish the presence of long-term cognitive neurological complications, such as altered learning and neurolinguistic abilities. Most pathologies that affect tyrosine catabolism produce hypertyrosinemia, which has also been found in cases of severe hepatocellular dysfunction.[1]

The pathologies associated with 4-HPPD include hereditary 4-HPPD dysfunction (OMIM 276710), also known as type III tyrosinemia, Hawkinsinuria (OMIM 140350), and TNT (OMIM 276500). Other diseases that might course with hypertyrosinemia are fumarylacetoacetate hydrolase deficiency (OMIM 276700), also known as tyrosinemia type 1a or hepatorenal tyrosinemia, and tyrosine aminotransferase deficiency (OMIM 276600), which is also known as Richner Hanhart syndrome (or type II tyrosinemia).

The clinical manifestations of TNT are variable, since patients may be asymptomatic or present with lethargy, poor suction, prolonged jaundice, and hypotonia, which are all attributed to neonatal prematurity. Furthermore, hypertyrosinemia, as well as high urinary excretion of tyrosine and its

[1] Tecnologico de Monterrey, Escuela de Medicina y Ciencias de la Salud, Monterrey, Nuevo Leon, Mexico
[2] Genomi-k S.A.P.I. de C.V, Monterrey, Nuevo Leon, Mexico
[3] Tecnologico de Monterrey, Escuela de Biotecnología y Ciencias de la Salud Monterrey, Nuevo Leon, Mexico

Corresponding Author:
Consuelo Cantú-Reyna, MD, Department of Genetics, Genomi-k S.A.P.I. de C.V., Ave. Cerro de las Mitras, 2411, Obispado, 64060, Monterrey, Nuevo Leon, Mexico.
Email: cocantu@genomi-k.com

metabolites (including hydroxyphenylpyruvic acid), are also present in TNT.[2]

There is no international consensus that currently defines the method of quantification and the limit values of detection for TNT; however, whereas normal serum tyrosine levels have reportedly ranged from 0.50 to 2.20 mg/dL, clinical significance is regarded as >3.60 mg/dL,[3] although some authors consider it to be >5 mg/dL.[4,5] These differing values were obtained using thin-layer chromatography, liquid chromatography, and gas chromatography tandem mass spectrometry (GC/MS/MS).[6]

The defect is more frequent in preterm infants (PI, <37 weeks of gestational age) than in full-term infants (FTI, 37 $\leq$ weeks of gestational age < 42), as the former have increased serum tyrosine levels between the second and third weeks of life; tyrosine levels return to normal values 2 to 3 weeks later.[7–9] The incidence of TNT has ranged from 0.2% to 10%.[10] Other sources reported that TNT affects as many as 0.5% to 5% FTI and up to 30% of PI.[11] In PI with high-protein milk intake, tyrosinemia may still be present, even when infants consume up to twice the recommended daily intake of ascorbic acid for infants and children (30 mg).[12,13]

Frequently, patients with TNT do not exhibit long-term complications, but some authors have reported the presence of cognitive dysfunction at 8-year follow-ups, especially in those with tyrosine levels >20 mg/dL.[13–18] Menkes et al.,[17] Partington et al.,[19] and Light et al.[20] found no difference in neurological assessment scores among children aged 1 to 8 years with a history of prematurity; however, some authors reported the presence of lethargy and decreased muscle tone.[20]

Transient neonatal tyrosinemia resolves without treatment in the first months of life.[21] However, some substances, such as ascorbic acid, can increase the activity of the immature 4-HPPD enzyme.[7] The administration of 200 to 400 mg/kg/d of vitamin C combined with a decreased protein intake of <2 g/kg/d has been described as a potential treatment for TNT.[2]

Aim

Our aim is to determine the incidence of TNT in Mexico compared to its frequency and correlation in various groups, depending on sex, gestational age (GA), and weight for gestational age (WGA); this was done to assess whether these parameters constitute risk factors that predict the development of TNT and to establish early treatment.

Methods

We obtained 177 004 newborn screening (NBS) reports within the Genomi-k S.A.P.I. de C.V. database, which were issued between January 2006 and August 2016. Those reports were issued after the analysis of dried blood spots processed by PerkinElmer Genetics (Bridgeville, Pennsylvania) via MS/MS. The laboratory classified presumed positives patients with cutoff tyrosine levels of $\geq$4.98 mg/dL.

Table 1. Characteristics of the Studied Population by Sex, GA, and WGA.

WGA	Sex	PI	FTI	Postterm	NR	Total
SGA	F	446	1134	16		1596
	M	368	1078	18		1464
AGA	F	8390	73 097	189		81 676
	M	9890	75 660	241		85 791
LGA	F	497	2233	2		2732
	M	466	2248	3		2717
Total		20 057	155 450	469	0	175 976
NR		75	540	2	411	1028

Abbreviations: AGA, appropriate for gestational age; F, female; FTI, full-term infant; LGA, large for gestational age; M, male; NR, not registered (sex, GA, or WGA was not included in the NBS report); PI, preterm infant; SGA, small for gestational age; WGA, weight for gestational age.

Table 2. Characteristics of the TNT Population by Sex, GA, and WGA.

WGA	Sex	PI	FTI	Postterm	Total
SGA	F	1	7	0	8
	M	3	0	0	3
AGA	F	79	150	0	229
	M	92	178	0	270
LGA	F	1	2	0	3
	M	1	1	0	2
Total		177	338	0	515

Abbreviations: AGA, appropriate for gestational age; F, female; FTI, full-term infant; LGA, large for gestational age; M, male; PI, preterm infant; SGA, small for gestational age; TNT, transient neonatal tyrosinemia; WGA, weight for gestational age.

Of the analyzed individuals, only 1 patient was excluded with the diagnosis of another type of tyrosinemia. Furthermore, 1028 reports were eliminated due to incomplete data (Table 1). A diagnosis of TNT was confirmed following a normal second NBS report. Descriptive statistics, Student *t* test, and logistic regression model were used to determine the relevance of the proposed variables.

Results

The 175 976 analyzed patients' reports were classified into 1 of 3 groups by sex, GA, and WGA. According to GA, there were 20 132 PI, 155 990 FTI, and 471 postterm infants. When we classified cases by sex, there were 86 004 female and 89 972 male newborns (Table 1). Once the population with TNT was identified, we classified those individuals into the same 3 groups (Table 2).

When examining the segmented sample among those with and without TNT, it was found that infants with TNT are, on average, 1.33 weeks younger than infants without TNT. Also, those with TNT tend to be classified as PI and SGA, with a WGA ratio smaller than that for the population without TNT (0.988 vs 1.014, respectively; Table 3).

Table 3. The Frequency and Probability (%) With Which the Segmented Population Develops TNT.[a]

TNT	GA	WGA	Frequency	*P* (%)
TNT	PI	SGA	4	1.32
		AGA	171	0.88
		LGA	2	0.58
	FTI	SGA	7	0.33
		AGA	328	0.22
		LGA	3	0.14
Without TNT	PI	SGA	810	98.7
		AGA	18 109	99.1
		LGA	961	99.4
	FTI	SGA	2239	99.7
		AGA	148 844	99.8
		LGA	4483	99.9

Abbreviations: AGA, appropriate for gestational age; FTI, full-term infant; GA, gestational age; LGA, large for gestational age; P, probability; PI, preterm infant; TNT, transient neonatal tyrosinemia; SGA, small for gestational age; WGA, weight for gestational age;
[a]The sum of the individuals plus the postterm infants (n = 15) is equal to 175 976.

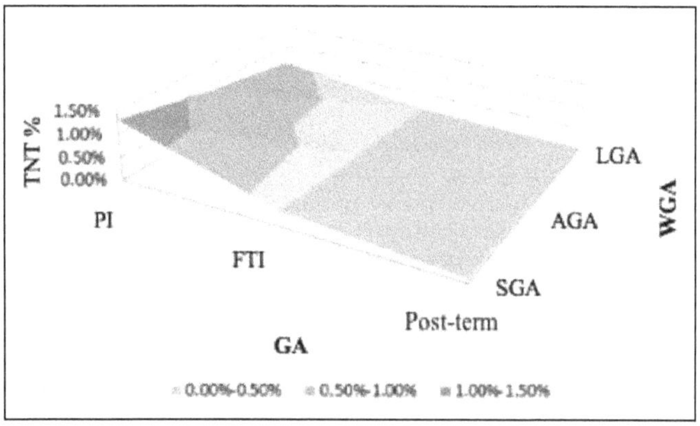

Figure 1. A representation of the probability with which TNT develops according to GA and WGA, based on the data in Table 4.
AGA indicates appropriate for gestational age; FTI, full-term infant; GA, gestational age; LGA, large for gestational age; PI, preterm infant, SGA, small for gestational age; TNT, transient neonatal tyrosinemia; WGA, weight for gestational age.

We reported that 1 in 342 newborns had indications of TNT from their NBS results at an incidence of 0.29% without segmentation. Our obtained incidence rates corresponded with the TNT incidence range from 0.2% to 10% reported by Martin et al.[11]

Our study showed that there is no correlation between sex and TNT, since 0.31% of males and 0.28% of females had TNT ($t_{513} = 1.032$; $P = .302$). The incidence rate increased to 0.36% in SGA and decreased to 0.09% in large for gestational age (LGA) newborns.

As shown in Figure 1 and Table 4, PI are 307% more likely than FTI to have TNT, whereas postterm newborns have a 75% lower probability of developing TNT. In the case of the WGA ratio, SGA infants have a greater probability for presenting

Table 4. Representation of the TNT Probability by GA and WGA.

WGA	PI	FTI	Postterm	*P* (%)
SGA	1.32	0.88	0.58	51%
AGA	0.33	0.05	0.14	0%
LGA	0.33	0.05	0.04	−34%
P (%)	307%	0%	−75%	

Abbreviations: AGA, appropriate for gestational age; FTI, full-term infant; GA, gestational age; LGA, large for gestational age; P, probability; PI, preterm infant; SGA, small for gestational age; TNT, transient neonatal tyrosinemia; WGA, weight for gestational age.

with TNT than appropriate for gestational age (AGA) infants. Conversely, LGA infants are 34% less likely to develop TNT.

Conclusion

We reported that TNT is present in 1 out 342 Mexican newborns, making it the most common amino acid defect. In addition, the frequency of TNT was much higher in PI infants (1:113) than in FTI and postterm infants (1:461), and there is an increased risk of developing TNT among SGA newborns compared with AGA newborns.

Transient neonatal tyrosinemia has a higher incidence rate than the other metabolic defects currently detected by NBS, such as congenital hypothyroidism (1:2 000), phenylketonuria (1:15 000), and cystic fibrosis (1:5 900).[22,23] Since neurological sequelae have been described, including alterations in learning and neurolinguistic abilities, we propose that clinicians should intentionally search for this pathology, so that timely treatments can be offered.

According to this study, the collaboration of a national-scale private company and a medical institution would strengthen NBS programs through follow-up strategies conducting new research to understand better the long-term neurological complications associated with this condition.

Acknowledgments

We thank the team at Genomi-k S.A.P.I. de C.V. for providing database access and for their kind support. English-language editing of this manuscript was provided by Journal Prep.

Declaration of Conflicting Interests

The author(s) declared no potential conflicts of interest with respect to the research, authorship, and/or publication of this article.

Funding

The author(s) received no financial support for the research, authorship, and/or publication of this article.

References

1. Mitchell GA, Grompe M, Lambert M, Tanguay RM. Hypertyrosinemia. In: Valle D, Beaudet AL, Vogelstein B, et al., eds. *The*

Online Metabolic and Molecular Bases of Inherited Disease (OMMBID). Chap 79. New York, NY: McGraw-Hill Companies, Inc.; 2014.

2. Kliegman R, Nelson WE. *Nelson Textbook of Pediatrics*. 19th ed. (Kliegman RM, ed.). Philadelphia, PA: Elsevier/Saunders; 2011.
3. Grompe M. Disorders of tyrosine metabolism. UpToDate. https://www.uptodate.com/contents/disorders-of-tyrosine-metabolism. Updated December 20, 2016. Accessed June 26, 2016.
4. Kaye CI; Committee on Genetics, Accurso F, et al. Newborn screening fact sheets. *Pediatrics*. 2006;118(3):e934-963. doi:10.1542/peds.2006-1783.
5. Levy HL, Shih VE, Madigan PM, MacCready RA. Transient tyrosinemia in full-term infants. *JAMA*. 1969;209(2):249-250. http://www.ncbi.nlm.nih.gov/pubmed/5819230.
6. Contreras RJ, Alonso JE, Viera Camayd I, Hernández CO, De la Peña D, Nogueras L. Transitory neonatal tyrosinemia: biochemical diagnosis of one case. *Rev Cuba Genética Comunitaria*. 2012; 6(1):57-60.
7. Mathews J, Partington MW. The plasma tyrosine levels of premature babies. *Arch Dis Child*. 1964;39(206):371-378. doi:10.1136/adc.39.206.371.
8. Goswami MND, Knox WE. Developmental changes of p-hydroxyphenylpyruvate-oxidase activity in mammalian liver. *Biochim Biophys Acta*. 1961;50(1):35-40. doi:10.1016/0006-3002(61)91056-3.
9. Hsia DY-Y, Litwack M, O'Flynn M, Jakovcic S. Serum phenylalanine and tyrosine levels in the newborn infant. *N Engl J Med*. 1962;267(21):1067-1070. doi:10.1056/NEJM196211222672104.
10. WHO Scientific Group on Screening for Inborn Errors of Metabolism, World Health Organization. *Investigación de Las Aberraciones Congénitas Del Metabolismo: Informe de Un Grupo Científico de La OMS*. Geneva, Switzerland: World Health Organization; 1968.
11. Martin HP, Fischer HL, Martin DS, Chase HP. The development of children with transient neonatal tyrosinemia. *J Pediatr*. 1974; 84(2):212-216. http://www.ncbi.nlm.nih.gov/pubmed/4810728.
12. Avery ME, Clow CL, Menkes JH, et al. Transient tyrosinemia of the newborn: dietary and clinical aspects. *Pediatrics*. 1967;39(3):378-384. http://www.ncbi.nlm.nih.gov/pubmed/6018968.
13. National Research Council (US) Subcommittee on the Tenth Edition of the Recommended Dietary Allowances. *Recommended Dietary Allowances*. 10th ed. Washington, DC: National Academies Press; 1989. doi:10.17226/1349.
14. Rice DN, Houston IB, Lyon ICT, et al. Transient neonatal tyrosinaemia. *J Inherit Metab Dis*. 1989;12(1):13-22. doi:10.1007/BF01805526.
15. Mamunes P, Prince PE, Thornton NH, Hunt PA, Hitchcock ES, Laupus WE. Intellectual deficits after transient tyrosinemia in the term neonate. *Pediatr Res*. 1976;8(4):344. doi:10.1203/00006450-197404000-00026.
16. Menkes JH, Jervis GA. Developmental retardation associated with an abnormality in tyrosine metabolism. Report of a case. *Pediatrics*. 1961;28:399-409. http://www.ncbi.nlm.nih.gov/pubmed/13769461.
17. Menkes JH, Chernick V, Ringel B. Effect of elevated blood tyrosine on subsequent intellectual development of premature infants. *J Pediatr*. 1966;69(4):583-588. http://www.ncbi.nlm.nih.gov/pubmed/5921333.
18. Auerbach VH, Digeorge AM, Brigham MP, Dobbs JM. Delayed maturation of tyrosine metabolism in a full-term sibling of a child with phenylketonuria. *J Pediatr*. 1963;62:938-940. http://www.ncbi.nlm.nih.gov/pubmed/13965496.
19. Partington MW, Delahaye DJ, Masotti RE, Read JH, Roberts B. Neonatal tyrosinaemia: a follow-up study. *Arch Dis Child*. 1968; 43(228):195-199. doi:10.1136/adc.43.228.195.
20. Light IJ, Sutherland JM, Berry KH. Clinical significance of tyrosinemia of prematurity. *Am J Dis Child*. 1973;125(2):243-247. doi:10.1001/archpedi.1973.04160020067013.
21. Buist N, Kennaway N, Fellman J. Disorders of tyrosine metabolism. In: Nyhan, ed. *Heritable Disorders of Amino Acid Metabolism: Patterns of Clinical Expression and Genetic Variation*. New York, NY: John Wiley & Sons, Ltd; 1974; 165.
22. Paz Valiñas L, Atienza Merino G. *Clinical Effectiveness of Neonatal Screening for Inborn Errors of Metabolism Using Tandem Mass Spectrometry. Systematic Review*. Madrid, Spain: Ministerio de Sanidad y Consumo. Avalia-t; 2006; 72-76.

20

Micronutrients: Speculation on Inborn Errors, Nutrigenomics, Evolution, the Microbiome, and Nutritional Immunity

Peter T. Clayton, MD[1] and Philippa B. Mills, PhD[1]

Abstract

Many micronutrients or cofactors derived from micronutrients are highly reactive, hence their role in catalysis of reactions by enzymes. The concentration of cofactors has to be kept low to avoid unwanted reactions while allowing them to bind to the (apo)enzymes that need them. A new disorder causing B6-responsive epilepsy (proline synthetase cotranscribed bacterial homologue deficiency) is probably due to the absence of an important intracellular pyridoxal phosphate chaperone. The availability of some micronutrients varies by orders of magnitude in different geographical areas. Selenium is both essential and toxic, and during evolution, different populations have had to adapt to this differing availability. An "inborn error of metabolism (IEM)" in a low selenium area of China may be a selective advantage in a high selenium area and vice versa; the concept of nutrigenomics is an important one for micronutrients. The gut flora may make an important contribution to vitamin synthesis. This is difficult to study, but experiments can be undertaken with the nematode, *Caenorhabditis elegans* (with or without an IEM) and a single clone of *Escherichia coli* (with or without an IEM) as food and gut flora. This model shows that the gut microbiome can have profound influences on the folate cycle and associated vitamins. Our innate immune system makes use of the micronutrient requirements of pathogens and can deprive a pathogen of essential micronutrient(s) or expose it to toxic levels. It is not surprising, therefore, that some mutations affecting the way the host handles micronutrients can confer an advantage in resistance to infection and this may have acted as a selective advantage during evolution. This will be discussed by reference to the relationship of inborn errors to resistance to malaria. Conversely, other inborn errors of micronutrient metabolism are likely to make it more difficult for the host to use nutritional immunity to fight infection; this probably accounts for the list of infections that are more serious in patients with hereditary haemochromatosis.

Keywords

vitamins, trace elements, pyridoxal 5'-phosphate, selenium, malaria, hemochromatosis

Introduction

The inborn errors affecting micronutrient metabolism are a very important group as they can often be treated effectively, for example, by increasing the intake of the micronutrient or speeding its elimination. There is accumulating evidence that micronutrient availability has led to evolutionary adaptations making man better able to survive as he has moved to areas with a lower or higher micronutrient availability. Furthermore, natural selection has favored genetic variants that improve our ability to use micronutrients in the fight against infection, variants that either restrict the availability of a micronutrient to a pathogen or subject it to toxic levels—"nutritional immunity." When considering the availability of micronutrients, it is important to remember that the gut flora can synthesize vitamins and so a dietary deficiency may be compensated in the holobiome. This review will focus on inborn errors and polymorphisms affecting micronutrient metabolism in the holobiome starting with a recently described inborn error that illustrates the need to carefully regulate the concentration of a highly reactive micronutrient in our cells.

[1] Genetics and Genomic Medicine, UCL, Great Ormond Street Institute of Child Health, London, United Kingdom

Corresponding Author:

Peter T. Clayton, MD, Genetics and Genomic Medicine, UCL, Great Ormond Street Institute of Child Health, 30 Guilford Street, London WC1N 1EH, United Kingdom.

Email: peter.clayton@ucl.ac.uk

The Reactivity of Pyridoxal Phosphate and Proline Synthetase Cotranscribed Bacterial Homologue Deficiency

Pyridoxal 5'-phosphate (PLP) is the active cofactor derived from all forms of vitamin B6 in the diet. It has a reactive aldehyde group, with the reactivity further enhanced by the phosphate group that prevents hydration of the aldehyde group (as occurs in pyridoxal) and by the aromatic ring that provides an electron sink. The aldehyde groups can react with amino and sulphydryl groups as well as the activated carbon atoms in Δ1-pyrroline-5-carboxylate (P5C) and Δ1-piperideine-6-carboxylate (P6C), compounds that accumulate in hyperprolinaemia type II and ALDH7A1 deficiency, respectively.[1-3] To prevent inappropriate reactions, it is estimated that the concentration of the free PLP is kept in the low micromolar range. Abundant proteins that can bind to PLP and keep the free PLP concentration low include albumin in plasma, hemoglobin in red cells, and glycogen phosphorylase in muscle. However, the cell must be able to deliver PLP to the apoenzymes that need it. We have found evidence to indicate that there is an intracellular protein that helps fulfill this role—proline synthetase cotranscribed bacterial homologue (PROSC) now renamed as pyridoxal phosphate binding protein.[4] Proline synthetase cotranscribed bacterial homologue was known to be a ubiquitously expressed protein that could bind PLP without any alteration in its quaternary structure and, while its structure was similar to that of alanine racemase, it had no apparent enzyme activity when tested with a range of amino acids. We had some discussions with Andrew Hanson as to whether it might prevent reaction of PLP with P6C and P5C. Then, at the 2012 SSIEM Meeting in Birmingham, Isa Holme and Niklas Darin told us of their studies on a family in which 2 siblings and a cousin had B6-responsive epilepsy and in whom mapping studies and exome analysis had shown a homozygous missense mutation in PROSC. We then sequenced PROSC in a cohort of 29 individuals with pyridoxine-responsive seizures of unknown cause and identified a further 4 patients with biallelic PROSC mutations.

The clinical features of the 7 patients thus identified[4] included features similar to those seen in other B6 disorders such as pyridoxamine phosphate oxidase (PNPO) deficiency—abnormal intrauterine movements (3/7), fetal distress (4/7), neonatal seizures (7/7) with burst suppression on electroencephalography (5/7), and a clear response to B6 (7/7). In addition, patients tended to have a birth head circumference below the 9th centile (4/7). Other features included systemic disease—lactic acidosis (4/7), anemia (2/7), and gastrointestinal dysfunction (3/7). Seizure control was somewhat better with PLP than pyridoxine (4/4), but most patients required an additional anticonvulsant for full seizure control (5/6). On follow-up, microcephaly was increasingly evident and most patients had a degree of developmental delay. Early computed tomography and magnetic resonance imaging (MRI) scans showed broad gyri and shallow sulci indicating an underdeveloped brain. Some patients had periventricular germinolytic cysts and others deep white matter edema and hemorrhages. Scans in childhood showed reduced myelination.

When we looked at the pretreatment cerebrospinal fluid (CSF) samples from the patients with PROSC mutations, we found low PLP levels and evidence of impaired activity of PLP-dependent enzymes such as aromatic amino acid decarboxylase (AADC)—elevated CSF concentrations of 3-orthomethyldopa, L-dopa, and/or 5-hydroxytryptophan—and urinary organic acid analysis showed raised vanillactate, also consistent with reduced AADC activity. These results confirmed the hypothesis that delivery of PLP to apo-AADC in the brain was impaired.

When PROSC-deficient fibroblasts were cultured in medium containing the usual amounts of fetal calf serum (a source of PLP) and supplementary pyridoxine, the cell content of PLP measured as nmol PLP per gram of cell protein was higher in the children with PROSC deficiency than in controls and a heterozygote. When the cell extract was fractionated into components with molecular weight below and above 3 kDa, the PLP content for PROSC-deficient patients was found to be increased in both fractions, suggesting that there was accumulation of PLP bound to both proteins and metabolites. This was compatible with the hypothesis that PROSC is an intracellular PLP binding protein preventing inappropriate reactions with both small and large molecules.

We then did some expression studies with Valerie de Crecy-Lagard, Laurence Prunetti, and Basma El Yacoubi from the University of Florida in Gainesville. They had shown that when *Escherichia coli* with a deletion of the PROSC homologue (ΔyggS) were cultured in a dish containing a pyridoxine-soaked disc, there was a ring of growth inhibition around the disc. Transfection with wild-type human *PROSC* abolished pyridoxine sensitivity. Human mutants affecting highly conserved regions of PROSC did not abolish *E coli* pyridoxine sensitivity. A missense mutant affecting an area not fully conserved across species did abolish *E coli* pyridoxine sensitivity. These studies provided further evidence that PROSC prevents toxic reactions of vitamin B6.

Plecko and colleagues have since shown that mutations in *PROSC* are also a cause of vitamin B6-dependent epilepsy in their cohort.[5] Onset of seizures in their patients was <10 days, and seizures were promptly controlled by pyridoxine in all patients, except one whose seizures had already been controlled by phenobarbitone. In contrast to our patients, all their patients were normocephalic with normal MRI scans and three out of four had normal IQ when assessed at 12.5, 15.5, and 30 years.

Geographical Variation in Micronutrient Availability

Deficiency of a micronutrient is a major world health problem. At least 2 billion people in the world are deficient in key vitamins and/or minerals, the commonest deficiencies being vitamin A, iodine, iron, and zinc.[6] In some areas of the world, there is also a risk of specific micronutrient toxicity. A good example of this is selenium; availability of this micronutrient varies by orders of magnitude between different geographical areas. Even within China, there are areas where people are at risk of deficiency and areas where there is a greater at risk of toxicity. Deficiency can give rise to an impaired immune response, infertility, cognitive decline, increased mortality, and specific forms of heart disease (Keshan) and bone disease (Kashin-Beck). Excess selenium, on the other hand, can cause nausea and vomiting, nail discoloration, brittleness, and loss, hair loss, fatigue, irritability, and a foul garlic breath odor. As man migrated out of Africa 60 000 to 100 000 years ago, he encountered both high and low selenium environments.

White and coworkers looked at variants in selenium-related genes in individuals living in high- and low-selenium areas.[7] They found that there was a glutathione peroxidase allele with increased catalytic efficiency of selenium that was more common in individuals living in low-selenium areas than in individuals from higher selenium areas. They found many other variants in genes regulating selenium and in selenoproteins in out-of-Africa migrants compared to ancestral African genes. This leads us to the conclusion that what is an inborn error of metabolism (IEM) in one geographical area might be a selective advantage in another!

The Gut Flora as a Source of Micronutrients; The Microbiome

The gut flora may be very important in micronutrient metabolism; bacteria are able to synthesize many vitamins. Unfortunately, the interaction between the host and the gut flora is complicated and difficult to study. We were fortunate to be invited to participate in a series of experiments on an elegant model system devised by Filipe Gomes Cabreiro and colleagues working in another part of UCL.[8]

For the nematode *Caenorhabditis elegans*, bacteria constitute both a food and a source of a gut flora. It is relatively straightforward to study the effect of the interaction between a worm with or without a knockout of an enzyme involved in micronutrient metabolism and fed a single *E coli* strain with or without a knockout of an enzyme involved in micronutrient metabolism. We can't go into detail for all combinations tested but will give 1 example. The worms were treated with the anticancer drug, 5-fluorouracil (5FU), at varying concentrations and the 5FU toxicity was measured by the fraction of the nematode's eggs that hatched at that concentration of 5FU. The main way in which 5FU prevents cellular replication is by inhibition of thymidylate synthesis leading to a deficient conversion of deoxyuridine monophosphate to deoxythymidine monophosphate for DNA synthesis. Reduced folates stabilize the 5FdUMP-TS complex that formed and enhance 5FU toxicity. When the worm was fed bacteria with a defect in the de novo pathway for PLP synthesis, the *pdxJ* strain, the worm's PLP level was virtually undetectable, and the toxicity of 5FU was markedly reduced compared to that in worms fed wild-type bacteria. When the worm was fed supplementary pyridoxal, its PLP level could be restored and the normal high toxicity of 5FU was also restored. This confirms previous work that indicates that 5FU toxicity is closely linked to the activity of the folate cycle and hence to PLP levels. 5-Fluorouracil toxicity is reduced by PLP deficiency. The important point here is that bacterial micronutrient metabolism can have a profound effect on host metabolism, including the metabolism of xenobiotics.

Conversely, there is increasing evidence that host metabolism can affect the species of bacteria present in the mammalian gut and their metabolic pathways. Vitamin D, acting on the vitamin D receptor, affects the production of antimicrobial peptides by the mouse including the cathelicidin antimicrobial peptides, β-defensins, and the autophagy regulator ATG16L1.[9] When the vitamin D receptor is knocked out in the mouse, there are changes both in the species of bacteria found in the large bowel and in the expression of their genes. The pathways upregulated in the bacteria in the caecum of the mouse include those affecting other micronutrients including riboflavin, retinol, and others.[9]

Inborn Errors and Carrier States That May Increase Resistance to Malaria

We have mentioned the fact that inborn errors of micronutrient metabolism might increase or decrease an individual's ability to use nutritional immunity to overcome an infection. It is believed that the ability to survive infection with the malarial parasite has been an important selective advantage in evolution. We have listed a few common inborn errors (and carrier states) affecting micronutrient metabolism that may confer resistance to malaria. These include the following.

Genetic Variants Leading to Low Free Pyridoxal Phosphate in Erythrocytes

Americans of Afro-Caribbean origin have a high incidence of a polymorphism in the erythroid-specific promoter of pyridoxal kinase.[10] This leads to low activity of pyridoxal kinase and this is thought to confer resistance to malaria. Sickle hemoglobin binds PLP more avidly than normal β-hemoglobin.[11] This may reduce the availability of free PLP to the parasites in the red cells. Children with sickle cell trait have protection against malaria morbidity and mortality.[12] The R116Q variant in PNPO markedly reduces the synthesis of PLP from pyridoxine phosphate in red cells.[13] We have suggested that the relatively high frequency of this mutation may be explained by resistance to malaria.[14] In the Ferrara Province of Italy, where malaria was endemic in the 12th century, there is a high incidence of individuals with a low activity of both PNPO and glutathione reductase and this cannot be explained by dietary riboflavin intake: the postulated reason for the high incidence is that reduced enzyme activity confers resistance to malaria.[15]

A Disorder of the Folate Cycle

In the mouse, methylene tetrahydrofolate deficiency confers resistance to malaria[16] and of course there is a common allele that reduces MTHFR activity in man, the C677T allele. Again resistance to malaria is suggested to be the selective advantage conferred by the C677T allele.

Evidence of Altered B6 and/or Folate Metabolism in Malaria

If we look at the metabolic profile of patients acutely infected with *Plasmodium falciparum*, one striking feature is hyperhomocysteinemia.[17] This suggests that the patient is trying to reduce the operation of the folate and remethylation cycles to impair 1-carbon metabolism in the parasite. This may indicate reduced availability of 1 of the 4 vitamins involved in the folate cycle.

Nutritional Immunity Affecting Other Micronutrients in Malaria

If we believe that the human host has improved the efficiency of its nutritional immunity during evolution where malaria acted as a selective pressure, we might expect evidence of upregulation of genes involved in micronutrient metabolism or transport during infection. Idaghdour and co-workers looked at whole-blood transcriptomes of *Plasmodium falciparum*-infected West African children.[18] Among the genes upregulated in the white cells of infected children were 2 genes affecting trace metal metabolism:

SLC39A8 is a transporter of manganese and zinc. It is known to be upregulated as a result of T-cell activation, especially at low zinc concentrations, and it is tempting to suggest that increased cellular uptake of zinc and/or manganese is playing a role in combating the infection with the parasite.

SCO1 is a copper chaperone, known to us because of its involvement in complex IV assembly. It is tempting to suggest that overexpression in response to *Plasmodium* infection exposes the parasite to either copper deficiency or copper toxicity.

Other Infections in Inborn Errors of Micronutrient Metabolism

We have tried to convince you that there is an important link between micronutrient metabolism and infection. If this is the case, we should see altered susceptibility to infection in our patients with inborn errors of micronutrient metabolism.

There is good evidence for this in hereditary hemochromatosis. Several papers have drawn attention to infections that appear to be more serious or more common in patients with hemochromatosis including those caused by *Listeria*, *Mucor*, and *Aspergillus* species.[19]

On the other hand, the Hfe knockout mouse is resistant to infection with the *Salmonella* that causes a typhoid fever-like illness in the mouse, *Salmonella typhimurium*. This has been attributed to impaired ability of the knockout mouse to restrict the parasite's access to intracellular iron.[20]

Conclusions

We hope we have convinced you that many micronutrients are reactive chemicals that the body handles with care, for example, through the use of binding proteins. Through evolution, we have learned to use micronutrients in the fight against infection. Ideally every individual (whether asymptomatic or with symptoms resulting from grossly deranged metabolism) should have a diet to suit their genome—"nutrigenomics." However, the dietary "prescription" needs to take account of geographical features; micronutrient availabilities differ in different parts of the world. The diet also needs to encourage the most beneficial gut flora. It may need to be modified to improve resistance to prevalent infections. Over long periods of time, evolution makes appropriate genomic adjustments to suit micronutrient availability and prevalent infections. An IEM can affect the individual's ability to use "nutritional immunity" to fight infection, for example, hereditary hemochromatosis confers resistance to some infections but susceptibility to others.

Authors' Note

All work done in our laboratory was performed with ethical approval. Specific approval details can be found in References 4, 8, 13 and 14.

Declaration of Conflicting Interests

The author(s) declared no potential conflicts of interest with respect to the research, authorship, and/or publication of this article.

Funding

The author(s) received no financial support for the research, authorship, and/or publication of this article.

References

1. Clayton PT. B6-responsive disorders: a model of vitamin dependency. *J Inherit Metab Dis*. 2006;29(2-3):317-326.
2. Farrant RD, Walker V, Mills GA, Mellor JM, Langley GJ. Pyridoxal phosphate de-activation by pyrroline-5-carboxylic acid. Increased risk of vitamin B6 deficiency and seizures in hyperprolinemia type II. *J Biol Chem*. 2001;276(18):15107-15116.
3. Mills PB, Struys E, Jakobs C, et al. Mutations in antiquitin in individuals with pyridoxine-dependent seizures. *Nat Med*. 2006; 12(3):307-309.
4. Darin N, Reid E, Prunetti L, et al. Mutations in PROSC disrupt cellular pyridoxal phosphate homeostasis and cause vitamin-B(6)-dependent epilepsy. *Am J Hum Genet*. 2016;99(6): 1325-1337.
5. Plecko B, Zweier M, Begemann A, et al. Confirmation of mutations in PROSC as a novel cause of vitamin B (6)-dependent epilepsy. *J Med Genet*. 2017;54(12):809-814.
6. WHO/WFP/UNICEF Statement. http://www.who.int/nutrition/publications/micronutrients/WHO_WFP_UNICEFstatement.pdf?ua=1. Accessed October 2017.

7. White L, Romagné F, Müller E, et al. Genetic adaptation to levels of dietary selenium in recent human history. *Mol Biol Evol.* 2015; 32(6):1507-1518.
8. Scott TA, Quintaneiro LM, Norvaisas P, et al. Host-microbe co-metabolism dictates cancer drug efficacy in *C. elegans*. *Cell.* 2017;169(3):442-456.
9. Jin D, Wu S, Zhang YG, Lu R, et al. Lack of vitamin D receptor causes dysbiosis and changes the functions of the murine intestinal microbiome. *Clin Ther.* 2015;37(5):996-1009.
10. Flanagan JM, Beutler E. The genetic basis of human erythrocyte pyridoxal kinase activity variation. *Haematologica.* 2006;91(6): 801-804.
11. Kark JA, Bongiovanni R, Hicks CU, Tarassoff PG, Hannah JS, Yoshida GY. Modification of intracellular hemoglobin with pyridoxal and pyridoxal 5'-phosphate. *Blood Cells.* 1982;8(2): 299-314.
12. Aidoo M, Terlouw DJ, Kolczak MS, et al. Protective effects of the sickle cell gene against malaria morbidity and mortality. *Lancet.* 2002;359(9314):1311-1312.
13. Wilson MP, Footitt EJ, Papandreou A, et al. An LC-MS/MS-based method for the quantification of Pyridox(am)ine 5'-Phosphate Oxidase activity in dried blood spots from patients with epilepsy. *Anal Chem.* 2017;89(17):8892-8900.
14. Mills PB, Camuzeaux SS, Footitt EJ, et al. Epilepsy due to PNPO mutations: genotype, environment and treatment affect presentation and outcome. *Brain.* 2014;137(Pt 5): 1350-1360.
15. Anderson BB, Giuberti M, Perry GM, Salsini G, Casadio I, Vullo C. Low red blood cell glutathione reductase and pyridoxine phosphate oxidase activities not related to dietary riboflavin: selection by malaria? *Am J Clin Nutr.* 1993;57(5):666-672.
16. Meadows DN, Pyzik M, Wu Q, et al. Increased resistance to malaria in mice with methylenetetrahydrofolate reductase (Mthfr) deficiency suggests a mechanism for selection of the MTHFR 677C>T (c.665C>T) variant. *Hum Mutat.* 2014;35(5): 594-600.
17. Chillemi R, Zappacosta B, Simporè J, Persichilli S, Musumeci M, Musumeci S. Hyperhomocysteinemia in acute Plasmodium falciparum malaria: an effect of host–parasite interaction. *Clin Chim Acta.* 2004;348(1-2):113-120.
18. Idaghdour Y, Quinlan J, Goulet JP, et al. Evidence for additive and interaction effects of host genotype and infection in malaria. *Proc Natl Acad Sci U S A.* 2012;109(42):16786-16793.
19. Khan FA, Fisher MA, Khakoo RA. Association of hemochromatosis with infectious diseases: expanding spectrum. *Int J Infect Dis.* 2007;11(6):482-487.
20. Nairz M, Theurl I, Schroll A, et al. Absence of functional Hfe protects mice from invasive *Salmonella enterica* serovar Typhimurium infection via induction of lipocalin-2. *Blood.* 2009; 114(17):3642-3651.

An Adapted Clinical Measurement Tool for the Key Symptoms of CLN2 Disease

Kathleen W. Wyrwich, PhD[1], Angela Schulz, MD[2], Miriam Nickel, MD[2], Peter Slasor, ScD[3], Temitayo Ajayi, MD[3], David R. Jacoby, MD, PhD[3], and Alfried Kohlschütter, MD[2]

Abstract

Neuronal ceroid lipofuscinosis type-2 (CLN2) disease is a rare, autosomal recessive, pediatric-onset, neurodegenerative lysosomal storage disease caused by mutations in the *TPP1* gene. Cerliponase alfa (Brineura®), a recombinant form of human tripeptidyl peptidase-1, was recently developed as a treatment for CLN2 disease. In clinical trials, the primary end point to evaluate treatment effect was the aggregate score for the motor and language (ML) domains of the CLN2 Clinical Rating Scale, an adaptation of the Hamburg scale's component items that include anchor point definitions to allow consistent ratings in multinational, multisite, clinical efficacy studies. Psychometric analyses demonstrated that the ML score of the CLN2 Clinical Rating Scale and individual item scores are well defined and possess adequate measurement properties (reliability, validity, and responsiveness) to demonstrate a clinical benefit over time. Additionally, analyses comparing the CLN2 Clinical Rating Scale ML ratings to the Hamburg scale's ML ratings demonstrated adequate similarity.

Keywords

CLN2 disease, neuronal ceroid lipofuscinosis type-2, Batten disease, cerliponase alfa, tripeptidyl peptidase-1, enzyme replacement therapy, intracerebroventricular, clinician-reported outcome, Hamburg Motor-Language scale, psychometric

Introduction

The neuronal ceroid lipofuscinoses (NCLs), also known as Batten disease, are discrete genetic lysosomal storage disorders characterized by pathologic autofluorescent cellular deposits, with the clinical hallmarks of progressive seizure disorder, ataxia, motor function loss, dementia, and blindness.[1–3] Neuronal ceroid lipofuscinosis type-2 (CLN2) disease is a rare, autosomal recessive, predominantly late infantile form of NCL caused by mutations in the *TPP1* gene (also referred to as the *CLN2* gene). The *TPP1* gene encodes tripeptidyl peptidase-1 (TPP1), which cleaves N-terminal tripeptides from polypeptides imported into lysosomes destined for cellular degradation. The TPP1 deficiency manifests as central nervous system neuronal cell dysfunction and death, reflected as a rapidly progressive neurodegeneration and loss of physical function.[1]

The clinical course of CLN2 disease is largely predictable.[4] In most cases, affected children appear healthy until age 2 to 4 years. Initial symptoms are typically new-onset seizures and inability to acquire new language milestones. This is rapidly followed by a period of active loss of function, characterized by ataxia, movement disorders, language regression, and cognitive impairment. After a period of 2 to 4 years, children become unable to walk and talk and eventually go blind. Severe neurological dysfunction occurs by age 4 to 8 years and death typically occurs by age 8 to 16 years.[1,2,5,6]

The Hamburg scale was developed to quantify the loss of function that occurs over the clinical course of CLN2 disease.[4] This 4-item instrument assesses motor function (walking ability), visual function, language, and seizures, with all items using 0 to 3 rating options and yielding a 0 to 12 total summed score. Worgall and colleagues[5] introduced a second CLN2 disease rating scale, the Weill Cornell Scale, which assesses

[1] Eli Lilly and Company, Indianapolis, IN, USA
[2] University Hospital Hamburg-Eppendorf, Hamburg, Germany
[3] BioMarin Pharmaceutical Inc, San Rafael, CA, USA

Corresponding Author:
Kathleen W. Wyrwich, PhD, Eli Lilly and Company, 3647 Hartford St, St. Louis, MO 63116, USA.
Email: wyrwich_kathy@lilly.com

Table 1. The Hamburg Motor and Language (HML) and CLN2 Clinical Rating Scale Motor-Language (ML) Domain Items.

HML Scale Items in Natural History Registry			ML Scale Items in Cerliponase Alfa Clinical Trials			Rationale for Adaptations
Motor	3	Walks normally[a]	Motor	3	Grossly normal gait. No prominent ataxia, no pathologic falls.	Clarification
	2	Frequent falls, clumsiness obvious		2	Independent gait, as defined by ability to walk without support for 10 steps. Will have obvious instability and may have intermittent falls	Added "step" criteria to clarify and harmonize the definition of gait changes across sites/investigators
	1	No unaided walking or crawling only		1	Requires external assistance to walk or can crawl only	Clarification
	0	Immobile, mostly bedridden		0	Can no longer walk or crawl	No changes
Language	3	Normal (individual maximum)[b]	Language	3	Apparently normal language. Intelligible and grossly age-appropriate. No decline noted yet.	Clarification
	2	Has become recognizably abnormal		2	Language has become recognizably abnormal: some intelligible words may form short sentences to convey concepts, requests, or needs. This score signifies a decline from a previous level of ability (from the individual maximum reached by the child).	Added the language baseline definition to loss of function
	1	Hardly understandable		1	Hardly understandable. Few intelligible words	No changes
	0	Unintelligible or no language		0	No intelligible words or vocalizations	No changes

[a]In some children, motor development was never really normal.
[b]In some children, normal language development was never present. In such cases, the best performance ever achieved was taken as a starting point and rated 3; when language then became recognizably worse, it was rated 2.

4 items: gait (walking ability), language, myoclonus (involuntary movements), and feeding/swallowing. Like the Hamburg scale, all Weill Cornell Scale items use 0 to 3 rating options and yield a 0 to 12 total summed score.

Brineura® (BioMarin Pharmaceutical Inc., Novato, CA) (cerliponase alfa), a recombinant form of TPP1, has been developed as a treatment for CLN2 disease.[7] Cerliponase alfa is administered directly into the central nervous system via an indwelling intracerebroventricular port. Determining the clinical efficacy of this new treatment required the use of a clinical outcome assessment (COA) tool capable of demonstrating (1) a clinically relevant shift in the course of disease compared to the natural history for children and adolescents with CLN2 disease and (2) the reliability, validity, responsiveness, and interpretability required for COA use in a multinational clinical trial.[8] An adapted scale, termed the CLN2 Clinical Rating Scale, was devised to include historically used motor and language (ML) anchor point definitions from existing natural history databases to enable prospective acquisition of clinical trial data comparable to existing historical data.

This report details the key measurement properties of reliability, validity, and responsiveness of the CLN2 Clinical Rating Scale and the 2 component scores (motor and language) for use in CLN2 clinical trials. Moreover, the process and results from testing the similarity with the Hamburg ML (HML) scale are described and reported, thus demonstrating the comparability of the HML scores, derived from a natural history cohort, to the CLN2 Clinical Rating Scale ML scores used in 2 cerliponase alfa clinical trials. This demonstration of comparability is an important aim of this report and provides assurance that the HML and the CLN2 Clinical Rating Scale ML scores are adequately similar for use in the interpretation of functional change over time in the clinical studies.

Methods

CLN2 Clinical Rating Scale ML Domain

The CLN2 Clinical Rating Scale ML domain was adapted from the common subscales of the Hamburg and Weill Cornell CLN2 clinical rating scales to be used as an assessment tool for multicenter efficacy studies supporting the development of cerliponase alfa. The ML functions are fundamental disease domains, decline rapidly and predictably as a function of age, and are relatively insensitive to standard of care.

The rating is structured so that a score of 3 indicates a *normal condition*, 2 is *a slight or just noticeable abnormality*, 1 is *a severe abnormality*, and 0 denotes a *complete loss of functioning*. Because of wording ambiguity and differences between scales, item wording and anchor point definitions were refined for the CLN2 Clinical Rating Scale. This adaptation was conducted to codify the historical transitions in the items such that the treatment study could be directly compared to natural history gathered at both the University Hospital-Eppendorf in Hamburg and the Weill Cornell Medical College. The changes used in the CLN2 ML scale and the rationale are shown in Table 1.

Differences in 1-point scoring on the ML domains are measurable and clinically important. For example, in the motor domain, a 1-point drop from a rating of 3 to a rating of 2 is the difference between a child who can walk normally and a child who is abnormal but retains independent ambulation of at least 10 steps. Further, 1-point drop to a score of 1 indicates a child who no longer independently ambulates but can still move by some self-process. The last 1-point drop to a score of 0 indicates a child who is no longer self-mobile. Similarly, it can be observed that each of the language domain ratings also represent clinically meaningful levels.

Patient Population

A dose-escalation, single-arm, multinational phase 1/2 study (Clinicaltrials.gov identifier NCT01907087) evaluated the efficacy and safety of cerliponase alfa in patients with CLN2 disease. It included a stable dose period of 48 weeks at a dose of 300 mg every 2 weeks (Q2W), administered via an intracerebroventricular catheter. An ongoing open-label extension study (Clinicaltrials.gov identifier NCT02485899) continues to evaluate the efficacy and safety of cerliponase alfa. Any patient who completed treatment in the phase 1/2 study was eligible. All patients continue to receive cerliponase alfa at 300 mg Q2W for up to 240 weeks. Patients enrolled in the DEM-CHILD-independent CLN2 natural history registry[9] served as an untreated comparison group.

Eligible patients were required to have documented *TPP1* deficiency and genotype. Children with CLN2 disease were eligible who were at least 3 years old and disease score ≥ 3 on the 0- to 6-point CLN2 Clinical Rating ML scale, with scores of at least 1 in each of these domains. Written informed consent from a parent/legal guardian and assent from the patient, if appropriate, were obtained. The studies were performed in accordance with the Declaration of Helsinki; approval was obtained from the institutional review board at each participating center.

Interrater Reliability

Clinical ratings were performed in-person every 8 weeks, and each assessment was videotaped. The prespecified methodology was as follows: 36 videotapes from 4 representative and regular time points (baseline, week 25, week 49, and week 73 [week 25 of extension study]) for 11 patients enrolled in the clinical studies who were/are being treated at the Hamburg clinic were independently rated by a nonstudy scale trainer. These ratings were then compared to the motor, language, and combined ML scale ratings given by the respective study clinicians. Weighted kappa (κ_w) statistics[10] assessed the level of rater agreement between the nonstudy trainer's ML scale ratings when compared to the study investigators' ratings to better understand interrater reliability using the Landis and Koch[11] classifications of agreement (0.00-0.20 indicates slight agreement, 0.21-0.40 indicates fair agreement, 0.41-0.60 indicates moderate agreement, 0.61-0.80 indicates substantial agreement, 0.81-0.99 indicates almost perfect agreement, and 1.00 indicates complete/perfect agreement).

Construct Validity

The validity of an assessment tool indicates how well it measures what it is designed to measure. Validity is supported when different methods of measuring the same or similar constructs produce similar results. To examine construct validity, the pattern and magnitude of the relationship between the scores for the motor, language, and combined ML scale scores were compared to other similar health measures using Spearman correlation coefficients in the baseline data. For all correlational analyses, the absolute value of the Spearman correlation coefficients assessed whether weak ($|r|$ <0.30), moderate ($0.30 \leq |r| < 0.60$), or strong ($|r| \geq 0.60$) relationships exist.[12]

Similar health measures compared to the motor score included the Physical Functioning Domain (8 items) and the Total Scale score from the 23-item Pediatric Quality of Life (PedsQL) Generic Core Scales, V4.0.[13] Due to the impact of the child's motor functioning on a parent's caregiving role, the motor scores were compared to 3 key domain scores (Physical Functioning, Emotional Functioning, and Social Functioning) and the Total Score of the PedsQL Family Impact Module.[14] In addition, the Daily Activities Scale score from the CLN2 Quality of Life Questionnaire (CLN2 QL) was also examined to support the construct validity of the motor item's score.

The language score was compared to other PedsQL Family Impact Module Domain scores for Social Functioning, Cognitive Functioning, and Communications reflecting the impact of the child's language abilities on these parenting roles. Finally, the combined ML scale score was compared to the PedsQL Total Score, the PedsQL Family Impact Module Total Score, and the CLN2 QL Daily Activities Score.

Responsiveness

The responsiveness (ie, the ability to detect change over time) of the motor, language, and combined ML scores was also examined using Spearman correlation coefficient. The ML scores for change from baseline to week 49 (Study 201 Completion/Early Termination) were compared to the change score from baseline to the respective visit on the CLN2 QL Daily Activities Score. The absolute value of the Spearman correlation coefficient assessed whether weak ($|r| < .30$), moderate ($.30 \leq |r| < .60$), or strong ($|r| \geq .60$) relationships exist.[12]

Comparison Study of HML and CLN2 Clinical Rating Scale ML Domains

Ensuring the adequate similarity of measurements using the HML and the CLN2 Clinical Rating Scale ML domains is key to the interpretation of clinical trial results. Ideally, all natural history assessments could be scored using the ML domains by clinical trial raters. However, due to the historical nature of these data, subsequent deaths from some of these children, and the fact that videotaping patients were not part of the clinical acquisition routine in the natural history registry, a sufficient supply of natural history patient videos was not feasible.

Therefore, to bridge the similarities of these 2 rating scales, videotaped assessments were reviewed and scored using the HML scale by a rater independent of the clinical studies, trained on the HML definitions. The goal of this bridging investigation was to understand the degree of variability in ratings in the analyses that is attributable to the slight changes in the study rating definitions. The videos were viewed in their entirety, and the videos were not transcribed for review due to the lack of meaning that comes from the transcription of videos of patients with CLN2, many with quite limited language abilities.

κ_w statistics[10] assessed the level of rater agreement between the HML scale ratings (motor, language, and combined ML scores) when compared to the clinical trial clinician ratings using the ML scale. The κ_w results were interpreted using the Landis and Koch[11] classifications of agreement (see "Interrater Reliability" section) to assess the similarity of the 2 rating scales.

In addition, slope estimates for the rate of decline over 48 months of treatment were produced for each of the original and ML scale scores using the same algorithm as specified in the phase 1/2 study. The slope for a patient was computed as a change from baseline, using the last observation >0 and scaled as a rate per units of 48 weeks. The analyses were also produced for the separate ML components. Summary statistics (mean, median, standard deviation [SD]) were produced for the HML and Clinical Rating Scale ML slope estimates.

Table 2. Baseline Demographic Characteristics (Phase 1/2 Study, Enrolled Population).

	All Patients, N = 24
Age at enrollment, years	
Mean (SD)	4.3 (1.24)
Median	4.0
Minimum, maximum	3.0, 8.0
Sex, n (%)	
Female	15 (63)
Male	9 (38)
Race, n (%)	
Asian	1 (4)
White	23 (96)
Ethnicity, n (%)	
Hispanic or Latino	1 (4)
Not Hispanic or Latino	23 (96)
Age at disease onset, years, n (%)	
<3	7 (29)
3-<5	12 (50)
≥5	4 (17)
Unknown	1 (4)
Mean (SD)	3.4 (1.07)
Median	3.0
Minimum, maximum	2.5, 6.3
Genotype, n (%)	
c.622C>T	5 (21)
c.509-1G>C	2 (8)
c.622C>T and c.509-1G>C	2 (8)
c.622C>T and other	4 (17)
c.509-1G>C and other	4 (17)
Other	7 (29)
Screening ML Scale score, n (%)	
Mean (SD)	3.7 (0.95)
Median	3
Minimum, maximum	3, 6
Baseline ML Scale score[a]	
Mean (SD)	3.5 (1.20)
Median	3
Minimum, maximum	1, 6

Abbreviations: ML, motor and language; SD, standard deviation.
[a]Study-eligibility criteria were based on the baseline rather than screening visit.

Results

Patient Population

A total of 24 patients were screened for the phase 1/2 study at 5 clinical sites. All screened patients were enrolled. One patient was discontinued after placement of the intracerebroventricular catheter and the first 300 mg infusion at the parents' request, due to the patient's unwillingness to continue with study procedures. The remaining 23 patients completed the phase 1/2 study and went on to enroll in the extension study.

The mean (SD) age of the study patients at enrollment was 4.3 (1.24) years (Table 2). Most patients were white (96%); 63% were female. The mean (SD) age of CLN2 disease onset was 3.4 (1.07) years (Table 2). One or both of the 2 most common CLN2 alleles (ie, c.622C>T and c.509-1G>C) were present in 17 (71%) patients. The mean (SD) baseline ML scale score was 3.5 (1.20) points. Three patients had baseline ML scale scores below the study enrollment minimum of 3; however, study eligibility was determined at the screening rather than baseline assessment. The protocol permitted a 1-month interval between the screening and baseline visits.

Interrater Reliability

In the formal interrater study of Hamburg clinic patients using patient videos, κ_w results for motor score ratings for all videos (n = 36) were .93, indicating near-perfect agreement.[11] Perfect agreement (κ_w = 1.00) were observed at week 25 (n = 11), week 49 (n = 10), and week 73 (n = 3). At baseline, 2 ratings were provided that were 1 level lower than the clinical study ratings (κ_w .76; n = 12), but nonetheless, these ratings demonstrated substantial agreement (Table 3).

Similarly, for the language score ratings across all videos, κ_w = .82, thus indicating near-perfect agreement. The κ_w estimates at each time point ranged from .67 at week 49 to .93 at baseline. Moreover, the combined ML scale scores (0-6) generated from the ML scale trainer's ratings were in almost perfect agreement with those of the clinician raters ($.89 \le \kappa_w \le .93$) for each time point and across all rating periods—supporting interrater reliability for the ML scale scores. Moreover, the demonstrated consistency between the clinical trial ratings made by each of the study clinicians and the study's ML scale

Table 3. Interrater Reliability Estimates[a] in Clinical Studies Among Hamburg Clinic Patients.[b]

	Baseline, n = 12	Week 25, n = 11	Week 49, n = 10	Week 73, n = 3	All 4 Time Points, n = 36
ML scale motor ratings	0.76	1.00	1.00	1.00	0.93
ML scale language ratings	0.93	0.79	0.67	0.80	0.82
Combined (0-6) ML scale scores	0.92	0.93	0.89	0.93	0.92

Abbreviation: ML, motor and language.
[a]Weighted kappa comparison between 2 raters.
[b]Conducted in 2016.

trainer supports the reproducibility of the ML ratings and procedures (Table 3).

Construct Validity

Construct validity analyses for the motor, language, and combined ML scale scores examined the magnitude of Spearman correlation coefficients at baseline. For the domains and total scores most closely related to the motor score, baseline correlations were generally moderate to strong, with the strongest observed relationships with the PedsQL Core Physical Functioning measure ($r = 0.64$) and Total Score ($r = 0.61$). For the domains scores most closely related to the language score, baseline correlations were generally moderate to strong with the PedsQL Family Impact Module's Communication ($r = .65$), Social ($r = .57$), and Cognitive Functioning ($r = .47$) Domain comparisons. The ML scale score demonstrated moderate relationships with the comparator instruments' Total Scores (PedsQL Total Score, $r = .35$; the PedsQL Family Impact Module Total Score, $r = .51$; the CLN2 QL Daily Activities Score, $r = .35$).

Responsiveness

The ML scale change scores (motor, language, and combined ML) from baseline to week 49 (end of study visit in Study 201) were compared to the change score from baseline to the respective visit on the CLN2 QL Daily Activities Score using the Spearman correlation coefficients. Both the ML and the motor change scores demonstrated a moderate level of responsiveness with the CLN2 QL Daily Activity Score ($r = 0.37$ and 0.41, respectively). The PedsQL Social Functioning measure's change score correlation with the language change score was 0.40—also achieving a moderate relationship to demonstrate the responsiveness of the ML combined and standalone items.

Comparison Study of HML and CLN2 Clinical Rating Scale ML Score

A bridging study using videotapes and ratings by an HML rater investigated whether adequate similarities exist between the ML scores of the HML and the CLN2 Clinical Rating Scale. The results demonstrate substantial-to-perfect agreement between the 2 corresponding motor scales ($.67 \leq \kappa_w \leq 1.00$), fair-to-substantial agreement between the language scales ($.34 \leq \kappa_w \leq .62$), and substantial agreement in the combined ML scores ($.67 \leq \kappa_w \leq .79$) at all of the investigated time points (baseline, week 25, week 49, and week 73). The mean slopes of ratings from baseline to week 49 computed for the HML and the ML scale ratings yielded nearly identical point estimates and variation for the Hamburg clinic patients in this investigation (Table 4). This was true for the mean slopes from the respective motor scales (0.14 ± 0.25 [HML] vs 0.17 ± 0.33 [ML]), language scales (0.00 ± 0.00 [HML] vs −0.02 ± 0.58 [ML]), and 0 to 6 ML combined score from each scale (0.05 ± 0.41 [HML] vs 0.17 ± 0.52 [ML]). These results provide assurance that the HML and the CLN2 Clinical Rating Scale ML scores are adequately similar for use in the interpretation of functional change over time in the clinical studies.

Table 4. Estimated Rate of Decline Over 48 Weeks in Phase 1/2 Study: Motor, Language, and Combined Scores Slope Estimates in the Scale Comparison Study.

Rate of Decline (Points/48 Weeks)[a]	CLN2 Rating Scale ML	HML
Motor scores	n = 12	n = 12
Mean (SD)	0.17 (0.33)	0.14 (0.25)
Median	0.00	0.00
Minimum, maximum	0.00, 1.01	0.00, 0.61
95% CI limit	−0.04, 0.39	−0.02, 0.30
Language scores[b]	n = 6	n = 6
Mean (SD)	−0.02 (0.58)	0.00 (0.00)
Median	0.00	0.00
Minimum, maximum	−0.61, 1.01	0.00, 0.00
95% CI limit	−0.62, 0.58	0.00, 0.00
ML combined score	n = 12	n = 12
Mean (SD)	0.17 (0.52)	0.05 (0.41)
Median	0.00	0.00
Minimum, maximum	−0.61, 1.01	−1.00, 0.61
95% CI limit	−0.16, 0.50	−0.21, 0.31

Abbreviations: CI, confidence interval; CLN2, neuronal ceroid lipofuscinosis type-2; HML, Hamburg Motor-Language; ML, motor and language; SD, standard deviation.
[a]Negative slopes denote improvement over time.
[b]Five patients were omitted from language slope estimation because the baseline language score was 0. One additional patient was omitted because there were no observations postbaseline with a language score >0.

Discussion

Clinical outcome assessments designed to demonstrate the benefits of a treatment must be well defined and possess adequate measurement properties.[8] The primary metric used to quantify a notable attenuation of CLN2 disease progression in clinical studies was the aggregate of the ML score in the CLN2 Clinical Rating Scale. In order to ensure measurement consistency across clinical trial sites, the CLN2 Clinical Rating Scale ML domain was adapted from the original Hamburg scale[4] to include anchor point definitions that would allow consistent ratings within the study conduct. The adapted CLN2 Clinical Rating Scale ML domain was intended to respect the historical application of the Hamburg scale and allow consistent and harmonized ratings in a multinational, multisite, clinical efficacy study.

The psychometric analyses of the ML rating scale with regard to reliability, construct validity, and responsiveness provide confidence in the measurement properties of this adapted instrument and the 2 component scores. Interrater reliability was assessed using Hamburg clinic patients in the clinical studies; the results are convincing and show that agreement for the motor, language, and combined ML scores was substantial to nearly perfect.[11] These results reflect the important success in achieving rater consistency in the clinical studies through strong and thorough rater trainings. Construct validity and ability to detect change were also demonstrated with moderate-to-strong correlations with key domains and total scores from quality-of-life instruments (PedsQL, PedsQL Family Impact Module, and CLN2 QL Daily Activities Score) measuring similar constructs.

Agreement with the ML scale, as assessed by κ_w values for single and combined ML scores, was near perfect for the motor score for all time points; there was fair-to-substantial agreement for the language scores.[11] External review of videotapes may pose challenges for precise language assessments that may contribute to the lack of strong agreement in the language score. In contrast to study raters, the external reviewer had no previous medical or social information such that previous maximum attained function was not known. Technical issues such as recording quality or sample bias that may limit the ability of the rater to accurately assess language capabilities may also confound results. However, the external video rating assessment of decline using the HML scale led to nearly identical values for progression slope point estimates and variability when compared to the individual and combined domains of the ML scale's rating changes over time, suggesting a strong relationship in the assessment of disease progression despite the lack of strong agreement in language scores. These results provide assurance that the ML scores from the 2 scales are adequately similar for use in the interpretation of the results from the clinical studies when compared to the natural history registry.

This study is not without limitations. First, no other known psychometric validation of this scale has been conducted outside these clinical studies; the use of the adapted instrument is encouraged to better understand the strength and durability of the conclusions in this report in other CLN2 disease investigations. In addition, no formal intrarater reliability study was conducted. However, the correspondence of ratings between the clinician's rating compared to the ratings by the rater trainer using the videotaped assessments was strong and demonstrated that each study clinician made his or her ratings in a manner that was strongly consistent with the opinion of the trainer on the study rating process—as may be expected by the use of well-trained physicians across these global academic medical centers.

Other limitations included the hampered ability to evaluate responsiveness (the ability to detect change over time) in these analyses given that few ML score shifts were observed in patients in the phase 1/2 study (Table 4). Nonetheless, moderate change correlations ($r \geq 0.37$) with key quality-of-life domains scores provide confidence in this measurement property. Finally, the scales' video-based ratings were subsequently compared to the primary source data for the clinical studies, which is the in-person rating by the patient's Hamburg clinic physician. The use of the videos introduced possibly important sources of error in comparing these ratings; namely, the rater was not present for any interactions between the patient and the study clinician prior to the start of videotaping (eg, patient walks up to greet the study physician in the clinic hallway) or any unobservable (on the video) details (eg, someone walking into the room, pictures in the room or the view outside the window, etc). In contrast, the study clinician often knew each patient was physically present throughout the clinic visit and assessment and was capable of making a comprehensive assessment that may not have been fully captured in the video. This limitation of video assessments may contribute to the lack of strong agreement between the raters' score of language ability, which may be more difficult to capture fully on video than motor ability, which had substantial-to-perfect agreement between the 2 corresponding motor scales. Importantly, this did not limit agreement in the assessment of change in language ability over time.

Conclusions

These results demonstrate that the ML domains of the CLN2 Clinical Rating Scale are objective, reproducible, valid, and responsive measures in children with CLN2 disease. These results also provide assurance that the HML and the CLN2 Clinical Rating Scale ML scores are adequately similar for use in the understanding of results from clinical trials. Moreover, change over time on the ML scores is interpretable.[8] That is, each unit difference on this scale measures a clinically meaningful change in a child's ML abilities. Indeed, anyone who has personally experienced a child's development knows that a change—especially a decline on this scale—is notable, relevant, and reflective of a meaningful change in a child's functioning in the clinical course of CLN2 disease.

Acknowledgments

The authors thank Janet Wittes at Statistics Collaborative, Inc, for statistical assistance with this research and Drs Lim Ming and Ruth

Williams for their participation in the discussions operationalizing the CLN2 Clinical Rating Scale items.

Declaration of Conflicting Interests

The author(s) declared the following potential conflicts of interest with respect to the research, authorship, and/or publication of this article: Peter Slasor, Temitayo Ajayi, and David R. Jacoby are employees and shareholders of BioMarin Pharmaceutical Inc.

Funding

The author(s) disclosed receipt of the following financial support for the research, authorship, and/or publication of this article: Kathleen Wyrwich was employed of Evidera Inc when this research was conducted, which received financial support from BioMarin Pharmaceutical Inc. in connection with the study development, execution, and manuscript development.

References

1. Kohlschutter A, Schulz A. CLN2 disease (classic late infantile neuronal ceroid lipofuscinosis). *Pediatr Endocrinol Rev.* 2016; 13(suppl 1):682-688.
2. Chang M, Cooper JD, Davidson BL, et al. CLN2. In: Mole SE, Williams RE, Goebel HH, eds. *The Neuronal Ceroid Lipofuscinoses (Batten Disease).* Oxford: Oxford University Press; 2011: 80-109.
3. Mink JW, Augustine EF, Adams HR, Marshall FJ, Kwon JM. Classification and natural history of the neuronal ceroid lipofuscinoses. *J Child Neurol.* 2013;28(9):1101-1105.
4. Steinfeld R, Heim P, von Gregory H, et al. Late infantile neuronal ceroid lipofuscinosis: quantitative description of the clinical course in patients with CLN2 mutations. *Am J Med Genet.* 2002;112(4):347-354.
5. Worgall S, Kekatpure MV, Heier L, et al. Neurological deterioration in late infantile neuronal ceroid lipofuscinosis. *Neurology.* 2007;69(6):521-535.
6. Williams RE, Aberg L, Autti T, Goebel HH, Kohlschutter A, Lonnqvist T. Diagnosis of the neuronal ceroid lipofuscinoses: an update. *Biochim Biophys Acta.* 2006;1762(10):865-872.
7. Schulz A, Ajayi T, Specchio N, et al; CLN2 Study Group. Study of intraventricular cerliponase alfa for CLN2 disease. *N Engl J Med.* 2018;378(20):1898-1907.
8. Walton MK, Powers JH 3rd, Hobart J, et al; International Society for Pharmacoeconomics and Outcomes Research Task Force for Clinical Outcomes Assessment. Clinical outcome assessments: conceptual foundation-report of the ISPOR clinical outcomes assessment – emerging good practices for outcomes research task force. *Value Health.* 2015;18(6):741-752.
9. Schulz A, Simonati A, Laine M, Williams R, Kohlschütter A, Nickel M. Abstracts of the 11th EPNS CongressOP48 – 2893: The DEM-CHILD NCL Patient Database: a tool for the evaluation of therapies in neuronal ceroid lipofuscinoses (NCL). *Eur J Paediatr Neurol.* 2015;19:S16.
10. Cohen J. Weighted kappa: nominal scale agreement with provision for scaled disagreement or partial credit. *Psychol Bull.* 1968; 70(4):213-220.
11. Landis JR, Koch GG. An application of hierarchical kappa-type statistics in the assessment of majority agreement among multiple observers. *Biometrics.* 1977;33(2):363-374.
12. Hinkle DE, Jurs SG, Wiersma W. *Applied Statistics for the Behavioral Sciences.* Boston: Houghton Mifflin; 1988.
13. Varni JW, Seid M, Kurtin PS. PedsQL 4.0: reliability and validity of the Pediatric Quality of Life Inventory version 4.0 generic core scales in healthy and patient populations. *Med Care.* 2001;39(8): 800-812.
14. Varni JW, Sherman SA, Burwinkle TM, Dickinson PE, Dixon P. The PedsQL family impact module: preliminary reliability and validity. *Health Qual Life Outcomes.* 2004;2:55.

22

Nutritional Status and Body Composition in Patients With Hepatic Glycogen Storage Diseases Treated With Uncooked Cornstarch

Bruna B. dos Santos, MSc[1], Tatiéle Nalin, PhD[2,3], Kamila C. Grokoski, MSc[4], Ingrid D. S. Perry, PhD[5], Lilia F. Refosco, MSc[2,6], Filippo P. Vairo, PhD[2], Carolina F. M. Souza, PhD[2], and Ida V. D. Schwartz, PhD[1,2,7]

Abstract

Hepatic glycogen storage diseases (GSDs) are genetic diseases associated with fasting hypoglycemia. Periodic intake of uncooked cornstarch is one of the treatment strategies available for those disorders. For reasons that are still not clear, patients with hepatic GSDs may be overweight. **Aims:** To assess nutritional status and body composition in patients with hepatic GSDs receiving uncooked cornstarch. **Methods:** The sample included 25 patients with hepatic GSD (type Ia = 14; Ib = 6; III = 3; IXα = 1; IXβ = 1), with a median age of 11.0 years (interquartile range [IQR] = 9.0-17.5), matched by age and gender with 25 healthy controls (median age = 12.0 years, IQR = 10.0-17.5). Clinical, biochemical, and treatment-related variables were obtained from medical records. Nutritional status and body composition were prospectively evaluated by bioelectrical impedance. **Results:** Patients and controls did not differ with regard to age and gender. Height was significantly reduced in patients (median = 1.43 m, IQR = 1.25-1.54) in comparison to controls (median = 1.54 m, IQR = 1.42-1.61; $P = .04$). Body mass index for age z-score and fat mass percentage were higher in patients (median = 1.84, IQR = 0.55-3.06; and 27.5%, IQR = 22.6-32.0, respectively) than in controls (median = 0.86, IQR = −0.55 to 1.82; $P = .04$ and 21.1%, IQR = 13.0-28.3; $P = .01$, respectively). When patients were stratified by type, those with GSD Ia had significantly higher adiposity (median fat mass = 28.7%, IQR = 25.3-32.9) than those with GSD III and GSD IXα/β (median fat mass = 20.9%, IQR = 14.9-22.6; $P = .02$). **Conclusions:** Our findings suggest that patients with hepatic GSD on treatment with cornstarch, especially those with GSD Ia, exhibit abnormalities in nutritional status and body composition, such as short stature and a trend toward overweight and obesity.

Keywords

hepatic glycogen storage diseases, nutritional status, body composition, adiposity, bioelectrical impedance

[1] Postgraduate Program in Genetics and Molecular Biology, Universidade Federal do Rio Grande do Sul, Porto Alegre, Rio Grande do Sul, Brazil
[2] Medical Genetics Service, Hospital de Clínicas de Porto Alegre, Porto Alegre, Rio Grande do Sul, Brazil
[3] Postgraduate Program in Medical Sciences, Universidade Federal do Rio Grande do Sul, Porto Alegre, Rio Grande do Sul, Brazil
[4] Postgraduate Program in Child and Adolescent Health, Universidade Federal do Rio Grande do Sul, Porto Alegre, Rio Grande do Sul, Brazil
[5] Postgraduate Program in Public Health, Universidade do Extremo Sul Catarinense, Criciúma, Santa Catarina, Brazil
[6] Nutrition and Dietetics Service, Hospital de Clínicas de Porto Alegre, Porto Alegre, Rio Grande do Sul, Brazil
[7] Department of Genetics, Universidade Federal do Rio Grande do Sul, Porto Alegre, Rio Grande do Sul, Brazil

Corresponding Author:

Tatiéle Nalin, Serviço de Genética Médica, Hospital de Clínicas de Porto Alegre, Rua Ramiro Barcelos, 2350, Porto Alegre, RS 90035-903, Brazil.
Email: tatinalin@gmail.com

Introduction

The glycogen storage diseases (GSDs), or glycogenosis, are a group of genetic diseases characterized by abnormalities in enzymes that regulate glycogen synthesis and degradation.[1] Glycogen, stored mainly in muscle and liver tissue, serves as a readily accessible source of energy[2] to maintain glucose homeostasis during fasting.[3]

Different GSD types exist and are classified accordingly to the organs affected, with a broad range of clinical manifestations, and gene/enzyme involved (Table 1). In hepatic GSDs, endogenous glucose production is impaired; thus, the main clinical consequence is fasting hypoglycemia.[1] Hepatomegaly is another common manifestation shared across nearly all GSD types. Symptoms vary depending on the specific form of GSD including hyperlactatemia, hyperlipidemia, hyperuricemia, cardiomyopathy, abnormal liver enzymes, hypotonia, and cirrhosis.[1,2,10,11]

The primary treatment goal in hepatic GSDs is to prevent hypoglycemia, avoid long-term complications, and ensure adequate growth.[12] One of the treatment approaches is dietary and may involve frequent, periodic administration of uncooked cornstarch (UCCS) and continuous nocturnal gastric drip feeding (CNGDF).[13] Liver transplantation can be considered in cases of severe hepatic cirrhosis, hepatic dysfunction, and/or hepatocellular carcinoma,[7] and kidney transplantation when there is renal insufficiency.[10]

Considering the clinical heterogeneity of hepatic GSD, dietary recommendations need to be adapted to the needs of each type of diseases and the age of the patient. The nutritional recommendations for GSD I, III, and IX are presented in Table 2. Daily caloric intake should be prescribed and monitored closely, as insufficient energy provision will be unable to correct metabolic derangements and, consequently, leads to

Table 1. Classification of Hepatic Glycogen Storage Diseases and Summary of Their Characteristics.[a]

Type (MIM)	Enzyme Involved	Gene	Inheritance Pattern	Clinical/Biochemical	Treatment
0, liver (240600)	Glycogen synthase (liver)	*GYS2*	AR	Fasting ketotic hypoglycemia; postprandial hyperglycemia, hyperlactatemia, and hyperlipidemia. No liver enlargement.	Protein-rich diet, low-glycemic index complex carbohydrates; bedtime uncooked cornstarch.
Ia (232200)	Glucose-6-phosphatase	*G6PC*	AR	Hypoglycemia, hepatomegaly, growth retardation, lactic acidosis, hyperuricemia, hyperlipidemia.	Uncooked cornstarch; galactose, fructose, lactose, and sucrose restriction.
Ib (232220)	Glucose-6-phosphate translocase	*SLC37A4*	AR	As in Ia, plus neutropenia, recurrent infections, inflammatory bowel disease.	Uncooked cornstarch; galactose, fructose, lactose, and sucrose restriction. Granulocyte colony-stimulating factor (filgrastim).
IIIa and IIIb (232400)	Glycogen debranching enzyme	*AGL*	AR	Hepatomegaly, hyperketotic hypoglycemia; growth retardation, hyperlipidemia, elevated AST, ALT, CPK. Muscle weakness and cardiomyopathy occur in subtype IIIa.	Uncooked cornstarch; protein-rich diet; sucrose restriction.
IV (232500)	Glycogen branching enzyme	*GBE1*	AR	Hepatomegaly, growth retardation, cirrhosis.	Liver transplantation in severe cases.
VI (232700)	Glycogen phosphorylase (liver)	*PYGL*	AR	Hepatomegaly, growth retardation; mild hypoglycemia, hyperlipidemia, hyperketosis.	If symptomatic: increased carbohydrate intake, frequent feedings, protein-rich diet.
IXα1 and IXα2 (306000)	Phosphorylase kinase	*PHKA2*	XLR	Hepatomegaly, fasting ketotic hypoglycemia, growth retardation, mild AST/ALT elevation, and hyperlipidemia.	Uncooked cornstarch; protein-rich diet; avoidance of large amounts of sucrose.
IXβ (261750)	Phosphorylase kinase	*PHKB*	AR	As in IXa.	Uncooked cornstarch; protein-rich diet; avoidance of large amounts of sucrose.
IXγ (613027)	Phosphorylase kinase	*PHKG2*	AR	As in IXa, plus cirrhosis.	Uncooked cornstarch; protein-rich diet; avoidance of large amounts of sucrose.
XI (227810)	Glucose transporter 2	*GLUT2*	AR	Hypoglycemia, failure to thrive, rickets, protuberant abdomen due to enlarged liver and kidneys.	Restricted galactose intake; uncooked cornstarch; supplementation of water, electrolytes, and vitamin D.

Abbreviations: AR, autosomal recessive; XLR, X-linked recessive; GYS2, Glycogen synthase 2; G6PC, Glucose-6-phosphatase catalytic subunit; SLC37A4, Solute carrier family 37 member 4; AGL, Amylo-alpha-1, 6-glucosidase, 4-alpha-glucanotransferase; GBE1, 1,4-alpha-glucan branching enzyme 1; PYGL, Glycogen phosphorylase L; PHKA2, Phosphorylase kinase regulatory subunit alpha 2; PHKB, Phosphorylase kinase regulatory subunit beta; PHKG2, Phosphorylase kinase catalytic subunit gamma 2; GLUT2, Solute carrier family 2 member 2; AR, autosomal recessive; XLR, X-linked recessive; AST, Aspartato Aminotransferase; ALT, Alanine Aminotransferase; CPK, Creatine Phosphokinase.

[a]Adapted from Wolfsdorf and Weinstein,[1] Beauchamp et al,[4] Kishnani et al,[5] Hicks et al,[6] Dagli et al,[7] Chen et al,[8] Kishnani et al,[9] and Bali et al.[10]

Table 2. Dietary Recommendations for Hepatic GSD I, III, and IX.[a]

Type	Age Group	UCCS (g/kg/dose)	Dose Interval of UCCS (h)	CARB (%)	PTN (%)	LIP (%)	Additional Recommendations
I	Infants	1.6	3-4	60-70	10-15	The remainder of %kcal[b]	Restriction of lactose and fructose
	Small children-puberty	1.7-2.5	4-6				
	Adults	1.7-2.5	Variable				
III	>12 months	1.0-2.5	4-6	35-55	20-30	20-35	Meal 3/3 h up to 12 months. High-protein diet (3 g/kg)
	Adults	Variable	Variable				
IX	All	0.6-2.5	Variable	[c]	15-25	[c]	High-protein diet

Abbreviations: CARB, carbohydrate; GSD, glycogen storage disorder; LIP, lipid; PTN, protein; UCCS, uncooked cornstarch.
[a]Adapted from Kishnani et al,[5] Hicks et al,[6] Dagli et al,[7] Kishnani et al,[9] Bali et al,[10] Froissart et al,[12] Goldberg and Slonim,[14] and Sentner et al.[15]
[b]<30% for children over 2 years.
[c]Similar to recommendations for GSD III.

growth impairment. On the other hand, excessive UCCS intake may lead to obesity.[12]

There are several reports of overweight in patients with hepatic GSDs, particularly in GSD Ia,[9,16,17] however, the etiology of this finding remains incompletely elucidated. On the one hand, dietary treatment with a complex carbohydrate can reduce the risk of short-term and long-term complications,[18] on the other hand, it could be associated with overweight and, eventually, excess adiposity. Short stature has also been reported in GSD types I, III, and IXα/β.[2,4,6,11,19]

Although changes in nutritional status appear to be frequent among patients with hepatic GSDs, knowledge gaps remain regarding these aspects as well as regarding the body composition of these patients. Within this context, the present study sought to evaluate nutritional status and body composition in patients with hepatic GSDs in comparison to healthy controls, through a review of clinical data and bioelectrical impedance analysis (BIA), in an attempt to improve the current understanding of the association of these aspects with GSD.

Table 3. Nutritional Status and Body Composition in Patients With Hepatic Glycogenosis Receiving Uncooked Cornstarch Therapy and Controls—Summary of the Main Findings.[a]

	GSD (n = 25)	Controls (n = 25)	P Value
Gender (F/M)	13/12	13/12	–
Age (years)	11.0 (9.0 to 17.5)	12.0 (10.0 to 17.5)	.45
Weight (kg)	49.0 (29.8 to 66.9)	50 (36.2 to 62.5)	.95
Height (m)	1.43 (1.25 to 1.54)	1.54 (1.42 to 1.61)	.04[b]
BMI (kg/m^2)			
≤19 years	22.5 (18.3 to 26.0)	20.3 (16.3 to 25.2)	.22
>19 years	28.2 (25.0 to 38.9)	21.9 (19.9 to 23.5)	.01[b]
Phase angle (°)	6.2 (5.4 to 7.0)	6.5 (5.6 to 7.1)	.40
Fat-free mass (%)	72.5 (68.0 to 77.3)	78.9 (71.7 to 87.0)	.01[b]
Fat mass (%)	27.5 (22.6 to 32.0)	21.1 (13.0 to 28.3)	.01[b]
Height for age (z)	−1.31 (−1.92 to 0.13)	−0.06 (−0.63 to 0.58)	<.01[b]
Weight for age (z)	0.07 (−0.78 to 2.02)	0.22 (−0.56 to 0.86)	.86
BMI-for-age (z)	1.84 (0.55 to 3.06)	0.86 (−0.55 to 1.82)	.04[b]

Abbreviations: BMI, body mass index; F/M, female/male; GSD, glycogen storage disease.
[a]Fat mass expressed as percentage of total body weight. Data expressed as median (interquartile range).
[b]Statistically significant.

Methods

Study Design

This cross-sectional study used a convenience sampling strategy to enroll patients with hepatic GSDs and healthy controls matched for age and gender. All patients were recruited from the Medical Genetics Service at Hospital de Clínicas de Porto Alegre (SGM-HCPA), Brazil. The 25 healthy controls had a median age of 12.0 years (interquartile range [IQR] = 10.0-17.5) and were recruited from the community of the same hospital. This study was approved by the HCPA Research Ethics Committee (protocol number: 14-0120) and conducted in accordance with the provisions of the Declaration of Helsinki. All participants or their legal guardians signed an informed consent term.

Sample

The sample included 25 patients receiving UCCS treatment, with a median age of 11.0 years (IQR = 9.0-17.5), of whom 14 had GSD Ia, 6 had GSD Ib, 3 had GSD III, and 2 had GSD IXα/β (Tables 3 and 4). All patients included in this study had a diagnosis of hepatic GSD confirmed by enzymatic and/or genetic analysis (median age at diagnosis = 8.5 months; IQR = 6-21.5) and are seen at the Outpatient Metabolic Disorders Clinic at SGM-HCPA (median age at treatment onset = 12 months; IQR = 6-35.2) every 3 to 6 months. Clinical variables (GSD type and comorbidities), biochemical parameters (serum lactate, glucose, triglycerides, and cholesterol levels), and treatment parameters (dose of UCCS administered) were obtained through a review of the medical records for the patients' latest visits (up to 3 months before inclusion in the study).

Table 4. Nutritional Status and Body Composition According to the Type of Hepatic Glycogenosis—Summary of the Main Findings (N = 25).[a]

	GSD Ia (n = 14)	GSD Ib (n = 6)	GSD III or IXα/β (n = 5)	P Value
Gender (F/M)	9/5	3/3	1/4	–
Age (years)	13.5 (9.7 to 18.2)	11.0 (5.2 to 18.5)	9.0 (8.5 to 12.0)	.24
UCCS/day (g)	383.0 (287.5 to 510.0)	332.5 (228.0 to 438.7)	288.0 (207.0 to 376.0)	.36
UCCS/weight (g/kg)	5.98 (4.82 to 8.12)	7.61 (6.38 to 11.29)	9.46 (4.88 to 11.44)	.20
Weight (kg)	56.0 (41.3 to 87.1)	43.8 (18.1 to 68.9)	30.0 (27.0 to 50.3)	.17
Height (m)	1.49 (1.34 to 1.56)	1.37 (1.04 to 1.52)	1.29 (1.24 to 1.52)	.37
BMI (kg/m^2)	24.9 (22.0 to 33.1)	23.2 (18.1 to 28.0)	19.0 (16.7 to 21.1)	.06
Fat-free mass (%)	71.3 (67.0 to 74.6)[b]	69.8 (63.0 to 77.6)	79.1 (77.3 to 85.0)[b]	.02[c]
Fat mass (%)	28.7 (25.3 to 32.9)[b]	30.1 (22.4 to 36.9)	20.9 (14.9 to 22.6)[b]	.02[c]
Phase angle (°)	6.65 (5.32 to 7.27)	5.40 (4.42 to 6.55)	6.20 (5.95 to 6.90)	.21
Height for age (z)	−1.17 (−1.82 to 0.11)	−1.78 (−2.05 to −0.46)	−0.91 (−1.93 to 0.94)	.53
Weight for age (z)	0.62 (−1.92 to 2.10)	0.55 (−0.78 to 1.52)	−0.18 (−1.07 to 1.85)	.99
BMI for age (z)	2.54 (0.44 to 3.59)	2.50 (1.01 to 3.01)	0.97 (0.22 to 1.50)	.33

Abbreviations: BMI, body mass index; F/M, female/male; GSD, glycogen storage disease; UCCS, uncooked cornstarch.
[a]Fat mass expressed as percentage of total body weight. Data expressed as median (interquartile range).
[b]Denotes significant between-group difference.
[c]Statistically significant.

Anthropometric Measurements

Weight was measured using digital scales (resolution 0.1 kg; Model 2096PP/2; Toledo, São Paulo, Brazil), while height was measured with a wall-mounted stadiometer (precision 0.1 cm; Harpenden; Holtain, Crymych, Wales, United Kingdom). These measurements were obtained while participants were in standing position and wearing minimal clothing. Body mass index (BMI) was calculated as weight (kg) divided by height in meter square (m^2) and classified as underweight, normal weight, overweight, or obese, per the World Health Organization (WHO) criteria.[20,21] In patients aged <19 years, nutritional status was calculated using BMI for age *z* scores calculated in WHO Anthro version 3.2.2 and WHO Anthroplus version 1.0.4.[22,23]

Bioelectrical Impedance Analysis of Body Composition

To estimate body composition (fat mass and fat-free mass), a BIA system was used (Biodynamics 450, version 5.1; Biodynamics Corporation, Seattle, Washington), with resting-tab electrocardiogram electrodes (Conmed Corporation, Utica, New York), as described elsewhere in the literature. Participants were instructed to refrain from physical activity or intake of caffeine-enriched foods and beverages in the 8 hours preceding assessment as well as to empty their bladders and remove all metal objects before starting the test.[24] Due to the need to maintain normal glucose levels, patients could not be asked to fast for 8 hours. Therefore, a 3-hour fast was defined as standard for all patients. Controls underwent the same preparation and were given the same instructions but with an 8-hour fast. During the test, participants remained in the supine position, with the limbs outstretched away from the body, while 4 electrodes were applied in the following distribution: 1 on the wrist, 1 on the hand, 1 on the ankle, and 1 on the foot (all on the right side of the body). The adiposity (percentage fat mass) was calculated according to the Obesity Medicine Association[25] reference values for adults and McCarthy et al[26] reference values for children. Bioelectrical impedance analysis also provided data on phase angle (PA), a variable derived from the relationship between resistance (R), reactance (Xc), and impedance (Z) ($PA = arc^{tang}\ Xc/R$) to the passage of a low-amplitude, high-frequency (50 kHz) electrical current during the procedure.[27] The cutoff of Bosy-Westphal et al[28] was used to evaluate PA.

Statistical Analysis

All analyses were carried out using SPSS Statistics, version 21.0 (IBM Corp, Armonk, New York). Categorical variables were expressed as absolute and relative frequencies, and continuous variables, as medians and IQRs. The Mann-Whitney *U* test was used for comparison between the case and control groups. The Kruskal-Wallis test, followed by a post hoc analysis, was used for comparison between subgroups of patients with different GSD types. Spearman coefficients were used to test for correlation. The significance level was set at 5%.

Results

The 25 patients included belonged to 24 unrelated families. The rate of parental consanguinity was 20.8%. Four patients (16%) had clinical diagnosis of inflammatory bowel disease; all had a diagnosis of GSD type Ib and were overweight or obese at the time of assessment. Three patients (12%), all with GSD Ia, were being treated for hypothyroidism; of these, 2 (67%) had excess weight and 1 had normal weight.

Median daily UCCS intake was 6.48 g/kg body weight (IQR = 5.11-9.97), for a median total of 360 g/day (IQR = 265-447). The UCCS doses were administered every 3 to 6 hours. The median total cholesterol and triglyceride levels in plasma, available for 24 patients, were 167.5 mg/dL (IQR =

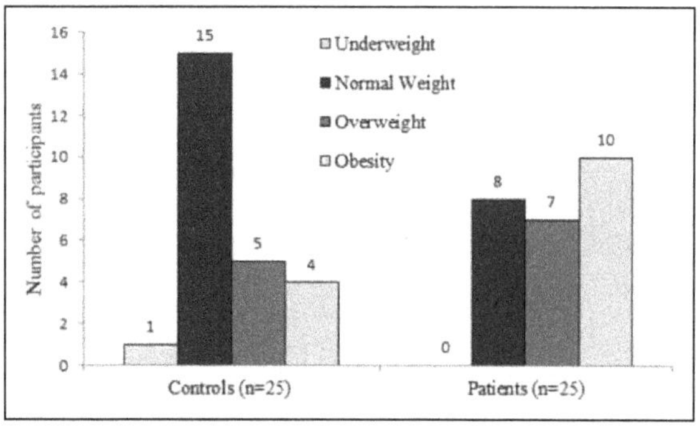

Figure 1. Classification of the nutritional status of patients with hepatic glycogen storage disease and controls, according to body mass index.[20,21]

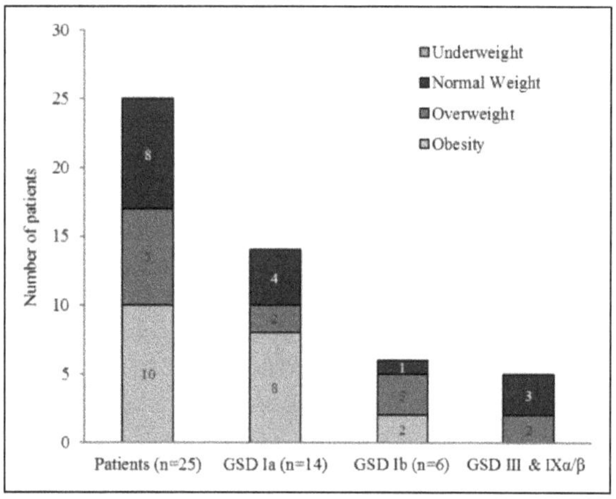

Figure 2. Classification of the nutritional status of patients with hepatic glycogen storage disease, according to body mass index.[20,21]

146.2-206.0) and 197.0 mg/dL (IQR = 119.7-407.5), respectively. The median serum glucose level was 86.5 mg/dL (IQR = 80.5-95.2, n = 22), while the median lactate level was 1.78 mmol/dL (IQR = 1.22-2.69, n = 20).

Table 3 reports anthropometric parameters and body composition data for patients and controls. Bioelectrical impedance analysis revealed that 16 (64%) patients (3 with normal weight, 3 overweight, and 10 obese) and 7 (28%) controls (1 with normal weight, 2 overweight, and 4 obese) had excess adiposity. Eight (32%) patients (6 with GSD Ia and 2 with GSD Ib) and 5 controls (20%) had PA values below the cutoff. Phase angle correlated strongly with fat-free mass in controls ($r_s = 0.7$; $P < .01$) and moderately in patients ($r_s = 0.4$; $P = .03$). Figure 1 shows the distribution of nutritional status in the sample, stratified by BMI classification.[20,21] High rates of excess weight (overweight = 28%; obesity = 40%) were found among patients. Conversely, most controls had normal weight (60%), while 9 had excess weight (overweight = 20%; obesity = 16%).

Stratification of patients by GSD type revealed a significant difference only for fat mass percentage; in this sample, patients with GSD Ia had greater adiposity than those with GSD III or IXα/β (Table 4).

Regarding stratification of nutritional status by GSD type (Figure 2), we found a heterogeneous distribution of BMI values: 2 of 5 patients with GSD III and IXα/β were overweight, while 5 out of 6 with GSD Ib and 10 out of 14 with GSD Ia had excess weight (overweight or obesity).

Discussion and Conclusion

This was the first study to evaluate body composition by BIA in patients with hepatic GSD on treatment with cornstarch. We chose BIA for evaluation of body composition because it is a noninvasive, low-cost, user-friendly method widely employed in clinical practice. Bioelectrical impedance analysis is a predictive technique for assessment of body composition whereby the passage of a low-amplitude, high-frequency electrical current through the body, particularly through the lowest-resistance compartment, allows direct measurement of resistance and reactance values, which are used to calculate impedance and PA; finally, it estimates total body water content, extracellular and intracellular water, fat-free mass, and fat mass.[29-31]

In a review, Andreoli et al[32] suggested that, compared to other techniques, BIA is a good tool for estimation of body composition in isovolemic patients. The estimated error for prediction of total body water content and fat-free mass by BIA is 2% to 4%. To achieve optimal precision or even improve the precision of this method, it is essential that measurement conditions be standardized.[33]

It is well-known that nonfasting state interferes with BIA findings. However, patients with GSD cannot be deprived of food for long periods without risking hypoglycemia. According to Kyle et al,[24] food and drink intake 2 to 4 hours before the test can reduce body impedance by 4 to 15 Ω, which represents an error of less than 3%. Thus, although an 8-hour fast is recommended, shorter periods can be acceptable both in clinical practice and in research settings.

A high frequency of obesity in patients with GSD was found by Chen et al[16] in a study of 13 GSD I patients in treatment (UCCS or CNGDF) for more than 5 years. The results of this evaluation showed that 10 of 13 patients were classified as obese according to percentage of ideal body weight for length percentile. Similar findings were described by Santos et al[17] in a cross-sectional study that evaluated patients with GSD I treated with UCCS, *z* scores of BMI for age showed that 16 of 21 patients were overweight. Short stature has also been reported by several authors as common problems in the hepatic GSD.[2,4,6,11,19]

In agreement with the literature, our findings showed that most patients had excess weight and adiposity, with higher BMI, BMI for age *z* scores, and body fat percentage than controls as well as lower median height than controls. Although anthropometric parameters revealed a stature deficit in the patient group, as in the Weinstein and Wolfsdorf[18] study, the median *z* score for height (−1.31; IQR = −1.92 to 0.13) was within the expected range according to WHO standards.[21] The pathophysiology of short stature in hepatic GSDs has yet to be elucidated. However, studies suggest that the carbohydrate overload for treatment can contribute not only to excess weight[5,10,12,34] but also to better height scores in these patients.[17,18] Although our treated patients had a short stature, suggesting that the use of UCCS does not heal the low height.

Comparison of body composition revealed that fat mass was significantly greater in patients than in controls overall and was significantly greater in patients with GSD Ia than in patients with GSD III and IXα/β (P = .02). Patients with GSD III and IXα/β were those who most resembled controls in terms of fat mass percentage.

Body mass index is widely used for assessment of nutritional status, but the underestimation of obesity is a major limitation of this method.[35] In 1 study, BIA was used to evaluate body composition in 1244 European children, from 2004 to 2006. The authors concluded that, in the pediatric population, fat-free mass and fat mass measurements provide a better understanding of growth and changes in body composition than BMI.[36] This discrepancy was also observed in our sample, in which excess adiposity was identified even in some patients classified as having normal weight by BMI.

Patients with GSD Ia, Ib, and III/IX were not found to differ regarding the daily amount of UCCS received (in g or in g/kg), but patients with GSD Ia were found to have higher fat mass than patients with GSD III/IX. So, although many authors suggest that excess weight and body fat in patients with GSD are associated with UCCS excessive intake,[5,10,12,34] our findings did not confirm this hypothesis. Another factor that may have been associated with excess weight, although not evaluated in this study, is the low engagement in physical activity. Uncertainty to whether physical activity is allowed and what dietary changes would be required may contribute to higher rates of sedentary behavior in this population.

Another BIA parameter that plays an important role in assessment of nutritional status is PA.[37–39] A positive correlation between PA and fat-free mass has been described both in healthy individuals and in pathological conditions.[40–42] We observed similar correlation in our control sample but not in patients with hepatic GSD, despite statistical significance (P = .03). Therefore, we suggest that PA is not a good predictor of fat-free mass in hepatic GSDs.

This parameter has also been associated with inflammation[43] and may be useful in the assessment of patients with hepatic GSDs, particularly GSD Ib, because of their greater susceptibility to inflammatory conditions.[44] There was no difference in PA between patients and controls, however, the median PA was lower in patients with GSD Ib than in patients with other types of GSD, suggesting possible predictive value in this subpopulation.

In conclusion, our findings suggest that Brazilian patients with hepatic GSDs have a shorter median height than healthy controls but still within normal range, and a tendency toward overweight and obesity, as demonstrated both by BMI (especially in patients with GSD type I) and by BIA-measured adiposity. Prospective studies with larger samples, taking into account measurement of anthropometric parameters as well as adiposity, may contribute to the further elucidation of the impact of these conditions on nutritional status and height. Furthermore, we believe greater research attention should be given to achieving a better understanding of the heterogeneous impacts of different GSD types on nutritional status, which could help prevent comorbidities associated with excess weight and adiposity and, thus, improve patient's quality of life.

Declaration of Conflicting Interests

The author(s) declared no potential conflicts of interest with respect to the research, authorship, and/or publication of this article.

Funding

The author(s) disclosed receipt of the following financial support for the research, authorship, and/or publication of this article: Funding for this study was provided by CNPq (Call for Proposals No. 31/2013—Metabolic and Endocrine Diseases), FAPERGS (PPSUS/2013), and the Hospital de Clínicas de Porto Alegre Research and Event Promotion Fund (FIPE/HCPA).

References

1. Wolfsdorf J, Weinstein DA. Glycogen storage diseases. *Rev Endocr Metab Disord*. 2003;4(1):95-102.
2. Gazzerro E, Andreu AL, Bruno C. Neuromuscular disorders of glycogen metabolism. *Curr Neurol Neurosci Rep*. 2013;13(3): 333.
3. Bhattacharya K. Investigation and management of the hepatic glycogen storage diseases. *Transl Pediatr*. 2015;4(2):240-248.
4. Beauchamp NJ, Dalton A, Ramaswami U, et al. Glycogen storage disease type IX: high variability in clinical phenotype. *Mol Genet Metab*. 2007;92(1-2):88-99.
5. Kishnani PS, Austin SL, Arn P, et al. Glycogen storage disease type III diagnosis and management guidelines. *Genet Med*. 2010; 12(7):446-463.
6. Hicks J, Wartchow E, Mierau G. Glycogen storage diseases: a brief review and update on clinical features, genetic abnormalities, pathologic features, and treatment. *Ultrastruct Pathol*. 2011; 35(5):183-196.
7. Dagli A, Sentner CP, Weinstein DA. Glycogen storage disease type III. 2016. http://www.ncbi.nlm.nih.gov/books/NBK26372/. Accessed September 12, 2017.
8. Chen Y, Kishnani PS, Koeberl D. Glycogen storage diseases In: Valle D, Beaudet AL, Vogelstein B, et al. eds. *The Online Metabolic and Molecular Bases of Inherited Disease*. 2014; chapter 71.
9. Kishnani PS, Austin SL, Abdenur JE, et al; American College of Medical Genetics and Genomics. Diagnosis and management of glycogen storage disease type I: a practice guideline of the American college of medical genetics and genomics. *Genet Med*. 2014; 16(11):e1.
10. Bali DS, Chen Y, Goldstein JL. Glycogen storage disease type I. 2016. http://www.ncbi.nlm.nih.gov/books/NBK1312/. Accessed September 12, 2017.
11. Özen H. Glycogen storage diseases: new perspectives. *World J Gastroenterol*. 2007;13(18):2541-2553.
12. Froissart R, Piraud M, Boudjemline AM, et al. Glucose-6-phosphatase deficiency. *Orphanet J Rare Dis*. 2011;6:27.

13. Chou JY, Jun HS, Mansfield BC. Glycogen storage disease type I and G6Pase-β deficiency: etiology and therapy. *Nat Rev Endocrinol.* 2010;6(12):676-688.
14. Goldberg T, Slonim AE. Nutrition therapy for hepatic glycogen storage diseases. *J Am Diet Assoc.* 1993;93(12):1423-1430.
15. Sentner CP, Hoogeveen IJ, Weinstein DA, et al. Glycogen storage disease type III: diagnosis, genotype, management, clinical course and outcome. *J Inherit Metab Dis.* 2016;39(5):697-704.
16. Chen YT, Bazzarre CH, Lee MM, Sidbury JB, Coleman RA. Type I glycogen storage disease: nine years of management with cornstarch. *Eur J Pediatr.* 1993;152(suppl 1):S56-S59.
17. Santos BL, Souza CF, Schuler-Faccini L, et al. Glycogen storage disease type I: clinical and laboratory profile. *J Pediatr.* 2014; 90(6):572-579.
18. Weinstein DA, Wolfsdorf JI. Effect of continuous glucose therapy with uncooked cornstarch on the long-term clinical course of type 1a glycogen storage disease. *Eur J Pediatr.* 2002;161(suppl 1):S35-S39.
19. Rake JP, Visser G, Labrune P, Leonard JV, Ullrich K, Smit GP. Glycogen storage disease type I: diagnosis, management, clinical course and outcome. Results of the European Study on Glycogen Storage Disease type I (ESGSD I). *Eur J Pediatr.* 2002;161(suppl 1):S20-S34.
20. World Health Organization. *Physical Status: The Use and Interpretation of Anthropometry.* Report of a WHO Expert Committee. Geneva, Switzerland: WHO; 1995.
21. World Health Organization. *WHO Child Growth Standards: Methods and Development: Length/Height-for-Age, Weight-for-Age, Weight-for-Length, Weight-for-Height and Body Mass Index-for-Age.* Geneva, Switzerland: WHO; 2006.
22. World Health Organization. *WHO AnthroPlus for Personal Computers Manual: Software for Assessing Growth of the World's Children and Adolescents.* Geneva, Switzerland: WHO; 2009.
23. World Health Organizations. *WHO Anthro for Personal Computers Manual: Software for Assessing Growth and Development of the World's Children.* Geneva, Switzerland: WHO; 2010.
24. Kyle UG, Bosaeus I, De Lorenzo AD, et al. Bioelectrical impedance analysis—part II: utilization in clinical practice. *Clin Nutr.* 2004;23:1430-1453.
25. Obesity Medicine Association. Obesity Algorithm®: Clinical Guidelines for Obesity Treatment. 2016. https://obesitymedicine.org/obesity-algorithm/. Accessed July 01, 2017.
26. McCarthy HD, Cole TJ, Fry T, Jebb SA, Prentice AM. Body fat reference curves for children. *Int J Obes.* 2006;30:598-602.
27. Kyle UG, Bosaeus I, De Lorenzo AD, et al. Bioelectrical impedance analysis—part I: review of principles and methods. *Clin Nutr.* 2004;23(5):1226-1243.
28. Bosy-Westphal A, Danielzik S, Dörhöfer RP, Later W, Wiese S, Müller MJ. Phase angle from bioelectrical impedance analysis: population reference values by age, sex, and body mass index. *J Parenter Enteral Nutr.* 2006;30(4):309-316.
29. Wells JCK, Fewtrell MS. Measuring body composition. *Arch Dis Child.* 2006;91(7):612-617.
30. Associação Médica Brasileira, Conselho Federal de Medicina. *Utilização da Bioimpedância para Avaliação da Massa Corpórea.* Projeto Diretrizes. 2009.
31. Fosbøl MØ, Zerahn B. Contemporary methods of body composition measurement. *Clin Physiol Funct Imaging.* 2015;35(2): 81-97.
32. Andreoli A, Garaci F, Cafarelli FP, Guglielmi G. Body composition in clinical practice. *Eur J Radiol.* 2006;85(8):1461-1468.
33. Kushner RF, Gudivaka R, Schoeller DA. Clinical characteristics influencing bioelectrical impedance analysis measurements. *Am J Clin Nutr.* 1996;64(suppl 3):423S-427S.
34. Derks TGJ, Martens DH, Sentner CP. Dietary treatment of glycogen storage disease type Ia: uncooked cornstarch and/or continuous nocturnal gastric drip-feeding? *Mol Genet Metab.* 2013; 109(1):1-2.
35. Peltz G, Aguirre MT, Sanderson M, Fadden MK. The role of fat mass index in determining obesity. *Am J Hum Biol.* 2010;22(5): 639-647.
36. Rush E, Reed PW, McLennan S, Coppinger T, Simmons D, Graham D. Tracking of body mass indices over 2 years in Māori and European children. *Eur J Clin Nutr.* 2012;66(2):143-149.
37. Nagano M, Suita S, Yamanouchi T. The validity of bioelectrical impedance phase angle for nutritional assessment in children. *J Pediatr Surg.* 2000;35(7):1035-1039.
38. Barbosa-Silva MC, Barros AJ. Bioelectrical impedance analysis in clinical practice: a new perspective on its use beyond body composition equations. *Curr Opin Clin Nutr Metab Care.* 2005; 8(3):311-317.
39. Kyle UG. Can phase angle determined by bioelectrical impedance analysis assess nutritional risk? a comparison between healthy and hospitalized subjects. *Clin Nutr.* 2012;31(6):875-881.
40. Selberg O, Selberg D. Norms and correlates of bioimpedance phase angle in healthy human subjects, hospitalized patients, and patients with liver cirrhosis. *Eur J Appl Physiol.* 2002;86(6): 509-516.
41. Visser M, van Venrooij LM, Wanders DC, et al. The bioelectrical impedance phase angle as an indicator of undernutrition and adverse clinical outcome in cardiac surgical patients. *Clin Nutr.* 2012;31(6):981-986.
42. Gonzalez MC, Barbosa-Silva TG, Bielemann RM, Gallagher D, Heymsfield SB. Phase angle and its determinants in healthy subjects: influence of body composition. *Am J Clin Nutr.* 2016; 103(3):712-716.
43. Stobäus N, Pirlich M, Valentini L, Schulzke JD, Norman K. Determinants of bioelectrical phase angle in disease. *Br J Nutr.* 2012;107(8):1217-1220.
44. Chou JY, Jun HS, Mansfield BC. Neutropenia in type Ib glycogen storage disease. *Curr Opin Hematol.* 2010;17(1):36-42.

23

High-Risk Screening and Diagnosis of Inborn Errors of Metabolism: A Practical Guide for Laboratories

Gabriel Civallero, PhD[1,2], Raquel de Kremer, MD, PhD[3], and Roberto Giugliani, MD, PhD[1,2]

Abstract

Inborn errors of metabolism (IEM) are a large and heterogeneous group of genetic diseases. In most of these conditions, the presence of variants in specific genes leads to enzyme deficiencies that affect a particular metabolic step. The number of laboratories dedicated to the study of IEM is very limited worldwide, and its multiplication is urgently required for a more effective diagnosis. With the scarcity of specialized centers, the diagnosis of affected individuals comes too late or does not happen at all. Moreover, the biological samples have to travel long distances, compromising its quality and delaying still more the diagnosis. In this work, we suggest a practical guide for a basic biochemical laboratory to get involved in the study of IEM. This proposal was based on already described metabolic tests and involves the need of just a few, simple, and affordable instruments that can give an enormous quantity of information about the possible metabolic defect faced, such as a spectrophotofluorometer and a gas chromatography/mass spectrometry (GC/MS) instrument. The procedures proposed can be customized and adapted to particular needs and situations, which make it especially useful for developing countries.

Keywords

inborn errors of metabolism, biochemical diagnosis, gas chromatography/mass spectrometry, spectrophotofluorometry, screening

Introduction

Inborn errors of metabolism (IEM) are a large and heterogeneous group of genetic diseases. In most of these conditions, the presence of variants in specific genes leads to enzyme deficiencies that affect a particular metabolic step. Depending on the metabolic error involved, the clinical presentation can be severe or lethal with neurodegenerative process, skeletal abnormalities, and/or physiologic dysfunctions.[1]

The global incidence of each particular IEM is low, but considered all together they represent more than 1 affected individual each 1000 births. The occurrence of each disease can be significantly different in particular regions. Based on clinical suspicions, the biochemical study of IEM generally begins with qualitative or quantitative tests involving metabolites related to sugars, organic acids, amino acids, sterols, fatty acids, complex lipids, porphyirins, pterines, purines and pyrimidines, and so on. These studies can be definitive or presumptive to define a specific IEM, and they are complemented with enzyme assays and/or molecular genetic testing.[2,3]

The analytical technology used by sophisticated laboratories for the diagnosis of IEM mainly includes gas chromatography/mass spectrometry (GC/MS), tandem mass spectrometry (MS/MS), amino acid analyzer, high-pressure liquid chromatography (HPLC), thin-layer chromatography, electrophoresis, and specific spectrophotometric or fluorometric enzyme assays.

In the last few years, an important strategy for early identification of IEM was initiated with the study of acylcarnitines and

[1] Medical Genetics Service, HCPA, Porto Alegre, Brazil
[2] Department of Genetics, UFRGS, Porto Alegre, Brazil
[3] Centro de Estudios de las Metabolopatías Congénitas, CEMECO, Facultad de Ciencias Médicas, Universidad Nacional de Córdoba, Argentina

Corresponding Author:
Gabriel Civallero, PhD, Medical Genetics Service, Hospital de Clinicas de Porto Alegre, Rua Ramiro Barcelos 2350, Porto Alegre, RS 90035-903, Brazil.
Email: gecivallero@yahoo.com

amino acids in newborn infants. With this simple analysis, made in dried blood spot (DBS) samples, it is possible to prevent the death or severe damage in affected babies, allowing immediate complementary studies to define the diagnosis and begin due therapy. Year after year, new countries or regions are joining to this scheme and also new metabolites are added to the screening.[4-6] The incorporation of DBS samples was also extended to perform diverse biochemical assays, especially focused on the study of lysosomal storage diseases (LSDs). The use of this type of samples facilitates its transportation from remote areas to specialized centers and could be extended to other metabolite studies, since their effectiveness was truly demonstrated.[7-20]

Despite these advances, an important deficiency is still evident. The number of laboratories dedicated to the study of IEM is very limited worldwide, and more laboratories performing IEM screening and diagnosis are required for a more efficient detection and therapy of patients. In the absence of specialized centers, the affected individuals are frequently undiagnosed, or their identification comes too late. Moreover, the biological samples have to travel long distances to reach a suitable laboratory, being exposed to deterioration during shipment and delaying still more the diagnosis.

Here, we present a practical guide for a basic biochemical laboratory to become involved in the study of IEM. This proposal was based on already described metabolic tests involving a few, simple, and affordable instruments that can give an enormous quantity of information about the possible metabolic defect faced, such as a spectrophotofluorometer and a GC/MS system. The next section describes the scope of tests that can be performed and the possible or definitive IEM involved.

Basic Biochemical Laboratory for IEM Study

Detailed biochemical procedures and its limitations can be found in the references cited in this section.

Screening Tests

Screening tests can be performed with a reactive strip or simple qualitative procedures as indicated subsequently. Despite being less used in the present days, these preliminary tests can be useful to guide the metabolic study, especially in emergency situations.[2,3]

Reactive Strips. Different reagent strips are commercially available for quick and qualitative analysis of several intermediates in urine, including protein, blood, leukocytes, nitrite, glucose, ketones (acetoacetic acid), pH, specific gravity, creatinine, bilirubin, and urobilinogen. Other strips allow the quick determination of reducing substances (glucose, lactose, fructose, galactose, pentoses, sulfite, etc). The interpretation of the results can be made by visual observation.

Qualitative tests. Complementing the reactive strip tests, there are simple qualitative assays that could bring useful information about the possible metabolic error present. The interpretation of the results can be made with simple sight, except the Ehrlich test and Bratton-Marshall reaction where a spectrophotometer is required.[2,3] The most common tests are as follows:

- Benedict test for reducing substances,
- 2,4-Dinitrophenylhydrazine) for α-keto acids,
- Nitroprusside test for cystine and homocystine,
- Nitrosonaphthol test for tyrosine metabolites,
- Ferric chloride test for PKU, Histidemia, MSUD, Tyrosinemia, Alkaptonuria, etc,
- Ehrlich test for porphyrins,
- Urine thiosulfate determination for defect of sulfite metabolism,
- Toluidine blue spot test for glycosaminoglycans (GAGs),
- Electrophoresis and thin-layer chromatography (TLC) of GAGs, oligosaccharides, sialyloligosaccharides, and
- Bratton-Marshall reaction.[21]

Spectrophotofluorometric Studies

These studies aim to determine total concentration of specific metabolites and to measure specific enzyme activities.[2,3,7-18,22-24] Chitotriosidase activity can be used for screening, as it is increased in plasma and DBS in several LSDs. Creatinine and protein determinations are generally performed as parameters to normalize other biochemical assays that refer its results to creatinine or protein concentrations, such as organic acids, GAGs, sialic acid, enzyme assays in tissues or leucocytes, and so on. Creatinine concentration is also an important parameter for the investigation of defects in the creatine metabolism. A summary of the most common spectrophotofluorometric measurements is presented in Table 1.

Gas Chromatography and MS

Organic acid assay (total ion chromatogram, TIC). This is one of the most informative assays that can be easily performed to investigate many IEM. Through a simple organic acid profile, it is possible to identify particular products related to a specific enzyme deficiency or to visualize "flags" that would help guide new studies. It is important to note that the organic acid profiles can be different in clinically sick and asymptomatic patients. As the number of new pathologies is growing fast, new key metabolites are being identified. Thus, it is not unusual reviewing old profiles, even those obtained years before. The organic acid profile also offers interesting information about enriched diet, drug intake, bacterial or plastic contamination, and so on.[2,3,25-28] A list of IEM that can be studied by organic assays is presented in Table 2.

Additional specific organic acid detection by GC and MS (simple ion monitoring, SIM). The extracted organic acids can also be analyzed by programming the mass spectrometer to detect only one or few isolated ions, allowing the identification and

Table 1. Details of Spectrophotoflurometric Assays and the IEM Studied.

Spectrophotoflurometric Assays	IEM
Carbohydrates and glycogen	
Total galactose test (P); Total fructose test (P);	Galactosemia
Total glycogen test and glycogen structure assay (P)[2,3]	Hereditary fructose intolerance
Enzyme assays[3]	Glycogenosis type Ia, II, IV, V, VI, VII, and IX
Galactose-1-phosphate, UDP-galactose-4-epimerase (P); fructose-bisphosphate aldolase, fructose-1,6-bisphosphatase (P); glucose-6-phosphatase (P); α-glucosidase (P); 1.4-α-glucan branching enzyme (P); phosphorylase (P); 6-hosphofructokinase (P); phosphorylase b-kinase (P)	
Pyruvate and ketone bodies	
Total Lactate, Pyruvate, and Ketone bodies tests (P)[2,3]	Pyruvate metabolism defects
Porphyrins	
Porphobilinogen test (P)[2,3]	Porphyrin metabolism defects
Pterins	
Dihydropteridine reductase assay (P)[2,3]	Pterin metabolism defects
Purine	
Bratton-Marshall reaction (P)[21]	Purine metabolism defect
Biotin	
Biotinidase enzyme assay (P)[2,3]	Biotinidase Deficiency
Lysosomal storage diseases (GAGs)	
Total urinary glycosaminoglycans (GAGs; P); plasma and urine free and total sialic acid test (P)[2,3,19,20]	Mucopolysaccharidoses (MPSs) Sialidosis, Galactosialidosis
Lysosomal Enzyme assays[2,3,7-18,22,24] β-galactosidose (F); β-glucosaminidase A (F); β-glucosaminidase A/ B (F); Arylsulfatase A (P); Galactocerebrosidase (F); α-galactosidose (F); β-glucosidase (F); Chitotriosidase (F); α-L-iduronidase (F); Iduro-2-sulfatase (F); Heparan-N-sulfatase (F); α-N-acetylglucosaminidase (F); Acetyl CoA:α-glucosaminide-N-acetyltransferase (F); N-acetylglucosamine-6-sulfate (F); N-acetylgalactosamine-6-sulfate (F); Arylsulatase B (P); β-glucuronidase (F); α-L-fucosidase (F); α-Mannosidase (F); β-Mannosidase (F); α-neuraminidase (F); Lipase (F); Ceramidase (F); α-N-acetylgalactosaminidase (F)	GM1 gangliosidoses; Mucolipidosis II/ III; B variant Tay-Sachs, B1 variant, Sandhoff disease; Metachromatic leukodystrophy; Multiple sulfatase Deficiency; Krabbe's disease; Fabry's disease; Gaucher's disease; Niemann-Pick disease types A/B/C; MPS types I, II, III-A, III-B, III-C, III-D, IV-A, VI, VII; Fucosidosis; α-Mannosidase; β-Mannosidase; Sialidosis; Galactosialidosis; Wolman disease. Cholesterol ester storage disease; Farber disease; Shindler Disease

Abbreviations: F, fluorometric assay; IEM, Inborn errors of metabolism; P, spectrophotometric assay.

quantification of metabolites at very low concentrations. The most important ions checked are usually succinylacetone (tyrosinemia type 1), orotic acid (urea cycle disorders), guanidinoacetoacetate (defects of creatine metabolism), methylmalonic acid (methylmalonic acidemia and disorder of cobalamin metabolism), mevalonic acid (mevalonic aciduria), and acetyl-N-aspartate (Canavan disease).[29-34]

Very long-chain fatty acids assay. Saturated and nonsaturated fatty acids and plasmalogens can be easily methylated and analyzed by GC/MS. The range of fatty acids to be screened include acids with medium-, long-, and very long-chain plasmalogens, along with pristanate and phytanate.[2,3] The fatty acid profile can give important information about possible peroxisomal disorder as described in Table 2.

Sterol profile assay. Sterols can be separated and identified by GC-MS (TIC and SIM modes). The range of pathologies studied is detailed subsequently. Similar to the organic acid profile, many "unknown metabolites" could be the future markers for novel enzyme deficiencies identified in the future, in the pre- or postsqualene steps of cholesterol synthesis.[2,3,35,36] A list of IEM that can be studied by the sterol profile is presented in Table 2.

Minimal Requirements for the Basic IEM Laboratory

Human Resources

Basically, the laboratory should count with qualified technicians for sample preparation, performance of the assays, and instrument operation. Inclusion of microtechniques with the use of multiwheel plate systems and/or microfluid-based enzyme assays[22] is recommended. Autosamplers for GC/MS or other robotic implements are also helpful. This means an enormous saving of expensive artificial substrates, buffers, reading times, and so on. Well-organized laboratories are more efficient, saving time, human effort, and chemical products.

Table 2. Details of GC/MS assays and the IEM studied.

GC/MS ASSAYS	IEM
Urine organic acid assay GC/MS, TIC[2,3,25–28] GC/MS, SIM[29–34]	Defects of aromatic amino acid metabolism Phenylketonuria, tyrosinemia, hawkinsinuria, alkaptonuria Defects of branched chain amino acids metabolism Maple urine syrup disease, dihydrolipoyl dehydrogenase (E3) deficiency, isovaleric acidemia, 3-methylcrotonyl-CoA carboxilase deficiency, multiple carboxylase deficiency, 3-methylglutaconic aciduria, 3-OH-3-methylglutaric aciduria, 3-oxothiolase deficiency, propionic acidemia, methylmalonic acidemia, malonyl-CoA decarboxylase deficiency Defects of dibasic amino acids metabolism Glutaric aciduria type I, 2-Ketoadipic aciduria Defects of fatty acid oxidation/pyruvate/Krebbs cycle/ mitochondrial respiratory chain Long-, medium-, and short-chain acyl-coA dehydrogenase deficiency, multiple acyl-CoA dehydrogenase deficiency Lactic acidemia (pyruvate carboxylase deficiency, pyruvate dehydrogenase deficiency, multiple carboxylase deficiency, defects in oxidative phosphorylation), 2-ketoglutarate dehydrogenase deficiency, fumarase deficiency, Barth syndrome Other organic acidurias: 5-Oxo-prolinuria, D-2-OH-glutaric aciduria, 4-OH-butiric aciduria, Canavan disease, mevalonic aciduria, n-glyceric aciduria, glyceroluria, hyperoxaluria, ketosis, Reye's syndrome, thymine and uracil acidurias. Urea cycle disorders and defects of creatine metabolism
Plasma very long-chain fatty acid assay GC/MS, TIC/SIM[2,3]	X-ALD, defects of phytanic/pristanic acid metabolism, infantile Refsum disease, RCDP, Zellweger and Zellweger-like syndromes, dihydroxyacetone phosphate acyltransferase deficiency
Plasma Sterol profile assay GC/MS, TIC/SIM[2,3,35,36]	Mevalonate kinase deficiency, CHILD syndrome, CDPX2. Greenberg dysplasia, Smith-Lemli-Opitz syndrome, lathosterolosis, desmosterolosis, sitosterolemia, CTX.

Abbreviations: CDPX2, X linked dominant Conradi-Hünermann chondrodysplasia; CTX, cerebrotendineos xanthomatosis; GC/MS, gas chromatography/mass spectrometry system; IEM, inborn errors of metabolism; RCDP, rhizomelic chondrodysplasia punctata; SIM, simple ion chromatogram mode; TIC, total ion chromatogram mode; X-ALD, X linked adrenoleukodystrphy.

The technicians should be backed by professionals who have a background in inherited metabolic diseases to evaluate the results and to take the appropriate actions to confirm positive cases and direct the patients to quick management and therapy.

For the assessment of laboratory performance, it is very important to adhere to international schemes of quality control, such as ERNDIM, CDC, and others.

Installations and Instruments

The laboratory should have an appropriate size (around 100 m^2 is recommended), with adequate ventilation and temperature control. This last point is especially important due to the sensitive instrumentation required. Work benches, hermetic hood for manipulation of toxic gases, nitrogen and helium tanks, and a safe system for reagent storage and for discarding dangerous substances are also necessary.

A spectrophotoflurometer and a GC/MS are the major instruments required for the basic IEM laboratory. It is important to subscribe to maintenance programs. The first instrument is a single machine with UV-visible and fluorescence detectors. In the case that a spectrophotometer is already available, only a spectrofluorometer needs to be added.

Minor instruments also are required, and these are similar to the ones available in a basic biochemical laboratory, including vortex, pH meter, digital balance, water bath, plate incubator, TLC and electrophoresis systems, and so on.

Final Considerations

Figure 1 shows a flowchart for the biochemical study of IEM. It is clear that a vast number of IEM can be explored with this basic laboratory. Evidently, not all IEM will be covered, but the most important areas will be studied. The relatively low cost of the major equipment required to run this laboratory makes them quite affordable, especially when compared to the high cost of an MS/MS or other sophisticated equipment. This is essentially important in countries or regions where there is a lack of specialized centers to perform these studies. Once the basic laboratory is running, the range of the pathologies investigated can be expanded, incorporating new equipment, such as an amino acid analyzer, HPLC, MS/MS, and instruments for molecular genetic tests and for cell culture. Local or regional incidence of IEM and the availability of therapies should be considered for such expansion. If the resources are very limited, a GC/MS instrument should be the first option because of the large scope of IEM that can be studied through a simple chromatography profiling of organic acids, very long chain fatty acids, and sterols.

Finally, we should emphasize that the IEM are "rare diseases" when considered individually, but the entire group has a

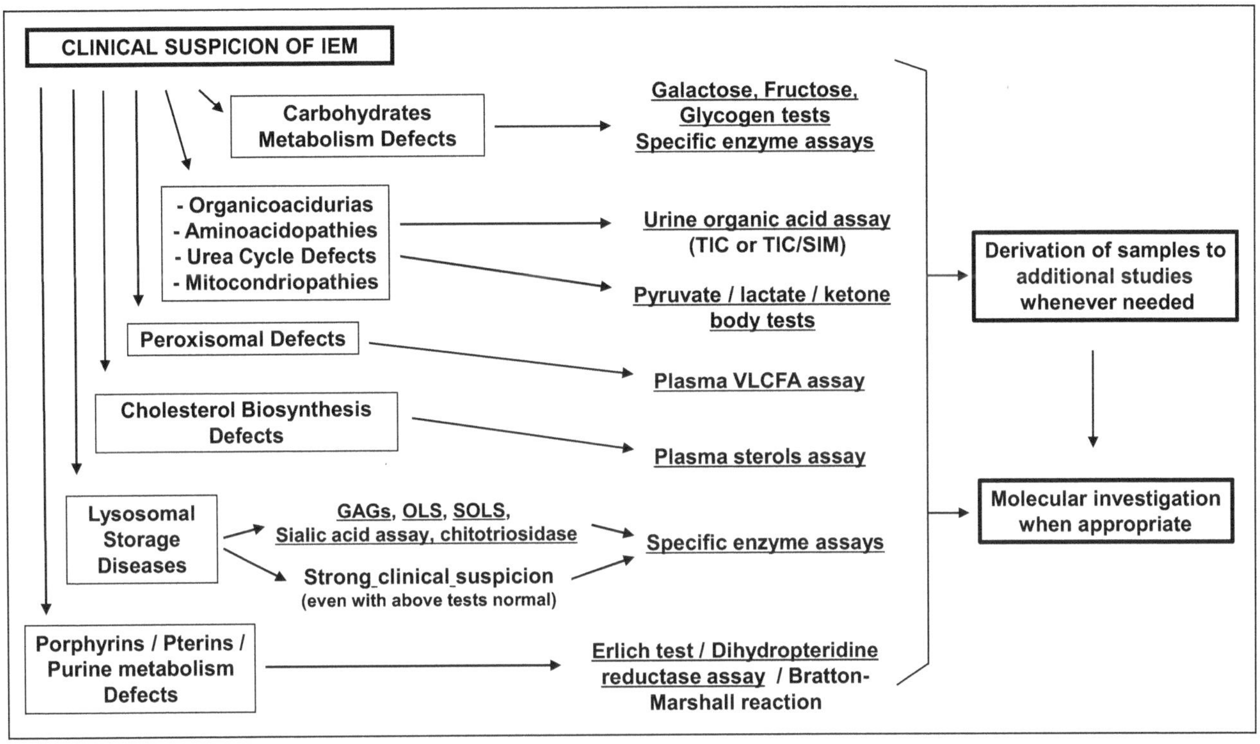

Figure 1. Proposed flow chart for the biochemical study of IEM.

frequency higher than 1 per 1000 births. Moreover, the number of patients detected and the definition of new IEM are continually expanding worldwide.[37-40] Many centers dedicated to the study of IEM are offering regular courses and training to physicians, biochemists, biologists, and related professionals, helping to extend the knowledge of these diseases and to encourage the health authorities and other international institutions to take appropriate actions to address these diseases.

Acknowledgments

This review was possible due to the continuous help and support provided along for many years by professionals from: (1) the Center for Study of Inherited Metabolic Diseases (CEMECO), Cordoba, Argentina; (2) Hugo and Ann Moser, Richard Kelley, Lisa Kratz, and professionals from the Kennedy Krieger Institute, Baltimore, USA; (3) professionals from the Medical Genetics Service of the Hospital de Clínicas de Porto Alegre, Brazil.

Declaration of Conflicting Interests

The author(s) declared no potential conflicts of interest with respect to the research, authorship, and/or publication of this article.

Funding

The author(s) received no financial support for the research, authorship, and/or publication of this article.

References

1. Scriver CR, Beaudet AL, Sly WS. *Metabolic and Molecular Basis of Inherited Disease, Eighth ed.* New York: McGraw Hill; 2001.
2. Hommes FA. *Techniques in Diagnostic Human Biochemical Genetics*. New York, NY: Wiley-Liss John Wiley & son; 1991.
3. Blau N, Duran M, Gibson KM. *Laboratory Guide to the Methods in Biochemical Genetics*. Heidelberg, Germany: Springer-Verlag Berlin; 2008.
4. Chace DH, Kalas TA. A biochemical perspective on the use of tandem mass spectrometry for newborn screening and clinical testing. *Clin Biochem*. 2005;38(4):296-309.
5. Haynes CA, De Jesús VR. Simultaneous quantitation of hexacosanoyl lysophosphatidylcholine, amino acids, acylcarnitines, and succinylacetone during FIA–ESI–MS/MS analysis of dried blood spot extracts for newborn screening. *Clin Chem*. 2016; 49(1-2):161-165.
6. Tortorelli S, Turgeon CT, Gavrilov DK, et al. Simultaneous testing for 6 lysosomal storage disorders and X-adrenoleukodystrophy in dried blood spots by tandem mass spectrometry. *Clin Chem*. 2016; 62(9):1248-1254.
7. Chamoles NA, Blanco MB, Gaggioli D, Casentini C. Hurler-like phenotype: enzymatic diagnosis in dried blood spots on filter paper. *Clin Chem*. 2001;47(12):2098-2102.
8. Chamoles NA, Blanco M, Gaggioli D, Casentini C. Gaucher and Niemann-Pick diseases-enzymatic diagnosis in dried blood spots on filter paper: retrospective diagnoses in newborn-screening cards. *Clin Chim Acta*. 2002;317(1-2):191-197.
9. Civallero G, Michelin K, de Mari J, et al. Twelve different enzyme assays on dried-blood filter paper samples to detection of patients with selected inherited lysosomal storage diseases. *Clin Chim Acta*. 2006;372(1-2):98-102.
10. Camelier MV, Burin MG, De Mari J, Vieira TA, Marasca G, Giugliani R. Practical and reliable enzyme test for the detection

of Mucopolysaccharidosis IVA (Morquio Syndrome type A) in dried blood samples. *Clin Chim Acta.* 2011;412(19-20):1805-1808.

11. Oemardien LF, Boer AM, Ruijter GJ, et al. Hemoglobin precipitation greatly improves 4-methylumbelliferone-based diagnostic assays for lysosomal storage diseases in dried blood spots. *Mol Genet Metab.* 2011;102(1):44-48.
12. Tolun AA, Graham C, Shi Q, et al. A novel fluorometric enzyme analysis method for Hunter syndrome using dried blood spots. *Mol Genet Metab.* 2012;105(3):519-521.
13. Ullal AJ, Millington DS, Bali DS. Development of a fluorometric microtiter plate based enzyme assay for MPS IVA (Morquio type A) using dried blood spots. *Mol Genet Metab Rep.* 2014;22(1):461-464.
14. Hamilton J, Jones I, Srivastava R, Galloway P. A new method for the measurement of lysosomal acid lipase in dried blood spots using the inhibitor Lalistat 2. *Clin Chim Acta.* 2012;413(15-16):1207-1210.
15. Civallero G, De Mari J, Bittar C, Burin M, Giugliani R. Extended use of a selective inhibitor of acid lipase for the diagnosis of Wolman disease and cholesteryl ester storage disease. *Gene.* 2014;539(1):154-156.
16. Civallero G, De Mari J, Viapiana Camelier M, Burin M, Giugliani R. Assay of heparan-N-sulfamidase in dried leukocytes impregnated in filter paper: a new tool for the identification of mucopolysaccharidosis IIIA and potentially other lysosomal diseases. *Mol Gen Metab.* 2013;108(4):267-268.
17. Camelier M, Civallero G, De Mari J, Burin M, Giugliani R. Galactocerebrosidase assay on dried-leukocytes impregnated in filter paper for the detection of Krabbe disease. *Clin Chim Acta.* 2015;438:178-180.
18. Camelier M, De Mari J, Burin M, Civallero G, Giugliani R. Extended use of dried-leukocytes impregnated in filter paper samples for detection of Pompe, Gaucher, and Morquio A diseases. *Clin Chim Acta.* 2015;446:218-220.
19. Whitley CB, Draper KA, Dutton CM, Brown PA, Severson SL, France LA. Diagnostic test for mucopolysaccharidosis. II. Rapid quantification of glycosaminoglycan in urine samples collected on a paper matrix. *Clin Chem.* 1989;35(10):2074-2081.
20. Civallero G, Bender F, Gomes A, et al. Reliable detection of mucopolysacchariduria in dried-urine filter paper samples. *Clin Chim Acta.* 2013;415:334-336.
21. Laikind PK, Seegmiller JE, Gruber HE. Detection of 5'-phosphoribosyl-4-(N-succinylcarboxamide)-5-aminoimidazole in urine by use of the Bratton-Marshall reaction: identification of patients deficient in adenylosuccinate lyase activity. *Anal Biochem.* 1986;156(1):81-90.
22. Sista RA, Wang T, Wu N, et al. Multiplex newborn screening for Pompe, Fabry, Hunter, Gaucher, and Hurler diseases using a digital microfluidic platform. *Clin Chim Acta.* 2013;424:12-18.
23. Bedia C, Camacho L, Abad JL, Fabriàs G, Levade T. A simple fluorogenic method for determination of acid ceramidase activity and diagnosis of Farber disease. *J Lipid Res.* 2010;51(12):3542-3547.
24. Vines DJ, Warburton MJ. Classical late infantile neuronal ceroid lipofuscinosis fibroblasts are deficient in lysosomal tripeptidyl peptidase I. *FEBS Lett.* 1999;443(2):131-135.
25. Tanaka K, West-Dull A, Hine DG, Lynn TB, Lowe T. Gas-chromatographic method of analysis for urinary organic acids. II. Description of the procedure, and its application to diagnosis of patient with organic acidurias. *Clin Chem.* 1980;26(13):1847-1853.
26. Tanaka K, Hine DG, West-Dull A, Lynn TB. Gas-chromatographic methods of analysis for urinary organic acids. I- Retention indices of 155 metabolically important compounds. *Clin Chem.* 1980;26(13):1839-1846.
27. Chalmers RA, Lawson AM. *Organic Acids in Man: Analytical Chemistry, Biochemistry and Diagnosis of the Organic Acidurias.* London, UK: Chapman and Hall; 1982.
28. Thompson JA, Miles BS, Fennessey PV. Urinary organic acids quantitated by age groups in a healthy pediatric population. *Clin Chem.* 1977;23(9):1734-1738.
29. Cyr D, Giguère R, Villain G, Lemieux B, Drouin R. A GC/MS validated method for the nanomolar range determination of succinylacetone in amniotic fluid and plasma: an analytical tool for tyrosinemia type I. *J Chromatogr B Analyt Technol Biomed Life Sci.* 2006;832(1):24-29.
30. McCann MT, Thompson MM, Gueron IC, Tuchman M. Quantification of orotic acid in dried filter-paper urine samples by stable isotope dilution. *Clin Chem.* 1995;41(5):739-743.
31. Struys EA, Jansen EE, ten Brink HJ, Verhoeven NM, van der Knaap MS, Jakobs C. An accurate stable isotope dilution gas chromatographic-mass spectrometric approach to the diagnosis of guanidinoacetate methyltransferase deficiency. *J Pharm Biomed Anal.* 1998;18(4-5):659-665.
32. Straczek J, Felden F, Dousset B, Gueant JL, Belleville F. Quantification of methylmalonic acid in serum measured by gas chromatography-mass spectrometry as tert.-butyldimethylsilyl derivatives. *J Chromatogr.* 1993;620(1):1-7.
33. Lindenthal B, von Bergmann K. Determination of urinary mevalonic acid using isotope dilution technique. *Biol Mass Spectrom.* 1994;23(7):445-450.
34. Kelley RI, Stamas JN. Quantification of N-acetyl-L-aspartic acid in urine by isotope-dilution gas chromatography-mass spectrometry. *J Inher Metab Dis.* 1991;15(1):97-104.
35. Kelley RI. Diagnosis of Smith-Lemli-Opitz syndrome by gas chromatography/mass spectrometry of 7-dehydrocholesterol in plasma, amniotic fluid and cultured skin fibroblasts. *Clin Chim Acta.* 1995;236(1):45-58.
36. He M, Kratz LE, Michel JJ, et al. Mutations in the human SC4MOL gene encoding a methyl sterol oxidase cause psoriasiform dermatitis, microcephaly, and developmental delay. *J Clin Invest.* 2010;121(3):976-984.
37. Ferreira CR, Gahl WA. Lysosomal storage diseases. *Transl Sci Rare Dis.* 2017;2(1-2):1-71.
38. Gilbert-Barness E, Farrell PM. Approach to diagnosis of metabolic diseases. *Transl Sci Rare Dis.* 2016;1(1):3-22.
39. Wanders RJ, Waterham HR, Ferdinandusse S. Metabolic interplay between peroxisomes and other subcellular organelles including mitochondria and the endoplasmic reticulum. *Front Cell Dev Biol.* 2016;3:83. https://doi.org/10.3389/fcell.2015.00083.
40. Corso G, Dello Russo A, Gelzo M. Liver and the defects of cholesterol and bile acids biosynthesis: rare disorders many diagnostic pitfalls. *World J Gastroenterol.* 2017;23(29):5257-5265.

24

Hematopoietic Stem Cell Transplantation in Mucopolysaccharidosis Type II

Anneliese L. Barth, MD, PhD[1] and Dafne D. G. Horovitz, MD, PhD[1]

Abstract

Mucopolysaccharidosis II (MPS II—Hunter syndrome) is an X-linked lysosomal storage disorder caused by a deficiency in iduronate-2 sulfatase. Enzyme replacement therapy does not cross the blood–brain barrier (BBB), limiting the results in neurological forms of the disease. Another treatment option for MPS, hematopoietic stem cell transplantation (HSCT) has become the treatment of choice for the severe form of MPS I since it can preserve neurocognition when performed early in the course of the disease. Even though the intravenous therapy does not cross the BBB, it has become the recommended treatment for MPS II, and HSCT was not often indicated. In an attempt to understand why this treatment modality is rejected by most specialists as a treatment option for patients with Hunter syndrome, we sought to raise all HSCT cases already reported in the scientific literature. Databases used were Medline/PubMed, Lilacs/BVS Cochrane Library, DARE, SciELO, and SCOPUS. Different combinations of the terms "mucopolysaccharidosis II," "Hunter syndrome," "hematopoietic stem cell transplantation," "bone marrow transplantation," and "umbilical cord blood stem cell transplantation" were used. A total of 780 articles were found. After excluding redundant references and articles not related to the theme, 26 articles were included. A descriptive summary of each article is presented, and the main features are summed up. The clinical experience with HSCT in MPS II is small, and most of the available literature is outdated. The available data reveal poor patient selection criteria, varied conditioning regimens, distinct follow-up parameters, and post-HSCT outcomes of interest, making impossible to compare and generalize the results obtained. Recently, after the development of new conditioning protocols and techniques and the creation of bone marrow donor registries and umbilical cord banks, HSCT has become more secure and accessible. It seems now appropriate to reconsider HSCT as a treatment option for the neuronopathic form of MPS II.

Keywords

mucopolysaccharidosis type II, hunter syndrome, hematopoietic stem cell transplantation, bone marrow transplantation, umbilical cord blood stem cell transplantation

Introduction

Mucopolysaccharidosis II (MPS II, Hunter syndrome, OMIM 309900) is an X-linked lysosomal storage disorder caused by a deficiency in the enzyme iduronate-2 sulfatase (I2 S), leading to the accumulation of the glycosaminoglycans (GAG) dermatan sulfate and heparan sulfate.[1] Mucopolysaccharidosis II affects multiple organs and systems with a variable age of onset of signs and symptoms. Two clinical presentations of Hunter syndrome have been reported, the mild, or attenuated, and the severe forms. The severe phenotype, with primary neural parenchymal disease, is referred as neuronopathic MPS II and the mild phenotype, without neural parenchymal involvement, as non-neuronopathic MPS II. The distinguishing factor between the 2 forms is the presence or absence of progressive intellectual deterioration. Both phenotypes exhibit cardiorespiratory and skeletal disease[2]

In 1968, Fratantoni et al[3] first established that substrate accumulation in the cells of patients with lysosomal enzyme deficiencies could be dramatically reduced by coculturing these cells

[1] Instituto Nacional de Saúde da Mulher, da Criança e do Adolescente Fernandes Figueira/Fiocruz – Rio de Janeiro, Brazil

Corresponding Author:

Anneliese L. Barth, Instituto Nacional de Saúde da Mulher, da Criança e do Adolescente Fernandes Figueira/Fiocruz – Rio de Janeiro, Brazil.

Email: anne.barth@iff.fiocruz.br

with cells producing the missing enzyme.[3] The principle of "cross-correction" was subsequently used to explore both exogenous enzyme replacement therapy (ERT) and allogeneic hematopoietic stem cell transplantation (HSCT) in numerous lysosomal disorders. As HSCT also enables engraftment of donor-derived microglial cells in the brain—serving as local enzyme production units—this treatment, contrary to ERT that does not cross the blood–brain barrier (BBB), has the potential to treat central nervous system (CNS) manifestations.[4]

Hematopoietic stem cell transplantation has been tested in various disorders and become the treatment of choice for the severe form of MPS I (Hurler syndrome) since it can preserve neurocognition when performed early in the course of the disease.[5–9] Compared to Hurler syndrome, the overall experience in the use of HSCT for treatment of other MPS types (II, III, IV, VI, and VII) is very limited, often evaluated only as part of large heterogeneous cohorts of transplanted patients with multiple metabolic diseases or as few case reports and with variable results.[10–12] Nevertheless, the scientific basis for the effectiveness of HSCT across the MPS spectrum remains the same: donor-derived cells would secrete the deficient enzyme, which would be recaptured by surrounding cells. The kinetics of cellular migration, differentiation, distribution, and effective enzyme delivery, however, may differ among MPS subtypes.

After 2006, with the approval of Elaprase (idursulfase, Shire Human Genetics Therapies, Inc., Cambridge, MA, USA), ERT has become the treatment of choice for patients with Hunter syndrome. Even though the intravenous therapy is known not to cross the BBB, being unable to prevent neurodegeneration in the neuronopathic form of MPS II, the HSCT was discouraged and no longer performed in most Western countries.[13]

In an attempt to understand why HSCT is rejected by most experts as a treatment option for MPS II, all articles and/or cases reported in the scientific literature were reviewed and analyzed.

Material and Methods

Controlled and randomized clinical trials are considered the gold standard of evidence on the effect of an intervention.[14] Due to the rarity of MPS II, controlled and randomized clinical trials evaluating the efficacy of HSCT on disease progression do not exist and are unlikely to occur. Therefore, in an attempt to evaluate the results obtained so far and to understand why HSCT has been rejected by most specialists as a therapeutic modality for MPS II, it was sought to raise all cases already reported in the scientific literature on the participant.

The study was divided into 3 stages:

- Phase 1—Search for primary studies.
- Phase 2—Selection of articles.
- Phase 3—Data analysis.

Phase 1—Search for Primary Studies

The electronic search was performed in the following databases: Medline/PubMed, Lilacs/BVS Cochrane Library, DARE, SciELO, and SCOPUS. The abovementioned databases were selected because they cover a large number of journals from different countries.

In an attempt to identify the largest possible number of articles for inclusion in the review, a more sensitive search strategy was performed, to the detriment of specificity. Different combinations of the terms "mucopolysaccharidosis II," "Hunter syndrome," "hematopoietic stem cell transplantation," "bone marrow transplantation," and "umbilical cord blood stem cell transplantation" were used in the various databases after consultation in the Medical Subject Heading and Subject Descriptor.

Case reports presented at congresses and published in special supplements of indexed journals were included, but there was no search in the gray literature (which comprises the literature not formally published) since there would be no guarantee as to the veracity and authenticity of data.

No date limit was set for the research since the objective was to find as many articles as possible in the literature. The searches were conducted until July 2017. The oldest article retrieved was from 1986.

Phase 2—Selection of Articles

Because MPS II is a rare condition, we did not expect to find a large number of articles and/or case reports. For this reason, all articles on HSCT in patients with Hunter syndrome were included in the evaluation, excluding only those whose transplantation was performed in patients with other MPS types than MPS II and those who evaluated the HSCT animal models of MPS II.

All studies identified in the initial search, respecting the exclusion criteria, had their summaries evaluated. When these were not available, the full article was studied.

Phase 3—Data analysis

The data were synthesized in a descriptive way, based on the results presented in each article.

Results

In the absence of formal studies evaluating HSCT as a therapeutic modality for MPS II, it was sought to collect all previously published articles on the subject and to briefly describe all cases of HSCT II already described in MPS II.

After defining the terms used in the bibliographic search and consulting the selected databases, 780 articles were found (Table 1). Many electronic databases index the same periodicals, and redundant references were retrieved. The fact we used more than one search mechanism on some databases, also contributed to redundancy. Of the total number of articles retrieved, 659 were excluded after reading the title and/or summary, remaining 121. After the exclusion of the repeated

Table 1. Synthesis of the Electronic Bases Used, Search Tools Used in Each Base and Number of References Found.

Database	Number of References
Search tool	
Medline/PubMed	
Mucopolysaccharidosis II [MeSH] AND hematopoietic stem cell transplantation[MeSH]	17
Mucopolysaccharidosis II [MeSH] AND cord blood stem cell transplantation [MeSH]	2
Mucopolysaccharidosis II [MeSH] AND bone marrow transplantation [MeSH]	20
Mucopolysaccharidosis II OR Hunter syndrome AND hematopoietic stem cell transplantation	57
Mucopolysaccharidosis IIOR Hunter syndrome AND cord blood stem cell transplantation	15
Mucopolysaccharidosis II OR Hunter syndrome AND bone marrow transplantation	7
LILACS/BVS	
Mucopolissacaridose II (DeCS) AND transplante de células-tronco hematopoiéticas (DeCS)	31
Mucopolissacaridose II (DeCS) AND transplante de medula óssea (DeCS)	29
Mucopolissacaridose II (DeCS) AND transplante de células-tronco do cordão umbilical (DeCS)	7
Cochrane Library	
Mucopolysaccharidosis II [MeSH] AND hematopoietic stem cell transplantation[MeSH]	0
Mucopolysaccharidosis II [MeSH] AND cord blood stem cell transplantation [MeSH]	0
Mucopolysaccharidosis II [MeSH] AND bone marrow transplantation [MeSH]	0
DARE	
Mucopolysaccharidosis II AND hematopoietic stem cell transplantation	0
Mucopolysaccharidosis II AND cord blood stem cell transplantation	0
Mucopolysaccharidosis II AND bone marrow transplantation	0
SciELO	
Mucopolysaccharidosis II AND hematopoietic stem cell transplantation	0
Mucopolysaccharidosis II AND cord blood stem cell transplantation	0
Mucopolysaccharidosis II AND bone marrow transplantation	2
Hunter syndrome AND hematopoietic stem cell transplantation	0
Hunter syndrome AND cord blood stem cell transplantation	0
Hunter syndrome AND bone marrow transplantation	2
SCOPUS	
Mucopolysaccharidosis II AND hematopoietic stem cell transplantation	67
Mucopolysaccharidosis II AND cord blood stem cell transplantation	118
Mucopolysaccharidosis II AND bone marrow transplantation	3
Hunter syndrome AND hematopoietic stem cell transplantation	143
Hunter syndrome AND cord blood stem cell transplantation	253
Hunter syndrome AND bone marrow transplantation	7

Abbreviations: DeCS, Subject Descriptor; MeSH, Medical Subject Heading.

articles, 37 articles were read in full. Of these, 11 were still excluded because they only referred to HSCT previously described or because they dealt with ethical issues regarding HSCT in Hunter syndrome, leaving 26 articles that were included in this review (Figure 1).

A descriptive summary of each article retrieved and included in this review is presented below. The main features of the articles are also summed up (Table 2).

The first patient with Hunter syndrome treated with HSCT who had clinical and biochemical data reported was described in 1986 by Warketin et al.[15] The patient underwent HSCT at 7 years and 5 months, had an initial intelligence quotient (IQ) of 87, which dropped to 73 (mainly due to language delay), and stabilized after transplantation. He presented reduction in skin lesions and hirsutism, improvement in joint stiffness and mobility, resolution of hepatosplenomegaly, and normalization of urinary and CSF excretion of GAG. The activity at I2 S normalized in leukocytes but remained well below normal range in plasma. After 3½ years of transplantation, the patient died suddenly and necropsy revealed GAG deposition of GAG in the heart valves and in the brain.

In 1994, Bergstrom et al[16] reported the results of HSCT in a 14-year non-neuronopathic patient. Three years after the procedure, the patient presented significant improvement, both subjectively and objectively, in the symptoms of the disease. There was resolution of cutaneous nodules and hepatosplenomegaly, attenuation of facial features, improvement in joint mobility, especially in the hands and the echocardiogram showed reduction in the valvular leaflets thickness with resolution of mitral insufficiency. The patient returned to school 7 months after the transplant and continued to have gains in his intellectual function.

Another case of HSCT in a patient with non-neuronopathic MPS II was described by Imaizumi et al[17] in 1994. The patient was transplanted at 9 years and 10 months, and 1½ year later, he showed improvements in his facial appearance, joint contractures, hepatomegaly, skin lesions, and height. Cardiac valve dysfunction did not progress, but there was no improvement in sensorineural hearing loss nor in bone deformities.

Miniero et al[18] also in 1994 reported the case of a 31-month patient with the neuronopathic form of MPS II who received granulocyte colony-stimulating factor (G-CSF) after bone marrow transplantation. Complete chimerism was confirmed at 11 and 80 days after transplantation. He had no complications or graft versus host disease. Two months after transplantation, skin and liver biopsies show stabilization of the disease. Six

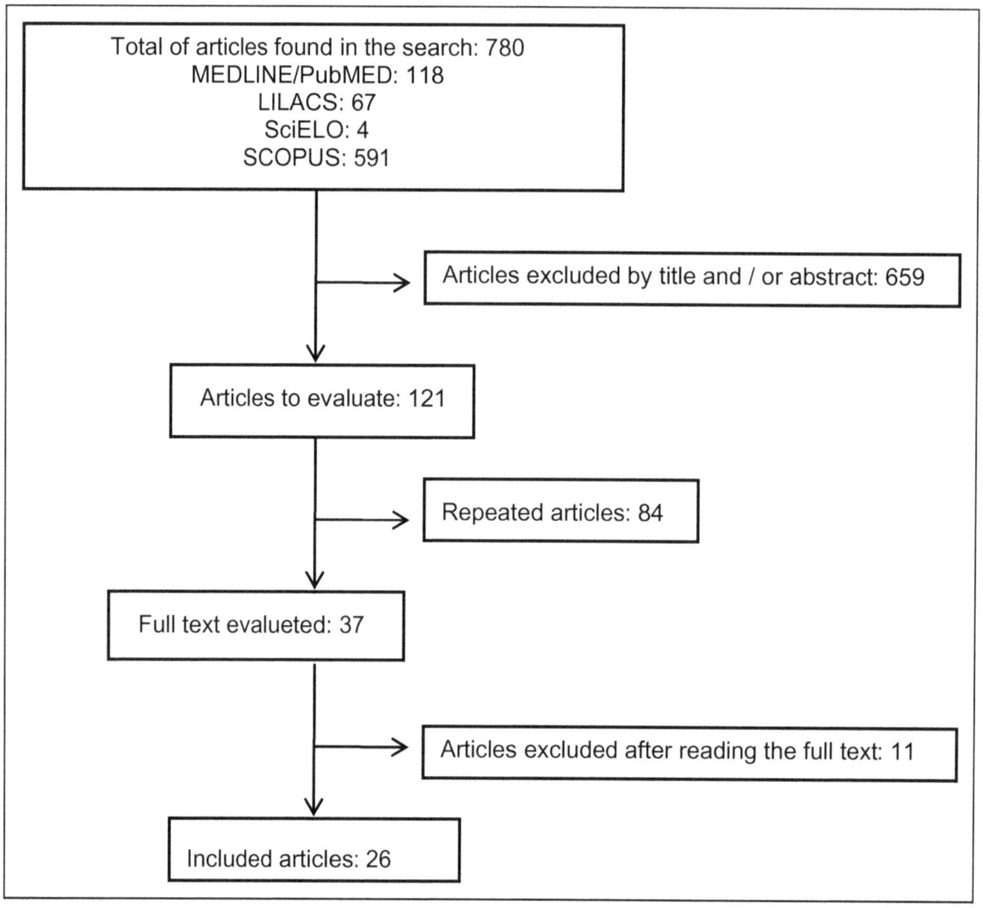

Figure 1. Flowchart of article selection.

months after transplantation, there was reduction in the urinary GAG excretion to near normal levels, and the activity of I2 S in leukocytes normalized, while in plasma remained undetectable. Administration of G-CSF did not induce proliferation of bone marrow histiocytes. This report suggested that G-CSF should be recommended for patients undergoing HSCT in order to reduce the period of neutropenia associated with the chemotherapy regimen preparatory to transplantation.

Coppa et al,[19] in 1995, reported the 2-year follow-up of a patient transplanted with 2 years and 9 months. During the period, there was normalization of hepatosplenomegaly, resumption of growth curve, reduction in skin thickness and hirsutism, and important improvement in joint mobility. The evaluation of the bone inventory showed stabilization of clinical condition in relation to the pretransplantation state, as well as brain magnetic resonance imaging (MRI) and audiometry. The echocardiogram showed ventricular size normalization; the urinary GAG excretion decreased progressively over the first 6 months and stabilized at levels close to normal. Enzymatic activity in leukocytes normalized but remained well below the normal range in plasma. The longitudinal neuropsychological evaluation showed significant worsening after the third month of transplantation, especially regarding verbal capacity. Twenty months after transplantation, there was partial recovery in motor and interpersonal skills, while verbal performance remained unchanged.

In 1996, McKinnes et al[20] reported the case of a transplanted patient in 1988 at 29 months of age. After 5½ years, leukocyte I2 S levels were normal whereas in plasma they were only 25% of normal. Urinary GAG excretion decreased to levels near to the upper limit of normal. Serial liver biopsies showed a significant reduction in deposited material in all cell types; however, serial rectal biopsies demonstrated GAG deposition in neural structures, with reduction in deposition in non-neural structures. There was improvement in some somatic symptoms such as the face and hair and in joint mobility, but skeletal deformities and auditory deficit did not improve, although did not progress either. Despite the clinical success of the transplant, with good grafting, normal levels of I2 S and physical improvement, the intellectual status continued to deteriorate. At 8 years of age, cognitive test results showed an IQ <20, compatible with a 6-month-old child. There was loss of intellectual capacity, adaptive functions, and language skills associated with behavior problems.

Also in 1996, Li et al[21] described the follow-up of a patient with the neuronopathic form of MPS II submitted to HSCT at 5 years. Liver and spleen returned to normal size and urinary GAG excretion normalized 1 year after transplantation. Three

Table 2. Summary of the Main Features of the Articles.

Author/Year	N° Pat.	Age at HSCT	Deaths	Phenotype	GAG	I2S	Neurol. Evaluation	Graft Failure	GVHD	Conclusion
Warketin et al, 1986	1	7 years 5 months	1		X	X	X			Necropsy: GAG deposits on heart and brain
Bergstrom et al, 1994	1	14 years		NN			X			Somatic and neurological benefit
Imaizumi et al, 1994	1	9 years 10 months		NN						Somatic benefit (except on hearing and bones)
Miniero et al, 1994	1	2 years 7 months			X	X				Uses of granulocyte colony stimulating factor
Coppa et al, 1995	1	2 years 9 months			X	X	X			Somatic and some neurological benefit
McKinnes et al, 1996	1	2 years 5 months			X	X	X			Somatic benefit but IQ reduction
Li et al, 1996	1	5 years		N	X	X	X			Somatic benefit and IQ stabilization
Vellodi et al, 1999	10	10 months-5 years 1 month	7				X			IQ reduction in 2 pat. and stabilization in the third
Coppa et al, 1999	1	3 years		NN	X	X	X			Somatic benefit and IQ stabilization
Mullen et al, 2000	1	10 months		NN						Somatic benefit but hemolytic anemia
Ito, 2004	5	4 years-11 years								Dermatological evaluation (papules)
Ochiai et al, 2005	3	5 years-8 years								Ultrastructural evaluation of peripheral nerves
Escolar et al, 2007	5	3 month-3 years 4 month	1				X	X (1)	X (1)	Neurological benefit. Uses of cord blood
Guffon et al, 2009	8	3 years-16 years	1	N(4)/NN(3)	X	X	X			Somatic benefit. Distinct neurological outcomes
Araya et al, 2009	1	6 years	1	N						Necropsy: I2 S activity in microglia
Poe et al, 2011	9	1.5 month-3 years 11 month	2				X			Neurological benefit but with some delay
Escolar et al, 2012	9	1.5 month-3 years 11 months					X			Continuous benefit, although slower
Tanaka et al, 2012	21	2 years-19 years		N/NN						Valid before cerebral atrophy and cardiac disease
Annibali et al, 2013	4	2 years 6 months-2 years 11 months		N			X			Neurological deterioration slower than expected
Patel et al, 2014	18									Only growth was evaluated
Tanjuakio et al, 2015	20			N/NN						Activities of daily living in MPS II
Cagle, 2015	1	3 years 1 month								No signs of regression until 4 years
Wang et al, 2016	12	2 years-6 years					X			Neurological benefit
Muschol et al, 2016	2	2 years 1 month-4 years 3 month			X	X				Neurological decline in 1 and stabilization in another
Barth et al, 2017	1	70 days		N	X	X	X			HSCT seems effective and can be considered
Kubaski et al, 2017	27			N/NN	X					HSCT seems effective and can be considered

Abbreviations: GAG, glycosaminoglycans; GVHD, graft versus host disease; HSCT, hematopoietic stem cell transplantation; I2 S, iduronate-2 sulfatase; IQ, intelligence quotient; MPS, mucopolysaccharidosis; N, neuronopathic; NN, non-neuronopathic; No. Pat, Number of patients.

years after HSCT, there was improvement in joint mobility and motor capacity and stabilization of the neurocognitive and cardiac functions. Plasma I2 S activity reached the normal limit 4 years after HSCT and remained around 60% of the normal value in leukocytes.

Vellodi et al[22] reported, in 1999, the long-term follow-up of 3 patients with MPS II undergoing HSCT from an initial cohort of 10 transplanted patients. Of these, 7 died after transplantation (performed between 1982 and 1985). Of the 3 patients who survived, 2 (1 transplanted at 20 months and another transplanted at 5 years and 1 month) showed progression of the neurodegenerative process. The third patient, submitted to HSCT at 10 months, presented stabilization of the neurological condition. After 7 years of transplantation, he had a borderline IQ of 78, a certain difficulty in concentration, but continued to attend regular school. The latter patient presented a positive family history for MPS II and comparatively post-HSCT presented a better outcome than his affected maternal uncle.

Also in 1999, Coppa et al[23] reported a 4-year follow-up of a patient with the non-neuronopathic form of MPS II submitted to HSCT at 3 years. There was attenuation of facial features, skin was less thick, abdominal ultrasonography showed resolution of hepatosplenomegaly, and he presented only small joint limitation. His IQ remained stable at 70, he spoke short phrases and knew some letters of the alphabet. Ultrastructural analysis of hepatocytes and fibroblasts showed only a few remaining vacuoles. Regarding the biochemical parameters, the urinary GAG excretion and the activity of I2 S in leukocytes normalized.

Mullen et al[24] described the long-term outcome of HSCT in a 10-month boy with non-neuronopathic MPS II. There was resolution of hepatomegaly, and his growth and development were normal; however, after 9 months, transplantation was complicated by the development of autoimmune hemolytic anemia. The patient required corticoid and other immunosuppressive treatment for 2 years and remained with positive direct Coombs test.

In 2004, Ito et al[25] evaluated 5 patients with MPS II, aged 4 to 11 years, submitted to HSCT. They found that the white-yellow papules characteristic of the disease disappeared completely within 35 days after transplantation (mean of 18 days) in all patients. They also observed that skin thickness tended to normalize after HSCT.

The ultrastructural assessment of cutaneous nerve involvement in 3 patients with MPS II before and after HSCT was published in 2005 by Ochiai et al.[26] Two patients underwent HSCT at 5 years and the third at 8 years. Electron microscopy studies showed that clear vacuoles were present in the cytoplasm of endoneurial fibroblasts and Schwann cells, 2 months and 2 years, respectively, after transplantation. On the other hand, only a few vacuoles remained in the dermal fibroblasts 2 months after HSCT and disappeared after 2 years of transplantation. The results suggested the existence of a hematoneural barrier (such as BBB in the CNS) that may be responsible for preclude enzymatic correction in the internal environment of cutaneous nerves and thus not preventing psychomotor degeneration in patients undergoing HSCT.

In 2007, Escolar et al[27] reported the neurological development of 5 children submitted to umbilical cord cell transplantation. The ages at the time of transplantation ranged from 0.26 to 3.4 years, and the follow-up period ranged from 1.7 to 3.9 years. Four patients presented complete grafting and 1 presented mixed chimerism. This patient died after a second HSCT due to complications related to graft versus host disease. The 4 patients who survived presented cognitive, motor, language, and adaptive skills gains. The older patient, who required the placement of ventriculoperitoneal shunt due to increased intracranial pressure, presented the slower rate of improvement. The authors concluded that, despite the mild auditory deficit present in all 4 patients, they continued to show neurological improvements in all areas. Long-term follow-up is needed.

A long series of cases of patients with Hunter syndrome treated with HSCT was reported in 2009 by Guffon et al.[28] The report involved 8 patients aged 3 to 16 years at the time of transplantation. Five boys had the neuronopathic form (diagnosis before 4 years of age and IQ <80), 2 had the non-neuronopathic form (diagnosis at 5 years and normal IQ), and 1 was considered to have an intermediate phenotype (diagnosis before 4 years and IQ ≥80 and <90). One of the patients with the neuronopathic form, transplanted at 3 years and 11 months, died suddenly at the age of 10 years of nontransplant-related cause. The remaining 7 patients were followed for periods ranging from 7 to 17 years and presented between 9 and 24 years in the last evaluation. All had normal I2 S activity in leukocytes and low in plasma. Urinary GAG levels were close to the upper limit of normal. There was resolution of hepatosplenomegaly and joint stiffness in all; there was also improvement in persistent rhinorrhea and upper airway obstruction. Valvular changes were detected in all of them before HSCT, but deterioration following transplantation was observed. Neuropsychological outcomes were distinct. The 2 boys with the non-neuronopathic form reached adulthood with normal IQ, normal school, and social development, without language impairment. Four patients with the neuronopathic form deteriorate after HSCT; 3 lost their ability to walk in early adolescence, 2 lost their language skills at 9 and 11, and 2 developed epilepsy. The other 2 patients required special education and had few social and language skills. Regarding auditory impairment, sensorineural deficit remained stable after transplantation and the transmission deficit improved. Four boys were using hearing aids at the last evaluation.

Araya et al,[29] in 2009, described the case of a 6-year-old patient with the neuronopathic form of MPS II submitted to HSCT. He died 10 months after the procedure due to laryngeal lymphoproliferative disease. During the posttransplant follow-up period, there was no improvement in hyperactivity, IQ, or brain MRI findings. Biochemical and histopathological analyzes on autopsied tissues showed the presence of distended cells with deposited material in the brain but not in the liver. Iduronate-2 sulfatase activity in the brain remained very low while in the liver it was 40% of the normal range. Tandem repeat analyzes showed weak bands, derived from the donor, not only in the liver but also in the brain. In addition, I2 S immunoreactivity was recognized not only in Kupffer cells but also in hepatocytes. Immunoreactivity of I2 S has also been found in microglial cells located predominantly in the perivascular spaces and some in the cerebral parenchyma. The efficacy of HSCT 10 months later was considered insufficient for the brain, but detection of donor-derived cells in the cerebral parenchyma suggests the potential of HSCT for the treatment neurological symptoms in patients with MPS II.

The neurodevelopment of 9 patients underwent HSCT was reported in 2011 by Poe et al.[7] Patients were between 1.5 and 47 months at the time of transplantation and were followed for periods ranging from 7 months to 7 years. Two patients died after transplantation. During the evaluation period, the patients performed between 3 and 12 neuropsychological evaluations. Of the 7 living patients, 5 continued to show gains in some or all of the developmental domains. One patient had normal development in 4 of the 6 domains evaluated. The study concluded that neurodevelopment was delayed after HSCT, although more research is needed to clarify the reason for this variability.

In 2012, Tanaka et al[30] published the results of a retrospective evaluation of the efficacy of HSCT performed between 1990 and 2003 in 21 patients with both forms of MPS II. The ages at the time of transplantation ranged from 2 to 19 years and 8 months (mean of 64.2 ± 30.2 months), and the 5-year survival rate was 88.5%. The authors concluded that HSCT is a valid treatment for patients with MPS II when performed before the onset of cerebral atrophy and heart valve disease.

Also in 2012, Escolar et al[31] reported the development of 9 patients with the neuronopathic phenotype of Hunter syndrome, transplanted with ages ranging from 1.5 to 47 months. They were followed up for 8 years and compared to 35 non-transplanted patients. The results showed that transplanted children aged <18 months had very close to normal cognitive, adaptive, and language skills. All early transplanted children showed continuous gains in these skills, albeit at a slower rate than normal children. The development of boys transplanted after 18 months of age reached a plateau and then declined to functional ages between 1 and 3 years. More consistent clinical data are not available.

The long-term follow-up of 4 patients with the neuronopathic form of MPS II undergoing HSCT was reported in 2013 by Annibali et al.[32] Patients were between 2 years and 6 months and 2 years and 11 months of age at the time of transplantation. Neuropsychological assessments showed IQ stabilization in 3 of the 4 patients in the first 5 years after transplantation, followed by a worsening in neurological status. Two patients who had mild mental retardation (MR; IQ = 70) before transplantation remained stable for 5 years and then had moderate MR until the last evaluation, 16 and 7 years after HSCT (IQ = 35 and IQ = 40), respectively. The third patient, who had moderate MR prior to transplantation (IQ = 49), presented neurological deterioration and 8 years later presented very severe MR (IQ = 15). The fourth patient, who had mild MR before HSCT (IQ = 80), remained stable up to 8 years after transplantation (IQ = 73). Patients with the neuronopathic form of MPS II submitted to HSCT showed improvement or stabilization of somatic symptoms while neurological impairment showed progression, albeit much slower than expected.

The impact of ERT and HSCT on the growth of 44 Japanese patients with Hunter syndrome was evaluated by Patel et al in 2014.[33] Twenty-six patients were treated with ERT, 12 with ERT, and 6 received ERT and HSCT. Weight and height were compared with those of untreated patients and controls from previous studies. Patients who received treatment with both ERT and HSCT had weights and heights higher than untreated patients. Enzyme replacement therapy and HSCT were equally effective in restoring growth in patients with MPS II. According to the authors, HSCT should be considered as one of the first therapeutic options for the early treatment of MPS II since positive effects on brain and heart valves have also been reported.

In 2015, Tanjuakio et al[34] tested a new questionnaire to assess the clinical phenotype and therapeutic efficacy of ERT and HSCT in patients with Hunter syndrome. The group developed a questionnaire of activities of daily living with 3 domains: "movement," "movement with cognition," and "cognition." The questionnaire was initially applied in 138 healthy controls (0.33 and 50 years) and successively in 72 patients with MPS II (4-49 years), 51 with the neuronopathic form, and 23 with the non-neuronopathic form. Twenty patients were treated with HSCT, 23 were treated with ERT initiated before 8 years of age, 25 started ERT after 8 years of age, and 4 patients never received specific treatment. The scores of patients with neurological impairment were lower than controls and patients with the non-neuronopathic form, in all categories. Among patients with the neuronopathic form, there was a tendency for transplant patients to present higher scores than patients who started ERT ≤ 8 years, and there was a significant difference in the score between the group that received ERT after age 8 and the group that performed HSCT, with the latter group achieving higher scores. The questionnaire showed the benefits of early treatment, with HSCT showing better results compared to ERT, although the differences were not statistically significant.

Cagle[35] briefly reported, in 2015, the case of a patient who underwent HSCT at 37 months. Up to 4 years of age, he showed no signs of neurological regression. The author mentions the need for the development of more reliable biomarkers for monitoring both disease and treatment.

In 2016, Wang et al[36] published an article on allogeneic HSCT in 34 Chinese patients with MPS. Of these, 12 patients had MPS II and were transplanted between the ages of 2 and 6 years. After HSCT, follow-up evaluations showed improvement in airway obstruction, recurrent episodes of otitis media, joint stiffness, and hepatosplenomegaly. The auditory deficit showed some improvement, the valve impairment showed improvement in some patients and progression in others, while there were no benefits in the bone disease. Regarding the CNS,

4 patients had significant improvement in motor skills and 2 patients showed small improvements in language skills. The results suggest that allogeneic HSCT is beneficial for the neurological development of patients with MPS II.

Muschol et al[37] also, in 2016, summarized the clinical outcomes of 2 patients undergoing HSCT at 2.1 and 4.25 years. Both patients presented good grafting, normalization of I2 S activity, and decline in urinary GAG excretion. After 2 years of transplantation, hepatosplenomegaly disappeared in both. One of the patients showed signs of hyperactivity and aggressive behavior 6 months after HSCT, lost the ability to talk 2 years later, and after 3 years of transplantation presented progressive cerebral atrophy. The other showed developmental delay but maintained the motor and language skills; imaging examinations revealed a reduction in white matter changes.

Recently, in 2017, Barth et al[13] reported the 7-year follow-up of a prenatally diagnosed MPS II boy with positive family history of severe MPS form, submitted to HSCT with umbilical cord blood cells at 70 days of age. Engraftment after 30 days revealed mixed chimerism with 79% donor cells; after 7 years, engraftment remains at 80%. The I2 S activity 30 days post-transplant was low in plasma and normal in leukocytes, and the same pattern is observed to date. At age 7 years, growth charts are normal, and he is very healthy, although mild signs of dysostosis multiplex are present, as well as hearing loss. The neuropsychological evaluation disclosed an IQ of 47. Despite this low measured IQ, the patient continues to show improvements in cognitive, language, and motor skills, being quite functional. The authors believe HSCT is a therapeutic option for patients with MPS II having the severe phenotype, as it could preserve neurocognition or even halt neurodegeneration when strict selection criteria are followed.

Also in 2017, Kubaski et al[38] compared the clinical and biochemical data of patients with MPS II who received HSCT and/or ERT. Demographics of 130 patients undergoing HSCT were compared to those of 54 patients treated with ERT and 11 untreated patients. Daily living activities were also evaluated in these patients. A greater number of transplanted patients presented improvement in somatic symptoms, joint stiffness, and daily living activities compared to those who received ERT. Both treatments provided significant reductions in GAG levels, but in general patients undergoing HSCT had lower GAG levels. Two patients with the non-neuronopathic form presented improvement in brain MRI after transplantation. The authors state that despite the need for controlled studies, HSCT seems to be effective and may be considered as a therapeutic option for patients with MPS II.

Discussion

Hematopoietic stem cell transplantation is the only currently available treatment capable of preventing progressive neurodegeneration that occurs in some metabolic diseases.[4,39,40,41] It has become the treatment of choice for the severe form of MPS type I since it is able to preserve neurocognition when performed early.[5,6,9,42] Since 1980, more than 600 HSCT have been performed in patients with Hurler syndrome.[4]

Clinical experience with HSCT in MPS II is small. Most of the available literature is outdated, and the few articles available refer to heterogeneous cohorts of patients transplanted with different metabolic diseases or to reports of isolated cases. The available data reveal poor patient selection criteria; many were already at advanced ages at the time of transplantation, some had the non-neuronopathic form while others presented the neuronopathic form of MPS II, already with neurological impairment. The conditioning regimens used were quite varied, as was the source of cells for transplantation. In addition, follow-up parameters and post-HSCT outcomes of interest were also varied, making it impossible to compare and generalize the results obtained.

After 2006, with the approval of Idursulfase alfa (Elaprase), ERT became the treatment of choice for MPS II. Although it is known not to cross the BBB, being unable to prevent the neurodegeneration that occurs in the neuronopathic form of MPS II, ERT has become the treatment of choice for patients diagnosed with Hunter syndrome, and HSCT was discouraged and no longer.[13]

It is important to remember that more than 10 years, HSCT was limited by the lack of available donors, high percentage of graft failure, and high rates of morbidity and mortality. In 2005, an international collaborative study developed guidelines for HSCT in patients with MPS, based on the identification of mortality predictors.[43] In 2012, the busulfan-based conditioning regimen was modified by replacement of cyclophosphamide with fludarabine leading to less toxicity with similar efficacy.[44] Other reduced toxicity regimens that improve patients survival presently being used include fludarabine/melphalan and treosulphan/fludarabina (EBMT/ESID Guidelines for HSCT, 2017).

The implementation of these new guidelines resulted in graft survival rates of more than 90%. Over the last decade, umbilical cord blood has been used with increasing frequency in the transplantation of children with metabolic diseases. Cord blood offers several advantages when compared to bone marrow as a source for transplantation, such as shorter time to donor searching, greater tolerance for human leucocyte antigen (HLA) incompatibilities, lower incidence and severity of graft versus host disease, and lower probability of viral infections transmission. Recent studies suggest that the highest event-free survival rates are achieved in patients receiving compatible sibling cords or fully compatibles cords (6/6) of related donors, followed by compatible 5/6 cords (or compatible cords 4/6 with high cell dosages) or with 10/10 compatibility of nonrelated donor. It is important to note that many of the related donors also carry mutations, which influence posttransplant enzyme levels. Lower enzyme levels appear to influence long-term outcomes, such as neurocognitive development. Patients with normal enzyme levels in leukocytes show better results such as higher growth, less need for orthopedic interventions, and respiratory care.[8,4]

It has already been proven that the results of HSCT in metabolic disorders (both transplantation outcomes and long-term outcomes) are better when it is performed earlier in the course of the disease. This has already been demonstrated in MPS I, metachromatic leukodystrophy, X-linked adrenoleukodystrophy, Krabbe's disease, and probably it is also true for other metabolic diseases.[4]

The high grafted survival rates observed after HSCT together with the low toxicity in patients with MPS would allow the indication of transplantation for other types of MPS, in addition to the severe form of MPS I. In addition, the scientific basis for its effectiveness remains the same: The donor cells would secrete the deficient enzyme that would be captured by surrounding cells, thus correcting the underlying enzyme deficiency.

Regarding the CNS, HSCT appears to be the only treatment capable of preserving neurocognitive function. Hematopoietic stem cell transplantation appears to be beneficial since monocytic/phagocytic cells are able to cross the BBB and host in the brain as microglia. Microglia derived from donor cells would be able to secrete the deficient enzyme that would be captured by receptor neurons correcting enzyme deficiency.[45] Araya et al[29] demonstrated the presence of donor cells in the microglia of patients with MPS II 10 months after transplantation. These cells were found not only in the perivascular spaces but also in the cerebral parenchyma, suggesting the potential of HSCT to treat the neurological symptoms of Hunter syndrome.[29]

The case reported by Barth et al showed favorable neurological outcome with early HSCT in the neuronopathic form of MPS II.[13] It is generally agreed that younger patients benefit most from HSCT. Thus, early diagnosis is fundamental to the success of transplantation since much of the morbidity associated with the disease is not reversed with HSCT. Because it takes a few months for the microglia to be replaced by cells from the donor, there seems to be some delay in the benefits of transplantation to the brain. Therefore, transplantation only offers clinical benefits when instituted in presymptomatic phases but may be as effective for MPS II as it is for MPS I when the patient is transplanted prior to the onset of neurological symptoms.[29]

Currently, with the high rates of graft survival and reduction in toxicity and complications related to HSCT with the new techniques and transplantation protocols, together with a superior metabolic correction when compared to ERT,[8,36] associated with the more careful selection of patients, HSCT should be considered as an alternative option to ERT.

In China and Japan, HSCT is a standard therapy, being even listed in the guideline for MPS II treatment in Japan.[30,34,38] In Brazil, a new guideline for HSCT has recently been approved, which will make it easier for patients with MPS II to have access to this procedure in a timely manner.[46]

In addition to a potentially more favorable effect on disease progression, there would be a gain in quality of life for patients and relatives who would not need to attend a hospital/infusion center weekly over 3 to 4 hours for lifelong infusions.

Economic evaluations of HSCT are difficult to compare between countries because of differences in health-care systems, transplantation coverage, and payment policies. However, US\$350 000 to US\$800 000 is a reasonable approximation for an allotransplant in the United States. Comparable cost in Latin America ranges from US\$25 000 to US\$75 000).[47] In Europe, in a single-institution study from Sweden, Svahn et al found costs for HCT with related donor transplantations compared with HSCT with unrelated donor transplantations of €129 133 versus €160 658.[48] In France, Cordonnier et al examining costs over a 12-month period found that myeloablative allogeneic transplantations cost less than reduced intensity conditioning transplants; €74 900 versus €78 700.[49] In Thailand, Ngamkiatphaisan et al[50] found a median cost for allogeneic HCT of €22.593 over 1-year posttransplantation.[50]

Regarding public health policy, the HSCT could be considered a very interesting option since the estimated mean annual cost of idursulfase for a 25Kg patient with MPS II is €290 000/ \$325 000; a lifelong cost much higher than that of the HSCT which is a procedure usually performed once.[51]

Conclusion

After little more than a decade of experience, the benefits and limitations of ERT for MPS II are known. Intravenous ERT is able to provide benefits for some of the somatic signs and symptoms of the disease, but, being incapable to cross the BBB, it does not improve or even halt the neurological symptoms and neurodegeneration that occur in patients with the neuronopathic form of Hunter syndrome.

Hematopoietic stem cell transplantation has become more secure and accessible after the development of new protocols and techniques and the creation of bone marrow donor registries and umbilical cord banks. Thus, HSCT should be considered as a treatment option to ERT in patients with MPS II. It is the only currently available treatment potentially capable of providing neurological benefits when rigid selection criteria are followed and it also should be thought for somatic treatment as it has lower cost compared to ERT for life and would provide better quality of life for the patients and their families. Longer follow-up and more reports of early transplanted patients are still necessary.

Declaration of Conflicting Interests

The author(s) declared no potential conflicts of interest with respect to the research, authorship, and/or publication of this article.

Funding

The author(s) disclosed receipt of the following financial support for the research, authorship, and/or publication of this article: AL Barth has received educational travel grants and/or speaker honoraria from Biomarin, Shire, and Sanofi Genzyme. DDG Horovitz has received educational travel grants and/or speaker honoraria from Biomarin, Shire, Sanofi Genzyme, and Ultragenyx.

References

1. Neufeld EF, Muenzer J. The mucopolysaccharidoses. In: Scriver CR, Beaudet AL, Sly WS, Valle D, eds, *The Metabolic and Molecular Bases of Inherited Disease*, 8th ed. New York, NY: McGrow-Hill; 2001.
2. Holt JB, Poe MD, Escolar ML. Natural progression of neurological disease in mucopolisaccharidosis type II. *Pediatrics*. 2011; 127(5):e1258-e1265.
3. Fratantoni JC, Hall CW, Neufeld EF. Hurler and Hunter syndromes: mutual correction of the defect in cultured fibroblasts. *Science*. 1968;162(3853):570-572.
4. Boelens JJ, van Hasselt PM. Neurodevelopmental outcome after hematopoietic stem cell transplantation in inborn errors of metabolism: current considerations and future perspectives. *Neuropediatr*. 2016;47(5):285-292.
5. Wraith JE, Beck M, Lane R, et al. Enzyme replacement therapy in patients who have mucopolysaccharidosis I and are younger than 5 years: results of a multinational study of recombinant human alpha-L-iduronidase (laronidase). *Pediatrics*. 2007;120(1): e37-e46.
6. de Ru MH, Boelens JJ, Das AM, Jones SA, et al. Enzyme replacement therapy and/or hematopoietic stem cell transplantation at diagnosis in patients with mucopolysaccharidosis type I: results of a European consensus procedure. *Orphanet J Rare Dis*. 2011;6:55.
7. Poe M, Escolar M, Kurtzberb J, et al. MPS II: developmental outcomes after hematopoietic stem cell transplantation. *Mol Genet Metab*. 2011;102(2):S36.
8. Aldenhoven M, Jones SA, Bonney D, et al. Hematopoietic cell transplantation for mucopolysaccharidosis patients is safe and effective: results after implementation of international guidelines. *Biol Blood Marrow Transplant*. 2015a;21(6):1106-1109.
9. Gosh A, Miller W, Orchard PJ, et al. Enzyme replacement therapyprior to hematopoietic stem cell transplantation in mucopolysaccharidosis type I: 10 year combined experience of 2 centers. *Mol Genet Metab*. 2016;117(3):373-377.
10. Peters C, Sterward CG; National Marrow Donor Program; International Bone Marrow Transplant Registry; Working Party on Inborn Errors, European Bone Marrow Transplant Group. Hematopoietic cell transplantation for inherited metabolic diseases: an overview of outcomes and practice guidelines. *Bone Marrow Transplant*. 2003;31(4):229-239.
11. Prasad VK, Mendizabal A, Parikh SH, et al. Unrelated donor umbilical cord blood transplantation for inherited metabolic disorders in 159 pediatricpatients from a single center: influence of cellular composition of the graft on transplantation outcomes. *Blood*. 2008;112(7):2979-2989.
12. Wynn RF, Wraith JE, Mercer J, et al. Improved metabolic correction in patientswith lysosomal storage disease treated with hematopoietic stem cell transplantcompared with enzyme replacement therapy. *J Pediatr*. 2009;154(4):609-611.
13. Barth AL, Magalhães TSPC, Reis AB, et al. Early hematopoietic stem cell transplantation in a patient with severe mucopolysaccharidosis II: A 7 years follow-up. *Mol Genet Metab Rep*. 2017; 12:62-68.
14. Sackett DL, Haynes RB, Guyatt GH, Tugwell P. *Clinical Epidemiology: A Basic Science for Clinical Medicine*. Boston/Toronto/London: Little, Brown and Company; 1992.
15. Warketin PI, Dixon MS, Shafer I, et al. Bone Marrow transplantation in Hunter syndrome: a preliminary report. *Birth Defects Orig Artic Ser*. 1986;22:31-39.
16. Bergstrom SK, Quinn JJ, Greenstein R, et al. Long-term follow-up of a patient transplanted for Hunter's disease type IIB: a case report and literature review. *Bone Marrow Transplant*. 1994; 14(4):653-658.
17. Imaizumi M, Gushi K, Kurobane I, et al. Long-term effects of bone marrow transplantation for inborn errors of metabolism: a study of four patients with lysosomal storage diseases. *Acta Ped Jpn*. 1994;36(1):30-36.
18. Miniero R, Busca A, Vassalo E, et al. Use of G-CSF in a patient with Hunter syndrome receiving bone marrow transplantation. *Am J Hematol*. 1994;47(1):59-60.
19. Coppa GV, Gabrielli O, Zampini L, et al. Bone marrow transplantation in Hunter syndrome (mucopolysaccharidosis type II): two-year follow-up of the first italian patient and review of the literature. *Pediatr Med Chir*. 1995;17(3):227-235.
20. McKinnes EJ, Sulzbacher S, Rutledge JC, Sanders J, Scott CR. Bone marrow transplantation in Hunter syndrome. *J Pediatr*. 1996;129(1):145-148.
21. Li P, Thompson JN, Hug P, Huffman P, Chuck G. Biochemical and molecular analysis in a patient with the severe form of Hunter syndrome after bone marrow transplantation. *Am J Med Genet*. 1996;64(4):531-535.
22. Vellodi A, Young E, Cooper A, Lidchi V, Winchester B, Wraith JE. Long-term follow-up following bone marrow transplantation for Hunter disease. *J Inherit Metab Dis*. 1999;22(5):638-648.
23. Coppa GV, Gabrielli O, Cordiali R, et al. Bone marrow transplantation in a Hunter patient with P266 H mutation. *Int J Mol Med*. 1999;4:433-436.
24. Mullen CA, Thompson JN, Richard LA, Chan KW. Unrelated umbilical cord blood transplantation in infancy for mucopolysaccharidosis type IIB (Hunter syndrome) complicated by autoimmune hemolytic anemia. *Bone Marrow Transplant*. 2000;25(10): 1093-1097.
25. Ito K, Ochiai T, Suzuki H, Chin M, Shichino H, Mugishima H. The effect of haematopoietic stem cell transplant on papules with 'pebbly' appearance in Hunter's syndrome. *Br J Dermatol*. 2004; 151(1):207-211.
26. Ochiai T, Ito K, Schichino H, Chin M, Mugishima H. Ultrastructural findings of cutaneous nerves in patients with Hunter's syndrome following hematopoietic stem cell transplant. *Med Mol Morphol*. 2005;38(2):118-122.
27. Escolar ML, Poe MD, Prasad V, et al. Neurodevelopmental outcomes of children with MPS II after unrelated umbilical cord blood transplantation. *Biol Blood Marrow Transplant*. 2007;13:63.
28. Guffon N, Bertrand Y, Forest I, et al. Bone marrow transplantation in children with hunter syndrome: outcome after 7 to 17 years. *J Pediatr*. 2009;154(5):733-737.
29. Araya K, Sakai N, Mohri I, et al. Localized donor cells in brain of a Hunter disease patient after cord blood stem cell transplantation. *Mol Genet Metab*. 2009;98(3):255-263.

30. Tanaka A, Okuyama T, Suzuki Y, et al. Long-term efficacy of hematopoietic stem cell transplantation on brain involvement in patients with mucopolysaccharidosis type II: A nationwide survey in Japan. *Mol Genet Metab*. 2012;107(3):513-520.
31. Escolar M, Poe M, Rajan D, et al. Long term outcomes of patients receiving umbilical blood stem cell transplantation for MPS II. *Mol Genet Metab*. 2012;108:S37.
32. Annibali R, Caponi L, Morganti A, et al. Hunter syndrome (mucopolysaccharidosis type II), severe phenotype: long term follow-up on patients undergone to hematopoietic stem cell transplantation. *Minerva Pediatr*. 2013;65(5):487-496.
33. Patel P, Suzuki Y, Tanaka A, et al. Impact of enzyme replacement therapy and hematopoietic stem cell therapy on growth in patients with Hunter syndrome. *Mol Genet Metab Rep*. 2014;1:184-196.
34. Tanjuakio J, Suzuki Y, Patel P, et al. Activities of daily living in patients with Hunter syndrome: impact of enzyme replacement therapy and hematopoietic stem cell transplantation. *Mol Genet Metab*. 2015;114(2):161-169.
35. Cagle S. Clinical outcomes and biochemical data following hematopoietic stem cell transplantation in a patient with Hunter syndrome. *Mol Genet Metab*. 2015;114:S28.
36. Wang J, Luan Z, Jiang H, et al. Allogeneic hematopoietic stem cell transplantation in 34 pediatric cases of mucopolysaccharidosis – a 10-year report from China Children Transplant Group. *Biol Blood Marrow Transpl*. 2016;22:2104-2108.
37. Muschol NM, Köhn AF, Ulrich K, et al. Clinical outcome after hematopoietic stem cell transplantation in two patients with Hunter syndrome. *Mol Genet Metab*. 2016;117:S84.
38. Kubaski F, Yabe H, Suzuki Y, et al. Hematopoietic stem cell transplantation for patients with mucopolysaccharidosis II. *Biol Blood Marrow Transplant*. 2017;23(10):1795-1803.
39. Krivit W. Allogenic stem cell transplantation for the treatment of lysosomal and peroxisomal metabolic diseases. *Springer Semin Immunopathol*. 2004;26(1-2):119-132.
40. Boelens JJ, Orchard PJ, Wynn R. Transplantation in inborn errors of metabolism: current considerations and future perspectives. *Br J Haematol*. 2014;167(3):293-303.
41. Aldenhoven M, Wynn RF, Orchard PJ, et al. Long-term outcome of Hurler syndrome patients after hematopoietic cell transplantation: an international multicenter study. *Blood*. 2015b;125(13): 2164-2172.
42. Poe MD, Chagnon SL, Escolar ML. Early treatment is associated with improved cognition in Hurler syndrome. *Ann Neurol*. 2014; 76(5):747-753.
43. Boelens JJ, Wynn RF, O'meara A, et al. Outcomes of hematopoietic stem cell transplantation for Hurler's syndrome in Europe: a risk factor analysis for graft failure. *Bone Marrow Transplant*. 2007;40(3):225-233.
44. Bartelink IH, Van Reij EM, Gerhardt CE, et al. Fludarabine and exposure-targeted busulfan compares favorably with busulfan cyclophosphamide-based regimens in pediatric hematopoietic cell transplantation: maintaining efficacy with less toxicity. *Biol Blood Marrow Transplant*. 2014;20(3):345-353.
45. Krivit W, Sung JH, Shapiro EG, Lockman LA. Microglia: the effector cell for reconstitution of the central nervous system following bone marrow transplantation for lysosomal and peroxisomal storagediseases. *Cell Transplant*. 1995;4(4): 385-392.
46. Protocolo Clínico e Diretrizes Terapêuticas da Mucopolissacaridose tipo II [internet]. Available: http://conitec.gov.br/images/Relatorios/2017/Recomendacao/relatorio_PCDT_MPS_II_CP_61_2017.pdf.
47. Gale RP, Seber A, Bomfim C, et al. Haematopoietic cell transplants in Latin America. *Bone Marrow Transplant*. 2016;51(7): 898-905.
48. Svahn BM, Alvin O, Ringdén O, Gardulf A, Remberger M. Costs of allogeneic hematopoietic stem cell transplantation. *Transplantation*. 2006;82(2):147-153.
49. Cordonnier C, Maury S, Esperou H, et al. Do mini transplants have mini costs? A cost comparison between myeloablative and nonmyeloablative allogeneic stem cell transplant in patients with acute myeloid leukemia. *Bone Marrow Transplant*. 2005;36(7): 649-654.
50. Ngamkiatphaisan S, Sriratanaban J, Kamolratanakul P, Intragumtornchai T, Noppakun N, Jongudomsuk P. Cost analysis of hematopoietic stem cell transplantation in adult patients with acute myeloid leukemia at King Chulalongkorn Memorial Hospital. *J Med Assoc Thai*. 2007;90(12):2565-2573.
51. Orofino J, Soto J, Casado MA, Oyagüez I. Global spending on orphan drugs in France, Germany, the UK, Italy and Spain during 2007. *Appl Health Econ Health Policy*. 2010;8(5):301-315.

Mimicking Ketonuria in the Ketogenesis Defect 3-Hydroxy-3-Methylglutaryl-Coenzyme A Lyase Deficiency: An Artefact in the Analysis of Urinary Organic Acids

Jörn Oliver Sass, Dr. rer. nat.[1], Malkanthi Fernando, Dr. rer. nat.[2], and Sidney Behringer, B.Sc.[2]

Abstract
3-Hydroxy-3-methylglutaryl-coenzyme A lyase (HMGCL, *HMGCL*) deficiency is a rare inborn error of ketogenesis. Even if the ketogenic enzyme is fully disrupted, an elevated signal for the ketone body acetoacetic acid is a frequent observation in the analysis of urinary organic acids, at least if derivatization is performed by methylation. We provide an explanation for this phenomenon and trace it back to degradation of the derivatized 3-hydroxy-3-methylglutaric acid and high temperature of the injector of the gas chromatograph.

Keywords
ketogenesis, ketone body synthesis, leucine degradation, fatty acid metabolism, organic aciduria, enzyme activity, organic acid analysis

Introduction

3-Hydroxy-3-methylglutaryl-coenzyme A lyase deficiency (HMGCLD) is a rare inborn error of ketone body synthesis and leucine degradation, caused by mutations in the *3-hydroxy-3-methylglutaryl-coenzyme A lyase* gene. It has first been described by Faull et al[1] in 1976; recently, we have reported the largest series so far of patients with this disease.[2]

3-Hydroxy-3-methylglutaryl-coenzyme A lyase deficiency patients present with a characteristic pattern of urinary organic acids that is dominated by leucine metabolites. Although HMGCLD impairs ketone body synthesis both from fatty acids and ketogenic amino acids, an elevated signal for the ketone body acetoacetic acid is a frequent observation in a laboratory where the derivatization in organic acid analysis is performed by methylation.[3,4] Although acetoacetate is normally interconverted enzymatically with 3-hydroxy-*n*-butyric acid, no alteration in 3-hydroxy-*n*-butyric acid levels is noted in such cases.

It has been speculated that the acetoacetate may be formed by bacterial degradation of 3-hydroxy-3-methylglutaric acid, but so far no evidence-based explanation of the origin of the acetoacetate has been given.[4] We have now tested the hypothesis that the formation of an acetoacetic acid signal is due to conversion of 3-hydroxy-3-methylglutaric acid during the analysis by gas chromatography-mass spectrometry (GC-MS) that is performed when patterns of urinary organic acids are obtained.

Methods

Most laboratories determine urinary organic acids by extraction from acidified urine followed by trimethylsilylation or methylation and subsequent GC-MS analysis.[5,6] Our methylation approach followed the description by Lehnert,[3] while the setup for trimethylsilylation using silylation agent (BSTFA + TMCS, 99:1, 33148 Supelco; Sigma-Aldrich,

[1] Bonn-Rhein-Sieg University of Applied Sciences, IFGA & Department of Natural Sciences, Inborn Errors of Metabolism, Rheinbach, Germany
[2] Department of General Pediatrics, Faculty of Medicine, Adolescent Medicine and Neonatology, Medical Center–University of Freiburg, Freiburg, Germany

Corresponding Author:
Jörn Oliver Sass, Bonn-Rhein-Sieg University of Applied Sciences, IFGA & Department of Natural Sciences, Inborn Errors of Metabolism, von-Liebig-Str. 20, 53359 Rheinbach, Germany.
Email: joern.oliver.sass@h-brs.de

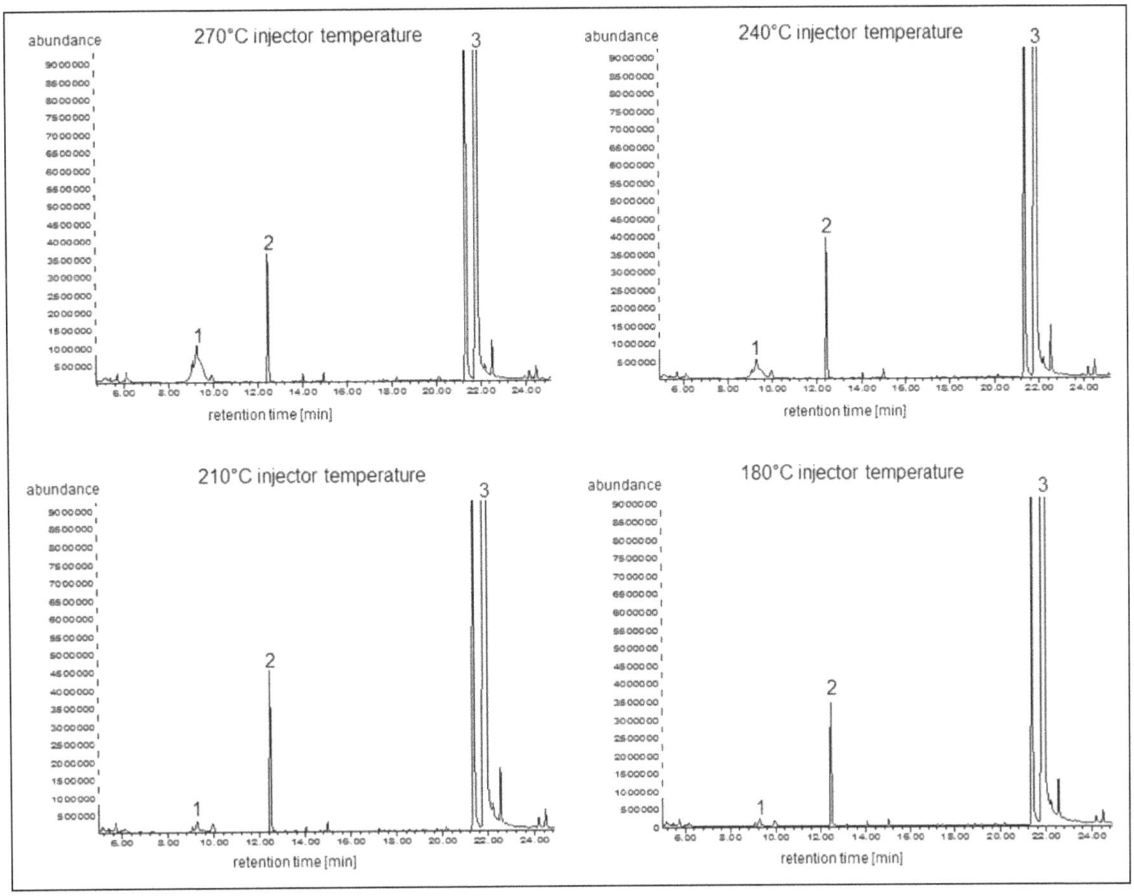

Figure 1. Impact of the injector temperature in GC-MS organic acid analysis (methylation) of 1 mM 3-hydroxy-3-methylglutaric acid. Signal 1 (acetoacetate methylester) increases with the injector temperature. Signal 2: Isopropylmalonic acid dimethylester (internal standard). Signal 3: 3-hydroxy-3-methyl glutaric acid dimethylester.

Taufkirchen, Germany) resembled that of Guneral and Bachmann,[7] although simple ethylacetate extraction was applied instead of solid-phase extraction. Internal standards were 0.04 mmol/L isopropylmalonic acid (for methylation) and 0.44 mmol/L tricarballylic acid (for trimethylsilylation), respectively.

For both types of derivatization, a 7890A gas chromatograph (Agilent) was used which was coupled to a 5975C mass-sensitive detector (Agilent, Waldbronn, Germany). Split injection was performed at a ratio of 1:5. New liners used were of the Ultra Inert Liner type (Agilent 5190-3168). For our experiments, different injector temperatures between 180°C and 270°C were applied.

For analysis after methylation, an FFAP column (25 m × 0.25 mm, 0.2 μm film; CP7717 Agilent) was used and a temperature program was started with 3 minutes constant temperature at 50°C, followed by rapid heating to 70°C. For separation, a gradient of 4°C/min has been used. The GC was then baked out at 260°C for 15 minutes.

For analysis after trimethylsilylation, a CP-Sil 5 CB column (25 m × 0.25 mm, 0.12 μm film; CP7710 Agilent) was used. The temperature program for separation started at initial 70°C and then heated with 4°C/min up to 200°C, followed by a gradient of 8°C/min up to 270°C and then baking out at the same temperature.

In order to avoid memory effects due to incomplete vaporization at low temperatures, we always inserted a blank run with the commonly used injector temperature (270°C) and injection of methanol or the silylation agent between 2 regular analyses.

In order to create stable, reproducible standard conditions and to avoid rapid contamination of the injector of the GC-MS system, aqueous solution of 1 mM 3-hydroxy-3-methylglutaric acid (Sigma H4392; Sigma-Aldrich, Taufkirchen, Germany) was studied instead of patient urine.

Results

Analysis of the methylated sample with the commonly used injector temperature of 270°C yielded a major signal of 3-hydroxy-3-methylglutaric acid dimethylester that was accompanied by a signal of acetoacetate methyl ester as it is known from urine of patients with HMGCLD (Figure 1). However, when the injector temperature was decreased, the signal of the acetoacetate methyl ester became smaller and almost disappeared at 180°C. This finding was reproducible in all 3 experiments performed.

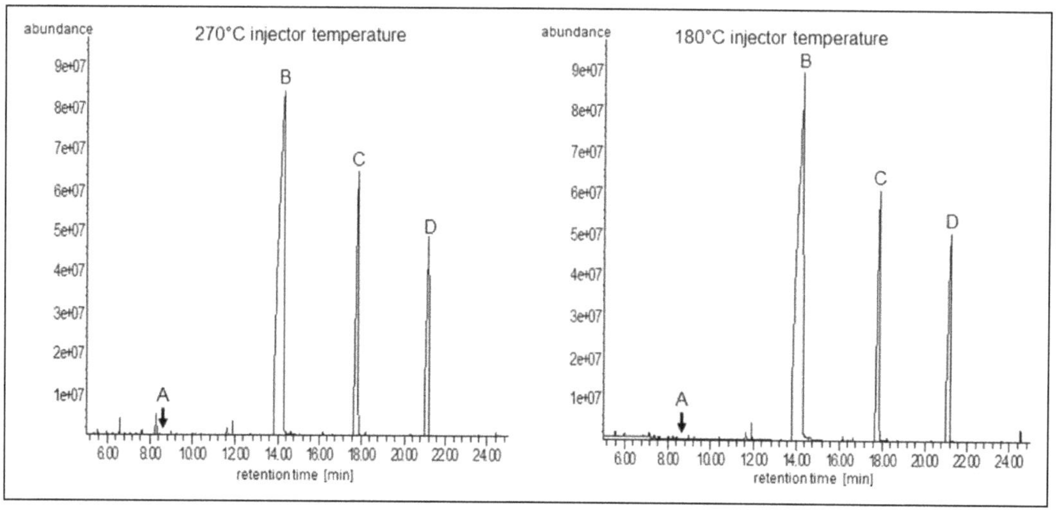

Figure 2. No effect of the injector temperature in GC-MS organic acid analysis (trimethylsilylation) of 1 mM 3-hydroxy-3-methylglutaric acid was noted. No signal was detected at the retention time of derivatized acetoacetate (signal A). Signal B: 3-methylglutaconic acid-bis(trimethylsilyl) ester. Signal C: 3-methyl-3-glutaric [(trimethylsilyl)oxy]-bis(trimethylsilyl) ester. Signal D: tricarballylic acid, tris(trimethylsilyl) ester (internal standard).

However, when a new Ultra Inert liner (Agilent 5190-3168) was inserted into the injector, initially, only a trace amounts of the acetoacetate methyl ester were detected. After just 10 regular injections with methylated urine samples, major formation of acetoacetate methyl ester was observed again. This suggests that the liner is soon activated and then catalyzes the degradation of dimethylated 3-hydroxy-3-methylglutaric acid at high temperatures.

In contrast, no derivatized acetoacetic acid was observed if trimethylsilylation was applied (Figure 2). However, a major signal of 3-methylglutaconic acid-bis(trimethylsilyl) ester was noted in addition to 3-hydroxy-3-methylglutaric acid ([trimethylsilyl]oxy)-bis(trimethylsilyl) ester and even exceeded the peak height and area of the latter. This is well-explained by dehydratation of 3-hydroxy-3-methylglutaric acid in analogy to that of 2-hydroxyglutaric acid.[8] In agreement with this and because the 3-hydroxy-group should have been protected from participation in the dehydration by trimethylsilylation, it is concluded that the dehydration occurs not in the injector, but already when the sample is derivatized. The extent of this conversion revealed no direct dependency on the injector temperature (270°C vs 180°C) or the age of the liner.

Discussion

Ketogenesis, the -mainly hepatic- formation of the ketone bodies acetoacetic acid and 3-hydroxy-n-butyric acid is the main path to the synthesis of ketone bodies[4]. Extrahepatic pseudoketogenesis based on reversal of ketone metabolism has especially been presented as an analytical problem for tracer studies.[9,10] Now, we present the formation of methylated acetoacetic acid as an artifact in the analysis of urinary organic acids. Its formation in the injector of the GC instrument can explain the unexpected signal of a ketone body in the organic acid patterns of patients with the ketogenesis defect HMGCLD. As a decrease of the injector temperature deteriorates the resolution of the chromatogram, one cannot simply reduce the injector temperature. However, now, after the mechanism that underlies the signal of methylated acetoacetic acid has been elucidated, it should not result in irritation any more when metabolite profiles are evaluated.

The production of 3-methylglutaconic acid during the sample preparation by trimethylsilylation might provoke questions regarding the biological origin of this metabolite in HMGCLD in general. However, the formation of this leucine metabolite has not only been observed by GC-MS (also after methylation), and is plausible in view of the pathway, but has also been observed by NMR spectroscopy where dehydratation of 3-hydroxy-3-methylglutaric acid can be excluded.[11,12] Thus, the production of some 3-methylglutaconic acid derivative during the sample preparation is not in contrast to its accumulation in vivo in HMGCLD.

Acknowledgments

Research of J. O. Sass in the ketone body field is supported by the program "FH Zeit für Forschung 2016" by the Ministry of Culture and Science of the German state of North Rhine-Westphalia (project 005-1703-0016, "KETOplus").

Declaration of Conflicting Interests

The author(s) declared no potential conflicts of interest with respect to the research, authorship, and/or publication of this article.

Funding

The author(s) received no financial support for the research, authorship, and/or publication of this article.

References

1. Faull K, Bolton P, Halpern B, et al. Patient with defect in leucine metabolism. *N Engl J Med.* 1976;294(18):1013.
2. Grünert SC, Schlatter SM, Schmitt RN, et al. 3-Hydroxy-3-methylglutaryl-coenzyme A lyase deficiency: clinical presentation and outcome in a series of 37 patients. *Mol Genet Metab.* 2017;121(3):206-215.
3. Lehnert W. Long-term results of selective screening for inborn errors of metabolism. *Eur J Pediatr.* 1994;153(suppl 1):S9-S13.
4. Sass JO. Inborn errors of ketogenesis and ketone body utilization. *J Inherit Metab Dis.* 2012. 35(1):23-28.
5. Sass JO, Sewell AC. Gas chromatography-mass spectrometry for selective screening for inborn errors of metabolism. In: Niessen WMA, ed. *Current Practice of Gas Chromatography-Mass Spectrometry.* New York, NY: Marcel Dekker; 2001:341-354.
6. Sass JO. Organoacidurien (Organic Acidurias). *J Lab Med.* 2011: 35(2):77-80.
7. Guneral F, Bachmann C. Age-related reference values for urinary organic acids in a healthy Turkish pediatric population. *Clin Chem.* 1994;40(6):862-866.
8. Scott ND. Preparation of glutaconic acid. US Patent 2,218,032. October 15, 1940.
9. Des Rosiers C, Montgomery JA, Garneau M, et al. Pseudoketogenesis in hepatectomized dogs. *Am J Physiol.* 1990;258(3 pt 1): E519-E528.
10. Fink G, Desrochers S, Des Rosiers C, et al. Pseudoketogenesis in the perfused rat heart. *J Biol Chem.* 1988;263(34):18036-18042.
11. Iles RA, Jago JR, Williams SR, Chalmers RA. 3-Hydroxy-3-methylglutaryl-CoA lyase deficiency studied using 2-dimensional proton nuclear magnetic resonance spectroscopy. *FEBS Lett.* 1986;203(1):49-53.
12. Lehnert W, Hunkler D. Possibilities of selective screening for inborn errors of metabolism using high-resolution 1H-FT-NMR spectrometry. *Eur J Pediatr.* 1986;145:260-266.

26

Overview of Approaches to Mitochondrial Disease Therapy

Diana Lehmann, MD[1,2] and Robert McFarland, PhD, MRCPCH[1]

Abstract

Mitochondrial respiratory chain diseases are the most prevalent group of inherited neurometabolic disorders and are clinically, biochemically, and genetically heterogeneous. They may present at any stage of life and often manifest with severe multisystem disease, although single organ involvement is characteristic of some conditions such as Leber hereditary optic neuropathy. As a result of these complexities, the diagnostic pathway is often challenging, so too is further advice, guidance, and therapy following diagnosis. Difficulties also occur with regard to genetic counseling, prognostic assessment, and treatment; there is still no cure or even agreed standards of treatment available for these debilitating diseases. Limited therapeutic options and a lack of curative treatment have led to physicians prescribing individual "trials of therapy" for which no evidence-based recommendations are available. However, new therapeutic options are the focus of active molecular genetic, biochemical, and clinical research, and some medicinal compounds have achieved international governmental approval. In this chapter, we summarize these advances and provide a broad overview of the treatment and novel approaches to preventing transmission of mitochondrial disease.

Keywords

mitochondrial disease, phenotype, genetic, therapy, mtDNA

Introduction

Mitochondrial disorders are frequently multisystemic and the most prevalent group of inherited neurometabolic diseases (prevalence: 1:4300).[1] The diseases are clinically, biochemically, and genetically heterogeneous so that recognition and diagnosis are often difficult. However, recent advances in next-generation sequencing (NGS) technology have led to vast improvements in genetic diagnosis for these patients. Improved diagnostic algorithms and the use of NGS have enabled an earlier diagnosis for many and, in rare cases, the early instigation of effective therapy. Due to the variability of clinical features and the particular nature of some of the biochemical or genetic defects, it is not easy for the lay practitioner to identify and screen for treatable aspects of mitochondrial disease and early referral to a specialized center is therefore recommended. There is still no cure available for the vast majority of these conditions, and though liver or hematopoietic stem cell transplant may offer hope for a few, clinical care is largely confined to managing the complications of these diseases (Newcastle Care Guidelines:www.newcastle-mitochondria.com) or assisting prevention through prenatal testing, preimplantation genetic diagnosis (PGD), and mitochondrial donation therapy. The limited therapeutic options and the lack of curative treatment options have led to increased individual therapy trials, particularly focused on optimizing oxidative phosphorylation (OXPHOS) and improving antioxidant capacity. Mostly, a combination of vitamins, commonly including coenzyme Q10 (ubiquinone), thiamine, and riboflavin is recommended. However, there are trials ongoing worldwide investigating potential therapeutic approaches.

Background of mtDNA and nDNA Mutations and Mitochondrial Disease

Primary mitochondrial diseases are genetic conditions that impair the process of intracellular energy conversion known

[1] Wellcome Centre for Mitochondrial Research, Institute of Neuroscience, Newcastle University, Newcastle upon Tyne, United Kingdom
[2] Department of Neurology, University of Halle-Wittenberg, Halle/Saale, Germany

Corresponding Author:
Diana Lehmann, MD, Wellcome Centre for Mitochondrial Research, Institute of Neuroscience, Newcastle University, Newcastle upon Tyne, United Kingdom.
Email: diana.lehmann@rku.de

as OXPHOS and may occur as a result of mutations in mitochondrial DNA (mtDNA) or nuclear DNA (nDNA). Mitochondrial DNA is a maternally inherited, circular double-stranded molecule of 16 569 base pairs, encoding 37 genes (13 proteins of the OXPHOS system, 2 rRNAs, and 22 tRNAs). The remaining mitochondrial proteins are nuclear-encoded and imported into the mitochondria. Mutations of mtDNA can be classified into (1) structural rearrangements (eg, large-scale single deletion of mtDNA), (2) quantitative disorders of mtDNA (reduction in mtDNA copy number, mtDNA depletion), and (3) point mutations.

All eukaryotic cells contain, depending on their lineage and differentiation, a variable number of mitochondria, which carry numerous copies of the mitochondrial genome (>100 000 copies in mature oocytes). During mitosis, wild-type mtDNA and mutant mtDNA are randomly distributed to the daughter cells (replicative segregation). A cell is deemed to be homoplasmic if all mtDNA copies are identical. However, a heteroplasmic state exists if wild-type and mutant mtDNA are coexistent in a cell. The level of heteroplasmy describes the percentage of mutant mtDNA and may vary over time. In general, the proportion of mutated mtDNA has to exceed a certain percentage (threshold) to cause biochemical defects leading to clinical symptoms and, above this threshold, the higher the level of heteroplasmy the greater the risk of disease. One clear exception occurs in the form of homoplasmic mutations where biochemical and clinical phenotype can be variably expressed.

Difficulties in "Genotype–Phenotype Correlations"

Defects of OXPHOS are one of the most common groups of inherited neurometabolic diseases, and with the advent of NGS technology, opportunities to make a genetic diagnosis in these disorders continue to grow. However, studying this disease remains problematic for a number of reasons. Firstly, the clinical manifestations of mitochondrial disease are protean and may present at any stage of life. Disease may involve a single (Leber hereditary optic neuropathy [LHON]) or multiple (Kearns Sayre Syndrome) organs, often with intermittent acute exacerbations punctuating a slowly progressive disease with extended periods of relative stability.[2,3] Moreover, the genotype–phenotype relationship in mitochondrial diseases can exhibit remarkable overlap, with the same clinical phenotype being caused by mutations in several different genes, and in contrast, the same genetic mutation can give rise to several distinct phenotypes.[1] For example, the m.3243A>G mutation is associated with mitochondrial encephalomyopathy, lactic acidosis, and stroke-like episodes (MELAS), maternally inherited diabetes and deafness (MIDD), chronic progressive external ophthalmoplegia (CPEO), and nonsyndromic clinical presentations. Aggravating the problem of "genotype–phenotype" correlations, there is a historical lack of genetic diagnosis and reliance on biochemical abnormalities detected in affected tissue.

Improvements in Clinical Research

During recent years, there has been an immense improvement in genetic diagnosis of patients with mitochondrial diseases due to advanced technologies including whole exome sequencing and whole genome sequencing. Improved diagnostic algorithms and the use of these new technologies have enabled an earlier diagnosis for many, and in rare cases, the early instigation of effective therapy.[4] The establishment of "orphan drug status" and other incentives, including tax respite and voucher exchange schemes, has made clinical research in mitochondrial disease rather more attractive to the pharmaceutical industry. A directive from the European Government requiring each member state of the European Union to produce a national strategy for rare diseases has also been helpful in mobilizing support from national governments. This area of research has been further assisted by the development of national cohorts and registries of patients, facilitating "deep" phenotyping and collection of natural history data. These initiatives have undoubtedly improved the "trial readiness" of the mitochondrial disease population in some countries at least.

Previous Therapeutic Approaches

Treatable Aspects

Due to the wide variability of phenotypes in mitochondrial diseases, early identification and screening for *treatable aspects* are necessary. If possible, the patient should be referred to a specialized mitochondrial center for initial diagnosis and coordination of investigation and treatment. Depending on the patient/parent preferences, subsequent care may be provided locally with input from the specialized center. Clinical care guidelines for managing various aspects of mitochondrial disease are available from the Wellcome Centre for Mitochondrial Research in Newcastle upon Tyne, United Kingdom. These clinical guidelines are updated every 2 years and can be found online: http://www.newcastle-mitochondria.com/clinical-professional-home-page/clinical-publications/clinical-guidelines/. Furthermore, handbooks for patients and parents of affected children are available for download from the Mitochondrial Medicine Society: http://www.mitosoc.org/toolkit/. Recently, the clinical guideline on management of stroke-like episodes in MELAS has been updated.[5]

Cardiac involvement is a common feature in mitochondrial diseases.[6] Both, conduction abnormalities and cardiomyopathy are observed in mitochondrial disease patients. Recent studies show an association of specific cardiac phenotypes with pathogenic mtDNA mutations (eg, heart block associated with large-scale mtDNA deletions, hypertrophic cardiomyopathy with mtDNA point mutations, and adult sudden death syndrome with the m. 3243A>G mutation).[7,8] General assessment of patients and seemingly asymptomatic carriers for possible cardiac involvement should include a standard 12-lead electrocardiogram and transthoracic echocardiogram. Cardiomyopathy can be managed with the use of angiotensin-converting enzyme inhibitors, which may prevent early hypertrophic remodeling, while coadministration of β-adrenergic receptor antagonists (βblockers) or calcium channel blockers will slow the heart rate and improve diastolic filling. Pacemaker implantation should be considered if patients are at risk of atrioventricular (AV) block (including first-degree AV block >300 milliseconds) or any fascicular block with or without symptoms. Clinical vigilance to identify heart block and prompt action with regard to implanting a pacing device can be lifesaving in mitochondrial disease.

Some mitochondrial diseases are defined by a severe *gastrointestinal* phenotype (eg, mitochondrial neurogastrointestinal encephalomyopathy [MNGIE]). Others, such as those caused by the m.3243A>G mutation, have significant gastrointestinal involvement which is often unrecognized and may lead to chronic intestinal pseudo-obstruction (CIPO), a potentially life-threatening complication in these patients. Acute presentations of CIPO can mimic mechanical obstruction of both, the upper gastrointestinal (GI) and the lower GI. In the acute phase, intravenous (IV) fluids (with avoidance of Ringers lactate solution) should be provided. Vomiting associated with CIPO can lead to serious complications, especially in patients who are not able to adequately protect their own airways. In any case of CIPO, surgical intervention should be the last option due to its high mortality rates.

Furthermore anorexia, nausea, and vomiting can cause difficulties in taking oral medication or even hamper fluid and calorie intake. Patients having chronic constipation may benefit from a low fiber diet and institution of simple measures such as increasing fluid intake and the use of osmotic laxatives. If these interventions are unsuccessful, then consideration should be given to referral for gastroenterological and dietetic opinions. Some patients with mitochondrial disease experience significant dysphagia or severe gastroesophageal reflux and surgical placement of a gastrostomy (with or without fundoplication) or jejunostomy may be necessary.

Diabetes Mellitus is one of the most common features in mitochondrial diseases and female patients harboring one of the commonest mtDNA mutations (m.3243A>G) appear to have an increased risk of gestational diabetes. Although a large proportion of patients with the m.3243A>G mutation have clinical features that do not conform with a specific syndrome, many do have a syndromic presentation that includes MELAS, CPEO, and MIDD. The clinical presentation ranges from ketone positive, insulin-dependent diabetes to classical non–insulin-dependent diabetes. Progression to insulin dependency as a result of pancreatic islet cell dysfunction is common and often rapid (<4 years).

Epilepsy is a regular feature of many mitochondrial diseases and particularly common in myoclonic epilepsy with ragged-red fibers (MERRF), MELAS, and *POLG1*-associated syndromes such as Alpers-Huttenlocher. The MELAS and MERRF seem to respond well to Levetiracetam and/or Clobazam, and early initiation/escalation of anticonvulsant therapy is crucial in managing stroke-like episodes with the aim of preventing cortical damage due to seizure activity. Sodium valproate should be avoided due to potential hepatotoxicity, particularly in patients with mutations in *POLG1*.

Central nervous system (CNS) involvement is a recognized feature of mitochondrial disease, with spasticity and dystonia being common CNS manifestations in both children and adults. Medical intervention with conventional treatments for spasticity and dystonia should be tailored to the individual and initiated early, in conjunction with appropriate physiotherapy. Baclofen or botulinum toxin injections should be considered in cases of spasticity while those having dystonia should be offered a trial of L-Dopa.

Exercise is known to improve functional capacity in patients with mitochondrial disease, and although exercise does not provide a cure for mitochondrial disease, it can greatly improve quality of life, prevent complications, and help with the management of ataxia.

Respiratory impairment, as a consequence of diaphragmatic weakness, is a common occurrence in mitochondrial myopathies though is often overlooked by both physicians and patients. Affected patients may develop chronic respiratory insufficiency or decompensate acutely as a result of cardiopulmonary disease, general anesthesia, or postoperative complications. Diaphragmatic weakness may also lead to nocturnal hypoventilation, which can be effectively treated by noninvasive positive pressure ventilation. Swallowing difficulties (usually due to bulbar weakness) can lead to aspiration pneumonia, and repeated episodes may contribute to chronic respiratory failure. Paradoxically, coughing can cause atelectasis, reduced lung volumes, and predispose to recurrent chest infections. Patients with respiratory involvement should be offered access to all relevant vaccinations (eg, influenza vaccine, pneumonia vaccine).

Otolaryngology and Psychological Support

Swallowing and speech difficulties can often be significantly improved by speech therapy. Hearing disorders can be improved with a hearing aid, and in individual cases, a cochlear implant may also be indicated. Many patients have difficulty coping with mitochondrial disease, and aspects such as fatigue are particularly challenging. Perhaps not surprisingly, the prevalence of psychological problems such as depression is high in this patient group, and psychotherapy is often appropriate.

Patient Groups

Patients, families, and carers affected by mitochondrial disease in many countries in Europe, North America, and Australasia have formed their own patient support groups. These, usually charitably funded groups provide practical and emotional support to families and often help with access to expert assessment and opinion. An international mitochondrial patient organization has been formed from representatives of individual mitochondrial patient groups across many different countries and, like the United Mitochondrial Disease Foundation (United States) and the Lily Foundation (United Kingdom), has campaigned for patients with mitochondrial disease at the highest levels of government.

Specific Therapies: Vitamins

Due to the clinical, biochemical, and genetic heterogeneity of mitochondrial diseases, there is still no standardized treatment available. Another limiting factor is the inaccessibility of the mitochondrion as a target for possible drugs: a potential treatment needs to enter the mitochondrial matrix, surrounded by 2 mitochondrial lipid membranes, having already traversed the cell membrane. A variable combination of vitamins, commonly including coenzyme Q10 (ubiquinone), thiamine, and riboflavin among others is often recommended on the basis that these may be helpful in optimizing OXPHOS and are very unlikely to cause harm at the doses prescribed.[9]

Vitamin cocktails: Coenzyme Q10 (ubiquinone) acts as a mobile electron carrier (complex I/II to complex III) and has, in addition, antioxidative properties. Although ubiquinone deficiency is a clear indication for treatment with high dose (500-1000 mg/d) coenzyme Q10,[10] this compound is also tried in many other mitochondrial diseases usually with more modest doses, in the range of 90 to 300 mg/d.[11] The side-effect profile of coenzyme Q10 is remarkably benign with even high doses producing few, if any, problems. Riboflavin (vitamin B_2) is a precursor of flavoprotein. It serves as a key building block in complex I and II and as cofactor in several other key enzymatic reactions involving fatty acid oxidation and the Krebs cycle. The main indication for treatment (50-100 mg/d orally) is complex I or complex II deficiency in relation to ubiquinone deficiency caused by *ETFDH* mutations.[10,12] Recently, a neonatal case of complex I deficiency (including hypotonia, cardiac hypertrophy, lactic acidosis) due to an *ACAD9* mutation has been reported. After treatment with large doses of Riboflavin, a favorable clinical response was observed. The patient had no cognitive impairment and normal psychomotor development at the age of 5 years.[13]

Carnitine transfers long-chain fatty acids across the mitochondrial inner membrane into the mitochondrial matrix where there are necessary for the mitochondrial β-oxidation. L-Carnitine is available for oral or intravenous use in mitochondrial diseases.[9] Individual therapy with acetyl-L-carnitine is often suggested; however, there is limited evidence to support this recommendation.[14]

Some vitamins, are mainly used as part of an antioxidant cocktail, for example, thiamine, vitamin C, and vitamin E. Thiamine, often used to treat patients with pyruvate dehydrogenase (PDH) deficiency, is known to enhance the activity of PDH and increase the availability of pyruvate for oxidation.[15] Biotin is a water-soluble vitamin that serves as an essential coenzyme for 5 carboxylases.[16] Both, biotin and thiamine are used in treatment of biotin-responsive basal ganglia disease caused by mutations in *SLC19A3* gene.[17] Furthermore, biotin is also used in patients with biotinidase deficiency mutations, which is known to mimic Leigh syndrome.

Many patients with mitochondrial disease are at risk of vitamin D deficiency due to their chronic ill health, lack of sun exposure (immobility), or/and dietary insufficiency. For this reason, frequent measurement of vitamin D levels in blood is recommended, and if applicable, vitamin D substitution should be ensured.

Idebenone

Leber hereditary optic neuropathy is most frequently caused by one of the following mtDNA mutations: m.11778G>A, m.3460G>A, and m.14484T>C though a number of "secondary" mutations have been described.[18] Most LHON patients remain asymptomatic until early adulthood when visual loss may be sudden and profound. Often asymmetric in onset, the visual loss can be triggered by smoking and possibly alcohol. The marked decrease in visual acuity experienced during the acute phase of LHON is thought to be a consequence of respiratory chain dysfunction in viable, but inactive, retinal ganglion cells.[19] Idebenone is known to preserve or reestablish retinal ganglion cell function during the acute phase and thus protects from irreversible retinal ganglion cell loss.[18] The first complete randomized, placebo-controlled, double-blind clinical trial in LHON, including 85 unselected patients with LHON ≥14 years of age, receiving 900 mg/d of idebenone or placebo in a 2:1 ratio for 24 weeks, provided clear evidence supporting the beneficial effects of idebenone in LHON.[20] Accordingly, the European Medicines Agency has subsequently licensed Raxone (idebenone) to treat adults and adolescents aged 12 years and older at a recommended daily dose of 900 mg. Treatment should begin immediately after diagnosis and continue, if possible, for at least 2 years.

L-Arginine and Citrulline

Stoke-like episodes in MELAS syndrome usually occur before the age of 40 years and are 1 cardinal clinical feature of this condition. Hemianopsia or cortical blindness are often the first focal neurological disturbances, and the episodes are often accompanied by migraine-like headaches with vomiting and epileptic seizures. Nitric oxide (NO) donors, such as L-arginine and citrulline, may be a therapeutic option for MELAS-related stroke-like episodes, and research studies are ongoing. These NO donors may reduce the severity of stroke-like episodes and reduce the frequency of the episodes.[21] However, there are only a few clinical trials investigating L-arginine, and the window of opportunity for treatment with L-arginine is limited (within 12 hours of onset).[21–25]

Dichloroacetate

Dichloroacetate (DCA) is a synthetic agent aimed to increase the respiratory chain substrate availability, so as to keep the PDH complex in an active state and reduce the accumulation of lactate in body tissues.[15] Dichloroacetate is used to treat lactic acidosis, a common problem in mitochondrial disorders. However, treatment with DCA leads to irreversible peripheral neuropathy. Controlled trials did not lead to conclusive evidence of the benefits of DCA in patients with mitochondrial disorders, but individual case reports suggest some benefit from using DCA as a treatment option.[9]

EPI-743 is a synthetic analogue of vitamin E (para-benzoquinone), targeting the repletion of reduced intracellular glutathione.[26] There are some studies showing that treatment with EPI-743 in patients with Leigh syndrome (subacute necrotizing encephalopathy) improved the clinical outcome.[26,27] EPI-743 is known to be a potent antioxidant (about >100× higher than CoQ10), but it failed to reach the end point in a recent double-blind randomized controlled trial, although an unblinded extension phase of the study is currently ongoing.

Potential Therapies

Heteroplasmy Shift

Mitochondrial DNA mutations tend to be present in a heteroplasmic state. Therefore, one therapeutic approach is the elimination or reduction of mutated mtDNA amount below the threshold at which the disease biochemically or clinically manifests. Several groups have recently developed cellular models by targeting to mitochondria recombinant restriction endonucleases,[28–30] zinc finger endonucleases,[31] or transcription activator-like effector nucleases (TALENs).[32] Bacman et al were able to reduce the level of heteroplasmy in cell lines of patients harboring a mtDNA deletion (human osteosarcoma cells heteroplasmic for the large 5 kb "common deletion") and a point mutation (osteosarcoma cybrids heteroplasmic for 14459G>A [LHON] in the *MT–ND6* gene).[32] The group engineered mitochondrial-specific TALENs. The expression of mitoTALENs led to permanent reductions in heteroplasmy levels in both cell lines. However, one limitation was the severe cellular depletion of mtDNA before repopulation with favorable heteroplasmy ratio.

Hypoxia

According to cell and zebra fish model studies, a genetic or small molecule activation of hypoxia response is protective against mitochondrial toxicity.[33] Limiting oxygen availability has been found to be a protective factor during respiratory chain inhibition. In a genetic mouse model of Leigh syndrome, it could be shown that chronic hypoxia leads to a marked improvement in survival, body weight, body temperature, behavior, neuropathology, and disease biomarkers.[33]

Bone Marrow and Liver Transplantation

MNGIE is clinically characterized by CPEO, severe gastrointestinal dysmotility leading to cachexia, peripheral neuropathy, and leukoencephalopathy, usually leading to death in early to mid-adulthood.[34] The genetic basis of this disease is a loss-of-function mutation in the *TYMP* gene encoding for the cytosolic enzyme thymidine phosphorylase (TPase), which leads to severe elevations of thymidine and deoxyuridine in blood and other tissues, likely disrupting the dinucleotide pool available for mtDNA synthesis and causing instability of the mtDNA that results in multiple deletions, depletion, and point mutations.[35,36] Approaches to eliminate thymidine and deoxyuridine in blood and other tissues only showed positive results transiently.[37–39] However, permanent restoration of TPase activity has been achieved by allogeneic hematopoietic stem cell transplantation.[40] Another approach of treatment to restore the TPase activity may be liver transplantation as a cellular source of TP.[41] A recent study investigated 11 patients who underwent hepatic resection for focal disorders. The overall results of Western blot, ELISA, immunohistochemistry, and qPCR showed that TYMP messenger RNA was expressed in the liver. Consequently, liver transplantation may be considered as a therapeutic alternative for patients with MNGIE.[41]

Ethylmalonic encephalopathy is caused by *ETHE1* mutations and leads to toxic accumulation of hydrogen sulfide and of its metabolites, including thiosulphate. Clinical features include diffuse microvasculature damage (petechial purpura, multiple necrotic brain lesions), orthostatic acrocyanosis, and hemorrhagic effusions of intestinal mucosa associated with chronic diarrhea. The early-onset brain damage leads to severe psychomotor delay with spastic tetraparesis.[42] Recently, the development of a liver-specific, adenovirus-mediated expression of human wild-type *ETHE1* as a therapy in an *Ethe1*$^{-/-}$ mouse model led to the hypothesis that liver transplantation could also ameliorate human ethylmalonic encephalopathy.[43] Recently, a 9-month-old girl underwent liver transplantation, with her mother as a living donor.[4] Eight months after liver transplantation, striking neurological improvement with remarkable achievements in psychomotor development, along with dramatic reversion of biochemical abnormalities, has been observed.

PGC1α

PGC1α is known to have neuroprotective effects by increasing mitochondrial biogenesis and its functioning.[44] Due to its role in regulation of mitochondrial function, PGC1α is emerging as an important player in ageing and neurodegenerative disorders.[44] Bezafibrate and resveratrol are known to be PGC1α stimulators, and the former already has supportive data from preclinical studies (cellular and mouse models) showing improvement in mitochondrial function and is already licensed as a treatment for high blood fat and has a well characterized side-effect profile. Currently, there is a phase II study of bezafibrate in people with mitochondrial myopathy ongoing in Newcastle upon Tyne, United Kingdom (Newcastle-upon-Tyne Hospitals NHS Trust).

MitoQ—Antioxidant Delivery

One major source of reactive oxygen species (ROS) are mitochondria. Consequently, the development of antioxidants, decreasing mitochondrial oxidative damage is one major approach in therapies of mitochondrial diseases.[45] To date, *MitoQ* is the best characterized mitochondria-targeted antioxidant, consisting of a quinone moiety linked to a triphenylphosphonium moiety and has been used in in vivo studies and in 2 phase II human trials, indicating that *MitoQ* can be successfully delivered orally to humans for up to a year and that these doses are effective in decreasing liver damage.[45]

Furthermore, there are several compounds under investigation. KH167 is an orally bioavailable small molecule, which is capable of reducing ROS in cells. Initial tests showed decreased intracellular ROS levels in a fibroblast patient cell line (mutation in the *NDUFS7* gene). A successful outcome after a phase I trial has been reported. Elamipretide as possible treatment for LHON—patients and RP103 reached a phase II trial. Fujii et al studied the effect of pyruvate in 4 bedridden pediatric patients with OXPHOS disorders.[46] The results showed a positive effect (evaluated with the Newcastle Paediatric Mitochondrial Disease Scale and the Gross Motor Function Measure with 88 items), at least in the short term. However, clinical trials with more patients and less severe disabilities are necessary to evaluate the long-term efficacy of this treatment.[46]

Prevention of Mitochondrial Diseases

The transmission of mitochondrial disease is dependent on the proportion of mutated mtDNA carried by the affected mother's egg. Homoplasmic mutations will be transmitted to each child in a homoplasmic state. However, in women with heteroplasmic mutation loads, the level transmitted to their children is more difficult to predict. The only methods to avoid transmission of mutated mtDNA are those dependent on egg donation, including mitochondrial donation where there remains a small risk of mutation carryover (see below). Other methods such as PGD are risk reduction procedures and are unlikely to completely prevent transmission of the mutated mtDNA.

Preimplantation genetic diagnosis and/or *prenatal diagnosis* are offered to women who have heteroplasmic mtDNA mutations, but are aiming to use their own eggs to have a baby, and women having a mitochondrial disease due to a nuclear mutation. Preimplantation genetic diagnosis may be offered as part of an in vitro fertilization (IVF) cycle prior to the pregnancy. Prenatal diagnosis will be carried out when the pregnancy has been established for some time (chorionic villus sampling at 11-12 weeks' gestation or amniocentesis at 15-17 weeks). However, none of these techniques can be offered to women with homoplasmic mutations.

Mitochondrial donation is a new approach to prevent the transmission of mutated mtDNA from mother to child.[47] The pronuclei, containing the nDNA of both parents, are removed from the fertilized egg and placed into a donor egg containing healthy mtDNA and from which the pronuclei have been removed, a technique known as pronuclear transfer. Alternatively, this IVF technique can be performed before fertilization using maternal spindle transfer and this may be ethically more acceptable to some couples.[48,49]

Authors' Note

Diana Lehmann is currently affiliated to Department of Neurology, University of Ulm, Ulm, Germany.

Declaration of Conflicting Interests

The author(s) declared no potential conflicts of interest with respect to the research, authorship, and/or publication of this article.

Funding

The author(s) received no financial support for the research, authorship, and/or publication of this article.

References

1. Gorman GS, Schaefer AM, Ng Y, et al. Prevalence of nuclear and mitochondrial DNA mutations related to adult mitochondrial disease. *Ann Neurol*. 2015;77(5):753-759.
2. Chinnery PF. Mitochondrial disorders overview. In: Pagon RA, Adam MP, Ardinger HH, Wallace SE, Amemiya A, Bean LJH, eds. *Gene Reviews(R)*. Seattle, WA. 1993.
3. McFarland R, Taylor RW, Turnbull DM. A neurological perspective on mitochondrial disease. *Lancet Neurol*. 2010;9(8):829-840.
4. Dionisi-Vici C, Diodato D, Torre G, et al. Liver transplant in ethylmalonic encephalopathy: a new treatment for an otherwise fatal disease. *Brain*. 2016;139(pt 4):1045-1051.
5. Koenig MK, Emrick L, Karaa A, et al. Recommendations for the management of strokelike episodes in patients with mitochondrial encephalomyopathy, lactic acidosis, and strokelike episodes. *JAMA Neurol*. 2016;73(5):591-594.
6. Chinnery P, Majamaa K, Turnbull D, Thorburn D. Treatment for mitochondrial disorders. *Cochrane Database Syst Rev*. 2006;(1): CD004426.
7. Ng YS, Grady JP, Lax NZ, et al. Sudden adult death syndrome in m.3243A>G-related mitochondrial disease: an unrecognized clinical entity in young, asymptomatic adults. *Eur Heart J*. 2016; 37(32):2552-2559.
8. Bates MG, Bourke JP, Giordano C, d'Amati G, Turnbull DM, Taylor RW. Cardiac involvement in mitochondrial DNA disease: clinical spectrum, diagnosis, and management. *Eur Heart J*. 2012; 33(24):3023-3033.
9. Parikh S, Saneto R, Falk MJ, et al. A modern approach to the treatment of mitochondrial disease. *Curr Treat Options Neurol*. 2009;11(6):414-430.
10. Gempel K, Topaloglu H, Talim B, et al. The myopathic form of coenzyme Q10 deficiency is caused by mutations in the electron-transferring-flavoprotein dehydrogenase (ETFDH) gene. *Brain*. 2007;130(pt 8):2037-2044.
11. Hanisch F, Zierz S. Only transient increase of serum CoQ subset 10 during long-term CoQ10 therapy in mitochondrial ophthalmoplegia. *Eur J Med Res*. 2003;8(11):485-491.
12. Ichiki T, Tanaka M, Nishikimi M, et al. Deficiency of subunits of Complex I and mitochondrial encephalomyopathy. *Ann Neurol*. 1988;23(3):287-294.
13. Haack TB, Danhauser K, Haberberger B, et al. Exome sequencing identifies ACAD9 mutations as a cause of complex I deficiency. *Nature Genet*. 2010;42(12):1131-1134.
14. Parikh S, Goldstein A, Koenig MK, et al. Diagnosis and management of mitochondrial disease: a consensus statement from the mitochondrial medicine society. *Genet Med*. 2015;17(9):689-701.

15. Avula S, Parikh S, Demarest S, Kurz J, Gropman A. Treatment of mitochondrial disorders. *Curr Treat Options Neurol.* 2014; 16(6):292.
16. Zempleni J, Hassan YI, Wijeratne SS. Biotin and biotinidase deficiency. *Expert Rev Endocrinol Metab.* 2008;3(6):715-724.
17. Flones I, Sztromwasser P, Haugarvoll K, et al. Novel SLC19A3 promoter deletion and allelic silencing in biotin-thiamine-responsive basal ganglia encephalopathy. *PLoS One.* 2016; 11(2):e0149055.
18. Klopstock T, Metz G, Yu-Wai-Man P, et al. Persistence of the treatment effect of idebenone in Leber's hereditary optic neuropathy. *Brain.* 2013;136(pt 2):e230.
19. Howell N. Leber hereditary optic neuropathy: respiratory chain dysfunction and degeneration of the optic nerve. *Vision Res.* 1998;38(10):1495-1504.
20. Klopstock T, Yu-Wai-Man P, Dimitriadis K, et al. A randomized placebo-controlled trial of idebenone in Leber's hereditary optic neuropathy. *Brain.* 2011;134(pt 9):2677-2686.
21. Koga Y, Akita Y, Nishioka J, et al. L-arginine improves the symptoms of strokelike episodes in MELAS. *Neurology.* 2005; 64(4):710-712.
22. Koga Y, Ishibashi M, Ueki I, et al. Effects of L-arginine on the acute phase of strokes in three patients with MELAS. *Neurology.* 2002;58(5):827-828.
23. Koga Y, Akita Y, Junko N, et al. Endothelial dysfunction in MELAS improved by l-arginine supplementation. *Neurology.* 2006;66(11):1766-1769.
24. Koga Y, Povalko N, Nishioka J, Katayama K, Yatsuga S, Matsuishi T. Molecular pathology of MELAS and L-arginine effects. *Biochim Biophys Acta.* 2012;1820(5):608-614.
25. Koga Y, Akita Y, Nishioka J, et al. MELAS and L-arginine therapy. *Mitochondrion.* 2007;7(1-2):133-139.
26. Martinelli D, Catteruccia M, Piemonte F, et al. EPI-743 reverses the progression of the pediatric mitochondrial disease – genetically defined Leigh syndrome. *Mol Genet Metab.* 2012;107(3):383-388.
27. Enns GM, Kinsman SL, Perlman SL, et al. Initial experience in the treatment of inherited mitochondrial disease with EPI-743. *Mol Genet Metab.* 2012;105(1):91-102.
28. Bacman SR, Williams SL, Hernandez D, Moraes CT. Modulating mtDNA heteroplasmy by mitochondria-targeted restriction endonucleases in a 'differential multiple cleavage-site' model. *Gen Ther.* 2007;14(18):1309-1318.
29. Bacman SR, Williams SL, Duan D, Moraes CT. Manipulation of mtDNA heteroplasmy in all striated muscles of newborn mice by AAV9-mediated delivery of a mitochondria-targeted restriction endonuclease. *Gen Ther.* 2012;19(11):1101-1106.
30. Srivastava S, Moraes CT. Manipulating mitochondrial DNA heteroplasmy by a mitochondrially targeted restriction endonuclease. *Hum Mol Genet.* 2001;10(26):3093-3099.
31. Gammage PA, Rorbach J, Vincent AI, Rebar EJ, Minczuk M. Mitochondrially targeted ZFNs for selective degradation of pathogenic mitochondrial genomes bearing large-scale deletions or point mutations. *EMBO Mol Med.* 2014;6(4):458-466.
32. Bacman SR, Williams SL, Pinto M, Peralta S, Moraes CT. Specific elimination of mutant mitochondrial genomes in patient-derived cells by mitoTALENs. *Nat Med.* 2013;19(9):1111-1113.
33. Jain IH, Zazzeron L, Goli R, et al. Hypoxia as a therapy for mitochondrial disease. *Science.* 2016;352(6281):54-61.
34. Hirano M, Silvestri G, Blake DM, et al. Mitochondrial neurogastrointestinal encephalomyopathy (MNGIE): clinical, biochemical, and genetic features of an autosomal recessive mitochondrial disorder. *Neurology.* 1994;44(4):721-727.
35. Valentino ML, Marti R, Tadesse S, et al. Thymidine and deoxyuridine accumulate in tissues of patients with mitochondrial neurogastrointestinal encephalomyopathy (MNGIE). *FEBS Lett.* 2007;581(18):3410-3414.
36. Lopez LC, Akman HO, Garcia-Cazorla A, et al. Unbalanced deoxynucleotide pools cause mitochondrial DNA instability in thymidine phosphorylase-deficient mice. *Hum Mol Genet.* 2009; 18(4):714-722.
37. Spinazzola A, Marti R, Nishino I, et al. Altered thymidine metabolism due to defects of thymidine phosphorylase. *J Biol Chem.* 2002;277(6):4128-4133.
38. la Marca G, Malvagia S, Casetta B, et al. Pre- and post-dialysis quantitative dosage of thymidine in urine and plasma of a MNGIE patient by using HPLC-ESI-MS/MS. *J Mass Spectrom.* 2006; 41(5):586-592.
39. Yavuz H, Ozel A, Christensen M, et al. Treatment of mitochondrial neurogastrointestinal encephalomyopathy with dialysis. *Arch Neurol.* 2007;64(3):435-438.
40. Schupbach M, Benoist JF, Casali C, et al. Allogeneic hematopoietic stem cell transplantation (HSCT) for mitochondrial neurogastrointestinal encephalomyopathy (MNGIE). *Neurology.* 2009;73(4):332.
41. Boschetti E, D'Alessandro R, Bianco F, et al. Liver as a source for thymidine phosphorylase replacement in mitochondrial neurogastrointestinal encephalomyopathy. *PLoS One.* 2014;9(5):e96692.
42. Mineri R, Rimoldi M, Burlina AB, et al. Identification of new mutations in the ETHE1 gene in a cohort of 14 patients presenting with ethylmalonic encephalopathy. *J Med Genet.* 2008;45(7): 473-478.
43. Di Meo I, Auricchio A, Lamperti C, Burlina A, Viscomi C, Zeviani M. Effective AAV-mediated gene therapy in a mouse model of ethylmalonic encephalopathy. *EMBO Mol Med.* 2012; 4(9):1008-1014.
44. Dabrowska A, Venero JL, Iwasawa R, et al. PGC-1alpha controls mitochondrial biogenesis and dynamics in lead-induced neurotoxicity. *Aging (Albany NY).* 2015;7(9):629-647.
45. Smith RA, Murphy MP. Animal and human studies with the mitochondria-targeted antioxidant MitoQ. *Ann N Y Acad Sci.* 2010;1201:96-103.
46. Fujii T, Nozaki F, Saito K, et al. Efficacy of pyruvate therapy in patients with mitochondrial disease: a semi-quantitative clinical evaluation study. *Mol Genet Metab.* 2014;112(2):133-138.
47. Craven L, Tuppen HA, Greggains GD, et al. Pronuclear transfer in human embryos to prevent transmission of mitochondrial DNA disease. *Nature.* 2010;465(7294):82-85.
48. Craven L, Herbert M, Murdoch A, Murphy J, Lawford Davies J, Turnbull DM. Research into policy: a brief history of mitochondrial donation. *Stem Cells.* 2016;34(2):265-267.
49. Hyslop LA, Blakeley P, Craven L, et al. Towards clinical application of pronuclear transfer to prevent mitochondrial DNA disease. *Nature.* 2016;534(7607):383-386.

27

Epilepsy and Mitochondrial Dysfunction: A Single Center's Experience

Russell P. Saneto, DO, PhD[1]

Abstract

Epilepsy is a common manifestation of mitochondrial disease. In a large cohort of children and adolescents with mitochondrial disease (n = 180), over 48% of patients developed seizures. The majority (68%) of patients were younger than 3 years and medically intractable (90%). The electroencephalographic pattern of multiregional epileptiform discharges over the left and right hemisphere with background slowing occurred in 62%. The epilepsy syndrome, infantile spasms, was seen in 17%. Polymerase γ mutations were the most common genetic etiology of seizures, representing Alpers-Huttenlocher syndrome (14%). The severity of disease in those patients with epilepsy was significant, as 13% of patients experienced early death. Simply the loss of energy production cannot explain the development of seizures or all patients with mitochondrial dysfunction would have epilepsy. Until the various aspects of mitochondrial physiology that are involved in proper brain development are understood, epilepsy and its treatment will remain unsatisfactory.

Keywords

epilepsy, seizures, mitochondrial disease, electroencephalogram, infantile spasms, Alpers-Huttenlocher syndrome, status epilepticus, treatment

Introduction

Mitochondria are essential organelles involved in the proper operation of the highly controlled cellular energetic processes of brain function, including amino acid and fatty acid synthesis and metabolism, heme synthesis, and control of intracellular calcium fluxes. Central to the cellular controls of these processes is mitochondrial energy production. Compromise of the organelle's ability to produce energy, adenosine triphosphate (ATP), can disrupt the intricate controls of the mitochondrial multiple functions and can lead to excitation and inhibition of communication between neurons and glia. The deficit in energy production alters the balance of neuronal excitation and inhibition, which can lead to seizures.

Mitochondria contain their own genome that gives rise to mitochondrial-specific protein translational components of 22 tRNAs, 2 rRNAs, and 13 polypeptides involved in the oxidative phosphorylation (OXPHOS) production of ATP.[1] However, the replication, maintenance, and expression of mitochondrial DNA (mtDNA) and the other mitochondrial processes are nuclear-encoded products from nuclear DNA (nDNA). The proper combination of mtDNA- and nDNA-encoded gene products is required for normal mitochondrial function.[2] When compromised, the unique properties of organelle-specific mtDNA and dependence of nDNA-encoded gene products can give rise to a wide variety of clinical phenotypes, including the high prevalence of seizures and encephalopathy in mitochondrial diseases. Several studies have shown that approximately 35% to 60% of individuals with biochemically confirmed mitochondrial disease have epilepsy.[3–7]

The available data suggest the prevalence of seizures is higher in the mitochondrial disease population compared to the general population in children.[3–9] However, the reasons for such a predominance of early-onset seizures is unclear. The literature is variable, with some studies describe few patients with early seizures, whereas others suggest early-onset seizures to be more common.[7–10] The aim of this study is to describe the age of onset, electroencephalogram (EEG), seizure semiologies, response to medical management, and outcomes in a large

[1] Division of Pediatric Neurology, Department of Neurology, University of Washington, Seattle, WA, USA

Corresponding Author:
Russell P. Saneto, DO, PhD, Division of Pediatric Neurology, Department of Neurology, University of Washington, 4800 Sand Point Way NE, Seattle, WA 98195, USA.
Email: russ.saneto@seattlechildrens.org

cohort of infants, children, and adolescents with mitochondrial disease from a single center.

Methods

This is a chart review cohort study from the years 2001 to 2016 of patients younger than 20 years who were diagnosed and managed at Seattle Children's Hospital. Our institutional review board (#11445) has approved this study. Mitochondrial disease confirmed whether the patient met the Bernier et al's criteria for definitive mitochondrial disease and/or possessed an mtDNA-encoded or nDNA-encoded pathological mutation.[11] When available and approved by insurance, mtDNA and nDNA gene sequencing was performed. All patients underwent 1 or more video EEG studies at Seattle Children's Hospital. Seizure semiologies were noted by video EEG and/or parental description of the events and adapted to the current International League Against Epilepsy (ILAE) classification, unless otherwise indicated.[12] Seizure frequency was determined by seizure diaries on sequential clinic visits. The author reviewed all studies and clinical reports.

Routine clinic appointments occurred at intervals of 3 to 6 months. Assessment of seizure types and their frequency and possible medication side effects took place at each visit. Seizure counts from patient seizure diaries were assessed at each visit. Families often would call the clinic's nurse line between clinic office visits to indicate seizure frequency changes and possible side effects. The author reviewed all notes recorded in the electronic medical record.

Prior to genetic testing, the determination of classically defined mitochondrial disease relied on the constellation of clinical, biochemical, and radiological signs and symptoms in the OXPHOS system. Over time, the enhanced knowledge of mitochondrial physiology, commercial availability in the identification of candidate genes involved in mitochondrial functioning, and a large number of defects outside the OXPHOS system that directly or indirectly affect mitochondrial energy production have been identified. Thus, any study examining patients described over time has bias to the diagnostic dilemma of imprecise diagnostic tools at the time of diagnosis and changing landscape of mitochondrial function elucidation.

Results

Patients

A total of 174 patients were identified as having primary mitochondrial disease, with 83 males and 91 females. Overall, the age of onset of symptoms was 3.72 years in patients without seizures (data not shown; 44.6 months; range: 1 week to 19 years). In those patients with epilepsy (n = 85; males = 41), the average age of symptom onset was earlier, as defined by seizures, with seizure onset at 2.86 years (34.3 months; range: 1 week to 19 years).

The age of onset of seizures: 40 (46%) patients had seizure onset during infancy, ≤1 year; 37 (44%) had onset during childhood, 1 to <10 years; and 8 (10%) had onset during adolescence, 10 to 19 years (Table 1). Seizures developed in 58 (68%) children younger than 3 years.

Earlier death was strongly associated in the seizure population compared to the nonseizure population. There were 5 patients who did not have seizures who died during the course of this study; average age of death was 25.4 months or about 2 years (data not shown; range: 5-60 months). In contrast, 26 patients had seizures and died (Table 1). The average age of death was 79.6 months or 6.6 years (data not shown; range: 7-168 months). Patients with infantile spasms or genetic etiologies of mitochondrial disease died earlier compared to patients with epilepsy outside these 2 categories. In patients with infantile spasms (n = 6), the time to death was earlier than the patient population with seizures (mean = 44 months; range: 8-60 months vs 79.6 months; Table 2). Only 2 patients with a history of infantile spasms were thought to have died due to sudden unexplained death due to epilepsy (SUDEP; Table 1). Patients with childhood Alpers-Huttenlocher syndrome who have died (n = 9) also had a shorter life span (Table 3). The mean time to death was 57 months (range: 9-103 months). Only 2 patients with Alpers-Huttenlocher syndrome died due to liver failure (mean = 216 months; range: 144-288 months). The other 7 patients died during status epilepticus, of which 6 died due to withdrawal of care by the parents. The other patient died of a cardiac arrest.

Twenty-six patients had pathological genetic mutations (Table 3). The most common genetic etiology of patients with epilepsy was *polymerase* γ *1* (*POLG*) mutations. Twelve patients had mutations in *POLG* and seizures. Those patients with childhood Alpers-Huttenlocher syndrome (n = 9) developed seizures at an average of 21.2 months (range: 8-36 months). Three patients with juvenile Alpers-Huttenlocher syndrome developed seizures at an average of 16 years (range: 14-17 years). Fourteen patients with other pathological genetic mutations in a variety of mtDNA or nDNA genes developed seizures at an average of 59.7 months (range: 3-228 months). Only 3 of these latter patients developed seizures before the age of 1 year. Ten of the other patients with genetic epilepsy developed seizures from 1 to 10 years, while a single patient developed seizures at the age of 19 years.

There were 56 patients without identified genetic mutations with electron transport chain (ETC) enzymatic defects and who met the Bernier et al's criteria for definitive mitochondrial disease (Table 1).[11] Forty patients had single ETC enzymatic defects. The most common single ETC defect was in complex I (n = 22). Thirteen patients had multiple ETC defects. There was a single patient with enzymatic defects suggesting an E3/lipoic acid dehydrogenase defect.[14]

Electroencephalogram Findings

The patient's age of the first EEG limited the EEG patterns of epilepsy onset. The timing of the initial study was dependent on the referral age or clinic discovery and time to arrange the initial EEG. However, once diagnosis occurred, all further evaluations occurred in 1 single center with multiple studies

Table 1. Demographics, Age of Seizure Onset, Seizure Semiology, Electron Transport Chain (ETC), and Molecular Abnormalities, and the Electroencephalograph Findings.[a]

Patient (Sex)	Age of Seizure Onset	Semiology	EEG Findings	ETC Abnormalities	Molecular Abnormality
1 (m)	1 month	Myo/tonic	MISD	IV	
2 (m)[b]	1 month	Myo/myoC/SE	SI	NA	*POLG*
3 (f)	1 month	F-motor	MISD	I, II/III	
4 (m)	1 month	ES > myo/F-motor	Hyps > MISD	III	
5 (m)	1 month	ES > myo/Tonic	Hyps > MISD	I	
6 (m)	2 months	F-motor	MISD	III	
7 (m)	2 months	ES > myo/tonic	Hyps > MISD	IV	*MTO1*
8 (f)	2 months	Myo/tonic/F-motor	MISD	I	
9 (f)[b]	2 months	ES > tonic	BS > MISD	NA	*E3/Lipoic acid*
10 (m)	2 months	Myo/tonic/clonic	MISD	NA	m.11778G>A
11 (m)	3 months	F-motor/dys	MISD	NA	m.8993T>G
12 (m)	3 months	ES > myo/tonic	Hyps > MISD	I	
13 (f)	3 months	ES > myo/tonic/myoC	Hyps > MISD	III	
14 (f)[b,c]	4 months	ES > myo/tonic	Hyps > MISD	I	
15 (f)	4 months	ES > myo/tonic	Hyps > MISD	II, III, IV	
16 (f)	4 month	ES > myo/tonic	Hyps > MISD	I	
17 (f)[b,c]	4 months	ES > F-motor	Hyps > MISD	I	
18 Female	4 months	Myo/tonic/F-motor	MISD	I	
19 (f)	4 months	ES > myo/tonic	BS > Hyps > MISD	IV	
20 (f)[b]	5 months	Myo	MISD	IV	
21 (m)	5 months	ES > myo/tonic	Hyps > MISD	I, IV	
22 (m)	5 months	Myo/tonic/F-motor	MISD	I	
23 (m)	6 months	Myo/tonic	MISD	I	
24 (m)	6 months	Myo/tonic/days	GSW	III	
25 (f)	6 months	Myo/tonic/atonic	MISD	I	
26 (f)	6 months	Myo/tonic	MISD	III	
27 (m)	6 months	Myo/tonic	MSID	I	
28 (m)[b]	7 months	Myo/tonic/GTC/myoC/EPC[c]	MISD	NA	*POLG*
29 (m)	8 months	F-motor	MISD	III	
30 (f)	8 months	Myo/2-GTC/F-motor	GSW	I	
31 (m)	8 months	Myo/2-GTC/F-motor	GSW	IV	
32 (f)[b]	9 months	Myo/EPC/F-Clonic/MyoC	MISD	NA	*POLG*
33 (m)[b]	9 months	Myo/F-clonic/myoC/EPC[c]	MISD	NA	*POLG*
34 (m)[b]	11 months	F-motor	MISD	I, III	
35 (m)	11 months	Myo/tonic/clonic	MISD	III, IV	
36 (m)[b]	12 months	ES/myo/tonic	Hyps > MISD	IV	*TANGO 2*
37 (m)	12 months	Myo/tonic	MISD	NA	m.8993T>G
38 (f)[b]	12 months	Myo/tonic	MISD	I	
39 (m)[b]	12 months	Myo/tonic	MISD	III	
40 (f)[b]	12 months	Myo/tonic/F-motor	MISD	NA	*PDHC* deficiency
41 (f)	15 months	Myo/tonic/F-motor	MISD	I, II/III	
42 (m)	15 months	ES/myo/tonic	Hyps > MISD	I	
43 (m)	18 months	Dys	MISD	IV	
44 (f)	18 months	Atonic/myo	MISD	IV	
45 (m)	20 months	F-motor/dys	Focal	I	
46 (m)	20 month	Myo/tonic	MISD	I	
47 (m)	2 years	Dys/myo	MISD	NA	m.8363G>A
48 (f)	2 years	Myo/tonic/F-motor	MISD	NA	*PDHA1*
49 (f)	2 years	Myo	MISD	I, III, IV	
50 (f)	2 years	Dys/atonic	GSW	II/III	
51 (f)	2 years	GTC (febrile)	SI	IV	
52 (f)	2 years	Dys/atonic	GSW	I	
53 (f)[b]	2 years	ES/tonic	Hyps > MISD	I, III, IV	
54 (f)	2 years	Myo/tonic/F-motor	MISD	I, IV	
55 (f)	2 years	Myo/tonic	MISD	I	
56 (f)	2 years	Myo/tonic	MISD	I, III, IV	

(continued)

Table 1. (continued)

Patient (Sex)	Age of Seizure Onset	Semiology	EEG Findings	ETC Abnormalities	Molecular Abnormality
57 (f)	2 years	EPC/myo/tonic	MISD	Normal	*RARS 2*
58 (f)[b]	2 years	Myo/F-clonic/EPC[c]	MISD	NA	*POLG*
59 (f)	3 years	F-motor	MISD	I	
60 (m)	3 years	F-motor/2-GTC	GSW > MISD	I/III, II/III	
61 (m)	3 years	Dys	MISD	I	
62 (m)	3 years	Myo/tonic	GSW	III	
63 (f)[b]	3 years	F-motor/F-clonic/myo/EPC[c]	MISD	NA	*POLG*
64 (f)	3 years	Myo/F-motor	MISD	IV	
65 (f)	4 years	Myo/2-GTC	MISD	I	
66 (f)	4 years	Tonic	MISD	I	
67 (m)	4 years	Dys/F-motor	GSW	I	
68 (f)[b]	4 years	F-motor/Myo/F-clonic/EPC[c]	MISD	NA	*POLG*
69 (m)	4 years	F-motor/myo/2-GTC/SE	MISD	NA	m.3243A>G
70 (m)[b]	5 years	F-motor/myo/F-clonic/EPC[c]	MISD > GSW > SI	Normal	*POLG*
71 (m)	5 years	F-motor/dys	MISD	III	
72 (m)	5 years	F-motor	Focal	I/III, II/III	
73 (m)	5 years	Myo/tonic	MISD	III, IV	
74 (f)[b]	6 years	F-motor/myo/SE	MISD	NA	*POLG*
75 (f)	7 years	Dys	MISD	NA	m.3243A>G
76 (f)	8 years	Dys	MISD	III	
77 (f)	9 years	Myo/F-motor	MISD	I	
78 (m)[b]	10 years	F-motor/myo	MISD	I	
79 (m)	10 years	F-motor/myo	MISD	NA	m.14478T>C
80 (m)[b]	11 years	Dys (NCS)	MISD	NA	m.14459A>G
81 (f)[b]	14 years	F-motor/myo/EPC+	MISD	III	*POLG*
82 (m)	14 years	F-motor/2-GTC	MISD	NA	m.3243A>G
83 (f)	17 years	F-motor/2-GTC/myo/SE	MISD	NA	*POLG*
84 (f)	17 years	F-motor/myo/SE	MISD	NA	*POLG*
85 (f)	19 years	Myo/tonic	MISD	NA	*SLC19A3*

Abbreviations: BS, burst suppression; dys, disconjugate; ES, epileptic spasm; EPC, epilepsy partialis continua; EPC[b], combination of epilepsy partialis continua; f, female; F-motor, focal motor; focal, epileptiform discharges over just a single region of 1 hemisphere; 2-GTC, secondary generalized tonic clonic; GSW, generalized spike and wave discharges; hyps, hypsarrhythmia; m, male; motor, minor motor movements that do not fall into category of focal or generalized; MISD, multifocal epileptiform discharges over the left and right hemisphere with background slowing; *MTO1*, mitochondrial-tRNA translation optimization factor; myo, myoclonic; myoC, myoclonus; NA, not tested for ETC activity; *PDHA 1*, pyruvate dehydrogenase alpha subunit gene; *PDHC*, pyruvate dehydrogenase complex gene; *POLG*, polymerase γ 1 gene; *RARS2*, arginyl-tRNA synthetase gene; SI, background slow for age; *SLC19A3*, solute carrier family 19 member 3 (thiamine transporter) gene; *TANGO 2*, transport and Golgi organization 2 homolog gene.
[a]After the age of 2 years, age of onset was rounded to the nearest year.
[b]Patients who have passed away.
[c]Patients who passed away to sudden unexplained death due to epilepsy.

obtained, which minimized the loss of EEG changes over time. The author reviewed all studies. The most common first EEG findings (n = 58) was an interictal pattern of multifocal spike discharges (MISD) over the left and right hemispheres with background slowing (Figure 1). Only a single patient presenting with MISD (n = 57) evolved into a different EEG pattern over the course of this study. Twenty-eight patients presented with other EEG patterns (see below). Sixteen of these patients evolved into an MISD pattern on EEG. Patients with *POLG* mutations initially presented with spikes/polyspikes over the occipital region (left and/or right), with slowing over the regions of epileptiform discharge. Only a single patient evolved from presenting with an MISD pattern to generalized slowing without epileptiform discharges. The MISD EEG pattern has also been described as multiple independent spike foci (MISF).[15] The MISD EEG pattern is epileptiform discharges arising from multiple cerebral lobes, including at least 1 area of both hemispheres.[13,15] The EEG pattern of MISD may or may not be associated with background slowing. All of the patients in this series who had MISD had background slowing, which corresponds to the Severe Epilepsy-MISF description.[13,15] To avoid confusion, the term used in this report to describe the pattern of multifocal epileptiform discharges over the left and right hemispheres with background slowing will be labeled MISD.

Fourteen patients had an EEG pattern of hypsarrhythmia, and all 14 evolved into the EEG pattern of MISD (Table 2). The onset of hypsarrhythmia on average was 6.75 months (range: 2.5 months to 2 years). Once the pattern of MISD was established, none of these patients developed other EEG patterns over time, with examination of repeat EEGs ranging from 1 to 12 years.

Generalized spike wave pattern was seen in 6 patients with their first EEG study. Interictal discharges did not evolve into the slow spike and wave pattern described in Lennox-Gastaut syndrome.[16] Most interictal discharges were single, with some

Table 2. Mitochondrial Patients With Infantile Spasms: Hypsarrythmia on EEG, Epileptic Spasms, and Developmental Delay.[a,b,c]

Patient (Sex)	Age Onset	ETC/Genetic Defect	Medications	Age of Death
1 (m)	2 months	C-IV; *MTO1*	ACTH, VGB, TPM, FBM, CLB, LEV, LTG, KD	
2 (m)	3 months	C-I	ACTH, VGB, LTG, TPM, LEV, GAN	
3 (m)	3 months	C-III	ACTH, KD, LTG, RFM, LEV	
4 (f)	3 months	E3/lipoic acid	VGB, Prednisone, ZNS	8 months
5 (m)	3 months	C-I	PB, ACTH, VGB, LAC, LTG, LEV, KD	
6 (f)	4 months	C-I	ACTH, ZNS, LTG	5 years
7 (m)	4 months	C-II, C-III, C-IV	ACTH, ZNS, LTG, RFM, LAC, VPA, CLB	
8 (f)	4 months	C-I	ACTH, ZNS, VGB	4 years
9 (f)	4 months	C-I	ACTH, VGB, LTG, CLB, RFM, GAN	
10 (f)	4 months	C-IV	PB, ZNS, B6/LEV/KD	4 years
11 (m)	5 months	C-I, C-IV	ACTH, ZNS, TPM, LEV, LTG, KD	
12 (m)	12 months	C-IV; *TANGO 2*	ACTH, ZNS, VPA, CLB, CBD	3 years
13 (m)	15 months	C-I	Prednisone, ZNS, LTG	
14 (f)	23 months	C-I, C-III, C-IV	ZNS, TPM, KD	5 years

Abbreviations: ACTH, adrenocorticotrophic hormone; B6, pyridoxine; C, electron transport chain complex; CBD, cannabidiol; CLB, clobazam; ETC, electron transport chain; f, female; FBM, felbamate; GAN, ganaloxone; KD, ketogenic diet; LAC, lacosamide; LEV, levetiracetam; LTG, lamotrigine; m, male; *MTO1*, mitochondrial-tRNA translation optimization factor 1 gene; PB, phenobarbital; RFM, rufinamide; E3/lipoic acid[13]; *TANGO 2*: transport and Golgi organization 2 homolog gene; TPM, topiramate; VGB, vigabatrin; VPA, valproic acid; ZNS, zonisamide.

[a]The demographic of sex, age of infantile spasms onset, electron transport chain or genetic defect, medications used and age of death (if occurred) are given.

[b]Patients 8 and 10 presented with an EEG pattern of suppression-bursts before evolving into hypsarrhythmia.

[c]Patient 3 became seizure free on monotherapy of ketogenic diet (4:1 ratio) but had to discontinue due to parental concerns.

occurring in runs of 3 to 4 Hertz with a short duration of 2 to 3 seconds. The spike pattern did not change over time, 4 to 10 years. The age of onset was 1.7 years (range: 6 months to 4 years). A single patient who presented with a generalized spike and wave pattern developed an EEG pattern of MISD over time. The other 5 patients continued to have generalized discharges over time.

There were 2 patients who presented with only independent focal discharges and did not meet the criteria of MISD. The interictal EEG pattern of focal discharges occurred in only 1 hemisphere. The age of presentation was 20 months and 5 years. Both patients' EEG pattern has remained with only focal discharges arising from the same hemisphere. Two patients presented with a suppression burst pattern. The age of onset was 2 and 4 months. Both patients evolved into the MISD pattern over time, with one of the patients evolving into hypsarrhythmia before MISD (patient 19: Table 1; patient 10: Table 2).

Those patients with *POLG* mutations (n = 12) all presented with independent focal discharges over the posterior head regions. Over time as the disease progresses, the EEG findings evolved into either a generalized spike and wave pattern, MISD pattern, generalized slowing of the background without epileptiform discharges; if frank liver failure occurred then a periodic epileptiform pattern occurred.[16–18] However, in some patients, care was withdrawn after genetic diagnosis was made, usually in the context of status epilepticus or severe neurological decompensation. In these patients, the natural history of EEG evolution could not be made.

Seizure Semiology

The 14 patients with hypsarrhythmia on EEG had epileptic spasms (Table 2). Spasms continued after the EEG had evolved into the interictal MISD pattern, but seizures eventually evolved into multiple seizure types. Patients progressed from epileptic spasms into tonic seizures. When captured on EEG, tonic seizures demonstrated background attenuation with overriding paroxysmal fast activity in a generalized distribution (Figure 1). In addition to tonic seizures, patients had both generalized and focal myoclonic seizures, the latter mostly involving the upper body. Focal myoclonic seizures were cortical in origin and seen with generalized and focal onset (Figure 1). The myoclonus events, when captured on video EEG, were not time-locked to EEG epileptiform discharges (data not shown).[19,20] Electrodiagnostic testing was not pursued to define etiology of spinal cord or peripheral nerve due to age of the population. Only 2 patients had persistent focal seizures arising from 1 hemisphere, either motor or dyscognitive (formerly described as partial complex or atypical absence).[14]

Six patients with interictal generalized spike discharges had a variety of seizure types. Four of the patients had periods of dyscognitive seizures. Two of the four patients had dyscognitive and atonic seizures. Another patient had dyscognitive and focal motor seizures. The 3 remaining patients had multiple seizure types, including generalized myoclonic seizures, tonic, and tonic–clonic seizures, and secondarily generalized tonic–clonic seizures. One of the latter patients also had focal motor seizures in addition to generalized seizures.

The seizure types in patients with MISD varied. Most patients presenting with this interictal EEG pattern had a combination of multiple seizure types (n = 57). In this population, the most common seizure type combination was generalized tonic and myoclonic seizures. Twelve of these patients only had tonic and myoclonic seizures, with another 12 patients having other seizure semiologies, in addition to tonic and myoclonic seizures. The next combination of

Table 3. Patients With Mitochondrial DNA- and Nuclear DNA-Encoded Mutations and Epilepsy.[a]

Patient (Sex)	Age Onset	Gene	Mutation	Status Epilepticus	Number Seizure Medications	Death
1 (m)	1 month	*POLG*	c.428C>T/c.679C>T	Yes	3	1 year
2 (m)	2 months	*ND5*	m.11778G>A	No	3	
3 (m)	2 months	*MTO1*	c.176C>G/c.922A>G	No	9	
4 (m)	3 months	*MT-ATP6*	m.8993T>G	No	4	7 years
5 (m)	7 months	*POLG*	c.2740A>C/c.3286C>T	Yes	4	2 years
6 (f)	9 months	*POLG*	c.1399G>A/c.2897T>G	Yes	5	
7 (m)	9 months	*POLG*	c.1399G>A/c.3313G>C	Yes	8	1 year
8 (m)	12 months	*TANGO2*	c.711-3C>G/del exon 3-9	Yes	5	4 years
9 (m)	12 months	*MT-ATP6*	m.8993T>G	No	4	
10 (m)	24 months	*MT-TK*	m.8363G>A	No	4	
11 (f)	24 months	*RARS2*	c.472_474delAAA/c.772C>A	Yes	7	
12 (f)	24 months	*PDHA1*	c.904C>A	No	2	
13 (f)	3 years	*POLG*	c.1399G>A/c.202C>T	Yes	5	3 years
14 (f)	3 years	*POLG*	c.2242G>C/c.2554C>T	Yes	4	8 years
15 (f)	4 years	*POLG*	c.2242G>C/c.2542G>A	Yes	6	7 years
16 (m)	4 years	*MTTL1*	m.3243A>G	Yes	4	
17 (m)	5 years	*MtDNA*	7.4 kb deletion	No	3	
18 (m)	5 years	*POLG*	c.1399G>A/c.2542G>A	Yes	5	12 years
19 (f)	6 years	*POLG*	c.229C>G/c.2243G>C	Yes	6	8 years
20 (f)	7 years	*MTTL1*	m.3243A>G	Yes	3	
21 (m)	10 years	*ND6*	m.14487T>C	Yes	3	
22 (m)	11 years	*ND6*	m.14459T>G	Yes	1	15 years
23 (f)	14 years	*POLG*	c.1399G>A/c.1399G>A	Yes	6	24 years
24 (f)	17 years	*POLG*	c.1399G>A/c.1399G>A	Yes	5	
25 (f)	17 years	*POLG*	c.1399G>A/c.1399G>A	Yes	6	
26 (f)	19 years	*SLC19A3*	c.1228A>G/c.223G>A	Yes	4	

Abbreviations: f, female; m, male; *MTO1*, mitochondrial-tRNA translation optimization factor 1 gene; *PDHA1*, pyruvate dehydrogenase E 1 gene; *POLG*, polymerase γ 1 gene; RARS 2, arginyl-tRNA synthetase gene; *SLC19A3*, solute carrier family 19 member 3 (thiamine transporter); *TANGO 2*, transport and golgi organization 2 homolog gene.

[a]After the age of 24 months, the age of onset was rounded up/down to reflect years.

seizure types was myoclonic and focal motor seizures (n = 6). The other 16 patients had multiple seizure types including mixtures of generalized atonic, tonic–clonic, and clonic seizures. Some patients also had secondarily generalized tonic–clonic seizures. There were patients who only had a single seizure type (n = 14). Four patients had dyscognitive seizures, 2 had myoclonic seizures, 6 had focal motor seizures, 1 patient had generalized tonic seizures, and 1 patient had generalized tonic–clonic seizures.

The most frequent overall seizure semiology in the cohort was myoclonic seizures (n = 61) followed by generalized tonic seizures (n = 39). Focal seizures were also common, and the most common was focal motor seizures (n = 34). Patients with mitochondrial disease demonstrate both generalized and focal seizures and the majority have multiple seizure types (n = 71).

Status Epilepticus

Twenty-one patients developed episodes of status epilepticus. Interestingly, 19 of these patients possessed either mtDNA-encoded or nuclear-encoded gene mutations (Table 3). The majority were patients with Alpers-Huttenlocher syndrome (n = 12), with 7 other patients having a mixture of mtDNA-encoded and nuclear-encoded mutations. Two patients without a molecular diagnosis had status events. One patient had the biochemical findings of E3/lipoic acid biosynthesis defects and the other patient had a complex I defect with magnetic resonance imaging (MRI) findings compatible with mitochondrial encephalomyopathy, lactic acidosis, and stroke-like syndrome (MELAS).

There were 12 patients with *POLG* mutations and Alpers-Huttenlocher syndrome. All 12 of these patients developed status epilepticus. Seven patients presented with epilepsy partialis continua (EPC) as their initial seizure.[21] Three of these 7 patients also later developed motor status epilepticus. The remaining 4 patients had motor status epilepticus that occurred after seizure onset.

Three patients with mtDNA-encoded mutations developed status epilepticus. Two patients developed EPC in the context of metabolic strokes, with 1 patient having the classic m.3243A>G mutation for MELAS, while the other had the overlap syndrome of MELAS and Leigh syndrome with the m.14478T>C mutation. The third patient developed nonconvulsive status epilepticus and carried the m.14459A>G mutation. A third patient with the m.3243A>G mutation did not evolve into status epilepticus.

Status epilepticus was seen in 2 patients who possessed a nuclear-encoded mutation. One patient had motor status epilepticus with compound heterozygous mutations in the

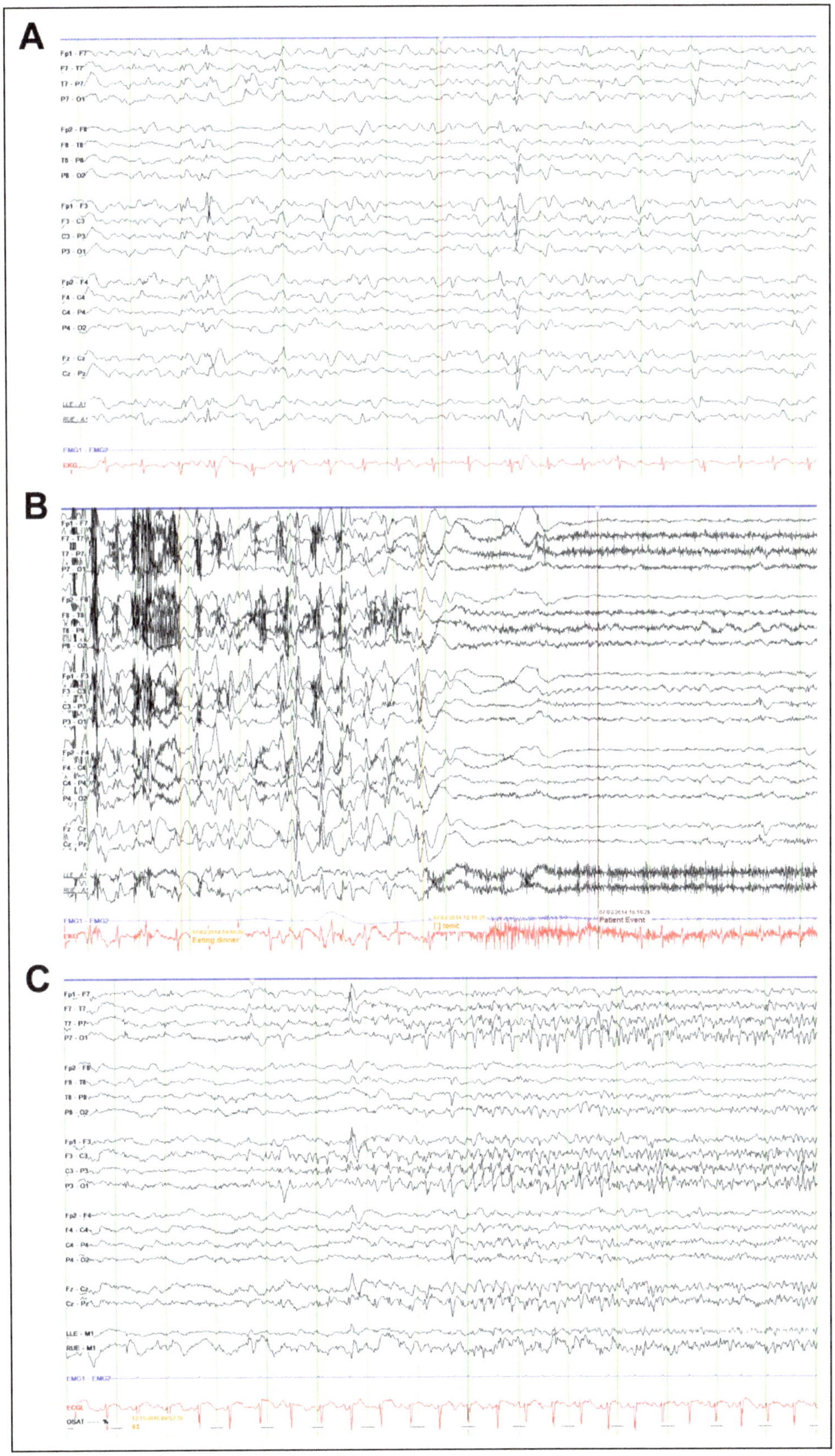

Figure 1. A, The electroencephalogram (EEG) pattern in panel A shows interictal epileptiform discharges over the left and right hemispheres with background slowing (multifocal spike discharges [MISD]). This EEG epoch is taken from a patient who had infantile spasms at 4 months of age. This EEG epoch represents the findings at age 12 years. Panel B: This EEG epoch is from the same patient at age 12 years showing a

Table 4. Seizure Medications Used for Seizure Control.[a,b]

Medication	Patients
Adrenocorticotrophic hormone	11
Carbamazepine	12
Clobazam	11
Ethosuximide	10
Felbamate	3
Ketogenic diet	21
Lacosamide	8
Lamotrigine	57
Levetiracetam	53
Oxcarbazepine	9
Phenobarbital	10
Prednisone	2
Phenytoin	4
Topiramate	24
Rufinamide	7
Valproic acid	18
Vigabatrin	9
Zonisamide	30

[a]This table indicates the individual seizure medications that each patient used during the course of this study.
[b]The range of seizure medications listed does not include those medications used to control status epilepticus or experimental medications used in clinical trials.

TANGO2 gene. The other patient developed nonconvulsive status epilepticus and had compound heterozygous mutations in the arginyl tRNA gene, *RARS 2*. Mutations were in trans for both patients with alterations segregating to biological parents.

Treatment

Treatment for seizure control is unsatisfying. No patient obtained seizure control with the initial seizure medication and multiple medications, both singly and in combination (Table 4). Currently, only 6 patients are in seizure control on medications with 0.5 to 14 years of seizure freedom. Two patients are taking monotherapy of lamotrigine. Both patients presented with MISD on the EEG. One of the patients had events described as dyscognitive with postictal behavioral changes, while the other had solely dyscognitive changes. The older patient has been seizure-free for 14 years. She initially failed ethosuximide and then transitioned onto topiramate therapy. Unfortunately, although seizures were controlled, she had behavioral side effects of cognitive slowing and regression in cognitive performance and subsequently switched to monotherapy of lamotrigine (Figure 2). She has remained in seizure control and her cognitive abilities greatly recovered. She has since won art contests, graduated from college, and is currently doing well in business. The second patient became seizure-free for the last 4 years on lamotrigine monotherapy. The third patient has been in seizure control on monotherapy of levetiracetam. This latter patient developed seizures at 1 month of age in the context of a fever and corona viral infection. Initially started on phenobarbital, he became-seizure free and switched to levetiracetam. He has been seizure-free for the last 6 months; he is currently 9 months of age. He was found to possess the mtDNA mutation, m.11778G>A. The other patients are on multiple antiseizure medications. Two of these latter patients are on the ketogenic diet and 2 traditional antiseizure medications. The other patient is on 3 antiseizure medications.

One patient was diagnosed with pyruvate dehydrogenase complex deficiency and was on the monotherapy of the ketogenic diet (4:1 ratio) until she died. She was already on the ketogenic diet when she transferred to our center. She was not completely seizure-free, but breakthrough seizures were infrequent, 2 to 3 per month.

The other 78 patients with seizures remain either uncontrolled or have died. Each has been on multiple medications, average of 4.3 + 0.9 (range: 3-5) at any one time (Table 4). The range of medication numbers trialed was 1 to 11. Alternative methods of seizure control occurred due to poor control with traditional seizure medications. Twenty-one patients tried the ketogenic diet (varying ratio: 2:1-4:1). Seven of the 21 patients on the ketogenic diet had a favorable response with >75% seizure reduction (as noted on seizure diaries). Three of the responders were seizure-free, but due to compliance or quality of life issues were withdrawn from the diet. Two of the patients remaining on the diet are to date seizure free as noted above, while 2 others remain with seizures but with a reduction in seizure frequency.

There were 8 patients implanted with the vagus nerve stimulator. Five of these patients were previously reported by our group.[22] Three additional patients were eventually implanted with this device in hopes of gaining seizure control. As with the other 5 patients, these 3 patients had a limited response to vagal nerve stimulation. All 3 patients had multiple electron transport complex deficiencies.

There were 14 patients with infantile spasms (Table 2). Video EEG captured epileptic spasms in all patients. Three patients had seizures prior to epileptic spasm onset and started phenobarbital as the initial medication. Eleven of the patients received adrenocorticotropic hormone (ACTH) when spasms and hypsarrhythmia started. Five of the patients had resolution of epileptic spasms and hypsarrhythmia on EEG; however upon weaning ACTH, epileptic spasms returned. In the other

Figure 1. (*Continued*) generalized tonic seizure. At the onset of the seizure, the background becomes attenuated with the evolution of low amplitude theta frequencies after several seconds. The total time of the tonic seizure was 25 seconds (not shown). During the seizure, the patient stiffened all limbs. Panel C: An epoch taken from a patient who developed infantile spasms at the same age of the patient whose EEG is shown in Panel A. The EEG epoch was from a video EEG study at 14 years of age and demonstrating a focal motor seizure that begins over the left frontocentral region with the seizure increasing the distribution to the left lateral hemisphere. The seizure remained focal throughout the course of the seizure. The patient developed right upper extremity stiffening with a head turn to the left. Prior to the seizure, the EEG demonstrated a similar background of MISD as the patient shown in A (data not shown).

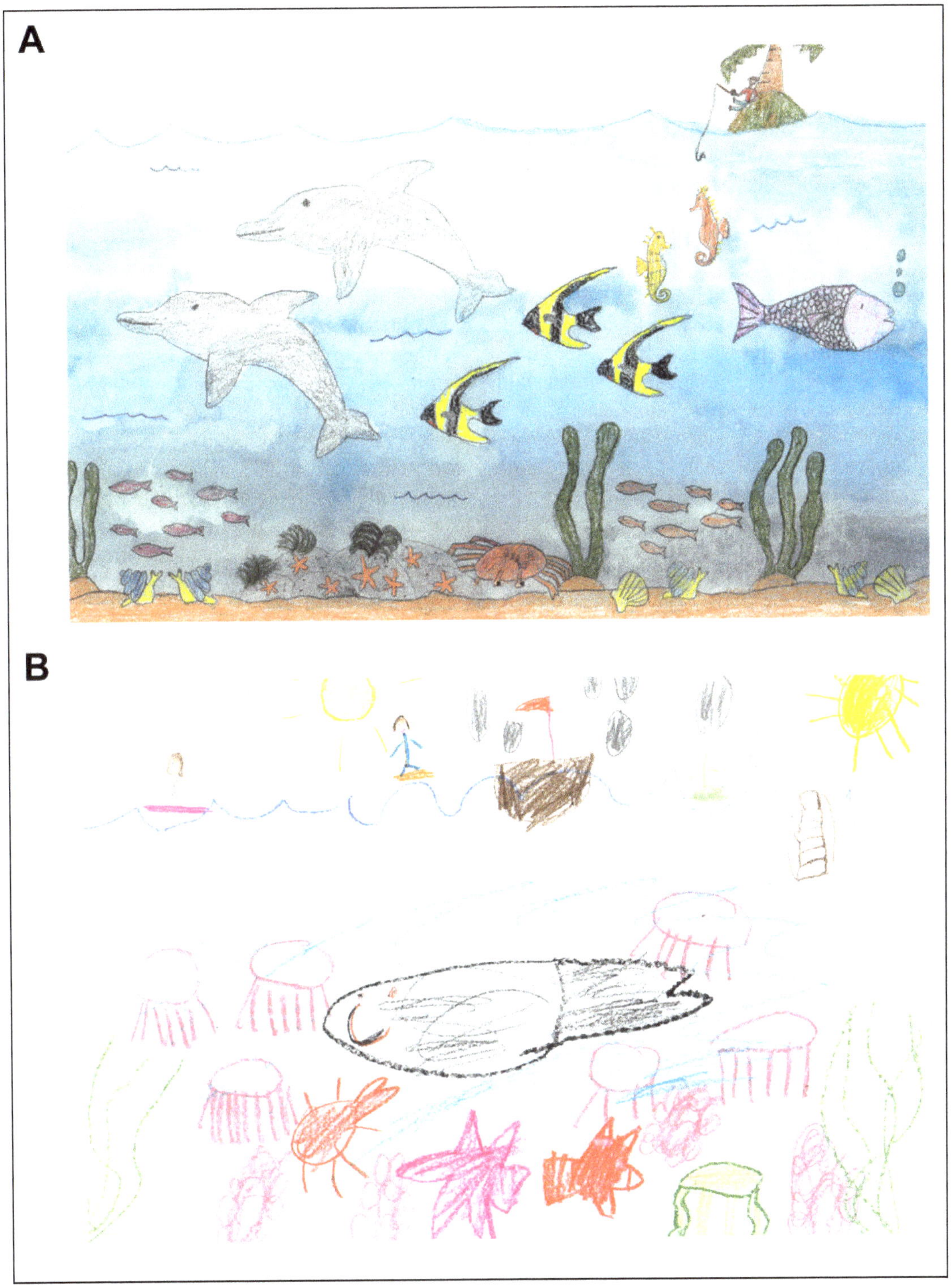

Figure 2. A, This picture shows a drawing by patient before being placed on topiramate monotherapy. At the time of this drawing, she was having dyscognitive seizures (atypical absence episodes with postictal changes). B, This picture shows a drawing by the same patient several months after starting topiramate monotherapy. Her seizures were well controlled at the time of the drawing. At the time of this drawing, the mother had noted that her daughter was cognitively slower and had difficulty in word finding.

6 patients given ACTH, there was no response. In all of these patients, vigabatrin was trialed without efficacy and was eventually withdrawn in all but a single patient, who had a mild reduction in seizure frequency. In the 3 patients who were not exposed to ACTH, vigabatrin, corticosteroids, zonisamide, and topiramate were initially trialed but without effect, and these medications were eventually stopped. Two patients enrolled in the Marinus Infantile Spasm Study, and neither patient responded to ganaxolone with epileptic spasm control. Six patients with epileptic spasms tried the ketogenic diet, with

currently only 2 patients on the diet. Of interest, 1 patient with complex III dysfunction became seizure-free on the monotherapy of the ketogenic diet for 5 years, but had to discontinue due to family issues (also described above). He, like all the other patients, currently remains with seizures. The average number of medications trialed was 6 (range: 3-9). Six patients in this population died during the course of this study, average age of death was 3.7 years (range: 1-5 years). The only patients who died of SUDEP were in the group with infantile spasms (Table 1).

The use of valproic acid is contraindicated in patients with Alpers-Huttenlocher syndrome.[17] Exposure to valproic acid can induce hepatopathy and progression to frank liver failure within as little as 4 to 6 weeks of exposure. Two patients with Alpers-Huttenlocher syndrome exposed to valproic acid died of liver failure. Another patient with Alpers-Huttenlocher syndrome progressed to liver failure without exposure to valproic acid. A second patient (Table 3; patient 1) with *POLG* mutations but with the syndrome of myocerebrohepatopathy spectrum died due to liver failure without exposure to valproic acid. Given the sensitivity to liver dysfunction with *POLG* mutations, valproic acid should be avoided in this patient population.

Discussion

In a single-cohort study of infants and children, of 174 patients with definite mitochondrial disease, over 48% had epilepsy. The prevalence of epilepsy was higher in the patients younger than 3 years compared to the older children and adolescents, 68% versus 32%. The high percentage of epilepsy and young age of seizure onset in mitochondrial disease have been seen in other studies.[4,5] Two studies have demonstrated rates of 65% (30 of 65 patients) and 55% (38 of 56 patients). Although in an adult cohort of patients with mitochondrial disease, only 23.1% had epilepsy with a mean age of onset at 29.4 years.[23] These data suggest that onset of epilepsy in patients with mitochondrial disease would follow the trend of other types of epilepsy presenting with higher prevalence during infancy and young childhood, compared to the adult population.[24]

There is a suggestion from the Seattle cohort that patients with epilepsy and mitochondrial disease have more severe disease. Earlier onset seizures coexisted with increased mortality compared to patients without epilepsy. Twenty-four patients with early-onset seizures died compared to only 5 patients without epilepsy. Using onset of seizures as the first clinical symptom, earlier onset of symptoms occurred in patients with epilepsy compared to patients without seizures, 2.9 versus 3.7 years, respectively. However, evidence exists that onset of other symptoms occurs earlier in patients with epilepsy than those without seizures.[5] Assuming the other symptoms besides epilepsy is occurring in our population, the likelihood for onset of disease is even more pronounced. Although our study had the limitation of insurance approval for obtaining genetic testing, more patients with early epilepsy onset had nuclear-encoded mutations compared to the overall group of patients with epilepsy (Table 3). Nuclear-encoded mitochondrial diseases are usually expressed earlier in life and are clinically more severe in nature.[7,25–27] Taken together, there is a strong suggestion that early-onset epilepsy in patients with mitochondrial disease portends more severe involvement of the disease. The more severe disease involvement early in life may be, in part, the decreased presence of epilepsy in the adult population.[23] Further investigations are needed to confirm this suggestion.

The age-dependent epileptic encephalopathy syndrome, infantile spasms, was seen in 14 patients (Table 2). The incidence in the general population has been estimated to be 1 per 3225.[28] It appears that this epilepsy syndrome is more common in mitochondrial disease than the general population. Infantile spasms was one of the most common of the classic epilepsy syndromes seen in the Seattle cohort; 17% of the patients with epilepsy developed infantile spasms. In this cohort, 13 patients had normal MRI scans of the brain; the exception was the patient with E3/lipoic acid deficiency with cortical dysplasia (data not shown). Although no mtDNA-encoded mutations were found, there were 2 nuclear-encoded pathological mutations found in our cohort. One patient had compound heterozygous mutations in *MTO1*, which has previously been reported.[29] The other patient had compound heterozygous mutations in *TANGO2*, which has been shown to be present in patients with seizures, but our patient would be the first one to be reported with infantile spasms.[30,31] Eleven of the other patients had defects in the ETC. Eight patients had single complex and 3 patients had multiple ETC complex defects (Table 2). One patient had an enzymatic profile and biochemical abnormalities consistent with E3/lipoic acid deficiency (noted above). Treatment was unsatisfying and all patients developed intractable seizures with an average of 5.4 medications per patient trialed. Mortality was high, and 6 patients died before the age of 6 years. Previous studies have been mixed with some showing a high percentage of patients with mitochondrial disease expressing infantile spasms, while others only limited numbers or none at all.[3,4,32] Given the data presented, as noted a decade ago, mitochondrial disease is most likely an underrecognized etiology of infantile spams and clinicians need to be aware of this possibility.[33]

The EEG pattern found in the cohort crossed genetic abnormalities, mtDNA or nDNA-encoded, seizure semiology, and age. The most common EEG pattern is MISD (84%), which in the vast majority remains a constant pattern over time and unchanging. Surprisingly, the EEG pattern seen in infantile spasms, hypsarrhythmia, evolved into the MISD pattern and did not change over time. Other studies have shown that the slow spike and wave pattern seen in Lennox-Gastaut syndrome can be seen in patients with mitochondrial disease; this was not seen in our cohort.[4] The reasons the slow spike and wave pattern not being seen in our cohort is unclear but suggests that Lennox-Gastaut syndrome is uncommon in mitochondrial disease. The patients in this study had mixed seizure types of focal seizures, generalized seizures, and noncerebral involuntary movements (eg myoclonus) with the same interictal pattern of MISD. The suggestion is that dysfunctional mitochondrial physiology within the brain produces a predictable electrical interictal EEG pattern that is capable of heterogeneous ictal clinical expression.

One of the striking findings of our cohort is the high frequency of status epilepticus. Both EPC and status epilepticus were common (~24%). A high percentage was found in patients with Alpers-Huttenlocher syndrome, which is well described.[16,17] Most patients with MELAS or MELAS overlap syndrome developed status epilepticus. The single patient with the m.3243A>G mutation who did not develop status was treated during the initial stroke-like episode with L-arginine therapy. As with patients with Alpers-Huttenlocher syndrome, patients with MELAS develop status epilepticus multiple times.[34] In the other 3 patients who developed status epilepticus, the etiology of status epilepticus is unclear but, likely in part, relates to acute energy deprivation.

Treatment of seizures in mitochondrial disease is unsatisfying. Only a few patients gained seizure control by medical management and high-fat diet, but most were not. No patient had significant benefit from vagus nerve stimulation in our study. Clearly, the medications and electrostimulation currently available have little benefit to control seizures completely. Furthermore, certain medications had organ-specific toxicity. Valproic acid has been shown to induce liver hepatopathy and can lead to frank liver failure in patients with Alpers-Huttenlocher syndrome.[16,17,25] Further research is needed in seizure management and awaits novel agents to be discovered and trialed.

Seizure semiologies varied; both focal and generalized events coexisted in the same patient. There were multiple seizure types in most patients, including myoclonic, tonic, epileptic spasms, focal motor, atonic, dyscognitive, and tonic–clonic. Most all of the patients in this study have cognitive delay/intellectual disability (data not presented, paper in preparation). Combined with the EEG pattern of MISD, the findings in this study are very compatible with the epilepsy syndrome named Markand-Blume-Ohtahara syndrome. This epilepsy syndrome has been described as demonstrating an EEG showing MISD, very frequent multiple types of seizures, mental retardation, and poor prognosis for seizure control.[35] This syndrome is not part of the current ILAE list of epilepsy syndromes but would be classified as "structural–metabolic."[14] There are few patients who have exclusively generalized or focal seizures, suggesting that the seizure phenotype of mitochondrial disease can be quite variable. The etiology of the differences between generalized and focal seizures remains unclear. However, the variation in energy demand likely plays a part of seizure semiology expression.

One of the dilemmas concerning epilepsy and mitochondrial disease is that not all patients have seizures. If seizures are strictly due to energy depravation, then all patients with mitochondrial disease would have seizures. The reasons for the variable expression of epilepsy within similar abnormalities and common biochemical and/or genetic mutations, remain unclear. Epilepsy has been related to multiple genetic mutations, both mtDNA- and nDNA-encoded, that are involved in the direct energy production machinery, calcium maintenance, oxidative radical formation, and immunological and vitamin deficiencies.[36] The other influences on phenotypic expression of epilepsy remain unclear, which are environmental, risk/permissive genes, and other yet undiscovered factors. How the combination of factors alters the vulnerability of the young developing brain remains unclear. Hopefully, as our understanding of how these factors are integrated in producing the epileptic state and with possible new therapeutic agents entering into the field, the control of seizures will get better.

Acknowledgments

The author would like to thank the families who allow him to care for their children.

Declaration of Conflicting Interests

The author(s) declared no potential conflicts of interest with respect to the research, authorship, and/or publication of this article.

Funding

The author(s) received no financial support for the research, authorship, and/or publication of this article.

References

1. Anderson S, Bankier AT, Barrell BG, et al. Sequence and organization of the human mitochondrial genome. *Nature*. 1981; 290(5806):457-465.
2. Chinnery PF, Hudson G. Mitochondrial genetics. *Br Med Bull*. 2013;106:135-159.
3. Canafoglia L, Franceschetti S, Antozzi C, et al. Epileptic phenotypes associated with mitochondrial disorders. *Neurology*. 2001; 56(10):1340-1346.
4. Lee YM, Kang HC, Lee JS, et al. Mitochondrial respiratory chain defects: underlying etiology in various epileptic conditions. *Epilepsia*. 2008;49(4):685-690.
5. El Sabbagh S, Lebre AS, Bahi-Buisson N, et al. Epileptic phenotypes in children with respiratory chain disorders. *Epilepsia*. 2010;51(7):1225-1235.
6. Chevallier JA, Von Allmen GK, Koenig MK. Seizure semiology and EEG findings in mitochondrial diseases. *Epilepsia*. 2014; 55(5):707-712.
7. Debray FG, Lambert M, Chevalier I, et al. Long-term outcome and clinical spectrum of 73 paediatric individuals with mitochondrial diseases. *Pediatrics*. 2007;119(4):722-733.
8. Verity CM, Winstone AM, Stellitano L, Krishnakumar D, Will R, McFarland R. The clinical presentation of mitochondrial diseases in children with progressive intellectual and neurological deterioration: a national, prospective, population-based study. *Dev Med Child Neurol*. 2010;52(5):434-440.
9. Scaglia F, Towbin JA, Craigen WJ, et al. Clinical spectrum, morbidity and mortality in 113 pediatric patients with mitochondrial disease. *Pediatrics*. 2004;114(4):925-931.
10. Garcia-Cozorla A, De Lonlay P, Nassogne MC, Rustin P, Touati G, Saudubray JM. Long-term follow-up of neonatal mitochondrial cytopathies: a study of 57 patients. *Pediatrics*. 2005; 116(5):1170-1177.

11. Bernier FP, Boneh A, Dennett X, Chow CW, Cleary MA, Thorburn DR. Diagnostic criteria for respiratory chain disorders in adults and children. *Neurology*. 2002;59(9):1406-1411.
12. Berg AT, Berkovic SF, Brodie MJ, et al. Revised terminology and concepts for organization of seizures and epilepsies: report of the ILAE commission on classification and terminology, 2005-2009. *Epilepsia*. 2010;51(4):676-685.
13. Burnstine TH, Vining EP, Uematsu S, Lesser RP. Multifocal independent epileptiform discharges in children: ictal correlates and surgical therapy. *Neurology*. 1991;41(8):1223-1228.
14. Mayr JA, Feichtinger RG, Tort F, Ribes A, Sperl W. Lipoic acid biosynthesis defects. *J Inherit Metab Dis*. 2014;37(4): 553-563.
15. Noriega-Sanchez A, Markand ON. Clinical and electroencephalographic correlation of independent multifocal spike discharges. *Neurology*. 1976;26(7):667-672.
16. Boyd SG, Harden A, Egger J, Pampligilone G. Progressive neuronal degeneration of childhood with liver disease (Alpers' disease): characteristic neurophysiological features. *Neuropediatrics*. 1986;17(2): 75-80.
17. Saneto RP, Cohen BH, Copeland WC, Naviaux RK. Alpers-Huttenlocher syndrome. *Pediatr Neurol*. 2013;48(3):167-178.
18. Saneto RP, Lee IC, Koenig MK, et al. *POLG* DNA testing as an emerging standard of care before instituting valproic acid therapy for pediatric seizure disorders. *Seizure*. 2010;19(3):140-146.
19. Gibbs FA, Gibbs EL, Lennox WG. The influence of the blood sugar level on the wave and spike formation in petite mal epilepsy. *Arch Neurol Psychiatry*. 1939;41:1111-1116.
20. Zutt R, van Egmond ME, Elting JW, et al. A novel diagnostic approach to patients with myoclonus. *Nat Rev Neurol*. 2015; 11(12):687-697.
21. Thomas JE, Reagen TJ, Klass DW. Epilepsia partialis continua. *Arch Neurol*. 1977;34(5):266-275.
22. Arthur TM, Saneto RP, de Menezes MS, et al. Vagus nerve stimulation in children with mitochondrial electron transport chain deficiencies. *Mitochondrion*. 2007;7(4):279-283.
23. Whittaker RG, Devine HE, Gorman GS, et al. Epilepsy in adults with mitochondrial disease: a cohort study. *Ann Neurol*. 2015; 78(6):949-957.
24. Helmers SL, Thurman DJ, Durgin TL, Pai AK, Faught E. Descriptive epidemiology of epilepsy in the US population: a different approach. *Epilepsia*. 2015;56(6):942-948.
25. Saneto RP, Naviaux RK. Polymerase gamma disease through the ages. *Dev Disabil Res Rev*. 2010;16(2):163-174.
26. Gibson K, Halliday JL, Kirby DM, Yaplito-Lee J, Thorburn DR, Boneh A. Mitochondrial oxidative physphorylation disorders presenting in neonates: clinical manifestations and enzymatic and molecular diagnoses. *Pediatrics*. 2008;122(5):1003-1008.
27. Rubio-Gozalbo ME, Dijkman KP, van den Heuvel LP, Sengers RC, Wendel U, Smeitink JA. Clinical differences in patients with mitochondriocytopathies due to nuclear versus mitochondrial DNA mutations. *Hum Mutat*. 2000;15(6):522-532.
28. Hrachovy RA, Frost JD Jr. Infantile epileptic encephalopathy with hypsarrhythmia (infantile Spasms/West syndrome). *J Clin Neurophysiol*. 2003;20(6):408-425.
29. Saneto RP. Defects in post-translational modification of mitochondrial transferase RNA: a patient with possible tRNA translation optimization factor 1, *MTO1* dysfunction. In: Saneto RP, Parikh S, Cohen BH, eds. *Mitochondrial Case Studies: Underlying Mechanisms and Diagnosis*. Amsterdam, the Netherlands: Academic Press; 2016:251-256.
30. Kremer LS, Distelmaier F, Alhaddad B, et al. Bi-allelic truncating mutations in *TANGO2* cause infancy-onset recurrent metabolic crises with encephaolcardiomyopathy. *Am J Hum Genet*. 2016; 98(2):358-362.
31. Lalini SR, Liu P, Rosenfeld JA, et al. Recurrent muscle weakness with rhabdomyolysis, metabolic crisis, and cardiac arrhythmia due to bi-allelic *TANGO2* mutations. *Am J Hum Genet*. 2016; 98(2):347-357.
32. Osborne JP, Lux AL, Edwards SW, et al. The underlying etiology of infantile spasms (West syndrome): information from the United Kingdom Infantile Spasms Study (UKISS) on contemporary causes and their classification. *Epilepsia*. 2010;51(10):2168-2174.
33. Shah NS, Mitchell WG, Boles RG. Mitochondrial disorders: a potentially under-recognized etiology of Infantile spasms. *J Child Neurol*. 2002;17(5):369-372.
34. Lee HN, Eom S, Kim SH, et al. Epilepsy characteristics and clinical outcome in patients with mitochondrial encehalomyopahty, lactic acidosis, and stroke-like episodes (MELAS). *Pediatr Neurol*. 2016;64:59-65.
35. Yamatogi Y, Ohtahara S. Severe epilepsy with multiple independent spike foci. *J Clin Neurophysiol*. 2003;20(6):442-448.
36. Rahman S. Pathophysiology of mitochondrial disease causing epilepsy and status epilepticus. *Epilepsy Behav*. 2015;49:71-75.

28

Understanding the Early Presentation of Mucopolysaccharidoses Disorders

Lorne Clarke, MD[1], Carolyn Ellaway, MBBS, PhD[2], Helen E. Foster, MD, MBBS[3], Roberto Giugliani, MD, PhD[4], Cyril Goizet, MD, PhD[5], Sarah Goring, MSc[6], Sara Hawley, MSc[7], Elaina Jurecki, MS, RD[7], Zaeem Khan, MPH, BSc[6], Christina Lampe, MD[8], Ken Martin, MD[9], Suzanne McMullen, MHA, BSc[6], John J. Mitchell, MD[10], Fathima Mubarack, MSc, MHA[7], H. Serap Sivri, MD[11], Martha Solano Villarreal, MD, PhD[12], Fiona J. Stewart, MB, BS[13], Anna Tylki-Szymanska, MD, PhD[14], Klane White, MD, MSc[15], and Frits Wijburg, MD, PhD[16]

Abstract

As therapies are developed for rare disorders, challenges of early diagnosis become particularly relevant. This article focuses on clinical recognition of mucopolysaccharidoses (MPS), a group of rare genetic diseases related to abnormalities in lysosomal function. As quality of outcomes with current therapies is impacted by timing of intervention, minimizing time to diagnosis is critical. The objective of this study was to characterize how, when, and to whom patients with MPS first present and develop tools to stimulate earlier recognition of MPS. A tripartite approach was used, including a systematic literature review yielding 194 studies, an online physician survey completed by 209 physicians who described

---

[1] British Columbia Children's Hospital Research Institute, University of British Columbia, Vancouver, British Columbia, Canada
[2] Sydney Children's Hospital Network, Sydney University, Sydney, Australia
[3] Great North Children's Hospital and Newcastle University, Newcastle upon Tyne, United Kingdom
[4] Medical Genetics Service HCPA, Dep Genet UFRGS & INAGEMP, Porto Alegre, Brazil
[5] Service de Génétique, CHU Bordeaux, Laboratoire MRGM, INSERM U 1211, University of Bordeaux, Bordeaux, France
[6] ICON plc, Vancouver, British Columbia, Canada
[7] BioMarin Pharmaceutical Inc., Novato, CA, USA
[8] Centre for Rare Diseases, Clinic for Children and Adolescents, Helios Dr. Horst Schmidt Kliniken, Wiesbaden, Germany
[9] UCSF Benioff Children's Hospital Oakland, Oakland, CA, USA
[10] Montreal Children's Hospital, Montreal, Quebec, Canada
[11] Hacettepe University Children's Hospital, Ankara, Turkey
[12] Fundacion Cardioinfantil, Bogota, Colombia
[13] Belfast City Hospital, Belfast, United Kingdom
[14] Children's Memorial Health Institute, Warsaw, Poland
[15] Seattle Children's Hospital, Seattle, WA, USA
[16] Academic Medical Center, University Hospital of Amsterdam, Amsterdam, the Netherlands

Corresponding Author:
Lorne Clarke, MD, British Columbia Children's Hospital Research Institute, University of British Columbia, Vancouver, British Columbia, Canada.
Email: lclarke@bcchr.ca

859 MPS cases, and a global panel of MPS experts who distilled the findings. Red flag signs/symptoms were identified for cardiology, pediatric neurology, otorhinolaryngology, rheumatology, orthopedics, pediatrics, and general medicine and converted into simple, specialty-specific tools intended to facilitate early diagnosis of MPS, enabling improved patient outcomes.

Keywords
mucopolysaccharidoses, mucopolysaccharidosis I, mucopolysaccharidosis II, mucopolysaccharidosis III, mucopolysaccharidosis IV, mucopolysaccharidosis VI, mucopolysaccharidosis VII, diagnosis

Introduction

The mucopolysaccharidoses (MPS) are rare genetic conditions caused by a deficiency of 1 of 11 lysosomal enzymes involved in glycosaminoglycan (GAG) catabolism. MPS is characterized by the accumulation of partially degraded GAGs (heparan sulfate, dermatan sulfate, keratan sulfate, chondroitin sulfate, or hyaluronan) within lysosomes and by the subsequent increase in GAGs in urine, blood, and cerebral spinal fluid.[1,2] Progressive damage occurs as GAGs accumulate within the cells. As lysosomes are found throughout the body, MPS can manifest through a myriad of signs and symptoms. Over time, MPS may result in multiple organ failure, cognitive impairment, and premature death.[1] Typically, symptom onset occurs between infancy and childhood.[3] The overall birth prevalence for MPS is approximately 1 in 25000 and varies by region and ethnic background.[4–7]

Seven MPS types have been identified (I, II, III, IV, VI, VII, and IX); MPS III has 4 subtypes (A, B, C, and D) and MPS IV has 2 (A and B). Although the subtypes are clinically similar, each one is linked to a specific enzyme deficiency. MPS II is inherited as an X-linked disorder, whereas all others are autosomal recessive conditions.[1]

MPS is usually diagnosed through biochemical testing for deficient enzymes and can be confirmed through molecular genetic testing. However, early clinical recognition of potential cases with MPS, which is needed to trigger this diagnostic testing, continues to pose a substantial challenge.[8] This is largely due to the disease rarity, phenotypic heterogeneity, and the wide range of nonspecific early signs and symptoms.

Diagnostic delays often involve referrals from one physician to another and place a substantial burden on the patient and caregivers. Patients are also at risk of misdiagnosis and undergoing inappropriate interventions or receiving ineffective treatments. Timely referral for diagnostic testing allows for prompt initiation of definitive therapy such as enzyme replacement therapy or hematopoietic stem cell transplantation for some types of MPS as well as enabling the appropriate management of secondary complications.[9] Earlier recognition also allows patients to partner with a physician with expertise in their rare disease and facilitates support through a patient organization sooner. Furthermore, early recognition alerts at-risk carriers and enables them to seek accurate genetic counseling and pursue prenatal testing and preimplantation genetic diagnosis.

A better understanding of the initial presentation of MPS is needed to improve early recognition of potential cases with MPS and facilitate a timely diagnosis, enabling optimal patient management and treatment when available. Unfortunately, previous efforts made in this area have not met with success.[8] Thus, a new approach is needed. The objectives of this review were to use a novel, evidence-based, multimethod approach to characterize how, when, and to whom individuals with MPS first present, identify specialty-specific red flag signs and symptoms, and develop clinical awareness diagnostic tools that have the potential to shorten the current diagnostic delay. The effectiveness of the tools will depend on how well the information they contain is disseminated and retained by the target audiences. By making different tools for each subspecialist, we aim to present only the most relevant information to each. However, effective dissemination of the tools subsequent to publication will be the most challenging and critical factor for ultimate success.

Materials and Methods

To achieve the objectives of this study, a systematic literature review was conducted first, followed by a physician survey to supplement the published evidence with real-world clinical experience and compensate for the possibility of publication bias in the results of the literature review (ie, overrepresentation of rare signs and symptoms and under representation of common ones). The results from the systematic literature review and physician survey were then reviewed by a panel of 16 international clinical MPS experts in order to identify specialty-specific red flag signs and symptoms evident in the early stages of the disease and generate specialty-specific tools to increase clinical awareness of potential cases with MPS.

Systematic Literature Review

Search strategy and study selection. The following electronic databases were searched: Embase (1970 to 27 June 2016) and MEDLINE via PubMed (1970 to 27 June 2016). Handsearches for registry studies, clinical surveillance, natural history, and genotype–phenotype correlation studies were also conducted in PubMed using a key word search. A transparent and reproducible search strategy (Supplemental Files 1 and 2) was developed in accordance with best practice guidelines.[10,11] Searches

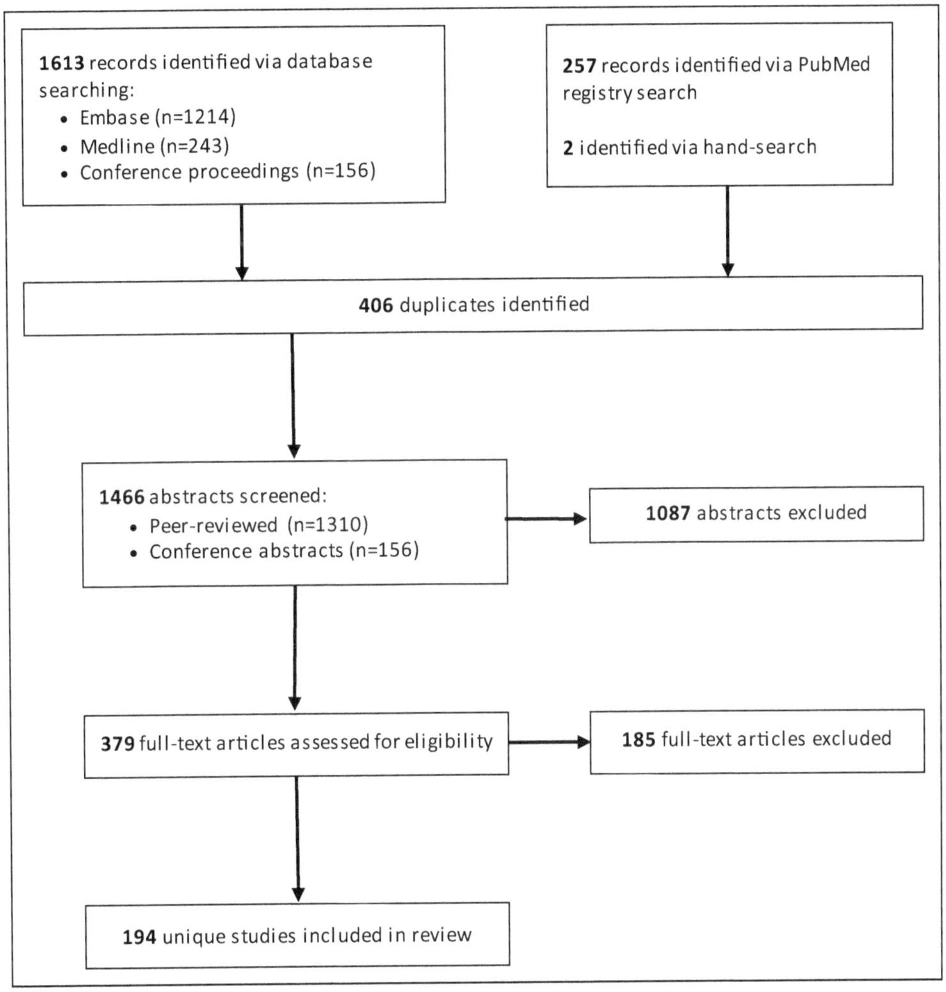

Figure 1. Literature review: PRISMA diagram.
N indicates number; PRISMA indicates Preferred Reporting Items for Systematic Reviews and Meta-Analyses.

were limited to English language and human studies only and were run on June 27, 2016.

Titles and abstracts of all articles obtained by the search were reviewed by a single reviewer (F.M.) against prespecified eligibility criteria. Titles and abstracts indicated as "unsure" were reviewed by a second reviewer (E.J.) for a final decision. Inclusion criteria were specified in terms of population, intervention and comparators, outcomes and study design (PICOS) framework. The population of interest was MPS (all types). No restrictions were placed on interventions, comparators, or study design. "Outcomes" included the clinical course leading to diagnosis, clinical presentation, presentation of signs and symptoms, clinical features, clinical assessment, phenotype, phenotype–genotype correlation, severity, or descriptions of slow or rapid progression of disease. All studies meeting the eligibility criteria were included in this review. Studies were excluded if they lacked information on presenting signs and symptoms or if they focused on therapeutics, diagnostics, newborn screening, or biochemical or molecular assays. A Preferred Reporting Items for Systematic Reviews and Meta-Analyses (PRISMA) flow diagram (Figure 1) was developed indicating the numbers of studies included and excluded at each stage of the review.

Data extraction and analysis. For each study, MPS type-specific data were extracted, meaning that a single study describing signs and symptoms of 2 different types of MPS was extracted as 2 separate records. Data were captured in Microsoft Excel extraction tables, and extraction fields were spot checked for potential errors.

Extracted data included median age of symptom onset, median age of diagnosis, median diagnostic delay, signs and symptoms (including presence/absence at case presentation and role in triggering the diagnosis), reporting physician specialty, and diagnostic errors. As most publications reported findings in aggregate, the units for reporting of the systematic literature review results are records as opposed to patients. Data were synthesized in tabular format; clinical features of MPS were stratified according to MPS type, age-group (<1, 1-4, 5-9, ≥10 years), major symptom categories, reporting physician specialty, or date of publication. Median values and ranges were used to present the data in aggregate.

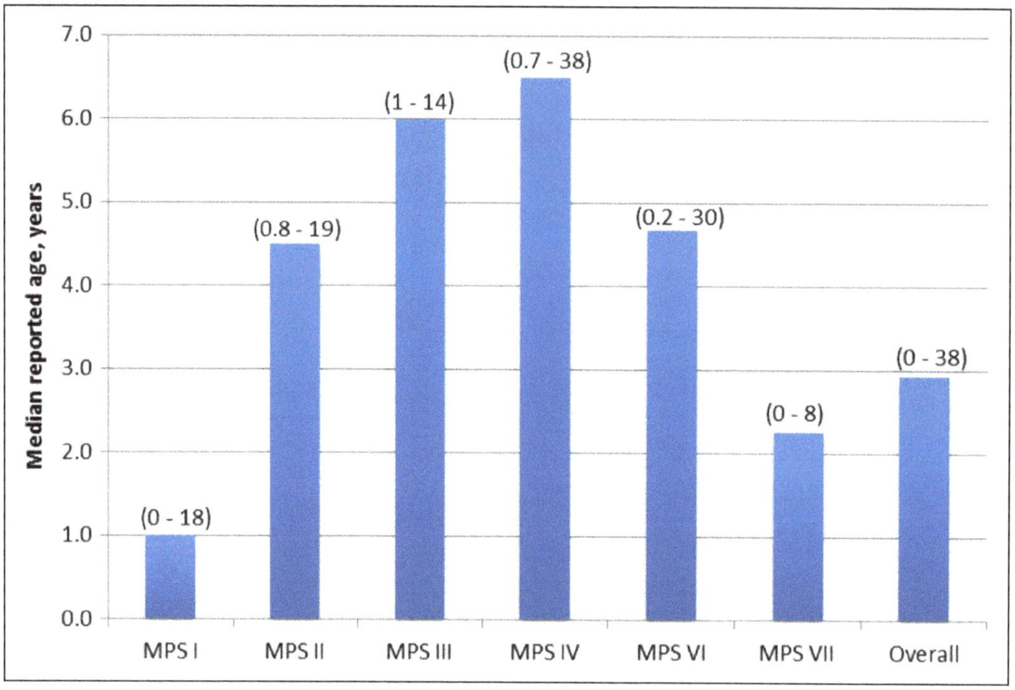

Figure 2. Literature review: duration of delays in diagnosis by mucopolysaccharidosis (MPS) type.
*Some studies excluded due to nonreporting. Age of diagnosis and duration of delay in diagnosis may not be consistent as results have been synthesized from different sources in the literature. Ranges are provided in brackets.

Physician Survey

Distribution and eligibility. The target population for the physician survey was physicians to whom potential patients with MPS first present. Physicians were recruited from an online research panel that had previously consented to participate in surveys. Eligibility criteria included physician specialty, country of practice, and a requirement to have currently or previously identified, diagnosed, or managed a minimum of 1 patient with confirmed or suspected MPS. Specialties were selected based on expert feedback of the most likely physicians to whom patients with MPS would present. Eligible specialties included general medicine, orthopedics, rheumatology, neurology, internal medicine, ophthalmology, cardiology, pediatrics, clinical genetics/metabolic genetics, and otorhinolaryngology. Eligible countries were selected based on where known MPS clinics were located to increase the likelihood of identifying eligible physicians and to provide geographic variability within the study sample. Eligible countries included Argentina, Australia, Brazil, Canada, Colombia, France, Germany, Italy, Japan, Malaysia, Singapore, South Korea, Spain, Turkey, the United Kingdom, and the United States. Eligible physicians completed the survey online.

Survey contents. The survey included questions regarding the physicians' demographics and clinical practice, as well as experience with MPS including specific presenting signs and symptoms, referral patterns and laboratory and radiology investigations; they may order for patients with suspected MPS. Physicians were asked to describe up to 10 potential cases with MPS they could recall, including the clinical features at presentation of the patient, the MPS type, the patient's age when symptoms first presented, and the duration that the patient had these presenting symptoms when they were either referred to them or referred on. The survey was available in 4 languages: English, Japanese, Portuguese, and Spanish. The survey took approximately 20 minutes to complete, and participants were compensated for their time. See Supplemental File 3 for the English version of the survey.

Data analysis. Data were synthesized in tabular format; clinical features of MPS were stratified according to MPS type, age-group (<1, 1-4, 5-9, $\geq$10 years), reporting physician specialty, and/or major symptom categories.

Clinical Expert Panel

An international panel of 16 physicians highly experienced in managing cases with MPS was convened. Members of this panel provided input into the systematic literature review and physician survey methods and reviewed the results. Using these findings, along with group discussion based on personal expertise and clinical experience, the panel members recommended key red flag early signs and symptoms with relatively good sensitivity and specificity for detecting MPS based on the physician survey and the panel's clinical experience. The panel members provided recommendations for key red flag signs and symptoms that would be suitable for specialist and nonspecialist physicians. The tools developed based on these

Table 1. Physician Survey: Number of Surveyed Physicians by Specialty.

	Physician Respondents (n = 209)	
	n	(%)
Specialty		
General practice/family medicine	42	(20.1)
Orthopedics	12	(5.7)
Rheumatology	18	(8.6)
Neurology	13	(6.2)
Internist	23	(11)
Ophthalmology	23	(11)
Medical genetics[a]	0	(0)
Cardiology	25	(12)
Pediatrics	25	(12)
Metabolic disease/metabolic genetics	18	(8.6)
Otorhinolaryngologist	10	(4.8)

[a]Physicians were recruited from specialist panels; however, a panel of pre-specified medical geneticists was not available

red flag signs and symptoms underwent iterative review cycles with the panel as well as cross-referencing with the physician survey and literature review results to ensure that each sign or symptom was common enough among patients with MPS to warrant inclusion and seen sufficiently infrequently by the physician type in question to be a realistic trigger for screening. The exact balance of specificity versus sensitivity determining inclusion/exclusion of an individual sign or symptom was based on the collective clinical judgment of the expert panel.

Results

Systematic Literature Review

A total of 1466 unique abstracts were identified. From these, 379 full-text publications were reviewed and 194 met the inclusion criteria (Figure 1). The majority (76%) of these studies reported on a single MPS type. A total of 330 MPS type-specific records, representing 194 unique studies, were identified.

Of the 194 studies included, 38% were reviews, 22% were case reports, and the remainder included case series, observational studies, surveys, and guidelines. MPS type-specific sample sizes ranged from 1 patient to 1041 patients; 42% of records contained fewer than 10 patients and only 3% of records contained 75 or greater patients. Overall, 44% of studies were European in origin, followed by Asian (15% of studies), and North American (14% of studies). Each MPS type was described in at least 1 study; descriptions of MPS I (39% of studies) and MPS IV (32% of studies) were most frequent.

In studies where the specialty of the diagnosing physician was described, it was most frequently geneticists, pediatricians, or metabolic specialists. Delays in diagnosis are reported in Figure 2 (additional data in Supplemental File 4). The typical delay in diagnosis, from time of symptom onset, was reported to be 2.9 years (ranging from 0 to 38 years). In approximately 20% of records, the median delay in diagnosis was reported to be at least 10 years. Some variability was observed across MPS types; the longest delays in diagnosis tended to be reported for MPS IV.

Coarse facial features, short stature, corneal clouding, hepatomegaly, and/or splenomegaly were the predominant signs and symptoms at presentation. Other frequently published presenting signs and symptoms included heart valve abnormality, neurological abnormality, joint abnormality, and varying levels of facial dysmorphism (additional data in Supplemental File 5).

Physician Survey

A total of 521 physicians were screened; 209 were eligible, and they participated in the survey. Between 5 and 20 participants were included per country, with general medicine being the most frequently represented specialty (20% of participants) and otorhinolaryngology the least frequent (5% of participants; Table 1). The majority of participants practiced in an academic setting (65%), and the study sample had a median of 16 years' experience postresidency (range: 2-56 years). Participants had experience with a median of 1 current MPS case (range: 0 to 200), and 3 previous MPS cases (range: 0 to 300). The majority (78%) of physicians had experience with MPS I. Participants reported having the least experience with MPS VII (14% reported any experience).

Physician participants described a total of 859 cases with MPS, with just over half of the cases being MPS I (n = 435) and only 17 cases being MPS VII. For all MPS types, 67% of cases described first presented under the age of 12 years, with 25% presenting under the age of 4 years.

Skeletal malformations and joint problems were the presenting signs and symptoms most frequently noted by the physicians, reported in more than 20% of cases across all MPS types (Figure 3). Gait disturbances, growth retardation, dysmorphic facial features, psychomotor retardation, and liver enlargement were also frequently reported, observed in more than 20% of reported cases for most MPS types. Corneal clouding was the most frequently observed ophthalmological sign for most MPS types (26% of all cases with MPS). Heart abnormalities and liver enlargement were observed at presentation in more than 20% of all cases with MPS reported, with heart abnormalities in over 30% of cases with MPS I, IV, and VI. MPS III was the type for which neurological signs and symptoms were most frequently reported at presentation.

Among cases presenting under the age of 4, just over half of patients presented with skeletal abnormalities or dysmorphic facial features (52% and 51%, respectively). Other frequently reported signs and symptoms in this age-group included developmental delay (45% of patients), growth retardation (38%), psychomotor retardation (36%), hypotonia (31%), and cognitive impairment (30%).

Forty-one percent of physicians reported that their patient had signs and symptoms that they did not know were associated

		MPS I (n=435) %	MPS II (n=42) %	MPS III (n=148) %	MPS IV (n=106) %	MPS VI (n=21) %	MPS VII (n=17) %	MPS IX (n=21) %	Unknown (n=69) %	Overall (n=859) %
Skeletal/muscular	Skeletal malformations	49.4	50	30.4	68.9	61.9	29.4	52.4	34.8	47.4
	Joint problems (stiffness or hypermobility)	33.8	28.6	37.2	34.9	42.9	35.3	52.4	30.4	34.7
	Gait disturbance	26.9	19	18.9	39.6	28.6	29.4	33.3	24.6	26.8
	Growth delays/short stature	30.6	26.2	27.7	42.5	57.1	11.8	23.8	27.5	31.2
	Knee deformities	18.4	26.2	12.8	28.3	28.6	23.5	23.8	13	19.1
	Hip deformities	17	4.8	16.9	27.4	19	5.9	14.3	11.6	17
	Gibbus deformity	10.1	14.3	2.7	15.1	14.3	5.9	14.3	7.2	9.5
	Other	1.1	0	0	0	0	5.9	4.8	1.4	0.9
Develop-mental	Dysmorphic/coarse facial features	40.2	35.7	37.8	36.8	38.1	29.4	19	27.5	37.4
	Psychomotor retardation	32	33.3	38.5	35.8	42.9	11.8	28.6	24.6	32.8
	Hypotonia	22.3	21.4	30.4	17	19	35.3	23.8	14.5	22.6
	Other	0.5	0	0	0	0	0	0	0	0.2
Organ system involvement	Heart abnormalities	30.6	16.7	12.8	36.8	42.9	5.9	14.3	17.4	26
	Breathing abnormalities	16.8	9.5	16.2	21.7	19	11.8	23.8	24.6	17.7
	Sleep apnea/sleep disordered breathing	13.1	9.5	18.9	13.2	28.6	11.8	23.8	17.4	14.9
	Liver enlargement	26.2	23.8	29.1	23.6	23.8	23.5	19	8.7	24.6
	Spleen enlargement	21.6	21.4	18.2	21.7	23.8	11.8	9.5	13	19.9
	Hearing deficits	11.3	16.7	16.9	10.4	14.3	5.9	4.8	15.9	12.6
	Multiple or recurrent hernia	5.3	14.3	4.1	10.4	14.3	17.6	4.8	4.3	6.5
	Other	0.2	0	0	0	0	0	0	0	0.1
Ophthalmo-logical	Clouding of the cornea	34	19	16.2	24.5	33.3	35.3	9.5	7.2	26.3
	Retinal degeneration	14.3	9.5	14.2	12.3	9.5	5.9	38.1	8.7	13.6
	Glaucoma/increased intraocular pressure	9.7	11.9	16.9	13.2	14.3	29.4	4.8	8.7	11.8
	Other	0.9	0	2	0	0	0	9.5	1.4	1.2
Neurological	Developmental delays	33.8	19	32.4	23.6	23.8	11.8	28.6	20.3	29.7
	Cognitive delays	22.1	9.5	34.5	13.2	28.6	11.8	28.6	18.8	22.4
	Hyperactivity	12	11.9	41.9	17.9	19	11.8	23.8	14.5	18.5
	Autism spectrum disorder	8.7	0	26.4	9.4	14.3	11.8	4.8	8.7	11.5
	Attention deficits	13.3	19	31.8	10.4	19	17.6	23.8	7.2	16.4
	Carpal tunnel syndrome	6.2	4.8	5.4	5.7	9.5	0	0	5.8	5.7
	Other	0.5	0	1.4	0	0	0	0	0	0.5
Otorhinolaryngo-logical	Frequent ear infections	20.2	21.4	10.8	19.8	9.5	11.8	28.6	15.9	18
	Frequent sinus infections	13.8	9.5	20.3	19.8	14.3	23.5	9.5	15.9	15.7
	Frequent tonsil infections	9.4	11.9	18.9	6.6	23.8	5.9	19	10.1	11.4
	Frequent placement of ear tubes	6	7.1	11.5	9.4	9.5	5.9	19	5.8	7.8
	Hearing impairment	9.4	9.5	15.5	12.3	23.8	0	14.3	4.3	10.7
	Other	0.2	0	0	0	0	0	0	0	0.1
Other	Skin abnormalities	12.4	26.2	11.5	14.2	14.3	11.8	14.3	10.1	13
	Hair abnormalities	12.6	11.9	16.9	7.5	19	17.6	9.5	1.4	12
	Hydrops fetalis	4.1	0	11.5	9.4	4.8	11.8	14.3	2.9	6.2
	Poor dentition/dental abnormalities	13.1	14.3	15.5	16	19	0	9.5	7.2	13.3
	Frequent colds/upper respiratory tract infections	9	2.4	10.8	9.4	9.5	23.5	33.3	10.1	10
	Macroglossia	12.2	7.1	15.5	13.2	19	0	9.5	11.6	12.5
	Family history of MPS	5.7	0	6.1	4.7	14.3	17.6	4.8	5.8	5.8
	Other	0.7	2.4	0.7	0	0	0	4.8	4.3	1

Figure 3. Physician survey: signs/symptoms present when mucopolysaccharidosis (MPS) first suspected or patient referred with suspected MPS*.

*Proportion among reported cases. Physicians were permitted to enter data for up to 10 patients; however, they were not asked to pull these data from patient charts—these are likely from memory. Cells are shaded if greater than 20%, with darkest shading for maximum values; "Other" fields within each subsection are populated by free-text fields. Ns in the column headers represent the number of patients entered where at least one symptom was also provided.

with MPS, including various behavioral abnormalities (5%), abdominal conditions such as hernias or hepatosplenomegaly (4%), skeletal manifestations (3%), and visual conditions (2%).

Large variation was observed in the duration that patients had MPS features prior to being referred or tested for MPS, ranging from 1 month to 5 years. The signs and symptoms that were present for the longest mean duration prior to referral included carpal tunnel syndrome, skin abnormalities, recurrent ear, nose, and/or sinus infection, gibbus, heart abnormalities, and a family history of MPS, all present for a mean of over 13 months prior to referral (Table 2).

Referral patterns demonstrated that a large number of specialties were involved in the pathway to an MPS diagnosis (Figure 4). General practice and pediatrics were the 2 specialties from which the surveyed physicians most frequently received referrals. Metabolic specialists and pediatricians were the specialties to which the surveyed physicians most frequently referred patients. Among the surveyed physicians, 27% indicated that they would order an initial screening test for MPS prior to referring a patient with suspected MPS. This highlights the need for better education of the medical community on MPS screening and testing.

Table 2. Physician Survey: Duration of Specific Signs/Symptoms at the Time of Decision to Test/Referral.[a]

		Duration of Symptom Prior to Testing or Referral (months)	
	Patients with symptom (n)	Mean (SD)	Median (Range)
Skeletal/muscular			
Skeletal malformations	407	12.2 (11.3)	10 (1-60)
Joint problems (stiffness or hypermobility)	298	12.8 (11.5)	9 (1-60)
Gait disturbance	230	10.4 (9.6)	6 (1-60)
Growth delays/short stature	268	11.6 (10.9)	7 (1-53)
Knee deformities	164	12.2 (10.6)	9 (1-48)
Hip deformities	146	12.9 (11.9)	10 (1-53)
Gibbus deformity	82	14.5 (12.8)	10 (1-60)
Developmental			
Dysmorphic/coarse facial features	321	11.0 (10.7)	7 (1-60)
Psychomotor retardation	282	10.2 (9.9)	6 (1-60)
Hypotonia	194	7.3 (6.4)	6 (1-30)
Organ system involvement			
Heart abnormalities	223	14.8 (11.8)	12 (1-53)
Breathing abnormalities	152	11.2 (9.8)	6.5 (1-53)
Sleep apnea/sleep disordered breathing	128	10.6 (9.0)	7 (1-60)
Liver enlargement	211	12.4 (12.1)	9 (1-60)
Spleen enlargement	171	12.5 (12.3)	10 (1-60)
Hearing deficits	108	11.3 (9.4)	7 (1-48)
Multiple or recurrent hernia	56	12.6 (11.9)	10 (1-60)
Ophthalmological			
Clouding of the cornea	226	11.9 (11.2)	10 (1-60)
Retinal degeneration	117	8.7 (5.8)	6 (1-24)
Glaucoma/increased intraocular pressure	101	10.5 (10.2)	6.5 (1-48)
Neurological			
Developmental delays	255	10.8 (10.8)	6 (1-60)
Cognitive delays	192	12.2 (11.4)	7 (1-60)
Hyperactivity	159	9.7 (10.8)	6 (1-60)
Autism spectrum disorder	99	10.6 (12.2)	6 (1-60)
Attention deficits	141	9.9 (8.7)	6 (1-40)
Carpal tunnel syndrome	49	15.1 (13.3)	13 (1-60)
Otorhinolaryngological			
Frequent ear infections	155	13.2 (10.9)	12 (1-60)
Frequent sinus infections	135	13.2 (11.3)	11 (1-60)
Frequent tonsil infections	98	9.6 (9.3)	6 (1-48)
Frequent placement of ear tubes	67	9.2 (7.0)	7 (1-30)
Hearing impairment	92	12.6 (10.5)	10 (1-48)
Other			
Skin abnormalities	112	14.9 (12.5)	12 (1-60)
Hair abnormalities	103	12.4 (11.0)	10 (1-60)
Hydrops fetalis	53	6.2 (4.0)	6 (2-20)
Poor dentition/ dental abnormalities	114	11.6 (10.1)	8 (1-48)
Frequent colds/ upper respiratory tract infections	86	12.3 (9.7)	12 (1-40)
Macroglossia	107	11.1 (9.7)	7 (1-48)
Family history of MPS	50	16.1 (14.1)	12 (1-60)

Abbreviations: MPS: Mucopolysaccharidosis; SD: Standard deviation.
[a]At time the surveyed physician decided to test for MPS or refer on or before the case was referred to the surveyed physician.

Clinical Expert Panel

The expert panel identified red flag signs and symptoms for consideration based on the systematic literature review, physician survey, and their own clinical experience. The red flag signs and symptoms were selected to be specific to physicians in pediatrics or general medicine as well as those in 5 subspecialty types to whom patients with early signs of MPS are likely to be referred: cardiology, pediatric neurology, otorhinolaryngology, rheumatology, and orthopedics. These specialties were selected based on the referral patterns reported in the physician survey, the early signs and symptoms identified in the systematic literature review and physician survey, and expert experience. One to 6 key red flag signs and symptoms were identified for each specialty type and were further augmented with lists of corroborating signs/symptoms to aid in the establishment of

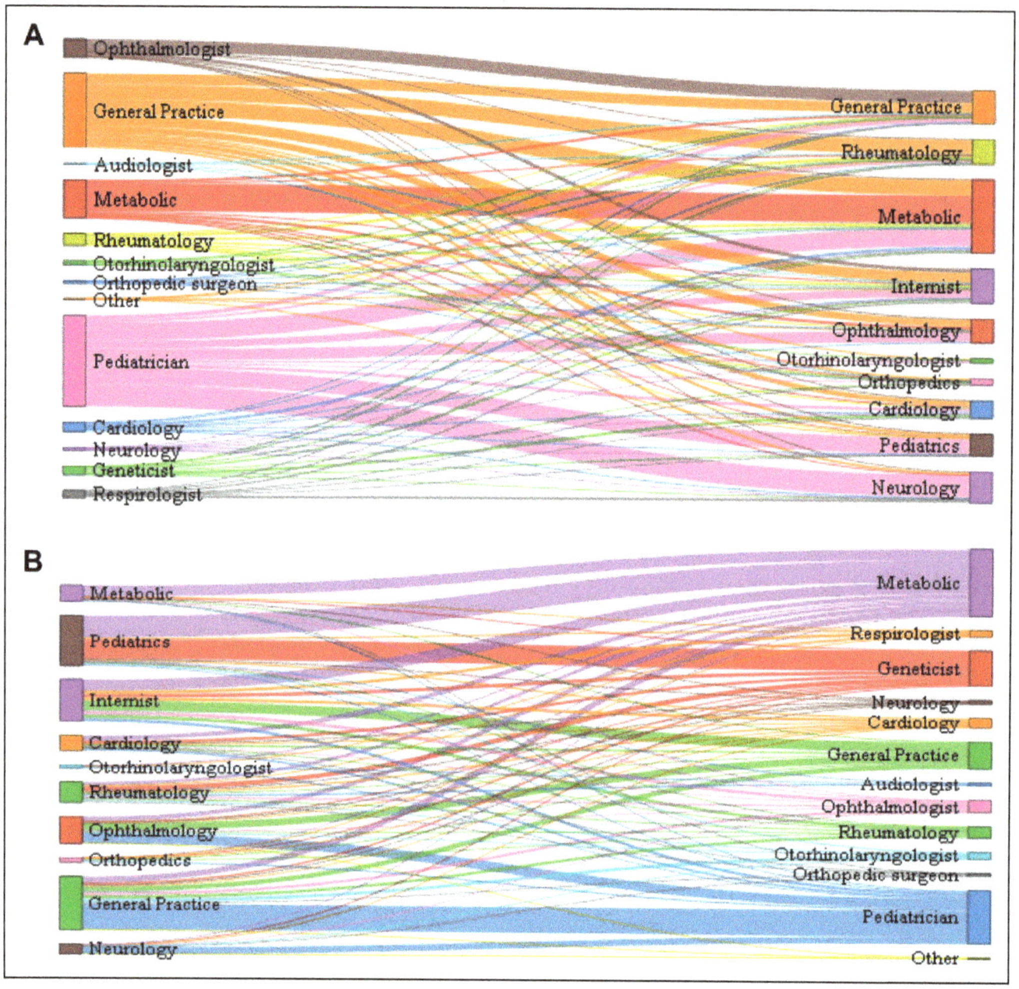

Figure 4. Physician survey: alluvial plots showing which specialties the surveyed physicians received the mucopolysaccharidosis (MPS) referrals from (A) and which specialties the surveyed physicians referred suspected MPS patients to (B).
Notes: The alluvial plot is weighted by the number of patients such that if a specialist said they had received 10 referrals from a general practitioner and 20 from a pediatrician, these weights are captured in the diagram.

clinical suspicion of MPS (Table 3). These red flag signs and symptoms were then converted into specialty-specific clinical awareness diagnostic tools (Supplemental Files 6, 7, 8, 9, 10, 11, and 12). The tools were developed to be simple and visual. They also highlight the incidence of MPS and urgency of early diagnosis, provide information on additional signs and symptoms to help establish stronger clinical suspicion of MPS and motivate testing, and list next steps.

While discussing next steps, the panel noted the differing availability of screening and diagnostic test options globally and the continuous improvement in testing technologies over time. These factors, combined with those previously noted highlight the need to better educate the medical community on MPS screening and testing, led to the identification of the need for a global MPS testing website with up-to-date, region-specific information. As a result, www.test4mps.com website was developed to provide information on how to test for MPS and to house a searchable database of laboratories that conduct MPS testing around the world.

Discussion

The largely unappreciated need for early diagnosis of MPS was evident in the physician survey and systematic review. Patient cases described in the physician survey were observed to have signs and symptoms for over a year prior to referral, ranging up to 5 years. Additionally, the observed referral patterns indicate that patients are presenting to a variety of specialists and are being referred on to a variety of other specialists. The systematic literature review reflected similar trends, with nearly 40% of records reporting a delay in diagnosis of 1 to 4 years and 20% reporting a delay of greater than 10 years. This clearly demonstrates a need to improve the early recognition of signs and symptoms to facilitate earlier MPS screening and referral to metabolic specialists or clinical geneticists.

Results of the survey and literature review also highlighted challenges of early MPS diagnosis: rarity and the varied and sometimes subtle nature of signs and symptoms at presentation. Forty one percent of physicians in the survey reported that their patient(s) had signs or symptoms that they were not initially

Table 3. List of Specialty-Specific Red Flag Symptoms for MPS Developed by International Panel of MPS Experts.

Specialty	Red Flag Symptoms						Corroborating Symptoms
Orthopedics	Bilateral hip dysplasia/ osteonecrosis (perthes-like)		Vertebral body abnormality (hypoplasia, beaking, platyspondyly, kyphosis/gibbus)				Abnormal skeletal features (such as gibbus, pectus, broad ribs, hypoplastic odontoid, enlarged sella turcica, genu valgus) Atypical Mongolian spots Carpal tunnel syndrome (bilateral) Chronic rhinorrhea Clawed hands Coarse facial features Corneal clouding Dental abnormalities Developmental delay Difficulty opening mouth Dilated Virchow-Robin spaces Enlarged tonsils/adenoids Glaucoma (bilateral) Hearing loss Heart valve disease Hernias, including previous hernia repair Hirsutism History of hernia repair Hydrocephalus Joint abnormalities (restriction/stiffness or hyper-mobility/laxity) Kyphosis Left ventricular hypertrophy Liver and/or spleen enlargement Macroglossia Multi-systemic involvement Nerve compression syndrome Psychomotor delay/regression Recurrent ear nose and throat infections Seizures Short stature Sleep apnea Spinal deformity Unexplained arthropathy, with/without pain
Cardiology	Cardiac valve thickening						
Otolaryngology	Recurrent ear, nose, or throat infection		Upper airway obstruction	Progressive hearing loss			
Pediatric Neurology	Developmental delay/regression		Language delay	Hyperactivity			
Rheumatology	Unexplained arthropathy (with or without pain)		No evidence of inflammation				
Pediatricians	Short stature/ Decreasing growth velocity	Gibbus	Developmental delay	Recurrent ENT-related symptoms or infections	Enlarged liver and/or spleen	Inguinal or umbilical hernia, especially recurrent/history of hernia repair	
General Practitioners	Unexplained arthropathy with or without pain	Early onset spinal disease	Joint restrictions/stiffness or laxity/ hypermobility		Cardiac valvular disease	Early corneal clouding	

Abbreviations: ENT, ear, nose, throat; MPS, mucopolysaccharidoses.

aware were associated with MPS. Even with increased awareness among those with little or no experience in managing an MPS patient, a further challenge lies in providing a description of a common presentation of MPS. While skeletal deformities and joint problems are the hallmarks of most of the MPS disorders, we compiled an extensive list of other clinical features with early onset that should make one consider MPS. For example, some of the early presenting signs and symptoms that were frequently reported in the literature and physician survey included growth retardation; recurrent ear, nose, and/or throat infections; coarse facial features; developmental delay; heart valve thickening; corneal clouding; progressive hearing loss; and hernias.

Although others have attempted to generate tools and/or algorithms based on presenting signs and symptoms to aid in the diagnosis of MPS, these efforts have resulted in no noticeable change in the average length of the diagnostic delay over time.[8] The difficulty in distributing this information and its very limited half-life with the target audiences are substantial contributing factors in the failure of these previous attempts. Unfortunately, we will be facing the same challenges with these tools. However, previous efforts have also had several notable limitations. They often targeted only a subset of the specialists likely to encounter undiagnosed individuals with MPS,[12–15] were limited to a particular MPS type[14,15] or a sub-group of the MPS population,[12,13] resulted in complex, multitiered algorithms with a high degree of specificity and inadequate sensitivity,[12,13] and relied solely on expert opinion.[12–15] Several steps were taken to overcome these previous limitations in the current project.

The majority of specialists to whom individuals with MPS present were included. All MPS disorders were targeted collectively, thereby increasing the incidence to within a range that may be more relevant for the target audience[8] and enabling physicians to proceed with the suspicion of MPS in general, without needing specific knowledge of the types of MPS. The proposed screening is based on simple red flags that are easier to recall than a complex algorithm. And importantly, the quality and quantity of data gathered through systematic review and physician survey provided a solid evidence-based foundation.

The literature review was conducted using systematic and reproducible methods and captured a broad range of study designs, including reviews, case reports, case series, and larger observational studies. The physician survey was internationally-based, multilingual, and included data collected from a wide range of specialties, thus reflecting the variation in symptom presentation and patterns of referrals across geographies and specialties. This multimethod approach is important for rare diseases where there is a paucity of large studies that capture the data needed to inform the research question.

Despite the extensive set of data collected, there were some notable limitations. For example, in the literature review, there is an inherent risk of publication bias (ie, there may have been a risk that particularly unusual presentations of MPS were included, as these were considered worthy of publication). However, given the large number of studies returned, and inclusion of several large observational studies, it is expected that these extremely unusual presentations would also be relatively infrequent in the synthesized data set. This limitation of the systematic literature review was also addressed by supplementing the review with a physician survey and by seeking clinical expert feedback on the generalizability of the results. A main limitation of the physician survey was that the data were, by the design of the study, based on physician recall rather than from a chart review. A sign or symptom not reported at presentation may have been due to it not being present, or alternatively, the physician may not have recalled the sign or symptom, or it may not have been identified at that time. Nonspecific signs and symptoms that could be identified by specialists outside of those included in this analysis may also have been missed. Furthermore, the MPS type was reported by the responding physician who may not have been the diagnosing physician, and thus, there may have been inaccuracies. Additionally, not all MPS types were equally represented; however, this limitation was mitigated by analyzing the data by MPS type and by including clinical experts to provide insight into all MPS types. To increase the likelihood of finding eligible physicians to participate in the survey, physicians were selected only from countries where there were known MPS clinics. Although this includes the majority of countries with a well-known population of patients with MPS, it is a limitation that not all countries with potential MPS patients were represented in the analysis.

The compilation of evidence from the systematic literature review and survey is extensive; however, through review and discussion with the international panel of clinical experts, the findings were distilled into targeted lists of specialty-specific red flag signs and symptoms, together with an additional list of corroborating signs and symptoms. These were synthesized into simple, specialty-specific tools that can help raise awareness while reducing the potentially overwhelming amount of information for practitioners who may only ever see 1 or 2 MPS patients in their entire career. The specialty-specific nature of these tools further maximizes their relevance. Importantly, these tools have also been coupled with real-world, up-to-date laboratory information to facilitate rapid action following initial suspicion of MPS.

The ability of these tools to have an impact for MPS patients and their families is completely dependent on what happens next. Due to the rarity of the disease, specialists may only see 1 patient with MPS during their career, perhaps years after this paper is published. The key knowledge we have assembled here will need to be available to physicians whenever they happen to encounter that patient. Using repetitive dissemination of our simple, evidence-based, specialty-specific tools and striving to ensure their continual presence (ie, tools posted on hospital walls, incorporation into guidelines, inclusion in an online application), we hope to have the critical information available at the right time for as many cases as possible. The effectiveness of our approach will need to be evaluated in a future study.

Ultimately, though these clinical awareness diagnostic tools will not completely close the diagnostic gap, we hope that they will help to narrow it until a more comprehensive solution, such as newborn screening, automated electronic medical record flagging, or mandatory subpopulation screening, is feasible.

Authors' Note

Sarah Goring, Suzanne McMullen, Sara Hawley, and Elaina Jurecki contributed to study design, and physician survey conduct. Fathima Mubarack and Elaina Jurecki designed the systematic literature review and Fathima Mubarack performed data extraction and Sarah Goring and Zaeem Khan contributed to the analysis of the systematic literature review. Lorne Clarke, Carolyn Ellaway, Helen E. Foster, Roberto Giugliani, Cyril Goizet, Christina Lampe, Ken Martin, John J. Mitchell, Martha Solano Villarreal, H. Serap Sivri, Fiona J. Stewart, Anna Tylki-Szymanska, Klane White, and Frits Wijburg were members of the clinical expert panel, and provided interpretation of the study results and selection of the relevant symptoms based on the study results. All authors read and approved the final manuscript.

Acknowledgments

We would like to acknowledge Dr Mira de Kruijf (Royal Manchester Children's Hospital), Dr Kuo Sheng Lee (Mackay Memorial Hospital), Dr Elizabeth Braunlin (University of Minnesota), Neil James, Tiffany Wong, Grace Chen, and Emanuela Izzo (BioMarin Pharmaceutical Inc.) for their contributions to this study.

Declaration of Conflicting Interests

The author(s) declared the following potential conflicts of interest with respect to the research, authorship, and/or publication of this article: Lorne Clarke receives honoraria and travel support from Sanofi, BioMarin, and Shire related to participation in disease registry boards and speakers bureaus. Carolyn Ellaway has received travel support and honoraria from BioMarin, Sanofi Genzyme, and Shire. Helen E. Foster on behalf of Newcastle University, United Kingdom has received speaker/chair honoraria and unrestricted educational bursaries from BioMarin and Sanofi Genzyme. Roberto Giugliani has received investigator fees, and/or travel grants, and/or speaker honoraria from Actelion, Amicus, Armagen, BioMarin, GC Pharma, JCR Pharmaceuticals, Lysogene, Sanofi Genzyme, Shire, and Ultragenyx. Cyril Goizet has received consulting fees from Sanofi Genzyme and BioMarin; honorarium for participation in advisory boards from BioMarin and Sanofi Genzyme; financial support for research activities from Sanofi Genzyme, Shire, and BioMarin; and funding for inscriptions and travels for congresses from Sanofi Genzyme, Shire, and BioMarin. Sara Hawley, Elaina Jurecki, and Fathima Mubarack are employees and stockholders of BioMarin. Christina Lampe has received honoraria/consultation fees from Shire, Alexion, Actelion, BioMarin and Genzyme, and has participated in company sponsored speaker's bureau for Shire, Alexion, Actelion, BioMarin and Genzyme. Ken Martin has accepted consulting fees or honoraria from the following companies engaged in developing MPS-related therapies: BioMarin, Sangamo, REGENXBIO, Ultragenyx, and Shire. John J. Mitchell has received speaker fees, consulting fees and research support from BioMarin and Shire, and receives funding support from the Harpur Foundation. H. Serap Sivri has received travel support and honoraria from BioMarin. Martha Solano Villarreal has received speaker fees and consulting fees from BioMarin. Fiona J. Stewart has received speaker fees and consultancy fees from BioMarin. Anna Tylki-Szymanska has received honoraria/consultation fees from Shire, BioMarin, Chiesi and Genzyme, and has participated in company sponsored speaker's bureau for Shire, BioMarin and Genzyme. Klane White has received honoraria/travel support from BioMarin, Genzyme, and Medicrea, and receives royalties from UpToDate.com and grant support from BioMarin. Frits Wijburg has received honoraria for presentations and board meetings, travel expenses to meetings and honoraria for consultancy work from Sanofi Genzyme, BioMarin, Actelion and Shire, and has received unrestricted educational grants and research grants from Sanofi Genzyme, BioMarin and Actelion. Sarah Goring, Zaeem Khan, and Suzanne McMullen declare that they have no competing interests.

Funding

The author(s) disclosed receipt of the following financial support for the research, authorship, and/or publication of this article: This study was funded by BioMarin Pharmaceutical Inc.

References

1. Muenzer J. Overview of the mucopolysaccharidoses. *Rheumatology*. 2011;50:v4-v12.
2. Bittar T. Mucopolysaccharidosis. In: Grogan DP, ed. Medscape. New York, NY: Medscape; 2013.
3. Neufeld EU, Muenzer J. The mucopolysaccharidoses. In: Scriver CR, Beaudet AL, Sly WS, Valle D, Childs B, Kinzler KW, Vogelstein B, eds. *The metabolic and molecular bases of inherited disease*. New York: McGraw-Hill; 2001: pp. 3421-3452.
4. Baehner F, Schmiedeskamp C, Krummenauer F, et al. Cumulative incidence rates of the mucopolysaccharidoses in Germany. *J Inherit Metab Dis*. 2005;28(6):1011-1017.
5. Meikle PJ, Hopwood JJ, Clague AE, Carey WF. Prevalence of lysosomal storage disorders. *JAMA*. 1999;281(3):249-254.
6. Poorthuis BJ, Wevers RA, Kleijer WJ, et al. The frequency of lysosomal storage diseases in the Netherlands. *Human Genet*. 1999;105(1-2):151-156.
7. Lin HY, Lin SP, Chuang CK, et al. Incidence of the mucopolysaccharidoses in Taiwan, 1984-2004. *Am J Med Genet A*. 2009; 149A(5):960-964.
8. Kuiper GA, Meijer OL, Langereis EJ, Wijburg FA. Failure to shorten the diagnostic delay in two ultra-orphan diseases (mucopolysaccharidosis types I and III): potential causes and implications. *Orphanet J Rare Dis*. 2018;13(1):2.
9. Wilson GN. Hunter syndrome (mucopolysaccharidosis II): diagnosis, genetic testing, treatment, and referral. *Consultant for Pediatricians*. 2015;14(5):206-212.
10. Centre for Reviews and Dissemination. *Systematic Reviews: CRD's Guidance for Undertaking Reviews in Health Care*. Layerthorpe, York: University of York. 2009. https://www.york.ac.uk/media/crd/Systematic_Reviews.pdf
11. Moher D, Liberati A, Tetzlaff J, Altman DG. Preferred reporting items for systematic reviews and meta-analyses: the PRISMA statement. *BMJ*. 2009;339:b2535.

12. Cimaz R, Coppa GV, Koné-Paut I, et al. Joint contractures in the absence of inflammation may indicate mucopolysaccharidosis. *Pediatr Rheumatol*. 2009;7:18.
13. Lehman TJA, Miller N, Norquist B, Underhill L, Keutzer J. Diagnosis of the mucopolysaccharidoses. *Rheumatology*. 2011;50(5):v41-v48.
14. Wood T, Bainbridge K, Beck M, et al. Diagnosing mucopolysaccharidosis IVA. *J Inherit Metab Dis*. 2013;36(2):293-307.
15. Wood T, Bodamer OA, Burin MG, et al. Expert recommendations for the laboratory diagnosis of MPS VI. *Mol Genet Metab*. 2012;106(1):73-82.

Quality of Life and Associated Factors in Japanese Children With Inborn Errors of Metabolism and Their Families

Keiko Yamaguchi, RN, PHN[1], Rie Wakimizu, PhD, RN, PHN[1], and Mitsuru Kubota, MD[2]

Abstract

To reveal the associated factors of quality of life (QoL) in children with inborn errors of metabolism (IEM), their siblings, and their primary caregivers and partners, we conducted an anonymous questionnaire survey in Japan. Descriptive, correlation, and multiple regression analyses were performed. Fifty-six children with IEM, 35 siblings, 143 primary caregivers, and 86 partners completed our questionnaires. There were significant positive correlations between higher QoL in children with IEM and lower disease influence ($r = 0.46$) and higher perceived emotional support ($r = 0.67$). We could not find any associated factor of siblings' QoL. Lower parental distress, higher family empowerment, and higher household income contributed to higher QoL in primary caregivers (adjusted $R^2 = 0.636$). Higher household income, lower anxiety about childrearing, and higher satisfaction in the relationship with the child and entire family contributed to higher QoL of partners (adjusted $R^2 = 0.398$). We concluded that developing effective interventions to improve QoL is needed for the entire family in future outpatient settings.

Keywords

inborn errors of metabolism, quality of life, children, family, questionnaire survey

Introduction

In 2013, around 19 000 cases of patients with inborn errors of metabolism (IEM) were reported in Japan.[1] Although there have been recent improvements in the early detection and treatment of these conditions in Japan,[2] patients will still have to live with this condition for the rest of their lives, even in cases in which early diagnosis and treatment were successful. During the process of coping with their conditions, patients will face the same variety of challenges as their parents.[3] As with other chronic childhood conditions, such as food allergies,[4] the different forms of dietary restriction involved in the treatment of IEM will affect not only child's quality of life (QoL) but the QoL of the entire family. Before considering effective means of support for these children and their families, it is essential to first understand their current QoL and associated factors.

In other countries, some studies on the QoL of patients with IEM and their parents have been conducted.[5-7] In Turkey, the researcher reported that children with IEM and poor dietary compliance had lower scores in 2 aspects of QoL: school life and disease perception.[5] In our previous literature review, we found that Japanese children with IEM and their parents faced various difficulties in daily life, through infancy to adolescence and young adulthood.[6] We then hypothesized that QoL would be affected and impaired by IEM for both children and their families.

On the other hand, Simon et al in Germany and Cazzorla et al in Italy reported that QoL scores among young adult and adult patients with phenylketonuria (PKU) were not significantly different when compared to those of healthy individuals.[7,8] This may imply that children with IEM somehow overcome their difficulties during maturation. During childhood, children with IEM and their families should be able to get support from the people around them. There have been some qualitative studies on QoL of these individuals,[9-11] but

[1] University of Tsukuba, Tsukuba, Ibaraki, Japan

[2] Kokuritsu Kenkyu Kaihatsu Hojin Kokuritsu, Seiiku Iryo Kenkyu Center, National Center for Child Health and Development, Setagaya-ku, Tokyo, Japan

Corresponding Author:

Keiko Yamaguchi, University of Tsukuba, 1-1-1 Tennodai, Tsukuba, Ibaraki 305-8575, Japan.

Email: yamaguchi.keiko.xa@alumni.tsukuba.ac.jp

currently, there are no quantitative studies assessing QoL and its associated factors among families impacted by IEM in Japan. We investigated the actual situation of the QOL of children with IEM and their entire families in Japan as the first step, although it is known that investigation of individual diseases is important. It would be helpful to clarify the common associated factors of QoL of such children and their families for policy making for supporting these families. Like in other international studies, it is important to report the QoL in every diagnosis; however, we believed that investigating the actual situation of the QOL of children with IEM and their entire family in Japan is the first step. It will be helpful to clarify the common associated factors of QoL of those children and families for policy making, regarding the support for those families at a national level.

Therefore, the purpose of our study was to report the QoL of children with IEM as well as that of their immediate family they live with and reveal the factors associated with QoL of these individuals. These findings will be the basis for providing effective support to the entire family from the perspective of medical professionals.

Methods

We conducted cross-sectional questionnaire survey among children with IEM, their siblings, their primary caregivers, and their partners. The study was conducted in Japan from August to October 2015. We have used the terms, "primary caregiver" and "partner" in this study rather than "mother" and "father" because the role of a primary caregiver might be undertaken by either the mother or father, depending on the family. Anonymous questionnaires were sent to 532 eligible families across Japan in July 2015. Participants sent the completed questionnaires back to our university voluntarily.

Participants

We recruited children with IEM and their families from Japan registration System for Metabolic & Inherited Diseases (JaSMIn). This voluntary self-registration system was established in 2013 as a way to improve the diagnosis and treatment of IEM by the National Center of Child Health and Development (http://jasmin-mcbank.com). Patients and families were registered in this system in order to participate in the studies aiming to improve the care they receive and to obtain information about the studies such as clinical trials. Patients and their families who are willing to cooperate with studies on IEM enroll in this system. There were 532 children aged between 0 and 20 years registered with JaSMIn in July 2015. The participants involved in this study were children with IEM aged 7 to 20 years, siblings aged 7 to 20 years, primary caregivers of children with IEM aged 0 to 20 years, and the partners of the primary caregivers. Children aged 0 to 20 years with special chronic diseases, including IEM, received medical aid in Japan. Even if a child with IEM was below 7 years of age, their older siblings and primary caregivers were included if they volunteered to participate in this study. We included only children and their families living together at the time of the investigation and excluded the data of siblings having IEM ($n = 3$) in our analysis.

Questionnaires

Questionnaire sheets and survey contents were prepared separately for each participant: children with IEM, siblings, primary caregivers, and partners of primary caregivers. All existing scales were calculated along with each instruction and analyzed by using raw scores without any transformation.

Children With IEM and Their Siblings

We used the Japanese version of the Kinder Lebensqualitats Fragebogen (KINDL) scale for assessing QoL of children. The scale was developed in Germany, and its reliability and validity have been confirmed in Japanese samples.[12,13] This scale has 24 items and consists of 6 subscales: physical, emotional, self-esteem, family, friends, and school. Total scores ranged between 20 and 100 in the KINDL scale. We also used the additional disease subscale of the KINDL, which comprises 6 general items related to the disease. The disease subscale of KINDL is conceptually divided from other subscales, and assesses how much their disease affects their daily lives.[12] The 6 items of the disease scales are "I was afraid that my illness might get worse," "I was sad because of my illness," "I was able to cope well with my illness," "My parents treated me like a baby because of my illness," "I wanted nobody to notice my illness," and "I missed something at school because of my illness." For the purpose of this study, we added 4 original items to assess the quality of emotional support received in daily life. Items included, "I have difficulty," "I have someone who helps me when I have a difficulty," "I have someone who I can talk to when I have a difficulty," and "I can talk to my parents when I have a difficulty." These study-specific items were scored the same way as the items of the original KINDL scale. If there were several siblings in a family, only 1 sibling answered the questionnaire. General characteristics were also recorded for children and their siblings.

Primary Caregivers

We used the Japanese version of the 26-item short form of the World Health Organization QoL (WHOQoL-26) questionnaire for assessing the QoL of primary caregivers.[14] The Japanese version's reliability and validity have previously been confirmed.[15] The WHOQOL-26 contains 24 items covering the 4 subscales of physical health, psychological health, social relationships, and environment and contains 2 items assessing global QoL.

For assessing parenting stress, we used the Parenting Stress Index–Short Form (PSI-SF).[16] The Japanese version was developed, and its reliability and validity have been established.[17,18] The Japanese version has 19 items and consists of 2 subscales: difficult child and parental distress. For assessing family

Table 1. Correlations Between QoL in Children With IEM and Their Siblings and Its Predictive Factors.

	Children With IEM (n = 56)					Siblings of a Child With IEM (n = 35)			
KINDL Scores	Age	Number of Siblings	Birth Order	Disease (KINDL)	Emotional Support Resources Score	Age	Number of Siblings	Birth Order	Emotional Support Resources Score
Physical	−0.268[a]	0.017	0.009	0.417[b]	0.417[b]	−0.325	−0.021	0.098	0.491[b]
Emotional	−0.23	0.008	−0.041	0.383[a]	0.415[b]	−0.069	0.098	−0.041	0.445[b]
Self-esteem	−0.071	−0.297[a]	−0.23	0.181	0.505[b]	−0.126	0.035	−0.011	0.155
Family	0.015	−0.058	−0.04	0.316[a]	0.443[b]	0.216	0.213	−0.068	0.505[b]
Friends	−0.107	−0.005	0.001	0.336[a]	0.492[b]	−0.469[b]	-0.126	0.058	0.164
School	−0.128	−0.081	−0.097	0.455[b]	0.426[b]	−0.15	-0.139	0.042	−0.047
Total	−0.153	−0.076	−0.054	0.460[b]	0.673[b]	−0.238	0.021	0.042	0.291

Abbreviations: IEM, inborn errors of metabolism; KINDL, Kinder Lebensqualitats Fragebogen; QoL, quality of life.
[a] $P < .05$.
[b] $P < .01$.

empowerment, we used the Family Empowerment Scale (FES).[19] The concept of family empowerment represents a family's ability to raise a child with disabilities independently and control their own lives and its process.[19] The reliability and validity of the Japanese version of Family Empowerment Scale (J-FES) have been established.[20] This scale has 34 items and consists of 3 subscales: family, service systems, and social politics. The J-FES was completed by the primary caregiver, and their answers were considered to represent the feelings of empowerment in the entire family.[20]

The questionnaire consisted of (1) characteristics of the primary caregivers and (2) predictive factors of their QoL. To assess the characteristics of primary caregivers and the factors predicting their QoL, our survey included items devised from both previous literature, studying QoL of other chronic conditions,[21-23] and our own literature review.[6] The characteristics of primary caregivers (1) are shown in Table 3. Predictive factors of primary caregivers' QoL (2) were described by the following 12 items: the age of IEM onset in children, number of IEM-related hospital visits per year, difficulties related to raising a child with IEM, anxieties related to raising a child with IEM, degree of distress related to caring for a child with IEM, information resource of their child's disease and treatment, satisfaction in the relationship with the child with IEM, satisfaction in the relationships within the family, household income, and degree of social acceptance and understanding shown to the child with IEM.

Partners of Primary Caregivers

We used the same WHOQOL-26 scale for assessing the QoL of partners.[15] The questionnaire consisted of (1) characteristics of partners and (2) predictive factors of QoL. Characteristics of partners (1) were the same 4 items as primary caregivers. Predictive factors of partners' QoL (2) were the following 7 items: current age of children with IEM, anxieties related to raising a child with IEM, degree of distress related to caring for a child with IEM, satisfaction in the relationship with the child with IEM, satisfaction in the relationships within family, household income, and the degree of social acceptance and understanding shown to the child with IEM.

Data Analysis

Data analysis was conducted using SPSS 21 for Mac (SPSS Inc). For inclusion in the analysis, all questionnaire scales and subscales were required to have been completed fully (KINDL, WHOQOL-26, PSI-SF, and FES), and additional sociodemographic information, such as age and sex, were required to be 90% complete. We excluded the responses from participants who were in the hospital at the time of the investigation, as their physical or mental condition while in the hospital would not be reflective of their daily life experience while living at home, which may have affected their answers. The descriptive statistics, means, standard deviations (SDs), and response weighting were calculated for each variable. Spearman rank-correlation coefficients were used to evaluate the relationships between QoL of children and predictive factors of QoL separately for both children with IEM and their siblings. Multiple regression analysis was conducted by stepwise selection for revealing the associated factors of QoL of primary caregivers and partners. We set WHOQOL-26 scores as the dependent variable and each of the 17 factors (primary caregivers) and 10 factors (partners) as explanatory variables. There was no multicollinearity.

Ethical Considerations

This study was conducted in accordance with the Declaration of Helsinki and was approved by the medical ethics review board of the University of Tsukuba (no 1101). Consent was implied if children with IEM, siblings, primary caregivers, and partners answered and returned the questionnaires. Participants only supplied their full names and addresses if they wanted to receive a completed report of this study after analysis, and at this point, participants were informed that their information would not be used for any other purpose.

Table 2. Characteristics of Children With IEM and Their Siblings.

	Children With IEM (n = 56)		Siblings of a Child With IEM (n = 35)	
	n/M (SD)	%/ range	n/M (SD)	%/ range
Age	12.0 (3.1)	7-20	12.4 (3.3)	7-20
7-12 years	31	54.4%	20	57.1%
13-17 years	23	41.0%	13	37.1%
18-20 years	2	3.6%	2	5.7%
Gender[a]				
Male	28	50.0%	11	31.4%
Female	28	50.0%	22	62.9%
NA	-	-	2	5.7%
Birth order				
First	27	48.2%	19	54.3%
Second	21	37.5%	14	40.0%
Third	8	14.3%	2	5.7%
The number of siblings				
Zero	11	19.0%	0	-
One	17	48.2%	17	48.6%
Two	17	30.4%	14	40.0%
Three	1	1.8%	3	8.6%
Four	0	0.0%	1	2.9%
Disease[b]				
With	56	100.0%	7	20.0%
Without	0	0.0%	31	88.6%
Diagnosis[c]				
Amino acid disorders	31	55.4%	-	-
Lysosomal storage disease	6	10.7%	-	-
Organic acidemias	9	16.1%	-	-
Carbohydrate metabolism disorders	4	7.1%	-	-
Metal metabolism disorders	4	7.1%	-	-
Fatty acid metabolism disorders	2	3.6%	-	-

Abbreviations: IEM, inborn errors of metabolism; M, mean; NA, not applicable; SD, standard deviation.
[a]Gender: male (boy) and female (girl).
[b]Comorbidities of children with IEM (n): heart disease (1) and atopic dermatitis (1).
[c]Siblings' diagnosis (n): allergic rhinitis (1), spina bifida (1), Basedow disease (1), and NA (1).

Table 3. Characteristics of Primary Caregivers of Children With IEM and Their Partners.

	Primary Caregivers (n = 143)		Partners (n = 86)	
	M (SD)	Range	M (SD)	Range
Age	42.4 (6.0)	27-58	43.3 (6.8)	26-59
20s	5	3.5%	2	2.3%
30s	36	25.2%	23	26.3%
40s	85	59.5%	45	51.5%
50s	17	11.9%	17	19.4%
Gender[a]				
Male	11	7.7%	76	88.4%
Female	132	92.3%	10	11.6%
Occupation				
Full-time housewife	65	45.5%	4	4.7%
Part-time job	29	20.3%	5	5.8%
Full-time job	34	23.8%	66	76.7%
Self-employed	10	7.0%	11	12.3%
Other	5	3.5%	0	0.0%
Disease				
With	27	18.9%	12	14.0%
Without	116	81.1%	74	86.0%

Abbreviations: IEM, inborn errors of metabolism; M, mean; SD, standard deviation.
[a]Gender: male (father) and female (mother).

Results

Of the 532 families who were sent the questionnaires, 143 participated in this study (response rate: 27.0%). Tables 2 and 3 show participant characteristics, Tables 4 and 5 show QoL scores, and Tables 1 and 6 show QoL associated factors. Details of predictive factors are available in Supplemental Tables 1 and 2.

Children With IEM

In total, 56 children with IEM answered the questionnaires. Table 2 shows their characteristics. To prevent the respondents being identifiable, we put the disease category names instead of disease names, for example, "amino acid disorders" instead of PKU and Maple Syrup Urine Disease (MSUD) (Table 2). The mean KINDL scores, additional disease subscale scores, and emotional support in daily life scores are shown in Table 4.

The mean age of the children was 12.0 ± 3.1 years (Table 2), and the mean score of their QoL was 69.2 ± 14.4 points (Table 4). There were significant positive correlations between QoL (total KINDL scores) and additional disease subscale scores ($r = 0.460$, $P < .01$) and between QoL and emotional support resources ($r = 0.673$, $P < .001$). All KINDL subscales were significantly and positively correlated with emotional support resources ($r = 0.415\text{-}0.505$, $P < .01$). The disease subscale was significantly correlated with the following 5 subscales of the KINDL: physical ($r = 0.417$, $P < .01$), emotional ($r = 0.383$, $P < .05$), family ($r = 0.316$, $P < .05$), friends ($r = 0.336$, $P < .05$), and school ($r = 0.455$, $P < .001$). There were negative correlations between the age of children with IEM and the physical subscale ($r = -0.268$, $P < .05$; Table 1).

Siblings of Children With IEM

In total, 35 siblings answered the questionnaires. Their characteristics are described in Table 2. Table 4 shows their mean KINDL scores, disease subscale scores, and our original scoring of emotional support resources in daily life.

The mean age of siblings was 12.4 ± 3.3 years (Table 2), and the mean score of their QoL was 71.7 ± 12.6 points (Table 4). There was no significant correlations between QoL (total KINDL scores) and other factors. Three KINDL subscales were significantly positively correlated with

Table 4. Current Status of QoL in Children With IEM and Their Siblings.[a]

Scores of the Japanese Version of the KINDL			Children With IEM (n = 56)		Siblings (n = 35)	
Subscales	No of Items	Score Range	M (SD)	Range	M (SD)	Range
Physical	4	0.0-100	75.9 (19.0)	25.0-100	77.1 (19.5)	18.8-100
Emotional	4	0.0-100	81.5 (14.2)	43.8-100	81.1 (13.1)	50.0-100
Self-esteem	4	0.0-100	51.8 (26.0)	0.0-100	58.8 (22.6)	0.0-100
Family	4	0.0-100	71.6 (20.7)	6.3-100	73.9 (17.3)	25.0-100
Friends	4	0.0-100	69.6 (20.7)	25.0-100	77.1 (16.1)	37.5-100
School	4	0.0-100	65.7 (19.3)	25.0-100	62.3 (18.9)	25-100
Total	24	0.0-100	69.2 (14.4)	29.2-100	71.7 (12.6)	28.1-90
Disease	6	0.0-100	75.0 (15.1)	37.5-100	79.2 (7.2) n = 4	71-83
Emotional support resources in daily life scores	4	0.0-100	76.0 (19.4)	0.0-100	80.7 (17.0)	37.5-100

Abbreviations: IEM, inborn errors of metabolism; KINDL, Kinder Lebensqualitats Fragebogen; M, mean; QoL, quality of life; SD, standard deviation.
[a]KINDL: higher scores indicate a higher QoL. KINDL disease scale: higher scores indicate less disease impact on their daily life. The emotional support resource in daily life (original questions): higher scores indicate higher levels of emotional support. Cronbach α: 0.80 (children with IEM) and 0.77 (siblings). All questions were answered on a 5-point Likert scale: 1 = never, 2 = rarely, 3 = sometimes, 4 = often, and 5 = all the time.

Table 5. Current Status of QoL in Primary Caregivers and Partners, Parental Stress of Primary Caregivers, and Family Empowerment.[a]

			Primary Caregivers (n = 143)		Partners (n = 86)	
	No of Items	Score Range	M (SD)	Range	M (SD)	Range
Scores of the Japanese version of WHOQOL-26	26	1.0-5.0	3.29 (0.62)	1.54-4.73	3.38 (0.48)	2.19-4.42
Physical health	7	1.0-5.0	3.33 (0.73)	1.29-4.86	3.50 (0.62)	2.14-4.71
Psychological health	6	1.0-5.0	3.27 (0.73)	1.17-5	3.44 (0.59)	1.67-5.00
Social relationships	3	1.0-5.0	3.38 (0.68)	1.0-5.0	3.29 (0.51)	2.00-4.33
Environment	8	1.0-5.0	3.27 (0.66)	1.25-4.75	3.32 (0.56)	1.75-4.50
Two items for total QoL	2	1.0-5.0	3.17 (0.74)	1.0-5.0	3.20 (0.670	1.50-5.00
Scores of the Japanese version of PSI-SF	19	19-95	45.2 (10.6)	22-82	-	-
Difficult child	9	10-50	21.6 (5.8)	9-40	-	-
Parental distress	10	9-45	23.6 (6.9)	10-44	-	-
Scores of the J-FES	34	34-170	103.3 (0.7)	14-60	-	-
Family	12	12-60	39.6 (7.6)	21-60	-	-
Service system	12	12-60	38.5 (7.5)	10-50	-	-
Social politics	10	10-50	25.1 (6.2)	45-170	-	-

Abbreviations: J-FES, Japanese version of Family Empowerment Scale; M, mean; PSI-SF, Parenting Stress Index–Short Form; QoL, quality of life; SD, standard deviation; WHOQOL-26, World Health Organization Quality of Life 26.
[a]WHOQOL-26: higher scores indicate a higher QoL; the answer way is a 5-point Likert scale: 1 = not at all, 2 = a little, 3 = moderately, 4 = mostly, and 5 = completely. PSI-SF: higher scores indicate a higher parenting stress; the answer way is a 5-point Likert scale: 1 = not at all, 2 = no, 3 = yes and no, 4 = yes, and 5 = definitely. J-FES: higher scores indicate a higher family empowerment; the answer way is a 5-point Likert scale: 1 = not true at all, 2 = mostly not true, 3 = somewhat true, 4 = mostly true, and 5 = very true.

emotional support resources: physical ($r = 0.491$, $P < .01$), emotional ($r = 0.445$, $P < .01$), and family ($r = 0.505$, $P < .01$). There were negative correlations between the friends subscale and their age ($r = -0.469$, $P < .01$; Table 1).

Primary Caregivers of Children With IEM

A total of 143 primary caregivers answered the questionnaires, 92.3% of them were mothers. Table 3 shows their characteristics, and Table 5 shows the scores of each scale. Supplemental Table 1 shows the details of predictive factors of primary caregivers' QoL.

The mean age of primary caregivers was 42.4 ± 6.0 years (Table 3), and the mean score of their QoL was 3.29 ± 0.62 points. The mean score of PSI-SF was 45.2 ± 10.6 points and that of J-FES was 103.3 ± 0.7 points. The mean score of WHOQOL-26 was 3.29 ± 0.62 points (Table 5). Multiple regression analysis was performed with the total WHOQOL-26 score as the dependent variable. Lower parental distress scores (standard partial regression coefficient [sb] = −0.586, $P < .001$), higher scores on the J-FES family subscale (sb = 0.248, $P < .001$), and higher levels of household income (sb = 0.147, $P = .006$) contributed to higher QoL of primary caregivers (adjusted $R^2 = 0.636$), as shown in Table 6.

Partners of Primary Caregivers of Children With IEM

In total, 86 partners answered the questionnaires. A total of 88.4% of partners were fathers. Their characteristics are shown

Table 6. Factors Associated With Primary Caregivers' and Partners' QoL While a Child With IEM.

Dependent Variable: QoL Scores Explanatory variables	Primary Caregivers (n = 143)		Partners (n = 86)	
	sb	*P*	sb	*P*
Current age of children with IEM	−0.033	.522	0.121	.166
Age of onset	−0.047	.377	-	-
The number of times visiting a hospital per year	−0.062	.23	-	-
Age of primary caregivers	−0.014	.784	0.171	.056
The number of difficult things related to raising a child with IEM	−0.05	.37	-	-
The number of anxieties related to raising a child with IEM	−0.015	.781	−0.273	.003[a]
The number of eligible information resource of their child's disease and treatment	0.052	.308	-	-
Degree of distress related to caring for a child with IEM (1 = strongly disagree, 2 = disagree, 3 = undecided, 4 = agree, 5 = strongly agree)	−0.062	.24	−0.163	.083
Satisfaction with the relationship with the child with IEM (1 = very satisfied, 2 = satisfied, 3 = neither, 4 = dissatisfied, 5 = very dissatisfied)	0.01	.848	0.259	.01[b]
Satisfaction with the relationships within the family (1 = very satisfied, 2 = satisfied, 3 = neither, 4 = dissatisfied, 5 = very dissatisfied)	−0.033	.545	0.208	.04[b]
Degree of understanding their child with IEM by people around them (1 = bad, 2 = not good, 3 = normal, 4 = good, 5 = very good)	−0.044	.428	-	-
Household income (1 = wealthy, 2 = slightly wealthy, 3 = average, 4 = slightly poor, 5 = poor)	0.147	.006[a]	0.282	.002[a]
PSI-SF				
Difficult child	0.029	.612	-	-
Parental distress	−0.586	<.001[c]	-	-
J-FES scores				
Family	0.248	<.001[c]	0.024	.794
Service system	−0.024	.721	0.016	.859
Social politics	−0.1	.103	0.009	.916
R^2	0.644		0.426	
Adjusted R^2	0.636		0.398	

Abbreviations: IEM, inborn errors of metabolism; J-FES, Japanese version of Family Empowerment Scale; PSI-SF, Parenting Stress Index–Short Form; QoL, quality of life; sb, the values are standardized partial regression coefficients.
[a]P < .01.
[b]P < .05.

in Table 3, and Table 5 shows their scores on each scale. Supplementary Table 2 shows the details of predictive factors of QoL.

The mean age of partners was 43.3 ± 6.8 years (Table 3), and mean score of their QoL was 3.38 ± 0.48 points. In total, 93% of partners had some anxieties related to raising a child with IEM, and the distribution was similar to that of primary caregivers. The mean score of WHOQOL-26 was 3.38 ± 0.48 points (Table 5). Multiple regression analysis was performed with the total WHOQOL-26 score set as the dependent variable. The J-FES score provided by primary caregivers were assigned to their respective partners in this analysis because the J-FES score provided by the primary caregiver represents the empowerment represented by the entire family. Higher levels of household income (sb = 0.283, *P* = .002), fewer anxieties related to raising a child with IEM (sb = −0.273, *P* = .003), higher levels of satisfaction in the relationship with the child with IEM (sb = 0.259, *P* = .01), and higher levels of satisfaction with relationships within the family (sb = 0.208, *P* = .04) contributed to higher QoL of partners (adjusted R^2 = 0.398), as shown in Table 6.

Discussion

This was the first study to reveal current QoL and its associated factors in children with IEM, their siblings, primary caregivers, and their partners in Japan. Medical professionals and government employees, especially those involved in policy making for pediatric chronic illness, can now better understand QoL of these individuals and refer to these results when devising effective support to improve their QoL. The response rate was quite small because the questionnaires were mailed, and no incentive payments for families to cooperate with this study.

Children With IEM

Previous studies reported that QoL of children with IEM was lower than those with other pediatric chronic diseases.[24,25] Our results suggest that QoL tends to be lower in Japanese children with IEM, compared to the results of healthy Japanese children (73.2 points).[26] Additionally, in accordance with the results of previous studies in other countries,[5,24] QoL of children with IEM in Japan was affected by their condition. According to a previous study in France, the physical dimension of QoL was more affected by IEM than the psychological dimension.[24] Similar results can be seen in our study: the mean scores on the physical subscale of the KINDL tended to be lower than those of the emotional subscale, compared to the siblings' mean score and the mean scores of healthy children (physical: 82.4 points, emotional: 88.0 points).[26] There are some possible explanations. One is respondent bias, as only children with IEM who were under stable conditions and not staying in hospital were enrolled in this study. Second is a considerable experience of physical symptoms: for example, it is well known that patients with citrin deficiency experience daily fatigue, even under stable conditions, which affected their QoL.[2,27] Third is that they had sufficient emotional support resources: the results by our questions. Interestingly, enough emotional support resources contribute to all dimensions of KINDL (QoL), and the number of siblings was negatively correlated with the self-esteem dimension of QoL of children with IEM. Generally, Japanese children's self-esteem is potentially low,[28] and pediatric diseases affect their self-esteem and QoL.[29,30] Our results imply that the traits of their child–parent relationship and child–sibling relationship in the family with IEM and their effects on their QoL.

Siblings of Children With IEM

Although studies on siblings of children with chronic conditions, such as pediatric cancer and disabilities, exist,[31,32] no previous research has focused on the QoL of siblings of children with IEM. In these previous studies, it was reported that siblings of children with chronic conditions have anxiety for their future and problems with family relationships. However, siblings' QoL was in the same range as that of healthy children[26] and tended to be slightly better than the QoL scores of children with IEM. Age was negatively correlated with the friends' dimension of QoL of siblings, possibly because the relationships between children become more complicated when growing up.[33] As a next step, the study of siblings of children with IEM by qualitative approach might be needed to understand their anxiety for their future and problems with family relationships.

Primary Caregivers of Children With IEM

The QoL scores in primary caregivers were similar to those of healthy Japanese women (3.32 ± 0.41 points) and mothers raising children with food allergy (3.4 ± 0.4 points).[15,22] A previous study of parents raising children with IEM in Germany revealed predictors of parents' QoL. Older age in parents was positively associated with QoL, specifically in the emotional dimension and self-development,[34] but the age of primary caregivers was not an associated factor in this study. It is difficult to conclude whether age affects the QoL due to the biased distribution of the primary caregivers' ages; about 60% of the primary caregivers in this study were in their 40s. The researchers also reported the predictors of QoL to be family stress and social support.[34] In the current study, parental distress was the most influential factor of QoL of primary caregivers. For primary caregivers of children with IEM, the responsibility of managing the child's health must be included in the parental role, and this might result in considerable distress for them. Referring to the results of our literature review,[6] we consider that the small number of clinical doctors specializing in IEM and the lack of information about raising a child with IEM are also related to parental distress. It is also known that parents feel guilty about passing on a genetic disease,[3] and this contributes to their distress. Additionally, more than half of the children with IEM were diagnosed as having amino acid disorder; therefore, many parents could be responsible for dietary therapies. In fact, this is supported by the fact that over 40% of the primary caregivers responded that they had difficulty with diet therapy (Supplementary Table 1). In the future, we should investigate the parental distress of primary caregivers of children with IEM and diet therapy, in order to help to think the concrete way to support their childrearing.

Family empowerment was the second most influential factor on primary caregivers' QoL. This was the world's first study to explore family empowerment in families raising a child with IEM. The family subscale represents their power and confidence in raising their child within the family.[19] We clarified that improving their family empowerment contributes to improving primary caregivers' QoL, while raising a child with IEM. Therefore, we considered that supporting families as a whole is a significant perspective not only individual family members.

Partners of Primary Caregivers of Children With IEM

Compared to the national data on healthy Japanese men (3.24 ± 0.43 points),[15] the QoL of partners raising their child with IEM was higher in this study. The most positive influential factor of partners' QoL was household income. As previously mentioned, all children with IEM receive medical aid for hospital admission and visits and therapeutic special milk in Japan.[35] However, this medical aid does not cover the cost of any low-protein diet food, and such foods are always priced higher than common foods. Low-protein diet food is necessary for their appropriate diet therapy.[36] We could not conclude the causal correlation between their household income and the burden of high-priced low protein food in this study. It might be needed to investigate the annual cost of low-protein food and reconsider the application of medical aid for those families. Anxiety negatively related to raising their child with IEM was the secondary associated factor of their QoL. One previous study reported that it was important for parents raising a child with special needs to express and share their anxieties.[37] A representative of a parental support group of patients with IEM suggested that the primary reasons for joining the group was having considerable anxiety and loneliness due to the rarity of the disease.[38] Medical professionals should introduce such families to peer groups such as parental support group for children with IEM and provide the environment where they can easily share their anxieties at the daily outpatient setting.

Conclusion

Our study was the first cross-sectional questionnaire survey, revealing QoL and associated factors in children with IEM, their primary caregivers, and other family members in Japan. We revealed that there are different associated factors of QoL or each participant group, and we believe that each group should be supported inclusively: from the perspective of individuality and the family as a whole. By effectively utilizing the registration system (JaSMIn), important outcomes for the development of new treatments and improving QoL will be reported in the future too. The next challenge would be the development of interventions for improving QoL for these individuals in an outpatient setting.

Acknowledgments

The authors would like to express our greatest appreciation to Editage for their courteous English proofreading.

Declaration of Conflicting Interests

The author(s) declared no potential conflicts of interest with respect to the research, authorship, and/or publication of this article.

Funding

The author(s) disclosed receipt of the following financial support for the research, authorship, and/or publication of this article: This study was supported by a research scholarship from the Pfizer Health Research Foundation, 2015 to 2016. The study was partially supported by the Practical Research Project for Rare/Intractable Diseases from the Japan Agency for Medical Research and Development (AMED).

References

1. The Japanese Ministry of Health Labour and Welfare. The implementation status of newborn mass screening. http://www.jsms.gr.jp/contents04-01.html. Accessed January 30, 2018.
2. Endo F, Yamaguchi S, Ooura T, Okuyama T. *The Handbook of Inherited Metabolic Disease*. Tokyo: Nakayama Shoten; 2013.
3. Fujiwara K. Suggestion for understanding of amino acid metabolism of nursing from heredity support group. *J Jpn Soc Genet Nurs*. 2013;11(2):23-28.
4. Hayashi N, Imai T, Hasegawa M, et al. Comparison of quality of life of food allergic children and non-food allergic children. *Jpn J Pediatr Allergy Clin Immunol*. 2009;23(5):643-650.
5. Eminoglu TF, Soysai SA, Tumer L, Okur I, Hasanoglu A. Quality of life in children treated with restrictive diet for inherited metabolic disease. *Pediatr Int*. 2013;55(4):428-433. doi:10.1111/ped.12089.
6. Yamaguchi K, Wakimizu E, Kubota M. Difficulties in daily life and associated factors, and QoL of children with inherited metabolic disease and their parents in Japan: a literature review. *JIMD Rep*. 2016;33:1-10. doi:10.1007/8904_2016_573.
7. Simon E, Schwarz M, Roos J, et al. Evaluation of quality of life and description of the sociodemographic state in adolescent and young adult patients with phenylketonuria. *Health Qual Life Outcomes*. 2008;26(6):25-31. doi:10.1186/1477-7525-6-25.
8. Cazzorla C, Cegolon L, Burlina AP, et al. Quality of life assessment in a cohort of patients with phenylketonuria. *BMC Public Health*. 2014;14:1243-1252. doi:10.1186/1471-2458-14-1243.
9. Abe S. The experience of the mother who had a child diagnosed by newborn mass-screening. *Jpn J Inherit Metab Dis*. 2012;28:183.
10. Sakoda M, Yamamoto K, Yamaguchi S, Kawame H. The life story of the mother who has children with propionic acidemia. *J Jpn Pediatr Soc*. 2013;117(2):293.
11. Taketa M, Fujiwara Y, Endou M, et al. Nursing for children with propionic acidaemia need lifelong treatment-focusing on education to mother independently and continually. *Jpn J Child Nurs*. 1991;14(11):1433-1437.
12. Ravens-Sieberer U, Gortler E, Bullinger M. Subjective health and health behavior of children and adolescents—a survey of Humburg students within the scope of school medical examination. *Gesundheitswesen*. 2000;62(3):148-155. doi:10.1055/s-2000-10487.
13. Shibata R, Nemoto Y, Matsuzaki K, et al. A study of Kid-KINDL questionnaire for measuring quality of life in elementary school children in Japan. *J Jpn Pediatr Soc*. 2003;107(11):1514-1520.
14. World Health Organization Group. Study protocol for the World Health Organization project to develop a quality of life assessment instrument (WHOQOL). *Qual Life Res*. 1993;2:153-159. doi:10.1007/BF00435734.
15. Tasaki M, Nakane Y. *WHOQOL26 Manual Improved Edition*. Tokyo: Kaneko Shobou; 2007.
16. Abidin RR. *Parenting Stress Index Manual*. 1st ed. Virginia: Pediatric Psychology Press; 1983.
17. Kanematsu Y, Araki A, Narama M. *PSI Child Care Stress Index Guide. An Issue of General Corporate Judicial Person Employment Meeting for the Study*. Tokyo; 2014.
18. Araki A, Kanematsu Y, Yokosawa S, Arayashiki A, Aizumi I, Hujishima K. A study for developing parenting stress-short form scale. *J Child Health*. 2005;64(3):408-416.
19. Koren PE, DeChillo N, Friesen BJ. Measuring empowerment in families whose children have emotional disabilities: a brief questionnaire. *Rehabil Psychol*. 1992;37(4):305-321. doi:org/10.1037/h0079106.
20. Wakimizu R, Fujioka H, Furuya K, et al. Development of Family Empowerment Scale Japanese version for measuring the empowerment of families rearing a child with disability. *J Health Welfare Stat*. 2011;57(13):33-41.
21. Adachi T, Kanaya E, Fujita M, Itoh M, Chiyo H, Mikami H. Effects of family relationship on the subjective well-being of the caregiver of a child receiving in-home medical care with high-technology devices. *J Jpn Acad of Commun Health Nurs*. 2000:2(1):61-68. doi:org/10.20746/jachn.2.1_61.
22. Aika S, Yamamoto Y, Taketani T, et al. Quality of life in the mothers of children with food allergy. *J Pediatr Allergy Clin Immunol*. 2015;29(2):169-180.
23. Wakimizu R, Yamaguchi K, Fujioka H, et al. Assessment of quality of life, family function and family empowerment for fam-

ilies who provide home care for a child with severe motor and intellectual disabilities in Japan. *Health*. 2016;8:304-317. doi:10.4236/health.2016.84032.

24. Fabre A, Baumstarck B, Cano A, et al. Assessment of quality of life of the children and parents affected by inborn errors of metabolism with restricted diet: preliminary results of a cross-sectional study. *Health Qual Life Outcomes*. 2013;11:158. doi:10.1186/1477-7525-11-158.
25. Hatzmann J, Valstar MJ, Bosch AM, Wiljburg FA, Heymans HS, Grootenhuis MA. Predicting health-related quality of life of parents of children with inherited metabolic diseases. *Acta Paediatr*. 2009;98(7):1205-1210. doi:10.1111/j.1651-2227.2009.01269.x.
26. Yamamoto E. A questionnaire study on the health-related quality of life in elementary school-age children. *Hum Dev Aichi Prefectural Univ*. 2010;1:37-52. http://ci.nii.ac.jp/els/110008434437.pdf?id=ART0009679850&type=pdf&&host=cinii&order_no=&ppv_type=0&lang_sw=&no=1485884347&cp=. Accessed January 30, 2018.
27. Okano Y, Kobayashi K, Ihara K, et al. Fatigue and quality of life in citrin deficiency during adaptation and compensation stage. *Mol Genet Metab*. 2013;109(1):9-13. doi:10.1016/j.ymgme.2013.01.020.
28. Furusyo J. *Why is Self-Esteem of Japanese Children Low?* Tokyo: Koubunsya; 2013. http://www.kobunsha.com/shelf/book/isbn/9784334035068. Accessed January 30, 2018.
29. Chaplin JE, Kriström B, Jonsson B, et al. Improvements in behaviour and self-esteem following growth hormone treatment in short prepubertal children. *Horm Res Paediatr*. 2011;75(4):291-303. doi:10.1159/000322937.
30. Ingulli EG, Mak RH. Growth in children with chronic kidney disease: role of nutrition, growth hormone, dialysis, and steroids. *Curr Opin Pediatr*. 2014;26(2):187-92. doi:10.1097/MOP.0000000000000070.
31. Sato I, Kamibeppu K. Provision and sharing of information with siblings of children with cancer: a review of explanations provided. *Jpn Soc Pediatr Hematol/Oncol*. 2009;46(1):31-38.
32. Abe M, Kanna M. Evaluation of a support program for siblings and parents of children with disabilities. *Jpn Assoc Spec Educ*. 2015;52(5):349-358.
33. Tsukahara T. Developmental problem and psychological education in infant and childhood: in the perspective social development. *Bull Ueda Women's Junior College*. 2011;34:131-142. http://ci.nii.ac.jp/naid/40019039254. Accessed January 30, 2018.
34. Fidika A, Salewski C, Goldbeck L. Quality of life among parents of children with phenylketonuria (PKU). *Health Qual Life Outcomes*. 2013;11:54. doi:10.1186/1477-7525-11-54.
35. Information Center for Specific Pediatric Chronic Diseases Japan. Medical Aid for children with specific pediatric chronic diseases. https://www.shouman.jp . Accessed January 30, 2018.
36. Ida S, Sakai N, Shintaku H T, Shintaku H, Tsukada S, Nagai N, Nishimoto Y. *Practice, Casebook of Education of Diet Therapy for Inborn Errors of Metabolism*. Tokyo: Shindan to Chiryosha; 2014.
37. Suzuki M. Recent trends of research papers about mothers who have children with food allergies in Japan. *Seisen J Nurs Stud*. 2013;2:103-110.
38. Kashiwagi A. The current situation and future issue of expanding newborn mass-screening. *J Jpn Soc Genet Nurs*. 2012;10(2):33-36.

Permissions

All chapters in this book were first published in JIEMS, by SAGE Publications; hereby published with permission under the Creative Commons Attribution License or equivalent. Every chapter published in this book has been scrutinized by our experts. Their significance has been extensively debated. The topics covered herein carry significant findings which will fuel the growth of the discipline. They may even be implemented as practical applications or may be referred to as a beginning point for another development.

The contributors of this book come from diverse backgrounds, making this book a truly international effort. This book will bring forth new frontiers with its revolutionizing research information and detailed analysis of the nascent developments around the world.

We would like to thank all the contributing authors for lending their expertise to make the book truly unique. They have played a crucial role in the development of this book. Without their invaluable contributions this book wouldn't have been possible. They have made vital efforts to compile up to date information on the varied aspects of this subject to make this book a valuable addition to the collection of many professionals and students.

This book was conceptualized with the vision of imparting up-to-date information and advanced data in this field. To ensure the same, a matchless editorial board was set up. Every individual on the board went through rigorous rounds of assessment to prove their worth. After which they invested a large part of their time researching and compiling the most relevant data for our readers.

The editorial board has been involved in producing this book since its inception. They have spent rigorous hours researching and exploring the diverse topics which have resulted in the successful publishing of this book. They have passed on their knowledge of decades through this book. To expedite this challenging task, the publisher supported the team at every step. A small team of assistant editors was also appointed to further simplify the editing procedure and attain best results for the readers.

Apart from the editorial board, the designing team has also invested a significant amount of their time in understanding the subject and creating the most relevant covers. They scrutinized every image to scout for the most suitable representation of the subject and create an appropriate cover for the book.

The publishing team has been an ardent support to the editorial, designing and production team. Their endless efforts to recruit the best for this project, has resulted in the accomplishment of this book. They are a veteran in the field of academics and their pool of knowledge is as vast as their experience in printing. Their expertise and guidance has proved useful at every step. Their uncompromising quality standards have made this book an exceptional effort. Their encouragement from time to time has been an inspiration for everyone.

The publisher and the editorial board hope that this book will prove to be a valuable piece of knowledge for researchers, students, practitioners and scholars across the globe.

List of Contributors

Mohamed Abd El Aal and Shaimaa Mahmoud
Department of Pediatrics, Faculty of Medicine, Sohag University, Sohag, Egypt

Elsayed Abdel kreem
Department of Pediatrics, Faculty of Medicine, Sohag University, Sohag, Egypt
Department of Pediatrics, Graduate School of Medicine, Gifu University, Gifu, Japan

Hiroki Otsuka, Hideo Sasai, Tomohiro Hori and Toshiyuki Fukao
Department of Pediatrics, Graduate School of Medicine, Gifu University, Gifu, Japan

Yuka Aoyama
Department of Biomedical Sciences, College of Life and Health Sciences, Education and Training Center of Medical Technology, Chubu University, Kasugai, Japan

Vincent C. Hsieh and Philip G. Morgan
Department of Anesthesiology and Perioperative Medicine, University of Washington, Seattle, WA, USA

Elliot J. Krane
Department of Anesthesiology, Perioperative and Pain Medicine, Stanford University, Stanford, CA, USA
Department of Pediatrics, Stanford University, Stanford, CA, USA

Alessandro Burlina
Neurological Unit, Department of Internal Medicine, St. Bassiano Hospital, Bassano del Grappa, Italy

Juan Politei
Fundación para el estudio de las enfermedades neurometabólicas (FESEN), Buenos Aires, Argentina

Michael Beck
Institute of Human Genetics, University Medical Center, Mainz, Germany

Graziela Schmitt Ribas, Jurema Fátima De Mari, Gabriel Civallero and Maira Graeff Burin
Medical Genetics Service, HCPA, and WHO Collaborating Center for the Development of Medical Genetic Services in Latin America, Porto Alegre, Rio Grande do Sul, Brazil

Heryk Motta de Souza
Faculdade de Farmácia, UFRGS, Porto Alegre, Rio Grande do Sul, Brazil

Carmen Regla Vargas
Medical Genetics Service, HCPA, and WHO Collaborating Center for the Development of Medical Genetic Services in Latin America, Porto Alegre, Rio Grande do Sul, Brazil
Departamento de Análises, Faculdade de Farmácia, UFRGS, Porto Alegre, Rio Grande do Sul, Brazil

Roberto Giugliani
Medical Genetics Service, HCPA, and WHO Collaborating Center for the Development of Medical Genetic Services in Latin America, Porto Alegre, Rio Grande do Sul, Brazil
Department of Genetics and Postgraduate Program in Genetics and Molecular
Biology, UFRGS, Porto Alegre, Rio Grande do Sul, Brazil
Instituto Nacional de Genética Médica Populacional—INAGEMP, Porto Alegre, Rio Grande do Sul, Brazil

Sara Poggiali, Daniela Ombrone, Giulia Forni, Sabrina Malvagia, Silvia Funghini and Massimo Mura
Newborn Screening, Biochemistry and Pharmacology Laboratory, Pediatric Neurology Clinic and Laboratories, Meyer Children's University Hospital, Florence, Italy

Elisabetta Pasquini
Metabolic and Muscular Unit, Pediatric Neurology Clinic, Meyer Children's University Hospital, Florence, Italy

Laura Santoro, Vincenzo Bellavia, Orazia Maria Granata, Tommaso Silvano Aronica
UOS Newborn Screening Center, UOC Pediatric Clinical Pathology, P.O.G. Di Cristina, Palermo, Italy

Cinzia Castana
UOC Pediatric Clinic, P.O.G. Di Cristina, Palermo, Italy

Kathleen S. McGreevy
Research, Innovation and International Relations Office, Meyer Children's University Hospital, Florence, Italy

Giancarlo la Marca
Newborn Screening, Biochemistry and Pharmacology Laboratory, Pediatric Neurology Clinic and Laboratories, Meyer Children's University Hospital, Florence, Italy
Department of Experimental and Clinical Biomedical Sciences, University of Florence, Florence, Italy

Viruna Neergheen and Annapurna Chalasani
Neurometabolic Unit, The National Hospital for Neurology and Neurosurgery, Queen Square, London, UK

Luke Wainwright
Department of Molecular Neuroscience, Institute of Neurology, University College London, London, UK

Delia Yubero, Raquel Montero and Rafael Artuch
Clinical Biochemistry department, Institut de Recerca Sant Joan de Déu and CIBERER, Barcelona, Spain

Iain Hargreaves
Neurometabolic Unit, The National Hospital for Neurology and Neurosurgery, Queen Square, London, UK
School of Pharmacy and Biomolecular Science, Liverpool John Moores University, Liverpool, UK

Gabriela Castro, Valerie Hamilton and Verónica Cornejo
Instituto de Nutrición y Tecnología de los Alimentos, Universidad de Chile, Santiago, Chile

Rachel D. Torok and Lisa K. Britt
Divisions of Pediatric Cardiology, Department of Pediatrics, Duke University Medical Center, Durham, NC, USA

Stephanie B. Wechsler
Divisions of Pediatric Cardiology, Department of Pediatrics, Duke University Medical Center, Durham, NC, USA
Divisions of Medical Genetics, Department of Pediatrics, Duke University Medical Center, Durham, NC, USA

Stephanie L. Austin and Priya S. Kishnani
Divisions of Medical Genetics, Department of Pediatrics, Duke University Medical Center, Durham, NC, USA

Jose E. Abdenur
Division of Metabolic Disorders, Children's Hospital of Orange County, Orange, CA, USA
Department of Pediatrics, University of California Irvine School of Medicine, Orange, CA, USA

Saida Ortolano
Group of Neonatal Pathology, Pediatrics and Rare Diseases, Instituto de Investigación Sanitaria Galicia Sur, Vigo, Spain

Adrián Fernández,
Favaloro Foundation University Hospital, Buenos Aires, Argentina

Juan Politei
Division of Neurometabolism, Department of Neurology, Foundation for Study of Neurometabolic Diseases (FESEN), Buenos Aires, Argentina

Johanna Acosta Guio
Instituto de Ortopedia Infantil Roosevelt, Bogotá, Colombia
Instituto de Genética, Universidad Nacional, Bogotá, Colombia

Gustavo Adolfo Giraldo-Ospina
Facultad de Medicina, Universidad Pontificia Bolivariana, Clínica Universitaria Bolivariana, Medellín, Colombia

Elizabeth D. Bacci and Katharine S. Gries
Evidera, Inc, Seattle, WA, USA

Kathleen W. Wyrwich
Evidera Inc, Bethesda, MD, USA

Yinpu Chen, Rishabh Jain, Laurel Konkol, Markus J. Merilainen and Haoling H. Weng
BioMarin Pharmaceuticals Inc, Novato, CA, USA

Ernesto Carlos González Reyes, Elisa M. Castells, Amarilys Frómeta, Lesley Del Río, Yileidis Tejeda, Pedro L. Pérez, Mary Triny Segura, Pedro Almenares, Yenitse Perea and René Robaina
Department of Newborn Screening, Immunoassay Center, Cubanacan, Havana, Cuba

Ana Luisa Arteaga
National Programs Department, TecnoSuma Internacional SA Cubanacan, Havana, Cuba

Niurka M. Carlos
Immunoassay Center, Cubanacan, Havana, Cuba

José L. Fernández-Yero
Center of Molecular Immunology, Atabey, Havana, Cuba

Cristiane Cecatto, Janaína C. da Silva and Alessandro Wajner
Programa de Pós-Graduação em Ciências Biológicas: Bioquímica, Instituto de Ciências Básicas da Saúde, Universidade Federal do Rio Grande do Sul, Porto Alegre, Rio Grande do Sul, Brazil

Alexandre U. Amaral
Programa de Pós-Graduação em Ciências Biológicas: Bioquímica, Instituto de Ciências Básicas da Saúde, Universidade Federal do Rio Grande do Sul, Porto Alegre, Rio Grande do Sul, Brazil
Departamento de Ciências Biológicas, Universidade Regional Integrada do Alto Uruguai e das Missões, Erechim, Rio Grande do Sul, Brazil

Moacir Wajner
Departamento deBioquímica, Instituto deCiênciasBásicas da Saúde,Universidade Federal do Rio Grande do Sul, Porto Alegre, Rio Grande do Sul, Brazil
Serviço de Genética Médica, Hospital de Clínicas de Porto Alegre, Porto Alegre, Rio Grande do Sul, Brazil

Miyono M. Hendrix, Stephanie L. Foster and Suzanne K. Cordovado
Centers for Disease Control and Prevention, Atlanta, GA, USA

Abel Santamaria
Laboratorio de Aminoácidos Excitadores, Instituto Nacional de Neurología y Neurocirugía, Mexico City, Mexico

Gabriela Aguilera
Laboratorio de Aminoácidos Excitadores, Instituto Nacional de Neurología y Neurocirugía, Mexico City, Mexico
Departamento de Ciencias Biológicas y de la Salud, Universidad Autónoma Metropolitana-Iztapalapa, Mexico City, Mexico

Soraia Poloni
Post-Graduation Program in Medical Sciences, Universidade Federal do Rio Grande do Sul, Porto Alegre, Brazil
Laboratory of Basic Research and Advanced Investigations in Neurosciences (BRAIN), Hospital de Clínicas de Porto Alegre, Porto Alegre, Brazil

Giovana W. Hoss, Fernanda Sperb-Ludwig and Taciane Borsatto
Laboratory of Basic Research and Advanced Investigations in Neurosciences (BRAIN), Hospital de Clínicas de Porto Alegre, Porto Alegre, Brazil
Post-Graduation Program in Genetics and Molecular Biology, Universidade Federal do Rio Grande do Sul, Porto Alegre, Brazil

Maria Juliana R. Doriqui
Complexo Hospitalar Materno-Infantil do Maranhaõ, Saõ Luis, Brazil

Emília K.E.A Leaõ and Ney Boa-Sorte
Complexo Hospitalar Professor Edgard Santos, Salvador, Brazil
Universidade do Estado da Bahia, Salvador, Brazil

Gerson Carvalho
Hospital de Apoio de Brasília, Brasília, Brazil

Hector Y. C. Wanderley
Escola Superior de Ciências da Santa Casa de Misericórdia de Vitória, Vitória, Brazil

Vânia D'Almeida
Department of Psychobiology, Universidade Federal de Saõ Paulo, Saõ Paulo, Brazil

Luiz C. Santana-da-Silva
Universidade Federal do Pará, Belém, Brazil

Henk J. Blom
Laboratory for Clinical Biochemistry and Metabolism, University Medical Center, Freiburg, Germany

Valeria M. Gutiérrez-García and Jesús Santos-Guzmán
Tecnologico de Monterrey, Escuela de Medicina y Ciencias de la Salud, Monterrey, Nuevo Leon, Mexico

Alexandra V. Zea-Rey and Diana L. Vazquez-Cantu
Tecnologico de Monterrey, Escuela de Medicina y Ciencias de la Salud, Monterrey, Nuevo Leon, Mexico
Genomi-k S.A.P.I. de C.V, Monterrey, Nuevo Leon, Mexico

Héctor Cruz-Camino
Genomi-k S.A.P.I. de C.V, Monterrey, Nuevo Leon, Mexico
Tecnologico de Monterrey, Escuela de Biotecnología y Ciencias de la Salud Monterrey, Nuevo Leon, Mexico

Consuelo Cantú -Reyna
Tecnologico de Monterrey, Escuela de Medicina y Ciencias de la Salud, Monterrey, Nuevo Leon, Mexico
Genomi-k S.A.P.I. de C.V, Monterrey, Nuevo Leon, Mexico
Tecnologico de Monterrey, Escuela de Biotecnología y Ciencias de la Salud Monterrey, Nuevo Leon, Mexico

Peter T. Clayton and Philippa B. Mills
Genetics and Genomic Medicine, UCL, Great Ormond Street Institute of Child Health, London, United Kingdom

Kathleen W. Wyrwich
Eli Lilly and Company, Indianapolis, IN, USA

Angela Schulz, Miriam Nickel and Alfried Kohlschütter
University Hospital Hamburg-Eppendorf, Hamburg, Germany

Peter Slasor, Temitayo Ajayi and David R. Jacoby
BioMarin Pharmaceutical Inc, San Rafael, CA, USA

Bruna B. dos Santos
Postgraduate Program in Genetics and Molecular Biology, Universidade Federal do Rio Grande do Sul, Porto Alegre, Rio Grande do Sul, Brazil

Filippo P. Vairo and Carolina F. M. Souza
Medical Genetics Service, Hospital de Clínicas de Porto Alegre, Porto Alegre, Rio Grande do Sul, Brazil

Tatíele Nalin
Medical Genetics Service, Hospital de Clínicas de Porto Alegre, Porto Alegre, Rio Grande do Sul, Brazil
Postgraduate Program in Medical Sciences, Universidade Federal do Rio Grande do Sul, Porto Alegre, Rio Grande do Sul, Brazil

Kamila C. Grokoski
Postgraduate Program in Child and Adolescent Health, Universidade Federal do Rio Grande do Sul, Porto Alegre, Rio Grande do Sul, Brazil

Ingrid D. S. Perry
Postgraduate Program in Public Health, Universidade do Extremo Sul Catarinense, Criciúma, Santa Catarina, Brazil

Lilia F. Refosco
Medical Genetics Service, Hospital de Clínicas de Porto Alegre, Porto Alegre, Rio Grande do Sul, Brazil
Nutrition and Dietetics Service, Hospital de Clínicas de Porto Alegre, Porto Alegre, Rio Grande do Sul, Brazil

Ida V. D. Schwartz
Postgraduate Program in Genetics and Molecular Biology, Universidade Federal do Rio Grande do Sul, Porto Alegre, Rio Grande do Sul, Brazil
Medical Genetics Service, Hospital de Clínicas de Porto Alegre, Porto Alegre, Rio Grande do Sul, Brazil
Department of Genetics, Universidade Federal do Rio Grande do Sul, Porto Alegre, Rio Grande do Sul, Brazil

Gabriel Civallero and Roberto Giugliani
Medical Genetics Service, HCPA, Porto Alegre, Brazil
Department of Genetics, UFRGS, Porto Alegre, Brazil

Raquel de Kremer
Centro de Estudios de las Metabolopatías Congénitas, CEMECO, Facultad de Ciencias Médicas, Universidad Nacional de Córdoba, Argentina

Anneliese L. Barth and Dafne D. G. Horovitz
Instituto Nacional de Saúde da Mulher, da Criança e do Adolescente Fernandes Figueira/Fiocruz - Rio de Janeiro, Brazil

Jörn Oliver Sass and Dr. rer. nat
Bonn-Rhein-Sieg University of Applied Sciences, IFGA & Department of Natural Sciences, Inborn Errors of Metabolism, Rheinbach, Germany

Malkanthi Fernando, Dr. rer. nat. and Sidney Behringer
Department of General Pediatrics, Faculty of Medicine, Adolescent Medicine and Neonatology, Medical Center–University of Freiburg, Freiburg, Germany

Robert McFarland
Wellcome Centre for Mitochondrial Research, Institute of Neuroscience, Newcastle University, Newcastle upon Tyne, United Kingdom

Diana Lehmann
Wellcome Centre for Mitochondrial Research, Institute of Neuroscience, Newcastle University, Newcastle upon Tyne, United Kingdom
Department of Neurology, University of Halle-Wittenberg, Halle/Saale, Germany

Russell P. Saneto
Division of Pediatric Neurology, Department of Neurology, University of Washington, Seattle, WA, USA

Lorne Clarke
British Columbia Children's Hospital Research Institute, University of British Columbia, Vancouver, British Columbia, Canada

Carolyn Ellaway
Sydney Children's Hospital Network, Sydney University, Sydney, Australia

Helen E. Foster
Great North Children's Hospital and Newcastle University, Newcastle upon Tyne, United Kingdom

Roberto Giugliani
Medical Genetics Service HCPA, Dep Genet UFRGS & INAGEMP, Porto Alegre, Brazil

Cyril Goizet
Service de Génétique, CHU Bordeaux, Laboratoire MRGM, INSERM U 1211, University of Bordeaux, Bordeaux, France

Sarah Goring, Zaeem Khan and Suzanne McMullen
ICON plc, Vancouver, British Columbia, Canada

Sara Hawley, Fathima Mubarack and Elaina Jurecki
BioMarin Pharmaceutical Inc., Novato, CA, USA

Christina Lampe
Centre for Rare Diseases, Clinic for Children and Adolescents, Helios Dr. Horst Schmidt Kliniken, Wiesbaden, Germany

Ken Martin
UCSF Benioff Children's Hospital Oakland, Oakland, CA, USA

John J. Mitchell
Montreal Children's Hospital, Montreal, Quebec, Canada

H. Serap Sivri
Hacettepe University Children's Hospital, Ankara, Turkey

Martha Solano Villarreal
Fundacion Cardioinfantil, Bogota, Colombia

Fiona J. Stewart
Belfast City Hospital, Belfast, United Kingdom

Anna Tylki-Szymanska
Children's Memorial Health Institute, Warsaw, Poland

Klane White
Seattle Children's Hospital, Seattle, WA, USA

Frits Wijburg
Academic Medical Center, University Hospital of Amsterdam, Amsterdam, the Netherlands

Keiko Yamaguchi and Rie Wakimizu
University of Tsukuba, Tsukuba, Ibaraki, Japan

Mitsuru Kubota
Kokuritsu Kenkyu Kaihatsu Hojin Kokuritsu, Seiiku Iryo Kenkyu Center, National Center for Child Health and Development, Setagaya-ku, Tokyo, Japan

Index

CPSIA information can be obtained
at www.ICGtesting.com
Printed in the USA
LVHW060852030122
707669LV00002B/105

9 781639 271191